The ECG
A Two-Step Approach to Diagnosis

Springer

Berlin
Heidelberg
New York
Hong Kong
London
Milan
Paris
Tokyo

MARC GERTSCH

The ECG
A Two-Step Approach to Diagnosis

Foreword by Christopher Cannon

With 1154 Figures and 54 Tables

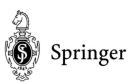 Springer

Professor Dr. MARC GERTSCH
Department of Cardiology
Swiss Cardiovascular Center Bern
University Clinic Inselspital
CH-3010 Bern
Switzerland

ISBN 3-540-00869-1-3

Library of Congress Cataloging-in-Publication Data

Gertsch, Marc, 1936-
    The ECG : a two-step approach to diagnosis / Marc Gertsch.
       p. ; cm.
    Includes bibliographical references.
    ISBN 3-540-00869-1 (hard cover : alk. paper)
     1. Electrocardiography. I. Title.
    [DNLM: 1. Electrocardiography--methods. 2. Arrhythmia--diagnosis. 3. Heart
    Diseases--diagnosis. WG G384e 2004]

    RC683.5.E5G477 2004
    616.1'207547--dc21

                                                        2003054780

Springer-Verlag Berlin Heidelberg New York
a member of BertelsmannSpringer Science+Business Media GmbH

http://www.springer.de

© Springer-Verlag Berlin Heidelberg 2004
Printed in Germany

Production Editor: Frank Krabbes, Heidelberg
Typesetting: wiskom e.K., Friedrichshafen
Cover design: D & P, Heidelberg
Printed on acid free paper   SPIN: 10911129   14/3109 - 5 4 3 2 1 0

I dedicate the book to my wife Ursula
and to our children Gustav, Natacha, Sonja and Anatol

Foreword

On this, the 100th anniversary of the electrocardiogram (ECG), it is a delight to welcome a new and comprehensive book on ECGs and arrhythmias. Professor Gertsch has compiled a wonderful book that covers all aspects of electrocardiography but with a very practical and clinically useful approach. In reading this book, I have been struck by its very straightforward layout and setup of each chapter, divided into sections for busy readers and advanced readers. This allows the reader to skim through the highlights of a particular section and, if he or she is more interested, can delve more deeply into that topic. The book has a very clear outline format so that one can follow the various issues on a topic. For example, in the ECG section, the various components of the ECG are divided into subsections and the various normal variants that can be seen are listed as subsections within each part of the chapter. The illustrations, figures, and tables in the book are very helpful. Within each chapter to explain vectors or mechanisms of arrhythmia are illustrations in color. Cataloged at the back of each chapter are example ECGs of all the topics discussed in each chapter.

This makes this book very useful for all levels of physicians and health-care professionals interested in ECGs, ranging from medical students who are first being exposed to electrocardiograms, to senior cardiologists who wish to find more detailed information about particular abnormalities. For all these reasons, I feel this book will be a welcome addition to the medical literature and should be very useful to cardiologists, electrophysiologists, internists, primary care physicians, nurses, medical residents, exercise physiologists and technicians, and all other health-care professionals caring for cardiac patients. Congratulations to Professor Gertsch on creating this important new book.

Christopher Cannon
Associate Professor of Medicine
Cardiovascular Division
Department of Medicine
Brigham and Women's Hospital
Harvard Medical School
Boston MA 02115
USA

Preface

Twenty-five years ago a publisher invited me to write an ECG book. I refused because I had no time, having a 120 percent job. This was a good decision. In the decades which followed I have learned much more about the ECG and about teaching. And so I have eventually created this book at the end of my professional life, taking a 50 percent time out for three years.

Being involved in non-invasive and invasive cardiology, I had the constant opportunity to compare the ECG patterns with hard facts, such as echocardiographic and angiographic findings, to name only the most important ones. I became acquainted with the significance of arrhythmias during the implantation of many pacemakers and attending intensive care and emergency stations.

In this book I have tried to differentiate between basically important and frequent ECG patterns and arrhythmias on one hand, and less important and rarer – but interesting – findings on the other. This has been achieved by dividing most chapters into a section *At a Glance* and a section *The Full Picture*. Moreover, I have taken up many suggestions by my colleagues, thus providing an extensive presentation of the normal ECG and its (normal) variants, and a large chapter about exercise ECGs. Other ideas were cooked in my own kitchen, such as the chapters 'Differential Diagnosis of Pathologic Q Waves' and 'Special Waves, Signs and Phenomena', as well as a list of the etiologies of electrolyte imbalances, and of pericarditis. With clinical data and the inclusion of about 50 case reports (also called 'short stories'), the clinical significance of 'the ECG' is highlighted and the reading experience thus enhanced.

The book is intended for cardiologists, internists and general practitioners, for the specialist team in intensive care units and for especially gifted and interested students.

Marc Gertsch

Introduction by Bernhard Meier

A single author book in any field of cardiology has become an exquisite rarity. It takes a super specialist to comprehensively review the large topic of electrocardiography in a fashion appropriate to cardiologists, internists, general practitioners, and medical students. Marc Gertsch meets that requirement as only few can. He is a professor of cardiology at the University of Bern, Switzerland, and he has devoted his professional life largely to the dwindling art of ECG interpretation. Keeping up a regular practise of clinical and invasive cardiology alongside has enabled him to correlate ECGs and real life at all times. At the dusk of his career he has sat down to convey his profound knowledge of electrocardiography to all those in the medical profession who use this key tool of the trade. Only few medical professionals have no interface whatsoever with electrocardiography. To all others who deal with the electrocardiograms occasionally or regularly, this book offers a unique opportunity to catch-up, to keep abreast, or even to excel in this domain.

The book is unique in its style as it is unique in its depth of practical information on carefully selected subheadings of the topic. The illustrations remain faithful to the saying that a picture is worth a thousand words. Yet, wherever needed, text and tables are interspersed and the clinical, physiological or etiological background of depicted electrocardiographic changes are elucidated, for example in a comprehensive list of etiologies of electrolyte imbalances.

The examples of electrocardiograms are carefully selected out of a gargantuan gamut of real life ECGs accumulated in a large tertiary center over years. They are crisply reproduced, succinctly explained, and very often rendered absolutely fascinating by the added history of the patient concerned.

The witty two-layer structure of the book allows the matter-of-fact reader to take home whatever is needed (and a little more) in virtually no time, while the wizard finds tasty tidbits, passion, and joy in digging into the deeper level.

This book is the next best thing to hovering over real ECGs, fresh from the machine, together with a master of the art such as the author Marc Gertsch.

Bernhard Meier, MD
Professor and Chairman of Cardiology
Swiss Cardiovascular Center Bern
University Hospital
CH-3010 Bern, Switzerland

Acknowledgements

I am grateful to:

- many colleagues in and outside of the hospital and my boss, Professor Bernhard Meier (Head of the Department of Cardiology, University Clinics, CH-Inselspital Bern), for continuous psychological support. Thanks also to Bernhard Meier for compiling an introduction for the book
- Professor Hein JJ Wellens (Utrecht/Netherlands), also for psychological support
- my colleagues Reto Candinas, Thomas Crohn, Andres Jaussi, Paul Dubach, Marc Zimmernmann, Verena Eigenmann, Martin Kägi, Benjamin Fässler, Guy de Sépibus, Felix Frey, Kerstin Wustmann, Christian Schüpfer, Christoph Noti, Beat Meyer, Etienne Delacrétaz, Jürg Fuhrer, Therese Sifeddine and the nurses of the intensive care and emergency units for providing ECGs
- Etienne Delacrétaz MD, for substantial and invaluable help in the chapter 'The WPW Syndrome'
- Paul Dubach MD, for having a glance at the chapter 'Exercise ECG'
- the 'Katharina Huber-Steiner Foundation' and Paul Mohacsi MD, for a grant of 7000 dollars.
- Pascal Meier MD, for valuable technical assistance
- Matthias Meier, student of architecture, for scanning about 50 percent of the ECGs
- Willi Hess, scientific illustrator, who put all my ideas into more than 50 splendid figures, with admirable endurance (and did more than this)
- Christoph Obrecht lic. biol., for most valuable assistance in many respects, including meticulous reading of the manuscript, asking uncomfortable questions, improving the English, scanning the other 50 percent of the ECGs, secretarial assistance, and repairing computers and other machines. Without his assistance I would not have been able to finish the book
- Benjamin Fässler, MD, and Christoph Obrecht for correcting the final manuscript, thus eliminating the last (?) errors
- Sandra Fabiani, Dr Thomas Mager, and Andrew Spencer of Springer-Verlag (Heidelberg/Berlin), with whom cooperation was extremely satisfying and pleasant
- Professor Christopher Paul Cannon (Brigham and Women's Hospital, Boston, USA) for writing the foreword.

August 2, 2003. Marc Gertsch

Contents

Section II   Pattern ECG

Chapter 3
The Normal ECG and its (Normal) Variants

Chapter 4
Atrial Enlargement and Other Abnormalities of the p Wave

Chapter 5
Left Ventricular Hypertrophy

Chapter 6
Right Ventricular Hypertrophy

Chapter 7

Biventricular Hypertrophy

Chapter 8

Pulmonary Embolism

Chapter 14

Chapter 15

Section IV Special Topics

Chapter 27

Chapter 28

Pacemaker ECG 505

Abbreviations

The following abbreviations are used regularly throughout the text.

AAI pacing	Atrial inhibited atrial pacing
ACE	Angiotensin-converting enzyme
acPE	Acute pulmonary embolism
AF	Atrial fibrillation
AJT	Automatic junctional tachycardia
AMI	Acute myocardial infarction
AP or acP	Action potential
APB	Atrial premature beat
ÅQRS$_F$	Mean QRS axis in the frontal plane
ASD	Atrial septal defect
AV	Atrioventricular
AVNRT	Atrioventricular nodal reentrant tachycardia
BVH	Biventricular hypertrophy
CABG	Aortocoronary bypass grafting
CAD	Coronary artery disease
CHD	Coronary heart disease
CK = CPK	Creatine kinase
CK-MB	Myocardial-bound creatine kinase
COPD	Chronic obstructive pulmonary disease
Coro	Coronary angiogram/coronary angiography. (In most cases 'Coro' also includes left ventricular angiography/-gram)
CPK	Creatine phosphokinase
CPR	Cardiopulmonary resuscitation
CT	Computerized tomography
CX	Circumflexa (circumflex branch of the left coronary artery)
DC	Direct current
DD	Differential diagnosis
DDD	Double chamber double inhibited (pacing)
ECG	Electrocardiogram
Echo	Echocardiogram/echocardiography (in most cases color Doppler is integrated)
EF	Ejection fraction (in most cases of the left ventricle)
EPI/EPS	Electrophysiologic investigation/study
HOCM	Hypertrophic obstructive cardiomyopathy

Htx	Xeno-transplantation of the heart
ICD	Implantable cardioverter defibrillator
INR	International normalized ratio (for oral anticoagulation)
LA	Left atrium/left atrial
LAD	Left anterior descending coronary artery = left anterior descending branch of the LCA
LAD	Left axis deviation ($\text{ÅQRS}_F < -30°$)
LAFB	Left anterior fascicular block (= left anterior 'hemiblock')
LBBB	(Complete) left bundle branch block
LCA	Left coronary artery
LPFB	Left posterior fascicular block (= left posterior 'hemiblock')
LV	Left ventricle/left ventricular
LVH	Left ventricular hypertrophy
MET	Metabolic equivalents
MET	Maximal exercise test
MI	Myocardial infarction
MRI	magnetic resonance imaging
NSAID	Nonsteroidal anti-inflammatory agent
PA	Pulmonary artery
PE	Pulmonary embolism
PET	Positron emission tomography
PJRT	Permanent junctional reciprocating tachycardia
PTCA	Percutaneous coronary transluminal angioplasty
RA	Right atrium/right atrial
RBBB	(Complete) right bundle branch block
RCA	Right coronary artery
RV	Right ventricle/right ventricular
RVD	Right ventricular dysplasia
RVOT	Right ventricular outflow tract
SA	Sinoatrial
SACT	Sinoatrial conduction time
SN	Sinus node
SNRT	Sinus node recovery time
SPECT	Single proton emission computed tomography
SR	Sinus rhythm
SVPB	Supraventricular premature beat
SVT	Supraventricular tachycardia
SVTab	Supraventricular tachycardia with aberration
VPB	Ventricular premature beat
VSD	Ventricular septal defect
VT	Ventricular tachycardia
VVI	One-chamber ventricular (pacemaker)
VVI(R)	Ventricular inhibited ventricular pacing with rate responsiveness
WPW syndrome	Wolff-Parkinson-White syndrome

Introduction and Concept of the Book

Introduction

The Value of 'the ECG' Today

During the last decades the so-called 'direct' and 'imaging' diagnostic methods, such as coronary angiography, echo/color Doppler, scintigraphy, computer tomography and magnetic resonance imaging, have contributed to improve diagnostic accuracy in cardiac diseases considerably. For several reasons 'the ECG' has not been trusted in view of these newer methods, but has remained the most used non-invasive diagnostic method worldwide. Why should this be?

Firstly, there is no method other than the electrocardiography for the diagnosis of *arrhythmias*. And in this field, the ECG is more accurate than all direct and imaging methods on their best performances. For the last 30 years – and even more recently – arrhythmias have gained even more importance due to enormous progress in diagnostic perfection and consecutive therapeutic procedures. The ambulatory (Holter) ECG has facilitated the indication for pacemaker implantations. Recording intracardiac potentials (measuring their time correlations and localizing special potentials inclusively) and inducing/interrupting supraventricular and ventricular tachycardias have proven to be compulsory conditions for the catheter-induced radio-frequency ablation of accessory pathways (in Wolf-Parkinson-White (WPW) syndrome) and other conduction substrates (atrial, AV nodal and ventricular tissue). Invasive electrophysiology has also helped to develop reliable implantable cardioverter defibrillators (ICD). However, *the initial diagnosis of arrhythmias is generally made with the help of a rhythm stripe or on the basis of a 12 lead routine ECG*.

Secondly, tremendous knowledge has been accumulated in the scalar or 'pattern' ECG, since its introduction by Einthoven in 1902. The diagnosis of *myocardial infarction,* in its acute, subacute and chronic phase, remained the cornerstone of 'pattern electrocardiography'. Can we imagine that a patient undergoes coronary angiography, percutaneous transluminal coronary angioplasty (PTCA) or coronary artery bypass grafting (CABG) before an ECG has been performed? In many cases an exercise ECG is required, although the potential of this test is limited in detecting ischemia. The immediate ECG diagnosis of acute infarction has become more urgent since the application of emergency PTCA and thrombolysis, the latter also in regional hospitals.

Conduction disturbances as second degree AV block, bundle branch block and fascicular blocks represent another unique domain of the ECG. These conduction block patterns have a major clinical significance as potential precursors of a complete AV block. Sometimes, a severe *electrolyte imbalance* (potassium, calcium) is first detected in the ECG. In 70–90% of cases *pericarditis* is confirmed or diagnosed by the ECG. Particular characteristics in the 12 lead ECG allow the distinction of ventricular tachycardia and supraventricular tachycardia with aberration in about 90%.

Many other ECG patterns of clinical significance are discussed in this book.

Thirdly, the ECG pattern may give *hints for tachyarrhythmias which are not yet present*.

Examples:

- Pre-excitation (shortened PQ interval with delta wave in the QRS complex → arrhythmias in the (WPW) syndrome.
- Prolonged QT interval ('long QT') → polymorphous ventricular tachycardia of the type 'torsades de pointes'.
- Incomplete right bundle branch block pattern combined with marked ST elevations in leads V_1/V_2 (Brugada syndrome) → ventricular tachycardias with possible fibrillation and sudden death.

Limitations of the Pattern ECG

1. Only 50–60% of acute and old myocardial infarctions can be diagnosed in the ECG on the basis of usual criteria. This is not surprising. On the contrary, the relatively high per-

centage is striking, considering that the routine ECG is a highly *indirect* method. Moreover, the study of more complex infarction patterns should allow a correct diagnosis in over 70% of cases.

2. It is obvious that the *echocardiogram* (by direct measurement) can better determine the dimensions and the wall thickness of all four heart chambers than the ECG. Famous indices for the detection of left ventricular hypertrophy as *Sokolow's, Lyon's* and *Romhilt's point score* indexes have revealed a very low sensitivity and good to moderate specificity. It is time to realize this.

3. 40 years ago even complex congenital heart diseases were diagnosed on the basis of clinical findings (especially auscultation), x-rays and, of course, the ECG. Heart catheterization, including angiography, has initiated a revolution. Today this field has become a domain of echo/Doppler.

4. The diagnosis of acute pulmonary embolism should most certainly not be based on an ECG alone.

5. Isolated alterations of the repolarization (T wave and ST segment) are unspecific and insensitive overall. The most important exception is the typical ECG pattern of an acute infarction. Generally, changes of ST and T segments should only be interpreted in the context of other ECG abnormalities (especially of the QRS complex) and clinical findings. This is true for every ECG, last but not least.

Conclusions

The advantages of the ECG by far outweigh its limitations. The ECG is rapidly registered, cheap and non-invasive, and provides important and also essential information about our patients, information that is often not available by other methods. About two million physicians throughout the world register and interpret ECGs, and indeed earn money by doing so. Is it not therefore appropriate for them to *study* this method?

Concept of the Book

After three *introductory chapters* ('Theoretical Basis', 'Practical Approach' and 'The Normal ECG and its Normal Variants') the common ECG patterns and arrhythmias are presented in Chapters 4 to 26.

In Chapters 27 to 32 *Special Topics* are presented more or less extensively, such as 'Exercise ECG', 'Pacemaker ECG', 'Congenital Heart Diseases and Acquired (Valvular) Heart Diseases' and 'Rare ECGs'.

About 50 *'short stories' or 'case reports'* highlight the clinical relevance of 'the ECG'.

Each chapter is subdivided into two sections, a section called *'At a Glance'* and a section called *'The Full Picture'*. The Section 'At a Glance' is intended for colleagues who wish to be confronted in a concise form with the most important and most frequent ECG patterns and arrhythmias. However, these colleagues will also want to be informed about newer opinions and current progress.

The section 'The Full Picture' is aimed at ECG readers who already 'know their ECGs' and intend to plunge deeper into more complex fields and who are also interested in more practical and theoretical details.

They will also want to invest time in thinking (occasionally) even in three dimensions.

A primary reader of the 'The Full Picture' sections may find his knowledge summarised by a glance or two into the 'At a Glance' sections. A primary reader of the 'At a Glance' sections may be stimulated and wish to know more about a certain subject by jumping into 'The Full Picture' section in some chapters.

A *therapy* is proposed whenever important and convenient.

References are provided in the 'The Full Picture' sections and are listed at the end of each chapter.

Chapter 1
Theoretical Basics

For All Readers

Some extensive and clinically oriented guides of electrocardiography, such as Chou's *Electrocardiography in Clinical Practice* [1], do not provide any chapters about the theoretical basis. It is thought that readers acquired this knowledge during their medical training. We have found it convenient to present some of the theory in the hope that it may enhance practical handling of the ECG. The special anatomic and pathophysiologic conditions are discussed in later chapters.

1 Anatomy of the Impulse Formation and Impulse Conduction Systems

Figure 1.1 shows the anatomy of the impulse formation and conduction systems. The normal cardiac electric impulse is created by the sinoatrial (SA) node, called the *sinus* node (SN), that is located in the superior and posterior wall of the right atrium. The peripheral cells of the sinus node are conduction fibers. Several intra- and interatrial conduction bundles have been described (such as the Bachman bundle) but their function has not been proven.

The *atrioventricular* (AV) node is situated just above the interventricular septum. The AV node is characterized by a functional longitudinal dissociation into two pathways, the alpha and the beta. These pathways have different conduction velocities and refractory periods and – like every conduction substrate – may also conduct retrogradely (these properties represent the condition for the circus movement of the electric impulse in AV nodal reentry tachycardia).

The AV node is directly connected to the *His bundle*, a 20-mm-long bundle running down the septum that divides into several branches. The first branch is the *left posterior fascicle*, which has a relatively large caliber and spreads out to the posterior and inferior portions of the left ventricle. Some millimeters further the remnant His bundle bifurcates into the *right*

bundle branch (the *right ventricular fascicle*), reaching the right ventricle, and the *left anterior fascicle*, responsible for the conduction to the high lateral portion of the left ventricle. The left posterior and left anterior fascicle together are called *left bundle branch*. In about half of the intraventricular systems in humans there is a fourth fascicle, called the *left medial fascicle*, or there is a plurifascicular left ventricular conduction system consisting of up to ten small fascicles [2]. All of the right and left fascicles are subdivided into smaller ramifications; the finest fibers that reach the working muscle cells are called *Purkinje* fibers.

2 Normal Impulse Conduction

The electric impulse of the sinus node is transmitted by its peripheral cells to the nearest atrial working cells. It then trav-

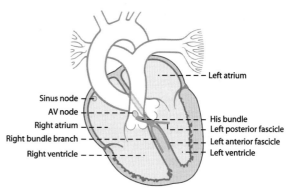

Figure 1.1

Anatomy of the impulse formation system and the impulse conduction system

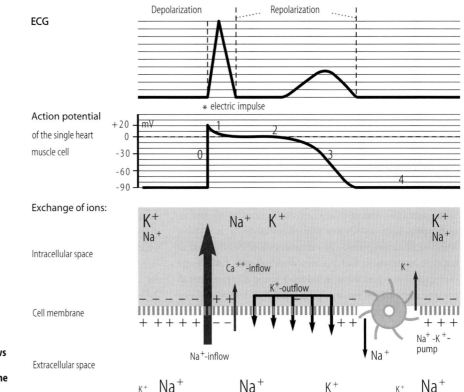

Figure 1.2
Correlation between ion flows and the intracellular action potential of a single cell of the working myocardium

els in concentric waves throughout the right atrium, reaching the left atrium and the AV node.

The impulse is slowed down for 60–120 msec in the AV node. Normally the impulse is conducted over the slow alpha pathway. This braking allows the atrioventricular valves to open and the ventricular walls to relax, thus enabling passive ventricular filling. This passive ventricular filling (during the ventricular diastole) is sustained by the atrial contraction (atrial kick) during the atrial systole. The electric impulse then spreads out very quickly (at a speed of 4 m/sec) down the His bundle, the ventricular fascicles, and the Purkinje fibers.

Its final ramifications are connected to the working muscle fibers in a network. The electric impulse induces contraction by an electromechanical coupling mechanism.

In about 1% of the population there is at least one (rarely more) *accessory conduction pathway*. Accessory conduction pathways are residual embryologic conduction bundles between the atria and the ventricles. An accessory pathway is a condition for the circus movement of reentry tachycardias in patients with the Wolff-Parkinson-White syndrome.

3 Action Potential of a Single Cell of Working Myocardium and its Relation to Ion Flows

Figure 1.2 shows the intracellular action potential of a 'working' heart muscle cell. At rest the myocardial cell is polarized at about – 90 mV. The electrical stimulus (symbolized as *) depolarizes the cell very fast, up to 0 mV; this is called phase 0 (with an 'overshoot' called phase 1). It is due to a quick shift of sodium ions from the extracellular space into the cell. Phases 0 and 1 correspond to the QRS in the ECG.

In phase 2, which is relatively flat, important and complex shifts of calcium occur. Phase 2 corresponds to the ST segment in the ECG. It is therefore understandable that calcium imbalances influence the duration of the ST segment.

During phase 3 the action potential slowly returns to its polarized state, mainly founded on shifts of potassium ions, transported from the cell to the extracellular space. Phase 3 corresponds to the T wave in the ECG.

In phase 4 the cell remains constantly polarized at – 90 mV until the next stimulus induces depolarization. However, in phase 4 there is an important (and essential) exchange between sodium ions (that are transferred out of the cell) and potassium ions (that are transferred into the cell) in order to restore the pre-existing extra- and intracellular ion content. This is performed with the help of the sodium–potassium (Na/K) ion pump. In the ECG, phase 4 corresponds to the isoelectric line between the end of the T wave and the beginning of the next ventricular cycle. Overall, the intracellular action potential shows a *monophasic* configuration, which strongly resembles the typical ECG pattern of acute myocardial infarction. In this condition the term 'monophasic deformation' is therefore used.

Figure 1.3 shows the main differences between the action potential of a) a working cell, b) a conduction cell, and c) a sinus node cell. In working fibers, the phase 4 of the action

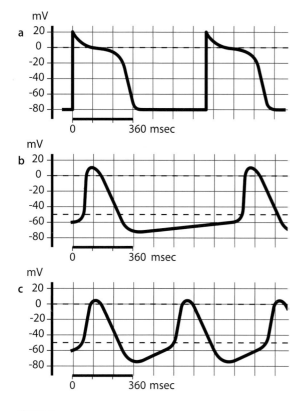

Figure 1.3
a) Action potential of a single working heart muscle cell; b) action potential of a single conduction cell; c) action potential of a single sinus node cell

potential remains stable (Fig. 1.3a). In contrast, in conduction fibers there is a slow depolarization during phase 4 that is called slow *spontaneous phase 4 (diastolic) depolarization*. This is an inherent characteristic also of a pacemaker cell, and it explains the potential capacity of a conduction cell to act as pacemaker. If the cell is not depolarized by an electrical stimulus before reaching the threshold at the level of about - 60 mV, it spontaneously depolarizes (Fig. 1.3b). This fact is important for understanding arrhythmias such as premature beats, escape beats, and escape rhythms.

A *ventricular premature* beat (VPB) is generated by a diseased Purkinje cell (or a group of fibers) that shows a faster spontaneous phase 4 depolarization than the sinus node. Thus the premature beat falls in *too early* (as the term describes it), disturbing the normal rhythm.

In contrast, an escape beat falls in *too late* (visually). For example, in the case of complete infra-Hissian atrioventricular block, asystole would occur – without a ventricular escape beat (or rhythm). As for the mechanism behind this, since no electric stimulus reaches the Purkinje fibers, their spontaneous phase 4 depolarization potential reaches the threshold and produces an action potential – an ordinary depolarization. The Purkinje fibers *substitute* the absent rhythm at a lower rate, in a beneficial manner.

The shape of the action potential between conduction cells and pacemaker cells does not differ, in principle. However, a relatively *fast* slow spontaneous phase 4 depolarization, associated with a *short* action potential (both resulting in a relative high rate), allows the pacemaker fibers to depolarize first. In normal conditions the fibers of the sinus node have the shortest action potential, thus dominating the heart rhythm (Fig. 1.3c).

4 Atrial Depolarization and Repolarization

In practice, the atrial depolarization occurs longitudinally. Because of its greater distance from the sinus node, the left atrium is depolarized 20–40 msec later than the right atrium. The depolarization of the atria lasts 80–110 msec and corresponds to the p wave in the ECG. The atrial repolarization, called Ta, follows the same way as the depolarization, and lasts about 300 msec (up to the apex of the ventricular T wave). The Ta wave is not visible in the ECG in normal conditions. In acute atrial infarction (a very rare condition) it may influence the segment between the end of the p wave and the beginning of the QRS complex, and eventually the beginning of the ST segment, by an elevation up to 1.5 mm. A depression of this segment is occasionally seen in elevated sympathetic tone. The alterations described are best visible in the limb leads.

The atrial vector lasts 90 msec and represents the sum of the right atrial vector and the left atrial vector (Figs 3.1a–b; Chapter 3 The Normal ECG and its Normal Variants). Because the sinus node is localized in the upper right atrium, the activation of the right atrium begins about 30 msec earlier than that of the left. Consequently, the activation of the right atrium terminates about 30 msec earlier than that of the left. Because the right atrium is localized anatomically anteriorly and more to the right, and the left atrium posteriorly and more to the left, the directions of these two atrial vectors are completely different. The right atrial vector points anteriorly, slightly inferiorly, and to the right, and the left atrial vector points posteriorly, slightly upwards, and to the left. The whole (sum) atrial vector is directed inferiorly, to the left, and anteriorly. The atrial vectors in pathologic conditions are described in Chapter 4 (Atrial Enlargement and Other Abnormalities of the p Wave).

5 Ventricular Depolarization and Repolarization

5.1 Vectors and Vectorcardiogram

Every depolarized heart cell produces an electric vector that has its amplitude, polarity, and (3-dimensional) direction. The sum of the vectors of all depolarized ventricular cells can be visualized with the ventricular *vectorcardiogram*. Figure 1.4 shows the spatial ventricular vectorcardiogram and its projection on the frontal and horizontal plane. The frontal ECG can be derived from the frontal vectorcardiogram (Fig. 1.5). This derived ECG is very similar to the directly derived ECG. The direct ECG in the horizontal plane is different from the ECG derived from the horizontal vectorcardiogram due to the 'magnifying glass' effect and the 'proximity' effect influencing voltage and polarity in the precordial ECG leads (see Section 7 below).

5.2 Simplified QRS Vectors

Figure 1.6 shows simplified QRS vectors. A vector is a theoretical model for an electric force. We distinguish between QRS vectors, ST vectors, and T vectors. The concept of vectors, especially QRS vectors with their amplitude and their directions in all three dimensions, is of great importance for understanding the scalar ECG in normal and some pathologic conditions

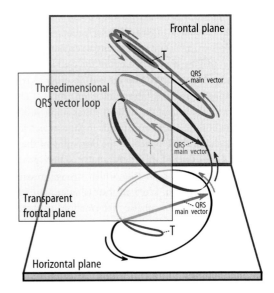

Figure 1.4
Ventricular vectorcardiogram

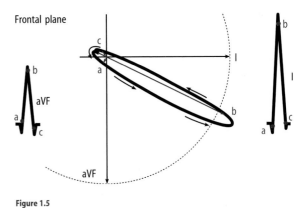

Figure 1.5
Frontal ECG derived from the frontal QRS vector loop

(such as bundle-branch blocks, fascicular blocks, left and right ventricular hypertrophy, and myocardial infarction). In addition, the instantaneous vectorial interpretation, as presented here (and later) in a *simplified* manner, considerably eases memorizing of the important ECG patterns. In normal and pathologic conditions (excluding left bundle-branch block and corrected transposition of the great arteries), ventricular excitation begins in the middle part of the interventricular septum on the left side and spreads out throughout the septum, from left to right. This first QRS vector (or septal vector) is known as

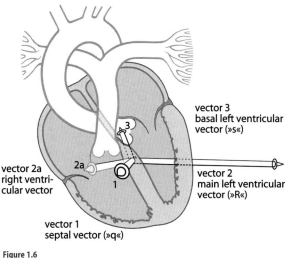

vector 3
basal left ventricular
vector (»s«)

vector 2a
right ventri-
cular vector

2a

vector 2
main left ventricular
vector (»R«)

vector 1
septal vector (»q«)

Figure 1.6
Simplified QRS vectors

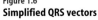

vector 1 and lasts about 15 msec; it is generally directed to the right, anteriorly, and slightly downwards, and corresponds to the small Q wave in leads I and V_5/V_6. In other leads (for instance in V_1/V_2) the same vector leads to a small R wave, due to projection.

Afterwards, the apical part of the left ventricle is depolarized, followed by excitation of the main portions of the left (and right) ventricle. The large second QRS vector (vector 2) lasts about 60 msec, is generally directed to the left, inferiorly, and mostly slightly posteriorly, and corresponds to the tall R waves in leads I and V_5/V_6, and the deep S waves in V_2/V_3. The large left ventricular main vector completely swallows the small simultaneous right ventricular 'vector 2a', produced by the depolarization of the right ventricle, with its muscle mass 15 times smaller than that of the left ventricle. With respect to ventricular depolarization (and repolarization) the human ECG represents a *levogram*. The right ventricular activation is only visible in the ECG in conditions that increase the RV vector (in right ventricular hypertrophy) or delays right ventricular excitation (in right bundle-branch block).

The remaining small upper ventricular parts (of the high lateral wall of the left and right ventricle and the upper part of the septum) are excited last. The third small QRS vector (vector 3) lasts about 15 msec, points generally superiorly, to the right, and posteriorly, and leads in the ECG to the small S wave in leads I/V_6 and to the last part of the S wave in leads V_2/V_3.

The QRS configuration in an ECG lead depends on the variations of the frontal QRS axis (the variations in the horizontal plane are of minor degree) on one hand, and, on the other, on the projection of the three ventricular vectors in the different ECG leads in the frontal and horizontal plane. A 'QRS' complex may also be an RS complex, a QS complex, or a simple R wave, and so on (Fig. 1.14).

The ventricular repolarization begins at the epicardium of the lateral ventricular walls and follows more or less the opposite direction to the depolarization. In the ECG it is represented by a part of the ST segment and by the T wave that again reflect *left* ventricular repolarization. The significance of the U wave is not clear. It may correspond to the repolarization of the Purkinje fibers.

6 Lead Systems

The 12 standard ECG leads are composed by six frontal leads and by six horizontal leads. The frontal plane is defined by the X and Y axes. The frontal bipolar leads contain leads I, II and III (Einthoven's bipolar leads) and leads aVR, aVL and aVF (Goldberger's so-called modified unipolar leads). The positions of the leads are presented in Figure 1.7.

Figure 1.8 shows Einthoven's triangle. A triangle with an asymmetric configuration, with the inferior apex pointing slightly to the right would, however, be more appropriate for the anatomical position of the heart.

In 'Cabrera's circle' the six frontal leads are integrated in the conventional system of coordinates in degrees (Fig. 1.9).

The *horizontal plane* is defined by the X and Z axes. The precordial leads were introduced by Wilson et al [3,4]. The localization of the six precordial unipolar leads V_1 to V_6 is shown in Figure 1.10. The additional dorsal unipolar leads V_7, V_8 and V_9 are important for direct detection of a *posterior* myocardial infarction and the additional right-precordial unipolar leads are indispensable for the detection of *right ventricular* myocardial infarction (Chapter 13 Myocardial Infarction).

Figure 1.11 shows the position of the Nehb leads (Nehb's triangle) that may, in some cases, better detect a posteroinferior infarction. The modified triangle of Sanz has added further aspects [5].

7 'Magnifying Glass' and 'Proximity' Effects

The distance from the heart to the exploring lead influences the amplitude of the ECG components. Evidently this is only valid for unipolar chest leads. A short distance (leads V_1 to

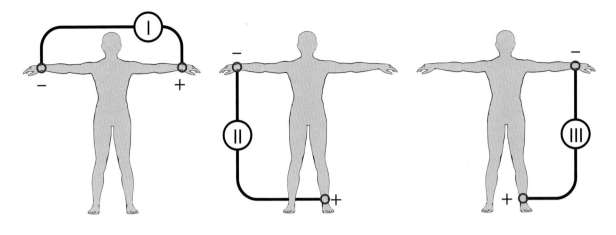

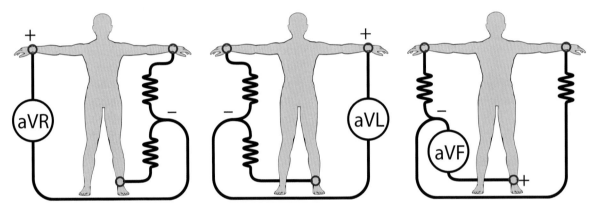

Figure 1.7
Position of the limb leads

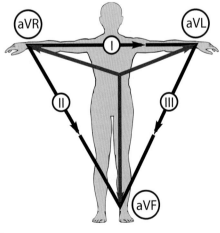

Figure 1.8
Einthoven's triangle

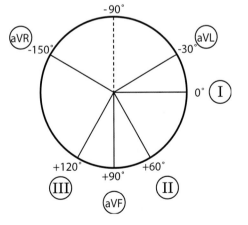

Figure 1.9
Cabrera's circle

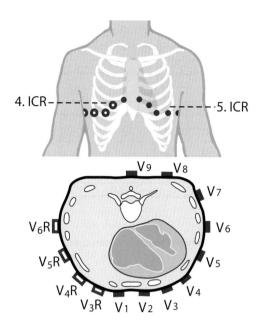

Figure 1.10
Position of the precordial leads

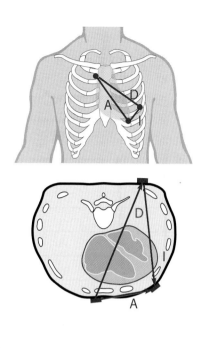

Figure 1.11
Nehb leads

V_3/V_4) enlarges the amplitude, a greater distance (leads V_5/V_6 to V_9) reduces the amplitude. Thus the S wave in V_2/V_3 is of greater amplitude than the R wave in V_6 to V_9. The amplitude in these leads is also decreased by the lung. The phenomenon is especially evident in the presence of a left bundle-branch block. Moreover, a precordial unipolar lead near the heart may better detect the vectors that are produced by myocardium just lying under the lead. This may produce an unexpected ECG pattern in certain special conditions (ECG 32.5a: Chapter 32 Rare ECGs).

8   Refractory Period

As illustrated in Figure 1.12 the heart muscle is not excitable during a period covered by the QRS complex, the ST segment, and a portion of the T wave (roughly at the apex). This period is called the 'absolute refractory period'. During the following short period – called the 'relative refractory period – the heart muscle is only excitable under special circumstances (such as ischemia) or by strong impulses (e.g. pacemaker impulses). This period is more or less identical to the so-called 'potential-

ly vulnerable' period. A ventricular premature beat falling into this 'vulnerable' period ('R-on-T' phenomenon) may induce ventricular fibrillation. Similarly, an atrial premature beat during the atrial repolarization (Ta) may induce atrial fibrillation ('p on Ta' phenomenon).

Another short period follows – the supernormal period – where a weak impulse *below* the normal stimulation threshold provokes depolarization. A ventricular premature beat falling in this period (covered by the last portion of the T wave and about 30 msec after the end of the T) never induces ventricular fibrillation, in contrast to that arising late in the ventricular cycle, in the region of the successive p wave. Besides the 'vulnerable period' there is another situation of membrane instability in this late ventricular period.

9   Nomenclature of the ECG

The descriptions of the electric heart cycle are presented in Figure 1.13 and the nomenclature of the QRS configuration in normal and pathologic conditions is shown in Figure 1.14. The nomenclature of the different grades of *ischemia* are shown in

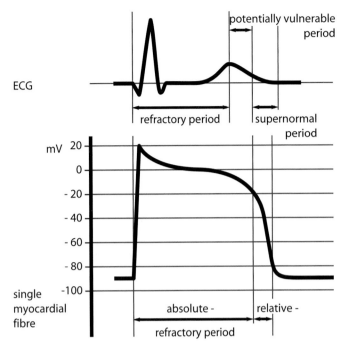

ECG

mV

single
myocardial
fibre

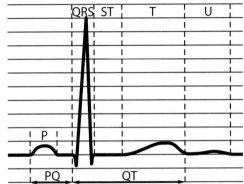

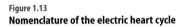

Figure 1.13
Nomenclature of the electric heart cycle

Figure 1.12
Refractory period

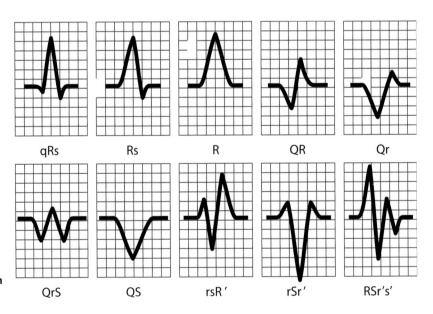

qRs Rs R QR Qr

QrS QS rsR′ rSr′ RSr′s′

Figure 1.14
**Nomenclature of the QRS configuration
in normal and pathologic conditions**

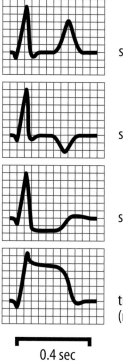

subendocardial ischemia

subepicardial ischemia

subendocardial lesion

transmural lesion
(monophasic deformation)

0.4 sec

Figure 1.15
T and ST alterations in the different stages of ischemia

Figure 1.15. The expressions for ischemia used below are electrocardiographic terms and represent the different grades of *hypoxia* of (mostly left) ventricular myocardium.

The slightest grade of ischemia manifests as *high and peaked T waves* and is called 'subendocardial ischemia'. The same morphologic alteration we find in moderate hyperkalemia. A higher grade of ischemia leads to the pattern of *symmetric negative T waves*. The term 'subepicardial ischemia' is sometimes used. The same alteration is found in many conditions besides ischemia (see Chapter 17 Alterations of Repolarization).

An even higher grade of ischemia leads to *depression of the ST segment* and is called 'subendocardial lesion'. This alter-

ation is also rather unspecific and is seen in conditions such as left ventricular hypertrophy and in patients receiving digitalis. ST depression is the best marker for ischemia during exercise.

These three grades of ischemia are reversible in many patients.

The highest grade of ischemia leads to extensive *elevation of the ST segment* ('monophasic deformation') and is called 'transmural lesion' or 'transmural injury'. This ECG pattern is only reversible in the case of vasospastic angina (Prinzmetal angina) and in other rare conditions. In about 99% of transmural lesions, ischemia persists and myocardial infarction (*necrosis*) develops, with appearance of new *Q waves*. Minor degrees of ST elevation are seen in pericarditis, early repolarization and other conditions, all in the absence of true ischemia (see Chapter 17 Alterations of Repolarization).

It has to be mentioned that theoretically in all grades of 'electrocardiographic ischemia' we find the highest grade in the subendocardial layers of the (left) ventricular myocardium.

For readers who are interested in more detail about the theoretical basis we would recommend the book by Bayés de Luna [6], and the work by Gettes [7], which is published as an admirable CD ROM.

References

1. Chou TC (ed). Electrocardiography in Clinical Practice. Adult and Pediatric, 4th edn. Philadelphia: WB Saunders, 1991
2. Demoulin JC, Kulbertus HE. Histopathological examination of concept of left hemiblock. Br Heart J 1972;34:807–14
3. Wilson FN, Hill IGW, Johnston FD. The interpretation of the galvanometric curves when one electrode is distant from the heart and the other near or in contact with its surface. Am Heart J 1934;10:176
4. Wilson FN, Johnston FD, Rosenbaum, et al. The precordial electrocardiogram. Am Heart J 1943;27:19–85
5. Saner H, Baur HR, Sanz E, Gurtner HP. Cardiogoniometry: a new noninvasive method for detection of ischemic heart disease. Clin Cardiol 1983;6:207–10
6. Bayés de Luna AJ. Clinical Electrocardiography. A Textbook. Armonk, NY: Furura Publishing, 1988
7. Gettes L. ECG Tutor (CD ROM). Armonk, NY: Futura Publishing, 2000

Chapter 2
Practical Approach

At a Glance

Some readers just taking a glance can be so fascinated by a special pattern on the ECG tracing (e.g. a bundle branch block or a striking Q wave) that they may overlook another abnormality; the best way to avoid such errors is to analyze the ECG systematically, step by step.

Before an ECG can be interpreted independently, it is necessary for the interpreter to know the basics of electrocardiography and rhythmology—the measurement of time intervals, the nomenclature, determination of the frontal QRS axis, definitions of pathologic Q or QS waves, differentiation between left and right bundle-branch block (BBB), and so on. The following requirements are valid:

i. Study of a short (good) ECG book.
ii. Interpreting hundreds of ECGs under the supervision of an experienced ECG reader. The 'New standards on electrocardiogram interpretations' of The American College of Cardiology and the American Heart Association [1] recom-

mend the following: reading a minimum of 500 tracings under expert supervision; ambulatory ECG training with supervised reading of an additional 150 tracings; and interpretation of at least 100 resting ECGs and 25 ambulatory ECGs per year.

Readers of either section of this chapter who find these approaches complex, or boring, should consider that:

i. knowing *only* how to measure 'ECG intervals' and to distinguish LBBB from RBBB does not make sense
ii. this chapter presents the author's own approach, which is roughly the same as that of every experienced ECG reader
iii. interpreting ECGs is not child's play.

The sections At a Glance and The Full Picture both contain reflections about differential diagnosis, and after some practice these reflections should come automatically to the reader.

1   The Practical Approach

Pathologic findings are shown in italics:

Table 2.1

1.	**Measurements (often done by the ECG machine)**

- rate (ventricular; and atrial in some cases); paper speed 25 mm/sec *or* 50 mm/sec
- P duration
- PQ interval
- QRS duration
- QT interval
- *plus* determination of the ÂQRS$_F$

2.	**Analysis of rhythm**

- Sinus rhythm (SR)?
- Other supraventricular rhythm?
    - Nonsinusal p waves: *atrial rhythm*
    - No p waves or retrograde atrial excitation: *AV junctional rhythm; AV reentry rhythms (tachycardias)*
    - Atrial flutter waves: *atrial flutter*
    - Atrial fibrillation waves: *atrial fibrillation*
    - *Additional aberration?* Broad QRS (≥ 120 msec): BBB
    - *Additional AV block 1°, 2° or 3°?* (possible in all supraventricular beats except in AV reentry tachycardias)
- Ventricular rhythm? (in most cases: AV dissociation)
    - Tachycardic: *ventricular tachycardia*
    - Bradycardic: *ventricular escape rhythm*
- Premature beats?
    - Small QRS: SVPBs
    - Broad QRS (> 120 msec): VPBs
    - Differential diagnosis: SVPBs with aberration
- Arrhythmias not fulfilling the criteria mentioned above

3.	**Morphologic analysis of components of the ECG (consider the calibration! Normal 1 mV = 10 mm; half calibration: 1 mV = 5 mm)**

- p wave (sinusal)
    - Normal
    - Signs for right, left or biatrial *enlargement*
- QRS (in SR)
    - Normal
    - Wide (> 120 msec): *RBBB, LBBB or bilateral BBB*
      Differential diagnosis: *pre-excitation*: delta wave and shortened PQ
    - Voltage criteria for *LVH or RVH* (or *BVH*)
    - (Formally) pathologic Q or QS waves: typical for *myocardial infarction*; typical for other conditions (normal variant, false poling of limb leads, LVH, pre-excitation, LBBB)
    - other criteria for LAFB or LPFB

continued on next page

Table 2.1
(continued)

- ST segment
    - ST elevation
        - a. Normal variant (V$_2$/V$_3$ or 'early repolarization')
        - b. Typical for *acute MI*
        - c. Typical for *acute pericarditis*
    - ST depression
        - a. *Ischemia*
        - b. *LVH*
        - c. due to *BBB*
- T wave
    - T negativity
        - a. Symmetric:
            - i. *ischemia*; other conditions (e.g. *subacute pericarditis*)
        - b. Asymmetric:
            - i. normal (due to projection: often in V$_1$, III/aVF)
            - ii. *LVH/LV overload*
            - iii. due to *BBB*
    - T positive, tall and peaked: *hyperkalemia*; *peracute ischemia* (rare)
- QT interval
    - QT prolonged: *long QT syndromes*; *hypocalcemia*
    - QT shortened: *hypercalcemia*
- U wave
    - Fusion of T and U: *hypokalemia*
    - U negativity: *ischemia*; *LVH*; *other conditions*

ÅQRS$_F$, frontal QRS axis; BBB, bundle-branch block; LAFB, left anterior fascicular block; LPFB, left posterior fascicular block; LVH, left ventricular hypertrophy; MI, myocardial infarction; SR, sinus rhythm; SVPB, supraventricular premature beat; VPB, ventricular premature beat; VT, ventricular tachycardia.

1.1 Definitive ECG Diagnosis

Take the important normal and pathologic findings from the analysis above and put them into the following scheme:

Table 2.2

	Example 1	Example 2
Rhythm/rate	SR, 72/min	*Atrial fibrillation*, medium rate 90 (max. 140, min. 40)
P	Normal	
PQ	Normal (0.16 sec)	
ÅQRS$_F$	Vertical (+ 80°)	LAD (− 60°): *LAFB*
QRS	Normal	0.12 sec, *LVH*
ST	Normal (elevation in V$_2$/V$_3$)	*Minor changes due to LAFB*
T	Normal (negative in III)	*Idem*
QT	Normal	Prolonged?
Special remarks		*Fusion of T and U*
Diagnosis	Normal ECG	*Atrial fibrillation, LAFB, LVH, hypokalemia?*

LAD, left axis deviation; LAFB, left anterior fascicular block; LVH, left ventricular hypertrophy; SR, sinus rhythm.

ECG Special

In our experience readers preferring the full picture may also have a lack of concentration during ECG interpretation, thus falling into the same traps as the glancers. The reasons for this are manifold.

Short Story/Case Report 1

About 10 years ago an ECG with obvious pre-excitation (ECG 2.1)—diagnosable by every dentist—was shown to the author by a very good-looking female colleague. The author's concentration was focused on the wrong subject and he interpreted the ECG as being normal.

2 Practical Approach

The practical approach includes:

i. analysis of rhythm
ii. morphologic analysis of p, QRS, ST and T (U) waves (measurement of the PQ interval and of the QT (QTc) interval are included)
iii. definitive ECG diagnosis.

2.1 Analysis of Rhythm

Typical pathologic findings are in italics (Table 2.3):

Table 2.3

Step 1
Regular or irregular?
• Regular: in most cases normal SR
pathologic regular rhythms: *escape rhythms; some forms of SVTs; VT*
• Irregular: the most frequent reason is regular SR *with SVPBs and VPBs;*
complete irregularity of the R–R intervals: atrial fibrillation

Step 2
Normal (sinusal p) wave present? >>> SR. If *not:*
• Abnormal (nonsinusal) p waves present: *atrial rhythm*
• No p waves: *AV junctional rhythm*
• Replacement of p waves by *other atrial waves: atrial flutter or atrial*
fibrillation

Step 3
Rate (of the ventricles)? Eventually rate of the *abnormal (nonsinusal)*
p waves or *flutter waves*?

Step 4
PQ interval? If we measure the PQ interval, we will not only recognise a
prolongation or shortening of the PQ time, but also that:
• p waves are partially conducted, and *partially not conducted*, in variable
manners: *in the three forms of AV block 2°*
• No p wave is conducted: *this means that the atria and ventricles are*
working independently from each other, in the presence of AV block 3°
(complete AV block)
• p waves are twisting around the QRS complexes *(in the special forms of*
AV dissociation)

Step 5
QRS duration normal (≤ 90 msec) or *prolonged?*
QRS ≥120 msec: *pattern of BBB*
• Supraventricular rhythm/tachycardia *with aberration*
• *Ventricular origin of the rhythm (with AV dissociation)*
– *Low rate (ventricular escape rhythm)*
– *Medium rate (accelerated idioventricular rhythm)*
– *High rate (VT)*

BBB, bundle-branch block; LVH, left ventricular hypertrophy; SR, sinus rhythm; SVPBs, supraventricular premature beats; VPBs, ventricular premature beats; VT, ventricular tachycardia.

2.2 Detailed Analysis of Morphology

Table 2.4

Step 1

P wave

1. Normal (sinusal)? (p duration 90–110 msec); note that a negative p in lead I means 'false poling' of the limb leads in 99% of the cases
2. Pathological p-waves
   - p duration ≥ 110 msec, accentuated terminal negativity in lead V_1: *LA enlargement*
   - p voltage ≥ 2.5 mm in leads III and aVF: *RA enlargement*
   - summation of both LA and RA enlargement: *biatrial enlargement*

Step 2

QRS

1. Frontal QRS axis = ÅQRS$_F$? (DD of different ÅQRS$_F$ see Chapter 3)
2. Broad QRS?
   - Typical configuration for aberration: *RBBB* (QRS ≥ 120 msec) or *LBBB* (≥ 140 msec); more or less typical BBB (≥ 160 msec): suspicious for *severe hyperkalemia*
   - Typical pattern of *bilateral BBB* (*RBBB+LAFB* or *RBBB+LPFB*)
   - Atypical BBB-like configuration (QRS ≥ 150 msec): suspicious for *ventricular origin of rhythm, generally with AV dissociation*
3. (Formally) pathologic Q or QS waves?
   - Typical for *old MI? (combined with symmetric negative T waves; typical history; risk factors for CHD)*
   - Atypical for old MI? (combined with asymmetric discordant T waves; atypical history; no risk factors for CHD)
   Differential diagnosis:
   - Artifact: Q/QS in lead I: false poling of limb leads (differential diagnosis: *situs inversus*)
   - Normal variant: QR or QS in lead III ('Q$_{III}$'): due to projection
   - *LVH* [QR or QS in lead III ('Q$_{III}$')]
   - *Pre-excitation (QS in III, aVF)*
   - *Hypertrophic (obstructive) cardiomyopathy*
   - *LBBB (QS in III, aVF, V_1 to V_4, with duration ≥ 140 msec)* (Formally pathologic Q waves see Chapter 14)
4. Signs for *LVH or RVH?* (Chapters 5 and 6)
5. Signs for *LAFB or LPFB?* (Chapter 9)
6. *Presence of delta wave?* (with shortened PQ: *pre-excitation*)
7. Presence of notching/slurring?
   - Normal variant (Chapter 3)
   - *Pathologic,* e.g. in *old MI* or *left fascicular block* (Chapters 9 and 13)

Table 2.4 *(continued)*

Step 3

ST segment

1. ST elevation?
   - Normal variants: ST (in V_2/V_3) 'early repolarization' (Chapter 3)
   - Pathologic: typical for *acute MI:* consider *other findings; symptoms, history, risk factors for CHD* (Chapter 13)
   - Pathologic: typical for *acute pericarditis: frontal ST vector about + 70°: ST elevations in leads aVF,* II and I (Chapter 15)
   - Pathologic: typical for *mirror image of ST depression:* e.g. in *LVH; systolic LV overload*
2. ST depression?
   - *Ischemic*
   - *LVH; LV overload*
   - *Related to BBB or other conditions* (Chapter 17)

Step 4

T (and U) waves

1. Asymmetric T negativity?
   - Normal in lead V_1; normal in vertical ÅQRS$_F$: in aVF, III(II); normal in left ÅQRS$_F$: in aVL
   - Pathologic in *LVH; LV overload; pre-excitation; BBB*
2. Symmetric T negativity?
   - Often *ischemic,* but extensive differential diagnosis: Later stage of *pericarditis; LVH; LV overload; acute pancreatitis; drugs; others*
3. High and symmetric T?
   - *Ischemia* (rare, because short-lasting)
   - *Hyperkalemia*
4. U negativity?
   - *Ischemic; other conditions*

Step 5

QT interval

1. QT prolonged
   - *'Long QT syndromes'* (Chapter 26)
   - *Hypocalcemia*
2. QT shortened: *hypercalcemia*
3. Fusion of T and U: *hypokalemia*

Step 6

Definitive diagnosis (see Table 2.2)

ÅQRS$_F$, frontal QRS axis; BBB, bundle-branch block; CHD, coronary heart disease; LA, left atrial; LAFB, left anterior fascicular block; LPFB, left posterior fascicular block; LVH, left ventricular hypertrophy; MI, myocardial infarction; RA, right atrial; SR, sinus rhythm; SVPBs, supraventricular premature beats; VPBs, ventricular premature beats; VT, ventricular tachycardia.

As mentioned above, an ECG must be interpreted in the context of the clinical findings of a patient; therefore in the ECGs in this book we give the age, gender, and clinical diagnosis of the patients, whenever convenient and possible.

References

1. Kadish AH, Buxton AE, Kennedy HL, et al. ACC/AHA clinical competence statement on electrocardiography and ambulatory electrocardiography: A report of the ACC/AHA/ACP-ASIM task force on clinical competence (ACC/AHA Committee to develop a clinical competence statement on electrocardiography and ambulatory electrocardiography) endorsed by the International Society for Holter and noninvasive electrocardiology. The American College of Cardiology/American Heart Association/American College of Physicians/American Society of Internal Medicine Task Force. The International Society for Holter and Noninvasive Electrocardiology. Circulation 2001;104:3169–78

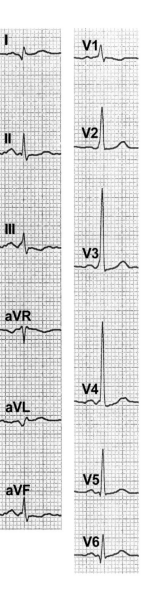

ECG 2.1
Pre-excitation with short PQ interval (0.10 sec). Obvious positive delta waves in III and aVF. Striking Q waves (negative delta waves) in I and aVL and abnormal R waves in V_1 and V_2. Note also biphasic (+/–) delta waves in V_5 and V_6.

At a Glance and The Full Picture

This chapter is not divided in two sections because the knowledge of the *normal* ECG and its *normal variants* is as essential for those readers choosing to glance as for those preferring the full picture. This chapter can be used as a dictionary by both types of readers.

When we interpret an ECG we compare it instantaneously with the *normal* ECG and *normal* variants stored in our memory; these memories are stored *visually* in the posterior parts of the cerebrum and *intellectually* in the frontal parts. If these reservoirs contain only question marks, we are as helpless and lost in our interpretation as someone wandering through a snowstorm without a compass. It is important therefore to fill, or reactivate, these reservoirs.

Normal ECG variants will be discussed extensively in this chapter, because their interpretation often leads to a wrong diagnosis. In contrast to pathologic ECG patterns, normal variants can be described as *constant ECG patterns that are neither linked to corresponding typical symptoms, nor to corresponding clinical and anamnestic findings, and not to drugs.*

As early as 1959, Goldman [1] demonstrated that misinterpretation of normal variants can lead to cardiac invalidism. Even today, ill-advised diagnostic and 'therapeutic' interventions may be based on normal variants.

The differential diagnoses of normal variants – the *pathologic conditions* – are presented in brief throughout this chapter.

1   Components of the Normal ECG

The *time intervals* of the ECG must be measured and the *whole* ECG must be examined *systematically* and with *caution* in order to avoid mistakes (Chapter 2 Practical Approach). In general, computers measure more precisely than the human eye.

However, computers can generate terrible errors, such as in determining rate – in the presence of high T waves, the computer may indicate double the real rate. For the patterns of *myocardial infarction* and *intraventricular conduction disturbance*, and for many *arrhythmias*, 'computer diagnosis' is unreliable.

1.1   Sinus Rhythm

The sinus node is the normal pacemaker of the heart. *Sinus rhythm* is an obligatory component of the normal ECG. If we diagnose sinus rhythm, we mean that the whole heart (the atria and the ventricles) is depolarized by the electrical stimulus originating in the sinus node and we use the abbreviation SR (ECG 3.1).

In some special conditions, such as complete atrioventricular (AV) block or in patients with a one-chamber ventricular pacemaker (VVI), the expression sinus 'rhythm' should be restricted to *atrial rhythm* only. A second rhythm that is responsible for the activation of the ventricles must be described separately. For example, ECG 3.2 shows complete AV block; *sinus rhythm of the atria*, rate 102/min; *ventricular escape rhythm*, rate 76/min.

The rate of normal sinus rhythm is 60–100/min (or better 50–90/min) [2]. Sinus rhythm with a rate below 50–60/min is called *sinus bradycardia;* sinus rhythm with a rate above 100/min is called *sinus tachycardia*. Generally, sinus rhythm is not completely regular, especially at lower rates. If the deviation exceeds more than 15% of the basic rate, the term *sinus arrhythmia* is used. In young healthy people the rate variability may exceed 50%.

Sinus bradycardia (ECG 3.3) is often seen as a normal variant in individuals at rest, and usually in athletes. Episodes of sinus bradycardia at a rate < 40/min were observed in young

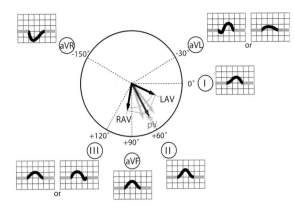

Figure 3.1a
Normal atrial vectors and corresponding p waves in the frontal plane. RAV=right atrial vector; LAV=left atrial vector; pV=p vector.

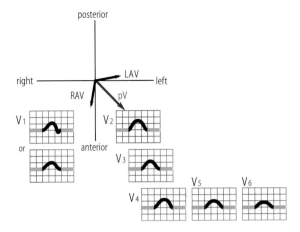

Figure 3.1b
Normal atrial vectors and corresponding p waves in the horizontal plane. RAV=right atrial vector; LAV=left atrial vector; pV=p vector.

healthy people, in 24% of men and 8% of women; with sinus pauses of up to 2.06 sec in men and 1.92 sec in women [3,4].

Differential diagnosis: Frequent organic disorders are hypothyreosis, cerebral diseases with elevated intracranial pressure, liver diseases, conditions following heart valve operations, and the sick sinus syndrome.

Sinus tachycardia (ECG 3.4) is normal during exercise and under conditions of mental stress.

Differential diagnosis: Includes febrile status, heart failure, hyperthyreosis, tumoral diseases, and cachexia.

Sinus arrhythmia is almost always normal (ECG 3.5). The rate variation depends on respiration, so that during inspiration the rate increases and during expiration the rate decreases, always with some delay. The rate deviation may reach 50% in children and +/− 15% in middle-aged people; in the elderly the deviation is small or absent.

Differential diagnosis: Atrial premature beats originating near the sinus node. Note: sinus arrhythmia is generally *not* a component of the sick sinus syndrome.

1.1.1 Atrial Vectors in Sinus Rhythm

Because the sinus node is situated in the right atrium, the activation of the right atrium begins about 30 msec before the activation of the left atrium. For the diagnosis of sinus rhythm it is not sufficient that after a normal PQ interval, a p wave is followed by a QRS. The activation of the atria by the electric stim-

ulus of the sinus node produces a *typical p vector* in the frontal and horizontal leads. The right atrium vector points inferiorly, anteriorly, and slightly to the right, whereas the left atrial vector points posteriorly, to the left, and slightly downwards (Figures 3.1a and 3.1b). The p vector in sinus rhythm is a *fusion* of the right atrial vector and the left atrial vector. In the limb leads, the fusion vector that corresponds to the p wave, has an axis of + 50° to + 80°, often about + 70°. As a consequence, the p wave is always *positive* in lead I and always *negative* in lead aVR (ECG 3.1). The p wave is mostly positive in II, aVF and III, but may also be biphasic (+/−) in these leads. In lead aVL, the p wave may be biphasic (−/+), positive or negative. If the p vector is not considered, one may mix up sinus rhythm with other atrial rhythms and especially with the most frequent kind of *false poling* (erroneous exchange of the upper limb leads). In this case, as the most striking sign, the p wave is *negative* in I. Of course, the QRS complex and the depolarization are also inverse in this lead (ECG 3.6), whereas the p and QRS configuration in the precordial leads is normal (for other false poling, see Chapter 32 Rare ECGs).

In the horizontal leads, the normal p wave is positive in all leads V_1 to V_6, with one frequent exception: in lead V_1 the p is often biphasic (+/−), with a first, positive portion and a (smaller) second, negative portion. The latter is due to activation of the left atrium that is placed dorsally in the thorax.

Differential diagnosis: There is no real differential diagnosis of sinus rhythm. Only a (rare) focus near the sinus node cannot be distinguished from one of sinusal origin.

The presence or absence of sinus rhythm of the atria should be examined carefully especially in cases of complete AV block (where only the atria follow a supraventricular rhythm).

Short Story/Case Report 1

In December 2002 we found ventricular pacemaker rhythm at a rate of 84/min in a 63-year-old woman who had been implanted with a one-chamber (VVIR) pacemaker for treatment of complete AV block with syncope in 1996. Yet the diagnosis of the arrhythmia was incomplete. She did not have sinus rhythm of the atria, but *atrial fibrillation* (ECG 3.7), thus needing additional therapy with an anticoagulation or aspirin. The correct and complete arrhythmia diagnosis is therefore: atrial fibrillation, complete AV block, ventricular pacemaker rhythm at a rate of 84/min.

The *scalar alterations* of the p wave concerning amplitude, form and duration are described in Chapter 4 Atrial Enlargement, and the p wave abnormalities due to *arrhythmias* are described in Chapters 18, 19, 23 and 24.

1.2 PQ Interval

The *normal* PQ interval is 0.13–0.20 sec. It is measured from the beginning of the P wave to the beginning of the QRS complex, being a Q wave or an R wave. Lead II is suitable for measuring this because the initial deflections of P and QRS are sharply defined in this lead. In some cases, the beginning of the P and QRS must be determined in another lead, or even in two different leads, registered simultaneously. In healthy individuals a shortened PQ (without a delta wave and without paroxysmal supraventricular tachycardia) is occasionally encountered (ECG 3.8). Also, there are AV blocks in normal individuals: AV block 1° in 8% (male) to 12% (female) [3,4] and intermittent AV block 2° type Wenckebach in 6% (male) to 4% (female) [3,4], especially in athletes, and during the night.

Early atrial premature beats may be completely AV blocked in normal individuals, especially in persons with AV block 1°, and during bradycardia.

Differential diagnosis: A PQ interval of more than 0.20 sec is defined as AV block 1°. A PQ interval of less than 0.13 sec associated with paroxysmal supraventricular tachycardias represents the so-called Lown-Ganong-Levine (LGL) syndrome. In the Wolff-Parkinson-White (WPW) syndrome a shortened PQ is linked to a delta wave of the QRS complex.

1.3 QRS complex

1.3.1 QRS Axis in the Frontal Plane (ÅQRS$_F$)

The normal QRS complex is very *variable* in the frontal leads and quite *uniform* in the horizontal leads.

In the *frontal leads* the direction of the QRS vector depends on habitus, body weight, body position, age (especially), and on unknown causes. The frontal QRS axis must be determined in a lying position. Generally, the mean QRS axis undergoes a rotation from right to left during aging. The reason is probably the increasing electric preponderance of the left ventricle compared to the right. Table 3.1 shows the common ÅQRS$_F$ axis (found in about 70% of normal individuals) in relation to age. ECGs 3.9a–3.9g represent such normal findings. Right-axis deviation or a left-axis deviation (ECG 3.9f shows near left-axis deviation) are very rare in middle-aged patients, and in these cases are often without explanation. Small changes of the QRS axis may be associated with the use of different ECG registration machines. A substantial change of ÅQRS$_F$ *within a short time* needs further evaluation.

Table 3.1
General behavior of QRS axis in the frontal plane (ÅQRS$_F$) in relation to age

Years	ÅQRS$_F$
0–2	+ 120°
2–10	+ 90°
10–25	+ 70°
25–40	+ 60°
40–70	+ 20°
70–90	– 20°

Differential diagnosis: a shift to the *right* is seen in some cases with pulmonary embolism, in emphysema, and chronic pulmonary hypertension. A shift to the *left* may be associated with inferior infarction or with left anterior fascicular block. The most spectacular alterations of the QRS axis without heart disease are seen in people with thoracic deformation, or after resection of one lung.

An S$_I$/S$_{II}$/S$_{III}$ configuration, generally with R waves greater than the S waves, is not a very rare finding in normal hearts (ECG 3.10) and may be associated with a frontal *sagittal* QRS axis.

Differential diagnosis: This S$_I$/S$_{II}$/S$_{III}$ pattern is rarely seen in right ventricular hypertrophy, or dilatation. In these cases the S wave generally has a greater amplitude than the R wave. Other signs are often also present of right ventricular hypertrophy or right ventricular dilatation, such as a tall R wave in lead V$_1$, or a pattern of incomplete or complete right bundle-branch block, and/or negative T waves in V$_1$ to V$_3$.

1.3.2 QRS Axis in the Horizontal Plane

The most common pattern in the horizontal leads is shown in ECG 3.1. In leads V_1 and V_2 there is a rS complex with small R waves and deep S waves. In lead V_3 (transition zone from a *negative* QRS to a *positive* QRS complex) the R wave is still smaller than the S wave. In lead V_4 the amplitude of the R wave is greater than that of the S wave, sometimes with a small Q wave. In leads V_5/V_6 a qR wave is generally seen, often without an S wave.

In *clockwise rotation* (ECG 3.11) the transition zone from negative to positive QRS is shifted to the *left*. This condition is also called 'poor R progression in the precordial leads'.

Differential diagnosis: Clockwise rotation may be seen, for example, in the presence of 'non-Q wave' anterior myocardial infarction, or in right and/or left ventricular dilatation.

Counterclockwise rotation (ECG 3.12) is characterized by a shift of the transition zone to the *right*. It is more common in *young* healthy individuals. In children up to 8 years of age a tall R wave in V_1 is frequent, and it occurs in 20% of children aged 8–12 years, and in 10% aged 12–16 years [5]. An R : S ratio of >1 in lead V_2 is rare in healthy adults (about 1%), whereas a R : S ratio >1 in lead V_2 is found in children in 10% [6].

Differential diagnosis: A prominent notched R wave, at least 0.04 sec broad, in V_2/V_3 (V_1) is seen in posterior infarction. An Rs complex in V_1 may be due to right ventricular hypertrophy. A tall R wave with delta wave in leads V_1 to V_3 (to V_6) is typical for one type of pre-excitation.

In some cases clockwise or counterclockwise rotation may be caused by erroneous placement of the precordial leads by one intercostal space too low or one space too high, respectively.

1.3.3 Two Special QRS Patterns

Two puzzling QRS patterns often provoke diagnostic difficulties (Chapter 14 Differential Diagnosis of Pathologic Q waves).

a. Q_{III} Type

The so-called Q_{III} *type* corresponds to a *QS* or *QR* pattern in lead III, sometimes combined with a significant Q wave, or very occasionally a QS pattern in aVF, and associated with a *positive asymmetric T wave* in most cases (ECGs 3.13a and 3.13b).

The QS or QR pattern in lead III is found in *normal* hearts and in various *pathologic conditions*.

Differential diagnosis: The pathologic conditions are: *inferior infarction*, often associated with a persisting symmetric negative

T wave; or the Q/QS wave is followed by a positive T wave, perhaps due to mirror image in *systolic overload* or *left ventricular hypertrophy*, to pre-excitation (with a negative delta wave) or *left bundle-branch block* (broad QRS and typical pattern in the other leads). In later stages of inferior myocardial infarction the T wave may also be positive in the inferior leads.

b. $QS_{V1/V2}$ Type

A *QS pattern* in leads V_1 and/or V_2 (ECG 3.14), found in healthy hearts, is a normal variant, or is due to misplacement of leads by one intercostal space (ICS) too high. In young people, there may be a negative T wave also in V_2, mimicking a small anteroseptal infarction with ischemia. In other cases we find a QS type only in V_2. The explanation is that on the thoracic wall, the lead V_2 is positioned superiorly compared with a line between V_1 and V_3, thus suppressing the initial R wave. The disappearance of QS and the appearance of an rS complex, respectively, after moving lead V_2 (and V_1) one ICS higher, is not a reliable criterion for absent infarction.

Differential diagnosis: An additional Q wave in lead V_3, or a QRS notching in more than two precordial leads, combined to a negative T wave in lead V_3, favors the diagnosis of old anteroseptal myocardial infarction.

The correct diagnosis in Q/QS_{III} and $QS_{V1/V2}$ is made not only by morphologic ECG criteria, but also by anamnestic and clinical findings. In cases of doubt, further examinations are necessary.

1.3.4 Other Normal Variants of the QRS Complex

a. Notching Versus Pseudo-Notching

Notching or a 'notch' is defined as a small (about 1–2 mm high) additional deflection with inverse polarity, within the Q, R, or S wave of the QRS complex (Figure 3.2a). In this book we do not distinguish between *notching* and *slurring* [that is defined

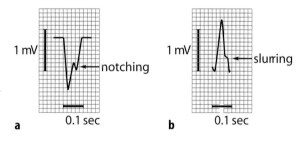

Figure 3.2
a. Notching of QRS. b. Slurring of QRS.

as 'slight' notching, without change of polarity (Figure 3.2b)]. Notching and slurring correspond either to a *localized disturbance (delay)* of conduction and excitation, or merely may be due to *projections* (known as *pseudo-notching*). In practice it is important to distinguish between *true* intraventricular conduction disturbance (notching) and a *harmless* functional alteration, based only on vectorial projection (pseudo-notching).

Differentiation between notching and pseudo-notching may be difficult. Slight pseudo-notching is frequently seen in the inferior leads III, aVF and II (ECGs 3.15a and 3.15b) and occasionally in lead aVL. A pseudo-notching in lead I is rare.

Differential diagnosis: Left posterior fascicular block: Often 'slurred R downstroke' in leads III, aVF and V_6. Left anterior fascicular block (always with left-axis deviation): Often 'slurred R downstroke' in leads I and aVL. Notching in the limb leads may also be seen in old myocardial infarction, with or without pathologic Q waves.

A pseudo-notching may also be present in the *transition zone* of the precordial leads, mostly in only one lead, and predominantly in V_3 (ECG 3.16a and 3.16b). Again, this is due to projection. The QRS complex cannot decide whether it should be negative or positive. ECG 3.16c shows notching in leads V_3 and III.

Differential diagnosis: In cases of notching in three or more precordial leads, an intraventricular conduction disturbance is probable, often due to an infarction scar (Chapter 13 Myocardial Infarction).

b. Pseudo-Delta Wave

Projections may also be associated with a positive *pseudo-delta wave* in leads III, aVF (II) and in leads V_2 and/or V_3 (ECGs 3.17a and 3.17b). Occurrence of a pseudo-delta wave in V_2/V_3 can be explained: the septal vector is (as normal) positive in these leads, but there is also a positive projection of the following 20–30 msec of the QRS complex, on leads V_2 and V_3. This pattern is often misinterpreted as ('abortive') pre-excitation. However, the PQ interval is *normal*. In highly doubtful cases, it is advisable to repeat the ECG or to perform a test with ajmaline. In pseudo-pre-excitation the delta wave persists, in true pre-excitation it should disappear.

c. QRS Low Voltage

A QRS voltage of less than 5 mm (0.5 mV) in up to three of the six frontal leads is not a rare finding. True *peripheral* low voltage is present if the QRS complex is smaller than 5 mm in five out of six or all six limb leads (ECG 3.18), a rare finding in normal individuals.

Differential diagnosis: True peripheral low voltage in pathologic conditions is found in lung emphysema, obese people, and rarely in patients with extensive pericardial effusion. Peripheral low voltage has little clinical importance. The same is valuable for the very rare *horizontal* low voltage defined as QRS voltage smaller than 7 mm in all precordial leads. A significant decrease of QRS voltage has been described after therapy with (overdosed) adrioblastine.

d. Incomplete Right Bundle-Branch Block (iRBBB)

An iRBBB (rSr' in lead V_1) is a frequent finding in healthy people, especially in young people. This pattern may lead to a notching or rSr' complex in lead III also. If r > r' (ECG 3.19a) a normal variant is probable. A notched S upstroke in V_1 often corresponds to iRBBB. In this case, there is a terminal R wave in lead aVR, as in common patterns of iRBBB. In addition, the QRS configuration with r < r' (ECG 3.19b) represents a normal variant in many cases. However, we have to exclude diseases of the right ventricle.

Differential diagnosis: iRBBB with r' > r is encountered in right ventricular systolic overload (as in pulmonary *embolism* and any disease with *pulmonary hypertension,* and/or *right ventricular hypertrophy*), in RV diastolic overload (as in *atrial septal defect*) or may represent a *precursor* of complete RBBB. iRBBB with r > r' is a rarer finding in these pathologic conditions. A new onset iRBBB may be a sign of acute right ventricular overload, or it can appear after different placing of lead V_1 – in which case it may be harmless.

1.4 ST Segment

For some physicians, an ST elevation of ≥ 2 mm in any ECG lead automatically means *acute ischemia*. This opinion needs to be revised: there is *one very common* normal ECG pattern with ST elevation, and *one very rare* normal variant.

1.4.1 Common Pattern of ST elevation: ST elevation in V_2/V_3

In about 70% of normal ECGs the so-called *junction (J) point* (the point that defines the end of the QRS complex and the beginning of the ST segment) is 0.5–1.5 mm above the isoelectric line in lead V_2 and often V_3, and consequently there is *elevation* of the ST segment (measured at rest 0.08 sec after the J point). Especially in *sinus bradycardia* the J point, and thus the ST segment, may be elevated up to 2–3 mm (ECG 3.20a), and rarely up to 4 mm. Vagal stimulation enhances the discordance of repolarization in the anteroseptal leads, and this phenomenon is magnified by the 'proximity effect'. The latter effect explains also the relative high amplitude of the S and

T waves in leads V_2 and V_3. This common pattern of repolarization *should not* be misinterpreted as acute ischemia.

Short Story/Case Report 2

A 38-year-old man with acute pain on the left side of the thorax was seen at the emergency station. He mentioned subfebrile body temperatures over the previous few days. The only risk factor for coronary heart disease (CHD) was that one of his uncles had a myocardial infarction at the age of 50 years. Blood pressure was 150/90 mmHg. The ECG showed sinus bradycardia with ST elevation of 2 mm in leads V_2 and V_3 (ECG 3.20b). Creatine kinase (CK) was slightly elevated (by 20%), and myocardial fraction of CK and troponin were normal. There was leukocytosis of $11 \times 10^9/l$. The diagnosis of acute anterior infarction was made and thrombolysis performed. The ECG remained unchanged. The pain disappeared after the first dose of morphine and blood pressure normalized. One day later the diagnosis was revised and an infectious disease of unclear origin with pain of chest skeletal muscle presumed. The patient insisted on a coronary angiography. The coronary arteries were normal. A day later the patient was dismissed without symptoms and with aspirin 500 mg for 7 days. On the basis of positive titers of coxsackievirus, the final diagnosis of coxsackievirus infection (Bornholm disease) was made. In conclusion, the chest pain was atypical and the ECG was normal. The slightly elevated CK was overestimated. It would have been better to observe the patient for some hours and to control the ECG and the enzymes.

1.4.2 Rare Pattern of ST Elevation: Early Repolarization

'Early repolarization' is characterized by a *marked, constant* elevation of the J point and the ST segment of 2–4 mm, emerging directly from the R wave downstroke, in the *anterior* precordial leads (accentuated more septally or more laterally) and/or the *inferior* leads III and aVF. It occurs more frequently in males than in females, but no less in white than in black people [7]. The pattern is very similar – even the same – as that of *acute infarction* or *Prinzmetal angina*. In these conditions the ST elevation varies within a short time and is mostly associated with chest pain. The correct diagnosis is based on anamnestic and clinical findings.

The ECGs presented in ECGs 3.21a–3.21d show examples of early repolarization in normal individuals, with an ST elevation of 2–3 mm in some leads.

Differential diagnosis: The most important differential diagnosis of ST elevation, arising from the R wave, is acute myocardial infarction and, rarely, vasospastic angina. Hypercalcemia may provoke a slight ST elevation of this type. ST elevations, generally arising from the S wave, are seen in acute pericarditis and as a mirror image of 'systolic left ventricular overload'.

If slight elevations of the ST segment in otherwise normal ECGs are included, early repolarization is not that rare. For differentiation between early repolarization and acute pericarditis see the paper by Spodick [8].

In some cases, an *Osborn wave* – a very short and small positive deflection within the ST segment (ECG 3.20a) – is seen in addition to the ST elevation [9]. In rare normal ECGs, without early repolarization, a *minimal* Osborn wave may be present in the inferior leads or in V_5/V_6 (ECG 3.22).

Differential diagnosis: An Osborn wave is regularly seen in hypothermia (ECGs 3.23a–3.23d) and sometimes in cases of acute pericarditis. For details, see Chapter 17 Special Waves And Phenomena.

1.5 T Wave and U Wave

1.5.1 T Wave

Besides the QRS complex (great variability of the axis in the frontal leads), the T wave is the most variable component of the ECG. There are some rules about normal T waves, however.

A normal T wave is *asymmetric*, with a slow upstroke and a more rapid downstroke.

In respect to polarity, T is positive in most leads and negative in some leads. In the *frontal leads* the T wave is positive in I and often positive in aVL, II, aVF, and III. The T wave is often negative in lead III (and aVF, occasionally also in II), independent of the frontal QRS axis (ECGs 3.24a and 3.24b). In a QRS axis of 0° or less, the T wave may be negative also in aVL, but *never* in lead I.

In the *horizontal* leads the T wave is negative or positive (or isoelectric) in V_1 and positive in V_2 to V_6. In rare cases there is a negative T wave in V_2 (and V_3), especially in young women (up to the age of 30 years). A negative T wave in any of the other precordial leads is very rare and should be interpreted as a normal variant only after exclusion of any pathology.

Differential diagnosis: T wave alterations alone, not with QRS abnormalities, have to be considered as *unspecific*. The reasons for pathologic T waves are manifold, but some general rules apply:

1. Coronary heart disease (CHD) is the most common origin of *symmetric* and *negative* T waves, so-called 'coronary' T waves

(ECG 3.24c). However, this type of T wave occurs in other conditions too, such as pericarditis, or severe anemia.

2. *Asymmetric, negative* T waves are generally associated with ventricular overload. In *left* ventricular overload we find discordant negative T waves in I, aVL, V_6 and V_5 (ECG 3.24d). It must be mentioned that often the distinction between left ventricular overload and coronary origin is impossible based on the morphology of the T wave. Furthermore, the combination of these two conditions is not rare. In *right* ventricular overload the T waves may be negative (concordant) in V_2 and V_3. T negativity in V_1 to V_3 is also found in cases of 'arrhythmogenic right ventricular dysplasia' and in funnel chest.

Tall, positive and even *symmetric* T waves may be seen in the precordial leads, especially in V_2 and V_3 (and V_4), often in younger people and associated with sinus bradycardia (ECGs 3.20a and 3.20b).

Differential diagnosis: Hyperkalemia. Very rare transitory sign of peracute ischemia.

1.5.2 U Wave

The U wave is a positive flat deflection after the T wave, visible best in leads V_5 and V_6. It is thought that the U wave represents the repolarization of the Purkinje fibers. The absence of the U wave is not rare and has no clinical significance.

Differential diagnosis: on one hand, negative U waves have been found (e.g. in acute ischemia or severe aortic valve incompetence) and even alternating U waves have been described. On the other hand, two conditions, not compromising the U wave alone, should be mentioned:

i.   The fusion of the T wave with the U wave, leading to a *TU wave*, is typical for *hypokalemia*.
ii. In the 'long QT syndromes' (see following section QT Interval) there is often a fusion of the T wave and the U wave. In fact, in many cases with this syndrome we do not know what we are measuring, whether it is the QT interval or the QTU interval.

1.6 QT Interval

The QT interval is measured from the beginning of the QRS complex to the end of the T wave, generally in lead II, where the end of the T wave is sharply determined in most ECGs. The QT time is rate dependent. The lower the rate, the longer the QT is, and the higher the rate, the shorter the QT. The time-corrected QT interval is called QTc. Today most ECG machines measure the QT interval automatically, the time-corrected QT (QTc) included. The QT interval and the QTc may also be calculated 'by hand', using the Bazett formula:

$$\left(QTc = \frac{QT}{\sqrt{60/f}} \text{ resp. } \frac{QT}{\sqrt{R-R}} \right)$$

Slightly shortened or slightly prolonged QT intervals are sometimes encountered in normal hearts. The QTc should *not* exceed 0.46 sec, however.

Differential diagnosis: A substantially prolonged QT interval is called long QT syndrome. The *acquired* type is more frequent and is generally due to drugs, to antiarrhythmic drugs of Class Ia or Class III (Vaughan-Williams), and due to ischemia. The *congenital* long QT syndrome (Romano-Ward syndrome, Jervell-Lange-Nielsen syndrome) is a rare condition. A pronounced prolongation of QT or QTU tends to a special form of fast polymorphic ventricular tachycardia, called torsade de pointes (for details see Chapter 26 Ventricular Tachycardias).

Some electrolyte disturbances influence the QT interval in a typical manner: A prolonged QT is also seen in *hypocalcemia* (in this case without disposition to torsade de pointes). A *TU fusion* is typical for *hypokalemia*, with possible consecutive torsade de pointes. A markedly shortened QT is very rare and is generally associated with *hypercalcemia* (Chapter 16 Electrolyte Imbalance).

1.7 Arrhythmias

It is quite difficult to classify certain arrhythmias into those that are *normal variants*, and those that are *pathologic* findings. We know, for example, that episodes of *ventricular tachycardia* (VT) [10] or a *slow ventricular escape rhythm* may be found in apparently healthy individuals, especially in athletes. However, a VT or a ventricular rhythm of 30/min would not be classified as a normal finding. Both examples represent common and clinically important and often dangerous arrhythmias, that may rarely arise in healthy individuals under special conditions, and in these cases they are (probably) harmless.

However, there are a substantial number of arrhythmias that occur so frequently in individuals without heart disease that they *may* represent normal variants. Three conditions must normally be fulfilled:

i.   Absence of any heart disease.
ii. Exclusion of many arrhythmias, *not* representing normal variants (Table 3.2).
iii. A 'normal-variant arrhythmia' should occur only rarely and should not be associated with very low or very high rates. However, a healthy individual may *feel* a normal-variant arrhythmia.

Table 3.3 reveals the arrhythmias that often represent *normal variants*. The number of normal *supraventricular* PBs, espe-

Table 3.2
Arrhythmias, *not* representing 'normal variants'

Complete AV block
AV block 2°, type Mobitz and type 'high degree'
Sinoatrial (SA) block 2° and 3°
Ventricular pauses of > 2 sec
Monomorphic ventricular tachycardia (VT: > three ventricular beats)
Polymorphic VT (torsade de pointes; other forms)
Ventricular triplets (three consecutive ventricular premature beats (VPBs)), multiple couplets
Multiple ventricular 'couplets'
Single ventricular VPBs if:
a. >200/24 h?
b. polymorphic
c. with true R-on-T phenomenon (ventricular PB *before* 90% of the preceding T wave: potential 'vulnerable period')
Most forms of atrial tachycardias (e.g. atrial flutter, atrial fibrillation, re-entrant atrioventricular (AV) tachycardias, re-entry tachycardias in the Wolff-Parkinson-White syndrome)
Supraventricular PBs in salvos (> 3 beats) and at a high rate (> 160/min)
Rare arrhythmias (e.g. parasystoly, accelerated idioventricular rhythm, AV dissociation with interference)
Ventricular fibrillation (of course)

Table 3.3
Frequent normal-variant arrhythmias

Sinus bradycardia: minimal rate about 45/min; minimal instantaneous rate during sleep about 35/min
Sinus tachycardia: maximal rate about 110/min
Sinus arrhythmia
Isolated ventricular pauses: < 2 sec during sleep
Isolated AV-junctional (AV-nodal) escape beats (during sinus arrhythmia or after a premature beat)
Short episodes of AV-nodal rhythm (with retrograde atrial activation)
Short episodes (< 10 beats?) of 'AV dissociation' (with accrochage, with synchronization)
Short episodes of accelerated idionodal rhythm
Episodes of normocardic ectopic atrial rhythm (e.g. so-called 'coronary sinus rhythm')
Supraventricular premature beats (PBs) (in most cases atrial PBs), if:
a) isolated (< 200/min?)
b) < 5 salvos (or < 20?) of maximal three beats
c) instantaneous rate (beat-to-beat interval) < 160/min
d) isolated *early* atrial PBs with functional complete AV block
Ventricular PBs (VPBs), if:
a) isolated (< 200/24 h?)
b) monomorphic
c) isolated 'couplets' (<20/24 h?), instantaneous rate < 160/min
d) isolated VPBs with 'pseudo-R-on-T phenomenon' (VPB *after* 90% of the preceding QT interval: 'supernormal period')

cially of normal *ventricular* PBs, is as arbitrary as it is questionable.

As mentioned above, there is no strict dividing line between pathologic arrhythmias and normal-variant arrhythmias, and there is no consent in the literature. The classification in Table 3.3 is based on 40 years of personal experience and on many discussions with other specialists in cardiology and rhythmology.

Principally, an arrhythmia should always be interpreted in the context of other clinical findings, considering also age and special conditions of a patient, including exercise capacity, psychological factors and drug abuse (ethyl, nicotine, medical drugs). Generally, 'normal-variant arrhythmias' should not be treated with antiarrhythmic drugs.

1.8 Day-to-Day and Circadian Variation

Day-to-day variation concerns the amplitude and axis of the QRS complex and variations of the T wave in particular. Willems et al [11] studied 20 healthy volunteers (7 women and 13 men aged 22–58 years; a total of 290 tracings) with the Frank leads ECG and vectorcardiogram. Several cases had marked changes of the frontal QRS axis, also with disappearance and reappearance of (small) Q waves. In one individual the anterior QRS forces in the transversal and sagittal planes disappeared. The authors believe *that such extreme changes occurring in normal subjects may be unusual, but should serve as a warning for too enthusiastic diagnostic and therapeutic interventions.* T wave changes were fairly common. Some variations could also be observed in tracings, recorded immediately one after the other ('circadian variation').

We have observed a young healthy individual with unexplainable T negativity in leads V_3 to V_5. Serial ECGs (two taken during the night) revealed that T negativity was only present between 11 A.M. and about 6 P.M.

General Conclusion

As mentioned at the beginning of this chapter, every 'unusual' ECG pattern should be interpreted in the context of the conditions of the person being investigated, including age, anamnesis, and other clinical findings and quality of symptoms.

References

1. Goldman MF. Normal variants in the electrocardiogram leading to cardiac invalidism. Am Heart J 1959;59:71–7
2. Spodick DH. Normal sinus heart rate: Sinus tachycardia and sinus bradycardia redefined. Am Heart J 1992;124:1119–21
3. Brodsky M, Wu D, Denes P, et al. Arrhythmias documented by 24-hour continuous electrocardiographic monitoring in 50 male medical students without apparent heart disease. Am J Cardiol 1977;39:390–5
4. Sobotka PA, Mayer JH, Bauernfeind RA, et al. Arrhythmias documented by 24-hour continuous ambulatory electrocardiographic monitoring in young women without apparent heart disease. Am Heart J 1981;101:753–9
5. James FW, Kaplan S. The normal electrocardiogram in the infant and child. Cardiovasc Clin 1973;5:294–311
6. Hiss RG, Lamb LE, Allen M. Electrocardiographic findings in 67 375 asymtomatic subjects: X. Normal values. Am J Cardiol 1960;6:200
7. Mehta M, Abnash CJ, Mehta A. Early repolarization. Clin Cardiol 1999;22:59–65
8. Spodick DH. Differential characteristics of the electrocardiogram in early repolarization and acute pericarditis. N Engl J Med 1976;295:523–7
9. Patel A, Getsos JP, Moussa G, Damato AN. The Osborn wave of hypothermia in normothermic patients. Clin Cardiol 1994;17:273–6
10. Bjerregaard P. Premature beats in healthy subjects 40–79 years of age. Europ Heart J 1982;3:493–503
11. Willems JL, Poblete PF, Pipberger HV. Day-to-day variation of the normal orthogonal electrocardiogram and vectorcardiogram. Circulation 1972;45:1057–64

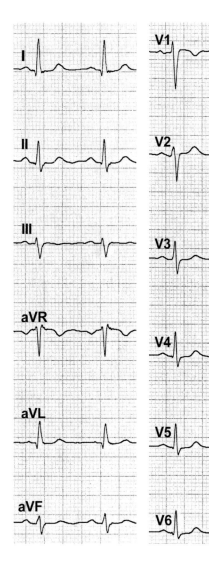

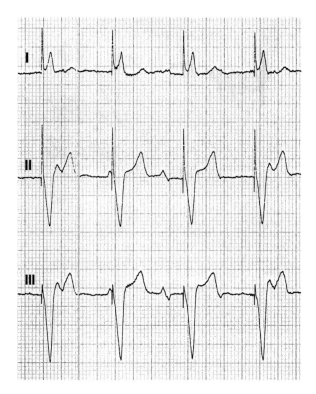

ECG 3.2
Sinus rhythm of the atria; ventricular pacemaker rhythm (complete AV block).

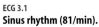
ECG 3.1
Sinus rhythm (81/min).

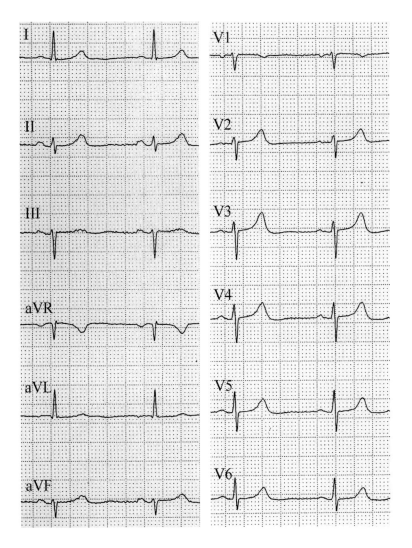

ECG 3.3
Sinus bradycardia, 49/min.

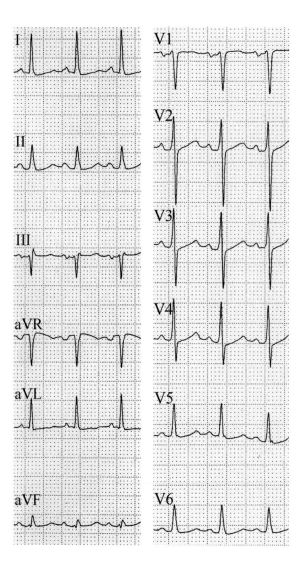
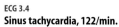

ECG 3.4
Sinus tachycardia, 122/min.

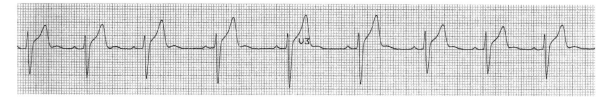

ECG 3.5
Sinus arrhythmia (minimal rate 42/min, maximal rate 67/min).

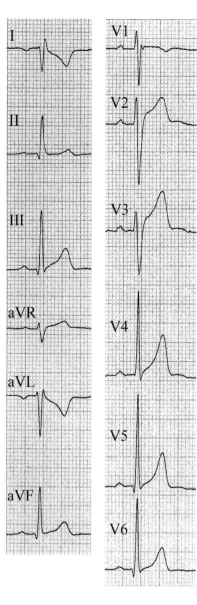

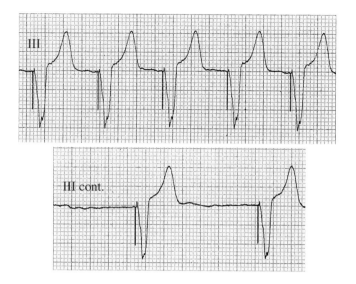

ECG 3.7
Ventricular pacemaker rhythm at a rate of 85/min. The U waves were misdiagnosed as p waves. Pacing at 44/min reveals fine f (fibrillation) waves.

ECG 3.6
False poling of the upper limb leads.

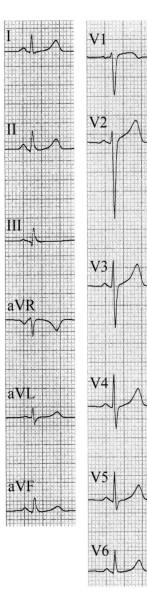

ECG 3.8
Short PQ interval, normal ECG, no episodes of tachycardia.

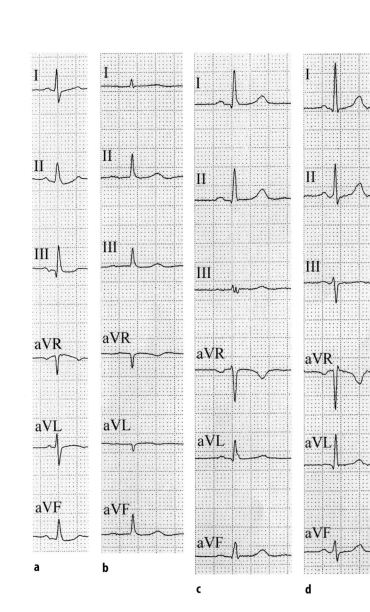

a   b   c   d

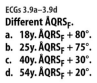

ECGs 3.9a–3.9d
Different ÅQRS_F.
a. 18y. $\text{ÅQRS}_F + 80°$.
b. 25y. $\text{ÅQRS}_F + 75°$.
c. 40y. $\text{ÅQRS}_F + 30°$.
d. 54y. $\text{ÅQRS}_F + 20°$.

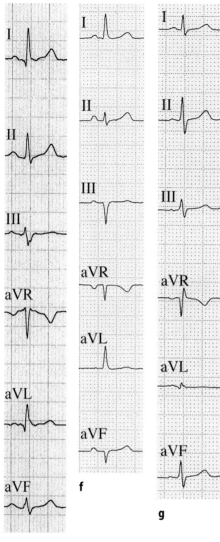

e

f

g

ECGs 3.9e–3.9g
Different ÂQRS$_F$.
e. 60y. ÂQRS$_F$ 0°.
f. 73y. ÂQRS$_F$ − 20°.
g. 25y. ÂQRS$_F$ not determinable. The positive and
    negative components of the QRS complex have
    almost the same amplitude in the individual limb
    leads. This frontal QRS axis is called *sagittal axis*.

ECG 3.10
S$_I$/S$_{II}$/S$_{III}$-type.

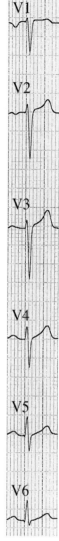

ECG 3.11
**Clockwise rotation of
QRS.**

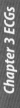

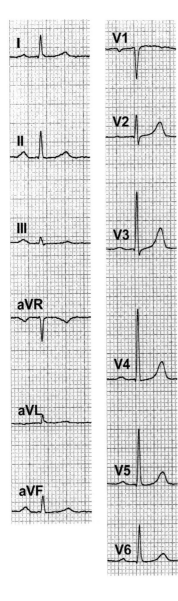

ECG 3.12
Counterclockwise rotation.

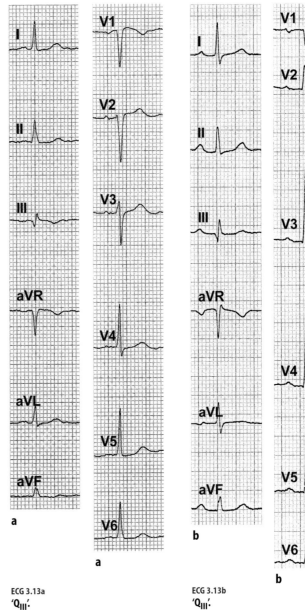

ECG 3.13a
'Q$_{III}$.'

a

ECG 3.13b
'Q$_{III}$.'

b

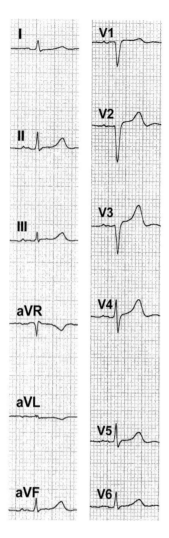

ECG 3.14
QS in lead V₁ and V₂, minimal
R wave in V₃.

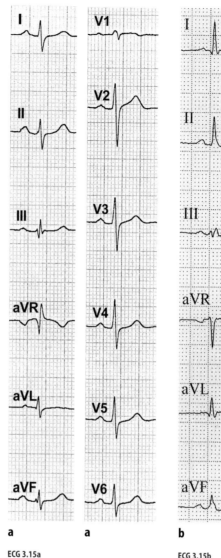

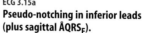

a   a

ECG 3.15a
**Pseudo-notching in inferior leads
(plus sagittal ÂQRS_F).**

b   b

ECG 3.15b
**Pseudo-notching in leads III/aVF (as
frequently seen in innocent incomplete right bundle-branch block, that
is *not* present in this case).**

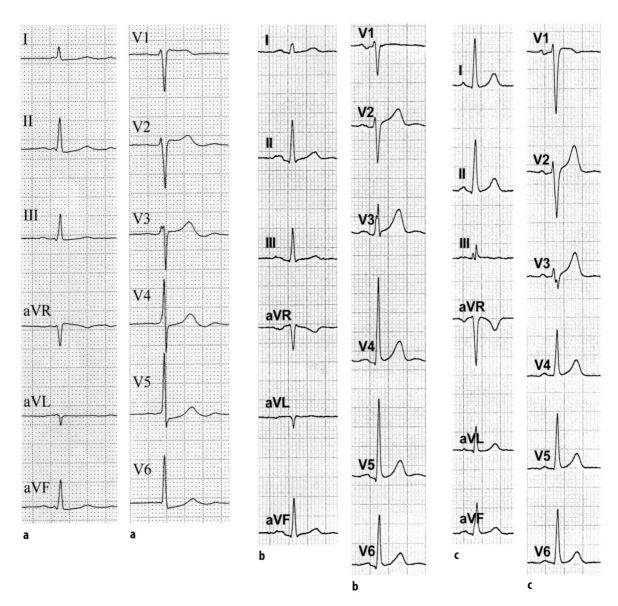

ECG 3.16a
Pseudo-notching in transition zone, lead V₃.

ECG 3.16b
Pseudo-notching in transition zone, lead V₃.

ECG 3.16c
Pseudo-notching in transition zone, lead V₃ *and* III.

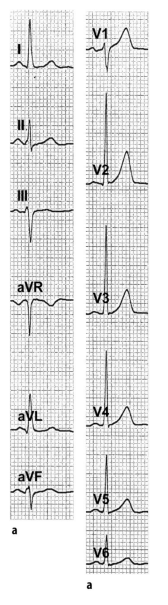

a

ECG 3.17a
Pseudo-delta wave in lead II.

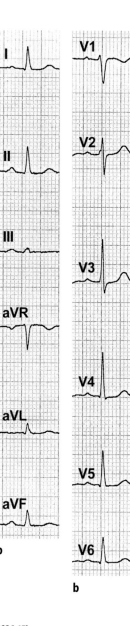

b

ECG 3.17b
Pseudo-delta wave in lead V$_2$.

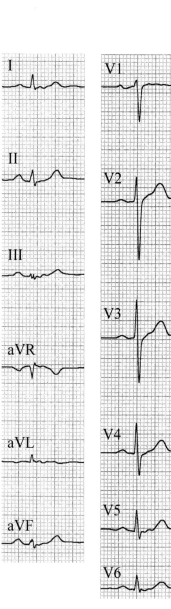

b

ECG 3.18
Peripheral QRS low voltage.

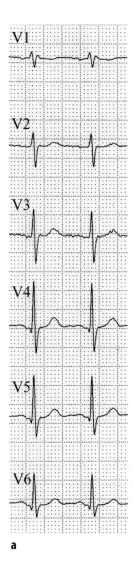

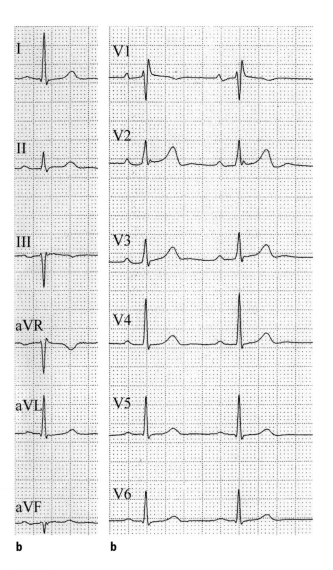

a   **b**   **b**

ECG 3.19a
Incomplete right bundle-branch block with r > r′ in V_1. It is better to consider the product of amplitude × duration of the r and r′ than the amplitude alone.

ECG 3.19b
Incomplete RBBB with r < r′ in V_1.

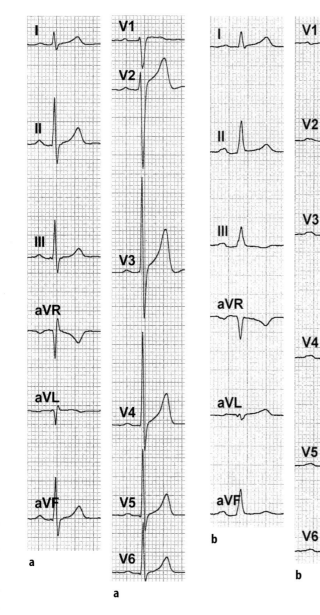

a

ECG 3.20a
ST elevation in V_2/V_3 (and V_1/V_4) with relatively high and peaked T waves in V_2 to V_6.

ECG 3.20b
**38y/m Short Story/Case Report 2.
ST elevation in V_2/V_3 (V_4).**

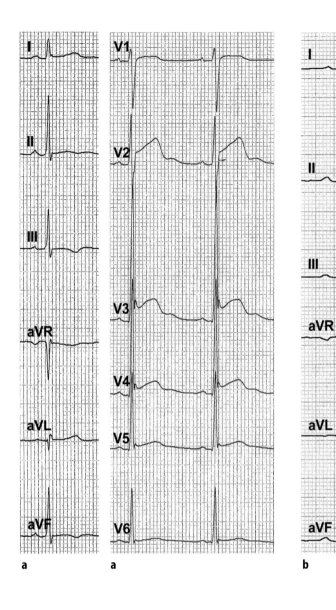

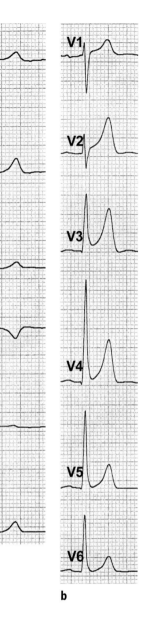

ECG 3.21a
28y/m. Early repolarization. The ST elevation (up to 4 mm) arises from the R wave in V₃ to V₄. Note the 'Osborn waves' in V₃ to V₆. Normal coronary arteries.

ECG 3.21b
31y/m. Early repolarization. ST elevation in (V₁) V₂ to V₄, with high, peaked and symmetroid T waves. Normal heart.

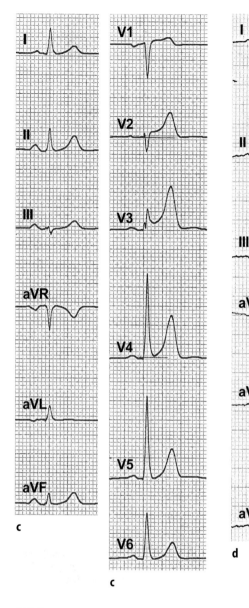

c

ECG 3.21c
45y/m. Early repolarization. ST elevation ≥ 2 mm in V₃, arising from the notched R wave. High T waves. Normal heart.

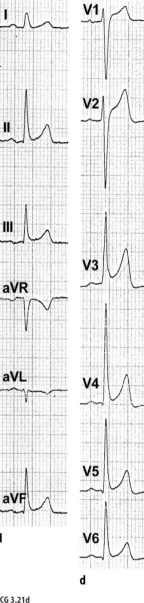

d

ECG 3.21d
Early repolarization. ST elevation of 2 mm, arising of the R waves in V₃ to V₄ (V₅/V₆).

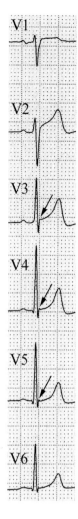
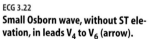

ECG 3.22
Small Osborn wave, without ST elevation, in leads V₄ to V₆ (arrow).

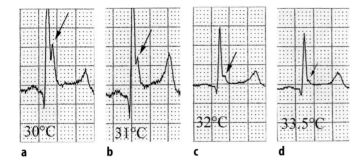

ECGs 3.23a–3.23d
ECG monitor lead: Osborn wave in a 53-year-old patient during open heart surgery. The Osborn wave and ST depression gradually diminishes during increasing body temperature.
a. Temperature 30 °C.
b. Temperature 31 °C.
c. Temperature 32 °C.
d. Temperature 33.5 °C.

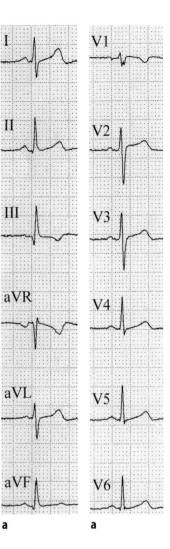

ECG 3.24a
Normal asymmetric (discordant) negative T wave in lead III (ÅQRS$_F$ + 75°) due to vectorial projection.

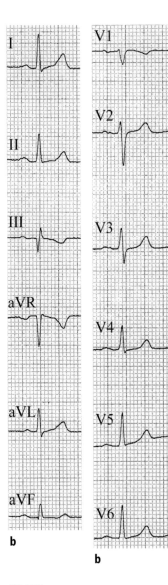

b

b

ECG 3.24b
Normal asymmetric (concordant) negative T wave in lead III, (ÂQRS_F + 30°) due to vectorial projection. Note also the Q wave in III (and aVF) in a normal heart.

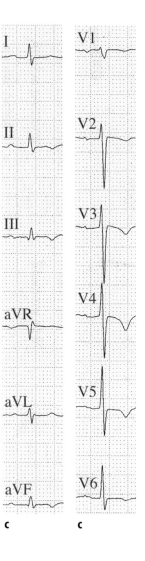

c

c

ECG 3.24c
Symmetrical discordant negative T waves in II, aVF, III and V$_3$ to V$_6$ with minimal ST depression in V$_4$/V$_5$. Those T waves are often caused by ischemia. This was the case in the 52 year old patient with coronary heart disease.

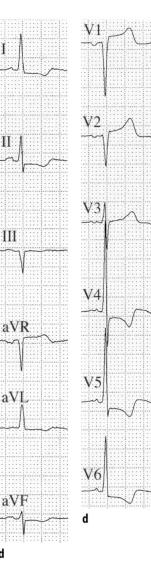

d

d

ECG 3.24d
Asymmetric (discordant) negative T waves in leads I, II (aVF, aVL) and V$_4$ to V$_6$, in some leads with significant ST depression. Those T waves are generally due to left ventricular overload and/or left ventricular hypertrophy (as in this case).

Chapter 4
Atrial Enlargement and Other Abnormalities of the p Wave

At a Glance

Pathologic p waves in sinus rhythm are not as important as QRS alterations. However, abnormal p waves may give some hint of hemodynamic abnormalities, especially if they are associated with pathologic QRS complexes.

ECG

The classical p mitrale, p pulmonale and p biatriale are due to chronic overload of the left atrium, the right atrium, or both, with consecutive hypertrophy *and* dilatation (>>> enlargement) of the respective atria.

In general *left* atrial enlargement is used as a synonym for *p mitrale* and *right* atrial enlargement as a synonym for *p pulmonale*.

1   Left Atrial Enlargement (p Mitrale)

The longer lasting activation of the hypertrophic left atrium provokes *prolongation* (≥ 0.110 msec) and sometimes *bifidity* of the p wave, especially in leads I or II and V_6, with an interpeak distance of > 40 msec. The second and negative portion of the p wave in lead V_1 (and often V_2) is accentuated (ECGs 4.1–4.3).

Some decades ago classical 'p mitrale' (often with clear bifidity) was commonly encountered in patients with *mitral stenosis*. For the decrease of rheumatic fever in many countries, the ECG pattern of left atrial enlargement (often with less clear bifidity) is more often found in severe mitral valve incompetence of any etiology, in aortic valve disease, and in hypertensive and other heart diseases with chronic left atrial overload. In recent publications, the ECG pattern of left atrial enlargement (p duration; the extent of terminal p negativity in V_1 (PTFV$_1$) see section 7) was compared with left atrial dimension, in mitral and aortic valve disease. The specificity of the ECG pattern was high (about 90%), whereas the sensitivity was modest (30%–60%). A bifid p wave was a rare finding and in patients with left atrial diameter ≥ 60 mm, atrial fibrillation was present in about 70%.

In the elderly, to a certain degree, p prolongation may be due to intra-atrial conduction block and is not necessarily associated with left atrial enlargement. However, major left atrial enlargement generally predisposes to atrial fibrillation, thrombosis in the left atrium, and consecutive cerebral strokes.

2   Right Atrial Enlargement (p Pulmonale)

As the activation of the right atrium begins earlier than that of the left atrium, an increase of the RA vector *does not prolong the p duration*. P pulmonale is characterized by *tall* and sometimes *pointed p waves* in leads II, aVF and III (ECG 4.4). The amplitude of the p waves is ≥ 2.5 mm in at least one of these leads. In the 'opposite' lead aVL, the p wave is completely negative. The p wave may be higher than normal and pointed in leads V_1/V_2 rarely in the other precordial leads (ECG 4.4).

Classical 'p pulmonale' (p > 2.5 mm in lead II) is rare and found in patients with lung diseases, especially in chronic obstructive pulmonary disease (COPD). A p wave amplitude of 2.0 to 2.5 mm in lead II is quite frequent and may represent right atrial enlargement of minor degree, or, more often, a normal variant especially in young asthenic individuals, and in elevated sympathetic tone (with sinus tachycardia).

3   Biatrial Enlargement (p Biatriale)

Biatrial enlargement is very rare and combines the criteria of left *and* right atrial hypertrophy (ECG 4.5); p biatriale may be seen in combined severe diseases of heart and lung, and in cases with a complex congenital heart disease.

4 Acute Left Atrial Overload

Although the borderline between left atrial overload without and with hypertrophy is not clearly established, it is reasonable to define the p pattern of left atrial overload *without hypertrophy*. Acute left atrial overload (or chronic overload without hypertrophy) is characterized by a *normal* p duration, combined with *accentuated p negativity* in lead V_1 (the negative component of the p wave being greater than the positive one). This pattern is common in many diseases leading to left atrial overload, such as hypertension, and moderate degrees of aortic and mitral valve diseases. It is often present during the acute stage of myocardial infarction (ECG 4.6) and generally regresses over days that follow. The pattern may also be due to the incorrect placement of lead V_1 (and V_2) by one intercostal space too high.

5 Acute Right Atrial Overload

Acute right atrial overload (e.g. in acute pulmonary embolism) leads to only minor (or no) alterations of the p wave, in most cases. A peaked p wave in lead V_1 or V_2 may be the only hint of it. Classical 'p pulmonale' in this condition is very rare.

6 Other Abnormalities of the p Wave

An abnormal p wave due to *rhythm disturbances* is of great interest. The conditions are discussed in Chapters 18, 19, 23 and 24.

The Full Picture

7 Etiology, Prevalence and Clinical Significance of Left Atrial Enlargement

Hazen et al [1] studied 411 patients (mean age 63 years) with acquired valve disease and left atrial enlargement, determined by echo. The correlation between p duration, especially the extent of terminal p negativity in V_1, termed $PTFV_1$ (the average area subtended by the terminal negative portion of biphasic p in V_1, measured in msec × mm), and left atrial diameter showed a specificity of about 90% and a sensitivity of 30% (to 60%). The same results were obtained in the bifid p wave with an interspike distance of ≥ 40 msec. Moreover, in patients with left atrial diameters of ≥ 60 mm, atrial fibrillation was present in 70%.

Fragola et al [2] published similar results in 1000 unselected consecutive patients (mean age 46 years) controlled by echo. (Definition of left atrial enlargement: left atrial dimension above the upper limit of the normal 95% predicted interval calculated as a function of age and body surface area.) They showed/used the following ECG criteria:

i. P wave duration ≥ 110 msec
ii. P terminal force in lead V_1 equal to or more negative than – 0.04 mm/sec

iii. P wave notching in a limb lead with a peak-to-peak interval ≥ 40 msec. The specificity was ≥ 97%, the sensitivity only 18%. For more details see the review article by Alpert and Munuswamy [3].

In older people, p prolongation (generally associated with flat p waves) may be due to interatrial block without left atrial enlargement (ECG 4.7). Recently, Spodick et al [4] emphasized the possible mechanical consequences. In fact, classic p mitrale (with a bifid p wave) is rarer today than it was decades ago because rheumatic fever has nearly been eliminated in countries with high levels of hygiene and medical care (probably related to the chronic 'intoxication' of meat stock with antibiotics, which (splendidly) induces general antibiotic prophylaxis in the population). Consequently, the incidence of mitral stenosis has declined. Nowadays, the ECG pattern of left atrial enlargement (not always with a bifid p) is found in severe disease of the mitral and aortic valves, of any etiology, and in hypertensive and chronic coronary heart disease. Congenital mitral stenosis is very rare. Alva et al [5] found only 16 cases during a 10-year period.

8 Etiology, Prevalence and Clinical Significance of Right Atrial Enlargement

Classical p pulmonale has become more rare, probably because of better therapy of the disease that is essentially responsible – chronic obstructive pulmonary disease. Often we find a relatively tall p wave of 2–2.5 mm in lead II in patients with lung diseases, as well as in normal individuals with sinus tachycardia.

Kaplan et al [6] studied 100 patients with right atrial enlargement, documented by echo, all associated with right ventricular enlargement (mild in 39%, moderate in 44% and severe in 17%). The patients had tricuspid regurgitation in 30%, pulmonary hypertension in 28%, cardiomyopathy in 14%, mitral valve disease in 11%, atrial septal defect in 9% and other diseases in 8%. Only 52 patients were in sinus rhythm; the others showed atrial arrhythmias, especially atrial fibrillation – in 41%! This high incidence indicates a substantial number of patients with associated left atrial enlargement, because in isolated right atrial enlargement – if not excessive – atrial fibrillation is relatively rare. Twenty-five patients with normal dimensions of the right atrium were the control group. 'p pulmonale' (p ≥ 2.5 mm in lead II) was identified in only 8% of the patients with right atrial enlargement. Out of 10 criteria studied, the following three proved to be the best (100% specificity preserved):

i. $ÅQRS_F > 90°$
ii. P wave height > 1.5 mm in lead V_2
iii. R/S ratio > 1 in lead V_1 (without RBBB).

The sensitivity was 24%–34%. As right atrial enlargement is generally combined with right ventricular enlargement in almost all cases, two of the three best criteria are based on alterations of the QRS complex. Also a qR pattern in V_1 has been described as highly specific for right atrial enlargement [6, 7, 8], often combined with dilatation of the right ventricle (Chapter 14 Differential Diagnosis of Pathologic Q Waves).

ECG Special

9 Vectors in Left Atrial Enlargement

In *sinus rhythm without atrial hypertrophy*, activation of the right atrium begins earlier than that of the left (the sinus node is in the upper part of the right atrium). The normal right atri-al p vector points to about + 60° in the frontal plane and anteriorly, the normal LA vector points to about + 30° in the limb leads, and posteriorly. In *left atrial enlargement* the RA vector is normal, whereas the hypertrophic left atrium produces a LA vector that is longer in duration and points more to the left (about 0°) and posteriorly. The consecutive p pattern is a prolonged p wave (> 0.11 sec, generally 0.12–0.14 sec), occasionally with a bifid form, best detectable in lead I or II and V_6 (ECGs 4.1–4.3). The first short 'hump' corresponds to the normal right p vector, and the second prolonged 'hump' to the prolonged LA vector. In addition, the negative second part of the p wave in V_1 (and often also in V_2) is prolonged and accentuated.

10 Vectors in Right Atrial Enlargement

In right atrial enlargement ('p pulmonale') the RA vector is prolonged with an orientation more inferiorly (to + 70°) and slightly more anteriorly. However, as right atrial activation occurs *before* left atrial activation, the prolonged RA vector never exceeds the end of the (normal) LA vector. Thus the whole p wave is *not* prolonged and the two components of the p wave (of right and left atrial origin) are completely fused. In the ECG we find normal broad and tall p waves in leads II, aVF and III. The amplitude of the p wave is ≥ 2.5 mm in these leads, with p negativity in lead aVL (ECG 4.4).

11 Special Alterations of the p Wave

11.1 So-called 'p Pulmonale Vasculare'

Severe pulmonary arterial hypertension (without emphysema) in chronic pulmonary embolism or in primary pulmonary hypertension leads to a p pattern different from that of classical p pulmonale. The p vector is less vertical, the highest p wave is present in lead II and sometimes more prominent in lead I than in lead III. In leads V_1/V_2 the p wave is generally somewhat peaky (ECG 4.8).

This p alteration has been called 'p pulmonale vasculare', in contrast to the classical p pulmonale (also called p pulmonale parenchymale).

The difference between the two p wave configurations in two different diseases – even with the same hemodynamic consequences – is unclear.

The pulmonary emphysema associated with COPD, that provokes a more vertical axis of the heart (and the right atrium), may be responsible for the more vertical p axis in p pulmonale parenchymale.

11.2 p Pseudo-Pulmonale

In rare cases, left atrial overload produces an increased p vector not only directed posteriorly, but also more *inferiorly* than to the left. In lead V_1 there is increased amplitude of the terminal negative portion of the p wave, whereas in leads II and aVF (and III) a tall p wave is observed. The first small hump of the slightly notched p wave corresponds to the first part of normal right atrial activation, while the second greater hump corresponds to the activation of the enlarged left atrium (ECG 4.9). This pattern is often misdiagnosed.

11.3 Imitation of p Pulmonale

Severe hyperkalemia often diminishes or even eliminates the p wave in the presence of sinus rhythm. On the contrary, in exceptional cases *hypokalemia* may enhance the p amplitude in the inferior leads, imitating p pulmonale. Also enhanced sympathetic tone and asthenic habitus may lead to p pulmonale-like patterns.

11.4 p Biatriale/Biatrial Enlargement

This is a very rare pattern, although it should be expected more frequently. The reason for this is the partial canceling of the middle and late portion of the enhanced RA vector by the enhanced LA vector, thus masking the p pulmonale.

11.5 Other Uncommon p Configurations in Sinus Rhythm

11.5.1 Negative p Wave in Lead I

A negative p wave in lead I combined with an 'inverse' QRS complex in this lead is typical for *false poling* in 99.9%, and for *situs inversus* in 0.1% (Chapter 32 Rare ECGs). In nonsinusal rhythm, a negative p wave in lead I is found in *left atrial rhythm* and also in some cases of *ectopic right atrial rhythm* (Chapter 19 Atrial Tachycardia).

11.5.2 Ebstein's Anomaly

In Ebstein's anomaly an extreme right atrial hypertrophy occasionally leads to extremely high and peaky p waves in the inferior leads, together with QRS and T abnormalities.

11.5.3 Atrial Infarction

In extremely rare cases, atrial infarction may provoke deformation of the p waves combined with changing alterations of atrial repolarization in serial ECGs (Chapter 13 Myocardial Infarction).

11.5.4 Tricuspid Atresia

Tricuspid atresia is an exotic rarity. From the book by Zimmerman et al [9] we have learned that in tricuspid atresia (an extreme presupposition for right atrial hypertrophy) the p wave may exceptionally be *negative in lead V_1.*

References

1. Hazen MS, Marwick TH, Underwood DA. Diagnostic accuracy of the resting electrocardiogram in detection and estimation of left atrial enlargement: an echocardiographic correlation in 551 patients. Amer Heart J 1991;122:823–8
2. Fragola PV, Calo L, Borzi M, et al. Diagnosis of left atrial enlargement with electrocardiogram. A misplaced reliance. Cardiologia 1994;39:247–52
3. Alpert MA, Munuswamy K. Electrocardiographic diagnosis of left atrial enlargement. Arch Intern Med 1989;149:1161–5
4. Spodick DH, Olds PA, Saad KM. Electromechanical disease of the left atrium – interatrial block. Preliminary observations on left atrial function. Europ Heart J 2000;2(Suppl K):76–7
5. Alva C, Gonzales B, Melendez C, Jimenez S. Estenosis mitral congenita. Arch Cardiol Mex 2001;71:206–13
6. Kaplan JD, Evans GT Jr, Foster E, et al. Evaluation of electrocardiographic criteria for right atrial enlargement by quantitative two-dimensional echocardiography. JACC 1994;23: 747–52
7. Reeves WC, Hallahan W, Schwiter EJ, et al. Two-dimensional echocardiographic assessment of electrocardiographic criteria for right atrial enlargement. Circulation 1981;64:387–91
8. Sodi Pallares D, Bisteni A, Herrmann GR. Some views of the significance of qR and QR type complexes in right precordial leads in the absence of myocardial infarction. Am Heart J 1952;43: 716–34
9. Zimmerman HA, Bersano E, Dicosky C. The Auricular Electrocardiogram. Springfield, IL: Charles S Thomas, 1968

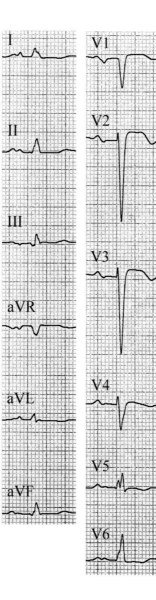

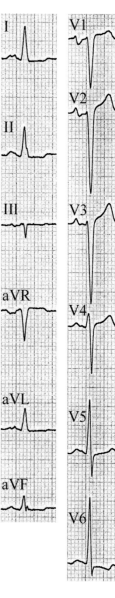

ECG 4.1

56 y/f. Severe mitral stenosis.
P mitrale/LA enlargement: PQ
duration 120 msec, bifidity of
p waves in limb leads, V_6 (V_2
to V_5). Accentuated and prolonged negative terminal
portion of p in lead V_1. Echo:
LA diameter 65 mm.

ECG 4.2

79 y/m. Old 'non-Q wave' lateral
infarction and left heart failure. *P
mitrale/LA enlargement:* p duration
150 msec, p bifidity in II, aVF and V_4
to V_6. Accentuated terminal p negativity in V_1 to V_3.

ECG 4.3

34 y/m. Hypertensive car-
diomyopathy. *P mitrale/LA
enlargement:* PQ duration
120 msec, p bifidity in aVL,
V_3 to V_5. Accentuated terminal p negativity in V_1/V_2.

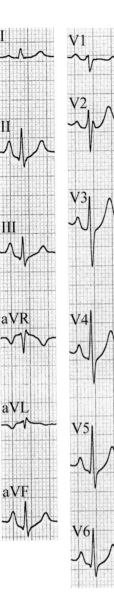

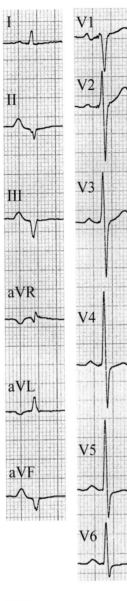

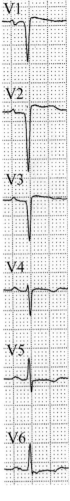

ECG 4.4

54 y/m. COPD. *P pulmonale/ RA enlargement:* prominent and peaked p waves in II (3 mm), aVF and III. Peaked p waves also in V_2/V_3 and atypically prominent in V_4 to V_6. Note the unusual 'PQ depression' (as in early acute pericarditis) due to the enhanced opposite atrial repolarization vector ('Ta').

ECG 4.5

58 y/m. CHD with old inferior and posterior MI, COPD. *P biatriale/ biatrial enlargement:* i) peaky and high p waves in inferior leads, p ≥ 2.5 mm in II; ii) p duration 120 msec, accentuated terminal p negativity in V_1. The QS (or rSr'?) configuration in the inferior leads and the broad/tall R waves in V_2 are due to infarction.

ECG 4.6

70 y/f. Two-day-old anteroseptal MI. *Acute left atrial overload:* p duration 100–110 msec. Slightly accentuated terminal p negativity in lead V_1, with normalization after two days (QS complexes and ST elevation in V_1 to V_3 due to MI).

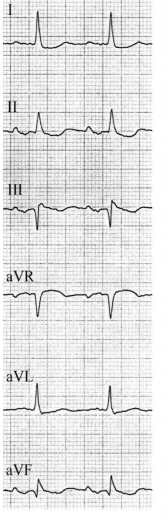
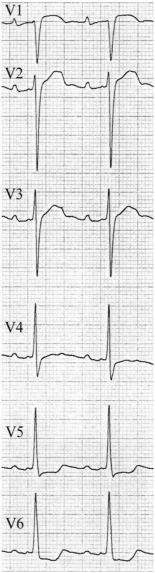
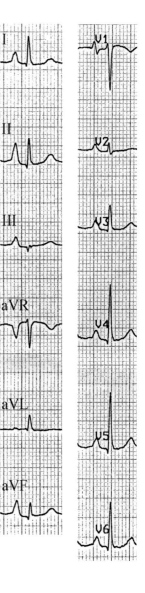

ECG 4.7

82 y/f. Psoriasis, mild hypertension. *Interatrial block:* **extreme prolongation of the p duration (200 msec), with p bifidity in leads I, II, aVR and V_2 to V_6 (interspike distance 140 msec). AV block 1°. Formally pathologic Q wave in lead III. Signs of LV strain in the lateral leads. Echo: mild LV hypertrophy (LV mass 110 g/m^2), normal LV ejection fraction without regional hypokinesia. LA dimension 40 mm.**

ECG 4.8

48 y/f. So-called *p pulmonale vasculare*: primary pulmonary hypertension. Giant p wave in lead II. Note that the p wave in lead I is higher than in lead III and that the p wave in aVL is flat positive. Peaked p waves in lead V_1 up to V_6. Surprisingly ÅQRS$_F$ is + 20° and signs of RV hypertrophy are lacking.

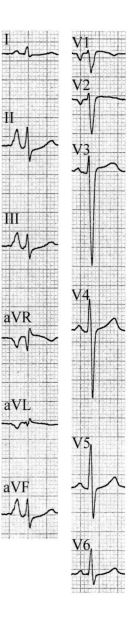

ECG 4.9

40 y/m. Hypertrophic and dilating LV cardiomyopathy with left heart failure. *P pseudo-pulmonale*: at a first glance classical p pulmonale in the limb leads, with a p of 4.5 mm in lead II. However, there is a slight notch 40 msec after the onset of the p wave, marking RA depolarization. The following 80 msec of the p wave are provoked by the LA vector, pointing abnormally downwards (and as usual posteriorly, see V_1/V_2); p duration 120 msec. Echo: dilated and hypertrophic LV; LV ejection fraction 30%. Normal dimension of RA and RV.

Chapter 5
Left Ventricular Hypertrophy

At a Glance

Left ventricular hypertrophy (LVH) is a common pathologic finding, occurring in about 20% of a population of 50-year-olds, and more in older people. It represents an independent predictor of premature death that is as important as frequent ventricular premature beats. The enhanced risk is due to consecutive malignant ventricular arrhythmias and to heart failure. It is possible to prevent or reduce LVH with drugs such as ACE inhibitors, thus eliminating or diminishing the fatal consequences. Therefore, reliable diagnosis of LVH has been the subject of increased interest during the last two decades.

ECG

Today the *echocardiogram* is generally acknowledged as the preferred diagnostic method. It has a specificity and sensitivity of about 90% (compared to anatomic evaluation using the left ventricular (LV) dissecting method as a gold standard). However, the ECG can and should be used as a *screening* method in modern times. Why is this the case?

First, the specificity of the old ECG criteria, which are used generally, is equivalent to that of the echocardiogram (90%–100%). However, this is at the expense of the sensitivity, which is poor at 20%–35%. It should be mentioned that the high level of specificity is only true for individuals aged over 40 years.

Second, ECGs are still performed at least six times more often than echocardiograms, albeit for *different* purposes. LVH may be detected when an ECG is used for such a different purpose.

Third, ECGs are registered by a technical assistant or a nurse in a short time, and are usually interpreted by the physician within minutes.

Fourth, the costs of an ECG are only about 20% of those of an echocardiogram.

Therefore, what is the best way to proceed in practice?

1 ECG Indices for LVH

If one or two of the older voltage ECG indices (summarized in Table 5.1) *and* the recently published Cornell index (Table 5.2) are *positive* in a patient older than 40 years, we can diagnose LVH with great accuracy.

If all these indices are negative, we cannot exclude LVH however. In patients with hypertension or other diseases disposing to LVH an echocardiogram must be performed. With this method LVH can be confirmed *or* excluded.

In *young* patients the ECG voltage criteria may be *false positive*. In doubtful cases, while respecting the clinical conditions, an echocardiogram is useful again.

Table 5.1

Old ECG voltage indices for detection of left ventricular hypertrophy

Limb leads
$R_{aVL} \geq 11$ mm (>12 mm) (Sokolow-Lyon 'II')
$R_{aVF} \geq 20$ mm
$R_I + S_{III} \geq 25$ mm (Gubner-Ungerleider)
$R_I - R_{III} + S_{III} - S_I \geq 17$ mm (Lewis 1914)
$R_{aVF} \geq 24$ mm

Precordial leads
$S_{V1} + R_{V5}$ (or R_{V6}) ≥ 35 mm (Sokolow = Sokolow-Lyon 'I')
R_{V5} (or R_{V6}) ≥ 26 mm
$S_{V2} + S_{V3} \geq 35$ mm
$S_{V1} \geq 24$ mm
$(R + S_{V3}) + (R + S_{V4}) \geq 32$ mm
$(R + S)_{maximal\ precordial} \geq 45$ mm

Other old ECG indices not mentioned in Table 5.1 that also respect T-wave negativity or the behavior of the p wave in lead V_1, have not improved at all the detection or exclusion of LVH (for example, the relatively complex 'Romhilt point-score index').

ECGs 5.1–5.3 show examples of LVH with positive voltage criteria, and ECG 5.4 shows a patient with LVH and negative voltage criteria. As mentioned before a false-negative result is a frequent finding, indicating low sensitivity. ECG 5.5 is an example of a false-positive Sokolow index. This is a rare finding at the age > 40 years and represents high specificity. However, it is not as rare in healthy young individuals, especially in men.

The Cornell index, a more recent voltage criterion, takes into account the gender of the patient: $R_{aVL} + S_{V_3} \geq 28$ mm in men, and ≥ 20 mm in women (Table 5.2; ECGs 5.1–5.6). The specificity of this index is 80%–90%, and the sensitivity about 35%. With the Cornell *product,* that is the product of the Cornell voltage and the QRS duration (Table 5.2), the sensitivity was improved from 36% to 51%.

2 Diagnosis of LVH in Intraventricular Conduction Disturbances

In the presence of left bundle-branch block (LBBB) and especially of left anterior fascicular block (LAFB) the diagnosis of LVH is markedly enhanced, for vectorial reasons. In contrast, the diagnosis is very much impaired in right bundle-branch block (RBBB), due to opposite vectors of the left and right ventricle.

Based on the Framingham study, LVH is responsible for 70% of the cases with LBBB. For the detection of LVH in LBBB

Table 5.2
'Cornell indices' for detection of left ventricular hypertrophy

'Cornell' index	
$R_{aVL} + S_{V3} \geq 28$ mm (male)	
$R_{aVL} + S_{V3} \geq 20$ mm (female)	
'Cornell' product (mm × sec)	
Male	$(R_{aVL} + S_{V3}) \times$ QRS duration
Female	$(R_{aVL} + S_{V3} + 8$ mm$) \times$ QRS duration
Corrected 'Cornell' product	
Male	$(R_{aVL} + S_{V3}) + \{0.0174 \times (age - 49)\} + \{0.191 \times (BMI - 26.5)\}$
Female	$(R_{aVL} + S_{V3}) + \{0.0387 \times (age - 50)\} + \{0.212 \times (BMI - 24.9)\}$

BMI: body mass index.

some indices have been published. The index $S_{V_1} + R_{V_5} > 45$ mm of Klein et al [1] is simple, whereas the 'index bundle' of Kafka et al [2] is very complicated. Based on our own data, the specificity of Klein's index is good-to-excellent but the sensitivity is significantly lower than that reported by Klein et al (ECG 5.7). LAFB results in a unique, uniform behavior of the QRS complex that facilitates the diagnosis of LVH. Consequently the index $S_{III} + (R + S)_{maximal\ precordial} \geq 30$ mm (male) or ≥ 28 mm (female) is very reliable, with a specificity *and* sensitivity of about 90% (ECGs 5.8–5.9).

RBBB reduces the R voltage in the precordial leads (generally 2–4 mm) by RV vectors opposite to LV vectors. Thus LVH is probable if the amplitude of R waves in V_4 to V_6 is greater than in a normal ECG (> 12 mm). However, an echocardiogram is better by far.

The Full Picture

Attempts to identify LVH in the ECG have not slackened during the last years. This is astonishing to a certain degree, because the superiority of the echocardiogram is generally acknowledged in this field. However, the ECG is a routine examination in the majority of patients and provides important information about rhythm abnormalities and conduction disturbances. Thus at the same time LVH can be identified in the ECG. However, LVH cannot be excluded in many cases. With the echocardiogram, LVH can be quantified by determining the LV mass in g/m². The echocardiogram is especially

important for long-term follow-up and for accurate measurement of LV function and dimensions.

3 Etiology and Prevalence

The most common etiology of LVH is arterial hypertension. Other etiologies include aortic valvular diseases, hypertrophic cardiomyopathies, and multiple rare diseases as metabolic disorders (hyperthyreosis, Cushing's disease, acromegaly). LVH probably represents the most common pathologic condition with potential severe consequences.

Echocardiographically diagnosed LVH is much more frequent than LVH detected by an ECG. In a general population sample of 5509 in Framingham, MA, the prevalence of LVH detected by ECG criteria was only 1.5% at the beginning of the study (another 1.7% had possible LVH) [3]. Based on an echocardiographic study of 4684 subjects in the Framingham population, Levy et al [4] detected LVH in 16% of men and 19% of women, with a dramatic increase in those aged of 70 years or more, to 33% of men and 49% of women. In a population of 3338 with uncomplicated hypertension, Hammond et al [5] found LVH in 12% of people with mild hypertension and in 20% of those with moderate hypertension.

ECG Special

4   Validation of the QRS Voltage Criteria

One of the main problems of LVH voltage ECG indices using the limb leads, alone or in combination with the precordial leads, is the wide variability of the frontal QRS axis. Although a frontal ÅQRS_F of $+ 30°$ to $- 30°$ is common at the age of 40 years or more, a substantial number of patients have a frontal QRS axis between $+ 30°$ and $+ 90°$. The difficulty then is to decide *what voltage* in *which lead* should be used for an index. The commonly used indices in limb leads – used from the time of Lewis in 1914 [6] – are listed in Table 5.1. Effectively, the index $R_I + S_{III} \geq 25$ mm [7] and the index $R_{aVL} \geq 11$ mm [8] are not sufficient, with high specificity of about 80%–95%, but low sensitivity of 30%. Schillaci et al [9] reported extreme values of 97% specificity and 12%–15% sensitivity.

The QRS variability in the precordial leads is far less pronounced with a common transition zone between V_3 (predominantly negative QRS) and V_4 (predominantly positive QRS). Some pathologic conditions such as funnel chest, pneumothorax, and dilatation of the right and/or left ventricle (see section 6.4) displace the transition zone; in the latter to the left, leading to deep S waves in leads V_5/V_6 at the expense of the R waves. Moreover, the ECG indices depending on the QRS voltage in the precordial leads are impaired by the 'proximity effect', whereby any precordial lead, especially a lead very near the heart, enhances vectors originating directly under the lead, and at the same time reduces heart vectors at a distance of more than 1 cm from the exploring lead. Thus local variations can alter the QRS amplitude; these variations include those of habitus or nutritional status, slight displacement or rotation of the heart, or minor changes in the placement of the leads. The latter is especially valid for leads V_2 and V_3 (V_4) that are nearest to the left ventricle. An unusual but instructive example of the 'proximity effect' in a patient with hypertrophic cardiomyopathy is shown in Chapter 32 Rare ECGs.

In fact, the indices based on the precordial QRS voltage, i.e. the Sokolow index, or the index $S_{V_3} \geq 25$ mm, show high specificity of 89% [9] and 94% [10], but a low sensitivity of 21% [9] and 20%–33% [10].

An attempt to summarize all Q, R and S amplitudes in the limb leads *and* the precordial leads seemed logical, considering that the human electric ventriculogram is a 'levogram'. However, the results were likewise disappointing. The QRS sum index has good specificity and low sensitivity. At a matched specificity of 95%, Molloy et al [11] reported a sensitivity of 31%. Multiplication with the QRS duration (=QRS sum-duration product) resulted in a slightly better sensitivity of 45% [11]. Koehler et al [12] found an insufficient specificity of 43%, but a high sensitivity of 74% with the Cornell index.

The index of the Cornell group respects the patient's gender: $R_{aVL} + S_{V_3} \geq 28$ mm for men and ≥ 20 mm for women. Schillaci et al [9] found a specificity of 97% and a sensitivity 16%. With a slightly modified Cornell voltage index $R_{aVL} + S_{V_3} \geq 24$ mm, instead of ≥ 28 for men, and additionally respecting a strain pattern or the Romhilt point-score index [13], the sensitivity was improved from 22% to 34%, at a preserved specificity of 93% [9]. This represents rather a complicated enterprise for a small improvement. In the study by Molloy et al [11], the sensitivity was increased with the Cornell voltage–duration product (Table 5.2) from 36% to 51%. Norman et al [14] reported a slightly better sensitivity in women than in men.

It has been shown that the inclusion of age and gender (in one of the first publications of the Cornell group [10]), and body mass index [14], as well as risk factors for LVH [15], improve the value of several ECG indices. However, the overall sensitivity could not be increased above 50%.

5   Detection of LVH in Ventricular Conduction Disturbances

Based on the behavior of the QRS vector it is easy to understand why a ventricular conduction disturbance may impair or enhance the diagnosis of LVH.

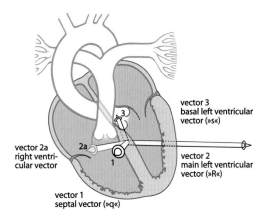

Figure 5.1a
Main QRS vectors in normal activation

vector 3
basal left ventricular
vector (»s«)

vector 2a
right ventri-
cular vector

vector 2
main left ventricular
vector (»R«)

vector 1
septal vector (»q«)

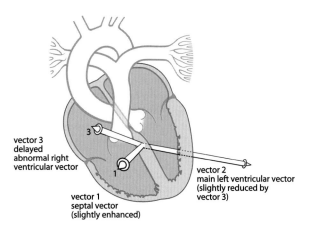

Figure 5.1b
Main QRS vectors in right bundle-branch block

vector 3
delayed
abnormal right
ventricular vector

vector 2
main left ventricular vector
(slightly reduced by
vector 3)

vector 1
septal vector
(slightly enhanced)

5.1 Right Bundle-Branch Block

As discussed in Chapter 10 (Bundle-Branch Blocks) the abnormal vectors produced by RBBB predominantly influence the last portion, but to a minor degree also the middle and even initial portions of QRS. The last, great and delayed RV vector 3 is responsible for the tall and broad R' wave in leads V_1 and aVR. This vector occurs predominantly *after* the end of LV excitation and does not influence the LV vectors. In contrast, RV vector 2a (that is *greater* than a normal RV vector, due to abnormal and slow excitation on a broad front of a portion of the RV) occurs at the same time as the normal main LV vector 2. As the RV vector 2a is opposite to the LV vector 2, the normal main LV vector is reduced (Figure 5.1b). This effect is measurable in the horizontal leads: The R waves in leads V_5/V_6 and also the S waves in leads V_2/V_3 are reduced by 2 mm to several millimeters. Additionally, vector 1 (the septal vector) is slightly altered in RBBB, compared to the normal ventricular activation (Figure 5.1a). This is only seen in a slightly increased R wave in the leads V2/V3.

Overall the ECG diagnosis of LVH is substantially impaired. All voltage indices using the horizontal leads (with or without limb leads) will reveal a higher specificity but an even lower sensitivity, compared to results in the absence of RBBB. This was proved in a publication by Vandenberg et al [16]. The authors investigated 100 patients with RBBB, using 32 ECG indices created for the detection of LVH. In the presence of left-

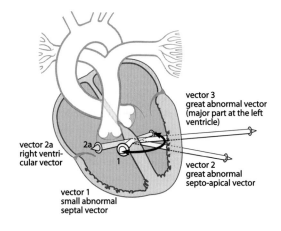

Figure 5.1c
Main QRS vectors in left bundle-branch block

vector 3
great abnormal vector
(major part at the left
ventricle)

vector 2a
right ventri-
cular vector

vector 2
great abnormal
septo-apical vector

vector 1
small abnormal
septal vector

axis deviation, the index $S_{III} + (R + S)_{maximal\ precordial} \geq 30$ mm proved to be 'probably the most useful criterion' with a specificity of 84% and a sensitivity of 54%. Of the other 31 indices, 27 had sensitivities below 30%, including 12 indices with a sensitivity of 0%–11%, but an excellent specificity of 98%–100%. Although the index mentioned above originates from our institution (it was specially created for the detection of LVH in the presence of (isolated) LAFB; see section 5.3 below), we do not recommend the use of this index in RBBB. The 100 patients of Vandenberg et al [16] with RBBB included several cases with associated LAFB that falsely improved the result. Moreover, the authors did not clearly define 'maximal R + S precordial' (for instance, were late RV vectors included?) and did not present an ECG example. So in this condition, and in cases of suspected LVH we propose that an echocardiogram is performed. In practice, LVH can be suspected if the R wave amplitude in V_5/V_6 (always reduced by RBBB) is strikingly high (ECG 5.10).

5.2 Left Bundle-Branch Block

The QRS vector is greatly altered in the presence of LBBB. Somewhat simplified, it consists of only *one great and prolonged vector,* directed to the left, and generally superiorly (in some instances inferiorly) and slightly posteriorly (Figure 5.1c). The normal small RV vector, although pointing to the opposite direction, is even more 'swallowed' by this great LV vector than in normal conditions. As the QRS vector is produced only by LV forces (including the septum) and points in only one direction, it seems obvious that the diagnosis of LVH should be enhanced, especially if an index is based on the precordial leads. Several publications seem to support this theoretical concept. Klein et al [1] applied the index $S_{V1} + R_{V6} \geq 45$ mm to 44 patients with LBBB (23 with LVH, 21 without), with the echocardiogram as control (LV mass > 260 g/m^2 or LV thickness of the posterior wall > 11 mm). The specificity was 100%, the sensitivity at 86% was also very high. Kafka et al [2] studied 125 patients with LBBB with the help of a complicated set of criteria:

i. $R_{aVL} > 11$ mm
ii. frontal QRS < − 40°
iii. $S_{V1} + R_{V5}$ (or R_{V6}) > 40 mm
iv. $S_{V2} > 30$ mm (or $S_{V3} > 25$ mm).

They compared the results with a LV mass of > 115 g/m^2 in the echocardiogram. The specificity was 90% and the sensitivity 75%. The index of Klein et al would be preferable in practice because of its simplicity (ECG 5.7). However, an unpublished study by the present author in 78 patients with LBBB (38 without LVH and 40 with LVH of various etiologies; 'gold standard': echocardiogram, discriminating LV mass index $\geq$ 124 g/m^2) revealed a sensitivity of only 28% and a specificity of 92% with the index of Klein et al. The index of Kafka et al resulted in a moderate specificity of 72%, and sensitivity of 52%. In the presence of LBBB, therefore, it seems preferable to apply only the excellent specificity of the Klein index [1].

5.3 Left Anterior Fascicular Block

In LAFB, where a frontal QRS left-axis deviation is mandatory, the frontal QRS is ideal for a voltage index. Lead III shows the greatest increase of the S amplitude in LVH. In the horizontal leads there is always a RS configuration. A clockwise rotation is most common but also a counterclockwise rotation may occur. However, with the criterion $(R + S)_{maximal\ precordial}$ all variations of the horizontal QRS vector loop are respected, the septum included (Figure 5.2, ECGs 5.8–5.9). With the combination of a frontal and horizontal voltage index, $S_{III} + (R + S)_{maximal\ precordial} \geq 30$ mm Gertsch et al [17] (Table 5.3) found in 50 patients with isolated LAFB (without myocardial infarction) a

Table 5.3

Index for the detection of left ventricular hypertrophy in left anterior fascicular block

Male
$S_{III} + (R + S)_{maximal\ precordial} > 30$ mm
Female
$S_{III} + (R + S)_{maximal\ precordial} > 28$ mm

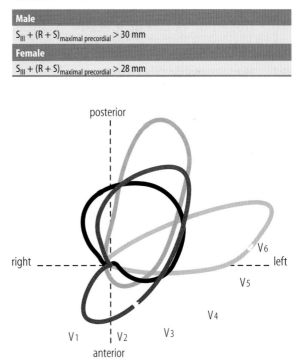

Figure 5.2
Variants of QRS vector loop (horizontal plane) in left anterior fascicular block

specificity of 89% and a very high sensitivity of 96% (echo criterion: LV mass $\geq$ 124 g/m^2). The authors suggested a value of 28 mm for females. The index proved to be superior to the criteria used hitherto by Milliken [18] and Bozzi and Figini [19].

5.4 Other Ventricular Conduction Disturbances

There are no data about the value of ECG indices for the diagnosis of LVH in *bilateral blocks*. However, based on the publication of Vandenberg et al [16] it can be assumed that for the combination RBBB + LAFB the index $S_{III} + (R + S)_{maximal\ precordial} \geq 30$ mm will have a specificity superior to 84% and a sensitivity superior to 54%.

In general, an *incomplete* RBBB does not influence the magnitude of the main LV vector, in the absence of RV hypertrophy. In some cases with a relative broad QRS complex and a tall r' wave in lead V_1, there is a slight reduction of the S amplitude in V_2/V_3, and of the R amplitude in V_5/V_6.

In all these conditions the echocardiogram will reveal reliable results.

6 Detection of LVH in Special Conditions

6.1 Hypertrophic Obstructive Cardiomyopathy

In hypertrophic obstructive cardiomyopathy (HOCM), LVH has different implications for the ECG that depend partially on the grade of unorganized anatomy of the LV muscle fibers, and partially on septal hypertrophy. The typical ECG pattern in HOCM is characterized by *deep and broad pathologic Q waves* reflecting septal hypertrophy.

In rare cases HOCM influences the whole QRS complex. The main QRS vector points to the *right* and *superiorly*. We had the opportunity to be confronted with this unusual ECG pattern under extraordinary circumstances.

Short Story/Case Report 1

On August 21 1965 a 22-year-old man was investigated as the last patient in the ambulatory section of our department. He complained of angina during strong exercise. He had a rough systolic murmur of grade 3/6 over the fourth left intercostal space. On x-ray his heart was slightly enlarged. His ECG was

most spectacular (ECG 5.11a) and was first interpreted as the atypical pattern of an old myocardial infarction. However, instantaneous and intensive research of the literature performed by all members of the department (only four at that time) revealed the likely presence of a recently described 'new' cardiac disease, a 'hypertrophic muscular subaortic stenosis', called hypertrophic obstructive cardiomyopathy today. Heart catheterization was planned for the following week.

The next morning we investigated a 27-year-old woman who had similar symptoms. Moreover, she had the strange feeling that there was not enough room for the blood in her heart. Her ECG (ECG 5.11b) was so similar to that of the young man that we first thought their ECGs had been confused. In both patients the diagnosis of severe HOCM was confirmed by heart catheterization and LV angiography, with an intraventricular gradient of 80 mmHg in both patients.

Overall we were confronted by strangely duplicated cases. Conversely, the follow-up in these two young patients was completely different. The woman died suddenly 4 months later while playing tennis. And astonishingly, the man is still alive, 37 years later, with no heart operation and with a minimal dose of propranolol (40 mg a day!). His obstructive cardiomyopathy converted over many years into a nonobstructive, modestly dilating cardiomyopathy.

The author has not seen such extreme ECG manifestations of HOCM during the next 35 years.

Such a QRS configuration can no longer be explained by septal hypertrophy alone (because the mass of the lateral wall often overweighs the septal mass); there will also be bizarre ventricular conduction disturbances due to the chaotic structure of the myocardial fibers.

ECG 5.12 shows another example of severe HOCM, with QS wave in lead V_3 and suspect Q waves in the inferolateral leads. A milder form of the disease can occasionally be detected, e.g. in the relatives of a patient with severe HOCM, on the basis of pronounced Q waves in the leads V_5 and V_6, and often in I and aVL (ECG 5.13).

However, it has to be mentioned that also severe cases of HOCM may not show any pathologic Q waves but a pattern of 'simple' LVH, with or without strain, an LBBB, or even a normal ECG. In the last case one may assume that the vectors produced by chaotic muscle fibers cancel themselves out. In ECGs with distinct Q waves a myocardial infarction can be excluded by the atypical localization of the Q waves, by the discordant positive and asymmetric T waves and especially by the clinical conditions.

6.2 Asymmetrical Apical LVH

Asymmetrical apical LVH [20] is an extremely rare condition outside of Japan [21]. The ECG is characterized by huge R waves and strikingly deep T waves in the precordial leads and some limb leads (ECG 5.14).

6.3 Systolic and Diastolic Overload

The terms *systolic overload* and *diastolic overload* were created by Cabrera and Monroy in 1952 [22,23]. The authors believed that in valvular and some congenital heart diseases a diastolic overload produces a distinct ECG pattern, compared to systolic overload. The pattern should consist of small and high R waves, slight ST elevations and tall symmetroid T waves in leads V_4 to V_6 (ECG 5.15). However, no reliable correlation could be found in other studies [24]. Moreover, a pattern of 'diastolic overload' generally turns into a pattern of 'systolic overload', when diastolic overload persists for years or decades. The QRS duration increases, the ST segment and the T wave become negative. In the early stage of diastolic overload, the respective patterns may occasionally be seen in patients with patent ductus arteriosus or aortic valve incompetence.

Short Story/Case Report 2

In May 1969 a 16-year-old girl was hospitalized for nausea and heavy vomiting. No diagnosis could be made. In the ECG the author found a sinus rhythm of 65/min, a slight ST elevation and tall, positive symmetroid T waves in the left precordial leads as a normal variant (ECG 5.16). The suggestion of diastolic overload (that occurs in the fourth to sixth months of pregnancy) and the proposal of a pregnancy test provoked enormous laughter from the author's colleagues. One day later everyone was amazed – the test was positive. This is an excellent example of an ECG interpretation that should *never* be applied (or only once) in a cardiologist's lifetime.

6.4 LVH Associated with Marked LV Dilatation

This is not a rare condition at all. Marked LV (and/or RV) dilatation leads to *QRS clockwise rotation* in the *precordial leads* and may change the $ÅQRS_F$, at the same time often diminishing the QRS voltage in some limb leads. This strongly impairs the detection of LVH in the ECG (ECG 5.17).

7 Factors Impairing the ECG Diagnosis of LVH

7.1 Gender and Race

Only recently has the reduced QRS voltage in white women compared to white men been accounted for in voltage indices. Black people, especially women, have significantly higher voltages than white people.

7.2 Age

In the young the QRS amplitude is significantly higher. As a rule, the ECG indices should only be used in individuals older than 40 years. Pipberger et al calculated a 6.5% decrease of the maximal spatial QRS vector per decade from the age of 20 years to 80 years [25].

7.3 Body Habitus and Body Weight

Body habitus and body weight strongly influence the QRS voltage, especially in the precordial leads. In obese patients, a voltage index is more often false negative; in slim people it is more often false positive. This may also occur in old patients with cachexia. Sometimes the voltage is diminished by strong thoracic muscles or by subepicardial fat.

7.4 Other Pathologic Conditions

Alterations of tissues near the heart (or surrounding it) are the main causes for the *reduction* of QRS voltage, especially pulmonary emphysema. Pulmonary edema and pneumothorax – and more often pericardial effusion – also diminish the voltage. 'Infiltrative' heart diseases, such as myocarditis, amyloidosis, or scleroderma, can reduce the amplitude of QRS, as can myocardial infarction. Right ventricular hypertrophy (RVH) and RBBB (also RBBB without RVH) reduce the amplitude of the R waves especially in leads V_4 to V_6 by simultaneous, opposite RV vectors. Hypothyreosis (myxedema) leads to reduction of the QRS (and T) voltage and a peripheral low voltage is seen in large pericardial effusion. *All of these conditions* impair the ECG diagnosis of LVH. As an exception, LBBB increases the voltage of the S waves in V_1 to V_3 (V_4). Occasionally a slight increase of precordial QRS voltage is observed in hyperthyreosis (without true LVH) that is reversible after treatment.

7.5 Variability of the Frontal and Horizontal QRS Vector

As mentioned before, variability of QRS configuration in the horizontal and especially in the *frontal* leads also makes it difficult to find accurate ECG indices.

8 Conclusions

In summary, the ECG detection of LVH seems to be reliable only in the presence of LAFB, due to the unique vectorial QRS behavior. For evaluation of ECGs without conduction disturbances (and without myocardial infarction) all QRS voltage criteria reveal good-to-excellent specificity, but low-to-very-low sensitivity. Probably the best criteria are the Cornell voltage index and the Cornell product, with a specificity of 85%–95% and a sensitivity of 30%–50%. In our experience, in LBBB, and especially in RBBB, the ECG is of little diagnostic value, although some good-to-excellent results have been reported in the literature. Especially in patients with clinically suspected LVH, and no or only one ECG voltage criterion indicating LVH, the accurate quantitative measurement with the echocardiogram is highly preferable.

9 Pathophysiology and Effects of LVH on the ECG

A slight dilatation of the left atrium is probably the first effect of hemodynamic LV overload. Then LVH begins to develop, usually in a concentric form, mainly leading to an increase of the left main LV vector.

Consequently the amplitudes of the R waves in V_5 and V_6 (V_4) increase and, as a mirror image, so do those of the S waves in leads V_2/V_3 (V_1). To a minor degree the R waves increase in leads I and aVL (in left QRS axis) or in III, aVF and II (in vertical QRS axis). As the conduction through the hypertrophied left ventricle takes longer, there is an *increase of QRS duration* and a *delay of the intrinsic deflection* that exceeds 0.055 sec (measured in V_5/V_6). At the same time the *frontal QRS axis is shifted to the left* in many cases of extensive LVH. However, an indifferent or even vertical QRS axis can also be observed in some patients with valvular aortic stenosis or in extracardiac conditions such as asthenic habitus and pulmonary emphysema. A prominent Q wave in lead III ('Q_{III}') and aVF, or even a QS complex in III (ECG 5.2), may be due to LVH (or a normal variant) and not to inferior infarction. In the case of LVH the T wave is generally positive; in case of infarction the T wave is generally negative and symmetrical in lead III.

Often the repolarization is also affected. The *depression of the ST segment,* mostly with an upward convex configuration, may reach 3 mm (measured at the J point or 0.08 sec after the J point). *Negative asymmetric* (discordant) T waves are quite common.

The useful ECG criteria for LVH respect the increase of QRS voltage. Some indices have been improved by multiplication of the voltage index with QRS duration, resulting in *products*. Additional inclusion of ST and T abnormalities have not much helped to improve LVH diagnosis due to the nonspecificity of repolarization changes.

10 Prognosis of LVH

LVH has been recognized as an independent factor for cardiovascular events and premature death.

LVH in hypertensive patients is associated with significantly increased mortality and with a threefold prevalence of coronary heart disease [3]. Sullivan et al [26] found a 5-year survival rate of 84.4% in patients with electrocardiographic LVH compared to 94.5% in patients without LVH. Haider et al [27] reported an increased incidence of sudden death, especially in men, based on the results in a cohort of 3661 patients enrolled in the Framingham study; LVH prevalence was 21.5%. A twofold mortality rate in black people compared with white people was found by Benjamin and Levy [28]. Based on a study in 6391 women and 5243 men (age 35–74 years, follow-up 7 years) Larsen et al [29] recently reported that the ECG pattern of LVH with negative T, with or without ST depression, are significantly associated with ischemic heart disease.

References

1. Klein RC, Zakauddin V, De Maria AN, Mason D. Electrocardiographic diagnosis of left ventricular hypertrophy in the presence of left bundle-branch block. Am Heart J 1984;108:502–6
2. Kafka H, Burggraf GW, Milliken JA. Electrocardiographic diagnosis of left ventricular hypertrophy in the presence of left bundle branch block: an echocardiographic study. Am J Cardiol 1985;55:103–6
3. Kannel WB, Gordon T, Offutt D. Left ventricular hypertrophy by electrocardiogram. Prevalence, incidence and mortality in the Framingham study. Ann Intern Med 1969;71:89–105
4. Levy D, Anderson KM, Savage DD, et al. Echocardiographically detected left ventricular hypertrophy: prevalence and risk factors. The Framingham Heart Study. Ann Intern Med 1988;108:7–13

5. Hammond IW, Devereux RB, et al. The prevalence and correlates of echocardiographic left ventricular hypertrophy among employed patients with uncomplicated hypertension. J Am Coll Cardiol 1986;7:639–50

6. Lewis T. Observation upon ventricular hypertrophy with especial reference to preponderance of one or other chamber. Heart 1914;5:367

7. Gubner R, Ungerleider HE. Electrocardiographic criteria for left ventricular hypertrophy. Arch Intern Med 1943;72:196–210

8. Sokolow M, Lyon TP. The ventricular complex in left ventricular hypertrophy as obtained by unipolar precordial and limb leads. Am Heart J 1949;37:161–86

9. Schillaci G, Verdecchia P, Borgioni C, et al. Improved electrocardiographic diagnosis of left ventricular hypertrophy. Am J Cardiol 1994;74:714–98

10. Casale PN, Devereux RB, Kligfield P, et al. Electrocardiographic detection of left ventricular hypertrophy: development and prospective validation of improved criteria. J Am Coll Cardiol 1985;6:572–80

11. Molloy TJ, Okin PM, Devereux RB, Kligfield P. Electrocardiographic detection of left ventricular hypertrophy by the simple QRS voltage–duration product. J Am Coll Cardiol 1992;20:1180–6

12. Koehler NR, Velho FJ, Bodanese LC, et al. Evaluation of QRS voltage in 12 derivations and Cornell criteria in the diagnosis of left ventricular hypertrophy. Arq Bras Cardiol 1994;63:197–201

13. Romhilt DW, Estes EH. A point-score system for the ECG diagnosis of left ventricular hypertrophy. Am Heart J 1968;75:752–8

14. Norman JE Jr, Levy D. Improved electrocardiographic detection of echocardiographic left ventricular hypertrophy: results of a correlated data base approach. J Am Coll Cardiol 1995;26:1022–9

15, Jaggy C, Perret F, Bovet P, et al. Performance of classic electrocardiographic criteria for left ventricular hypertrophy in an African population. Hypertension 2000;36:54–61

16. Vandenberg B, Sagar K, Paulsen W, Romhilt D. Electrocardiographic criteria for the diagnosis of left ventricular hypertrophy in the presence of complete right bundle branch block. Am J Cardiol 1989;63:1080–4

17. Gertsch M, Theler A, Foglia E. Electrocardiographic detection of left ventricular hypertrophy in the presence of left anterior fascicular block. Am J Cardiol 1988;61:1098–101

18. Milliken JA. Isolated and complicated left anterior fascicular block: a review of suggested electrocardiographic criteria. J Electrocardiol 1983;16:199–212

19. Bozzi G, Figini A. Left anterior hemiblock and electrocardiographic diagnosis of left ventricular hypertrophy. Adv Cardiol 1976;16:495–500

20. Sakamoto T, Tei C, Murayama M, et al. Giant T wave inversion as a manifestation of asymmetrical apical hypertrophy (AAH) of the left ventricle. Echocardiographic and ultrasonocardiotomographic study. Jap Heart J 1976;17:611–29

21. Suzuki J, Watanabe F, Takenaka K, et al. New subtype of apical hypertrophic cardiomyopathy identified with nuclear magnetic resonance imaging as an underlying cause of markedly inverted T waves. J Am Coll Cardiol 1993;22:1175–81

22. Cabrera E, Monroy JR. Systolic and diastolic loading of the heart. Part I. Physiologic and clinical data. Am Heart J 1952;43:661

23. Cabrera E, Monroy JR. Systolic and diastolic loading of the heart. Part II. Electrocardiographic data. Am Heart J 1952;43:669

24. Russo R, Rizzoli G, Stritoni P, et al. T-wave changes in patients with hemodynamic evidence of systolic or diastolic overload of the left ventricle: a retrospective study on isolated chronic aortic valve disease. Int J Cardiol 1987;14:137–43

25. Pipberger HV, Goldman MJ, Littmann D, et al. Correlations of the orthogonal electrocardiogram and vectorcardiogram with constitutional variables in 518 normal men. Circulation 1967;35:536–51

26. Sullivan JM, Vander Zwaag RV, el-Zeky F, et al. Left ventricular hypertrophy: effect on survival. J Am Coll Cardiol 1993;22:508–13

27. Haider AW, Larson MG, Benjamin EJ, Levy D. Increased left ventricular mass and hypertrophy are associated with increased risk for sudden death. J Am Coll Cardiol 1998;32:1454–9

28. Benjamin EJ, Levy D. Why is left ventricular hypertrophy so predictive of morbidity and mortality. Am J Med Sci 1999;317:168–75

29. Larsen CT, Dahlin J, Blackburn H, et al. Prevalence and prognosis of electrocardiographic left ventricular hypertrophy, ST segment depression and negative T wave; the Copenhagen City Heart Study. Eur Heart J 2002;23:315–24

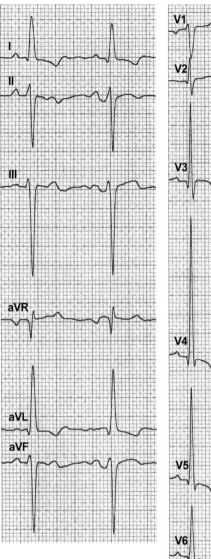
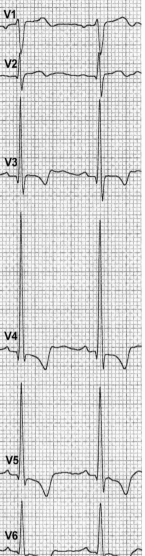
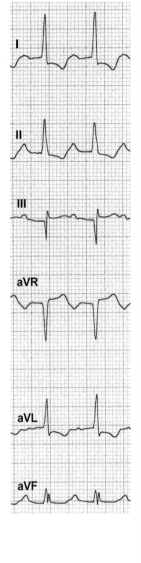
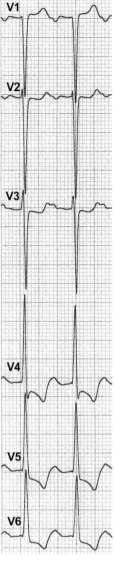

ECG 5.1

53y/m. Severe LVH 1 year after valve replacement for aortic valve incompetence. *Positive voltage indices*: R_{aVL} = 15 mm (> 11 mm); $R_I + S_{III}$ = 31 mm (> 25 mm). *Negative voltage indices*: Cornell: 21 mm (> 28 mm for male); Sokolow ($S_{V1} + R_{V5}$) = 29 mm (> 35 mm). Plus: negative T waves in leads with tall R waves. Left-axis deviation due to LVH, probably not due to LAFB. Echo: LV mass index 270 g/m².

ECG 5.2

69y/f. LVH, 2 months after aortic valve replacement.
Positive voltage indices: Sokolow: 41 mm; Cornell: 30 mm (20 mm for female). Negative voltage indices:
R_{aVL} = 9 mm; $R_I + S_{III}$ = 19 mm. Plus: significant
ST depression and T inversion in anterolateral leads.
Echo: LV mass index 150 g/m².

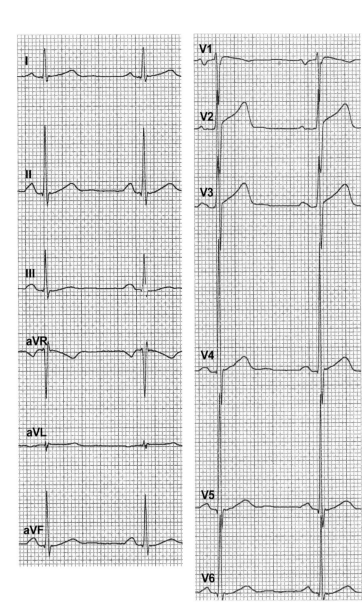

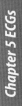
ECG 5.3

57y/m. Tall R waves in V$_4$/V$_5$ suggest LVH. Positive voltage criteria: Sokolow: 41 mm. Negative indices: R$_{aVL}$, Cornell, R$_I$ + S$_{III}$. No T inversion. Echo: LV mass 134 g/m^2.

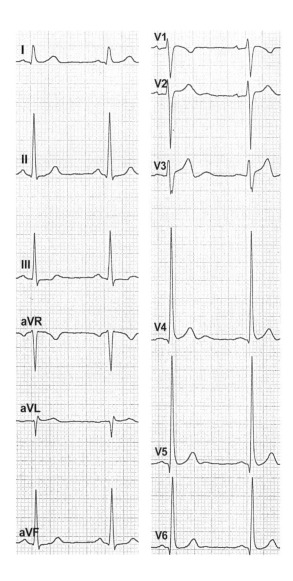

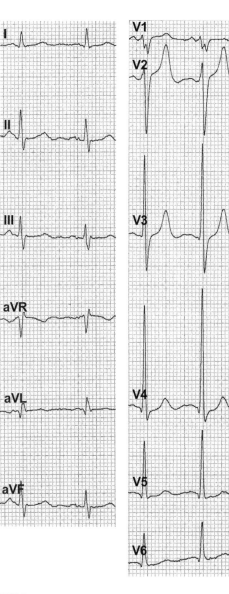

ECG 5.4
80y/m. All usual voltage criteria are negative. LVH may be suggested from the tall RS complexes in V_4/V_5, about 30 mm each. Hypertensive and coronary heart disease. Echo: LV mass 165 g/m^2.

ECG 5.5
24y/m. Positive Sokolow index (37 mm), all other voltage indices negative. Echo: No LVH. False-positive Sokolow index in a young healthy individual.

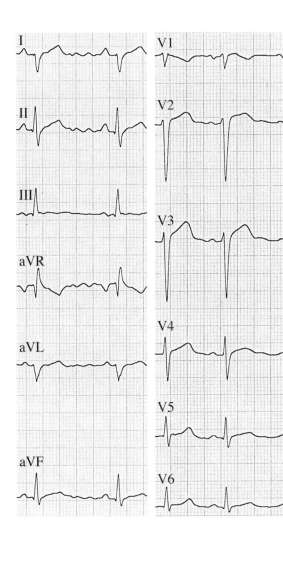

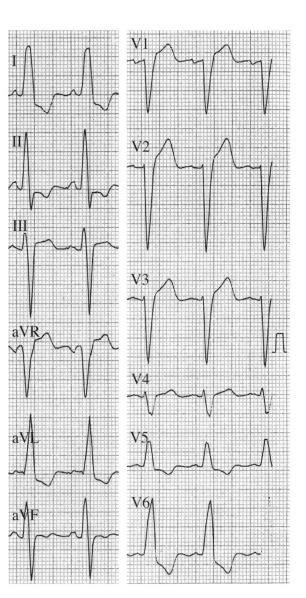

ECG 5.6

18y/m. Operated ventricular septal defect with rest-shunt. At first glance no LVH, but note calibration in precordial leads (1 mV = 5 mm!). Despite right-axis deviation and a minimal R wave in aVL, the Cornell index is positive: R_{aVL}=1 mm; S_{V3} = 34 mm; Sum = 35 mm (28 mm for male). All other indices are negative, partially due to right-axis deviation. Echo: LV mass 180 g/m^2.

ECG 5.7

79y/m. LVH with LBBB, showing striking QRS amplitudes in the precordial leads (see calibration 1 mV = 5 mm). However the index of Klein et al ($S_{V1} + R_{V5} \geq$ 45 mm) is negative, with 42 mm.

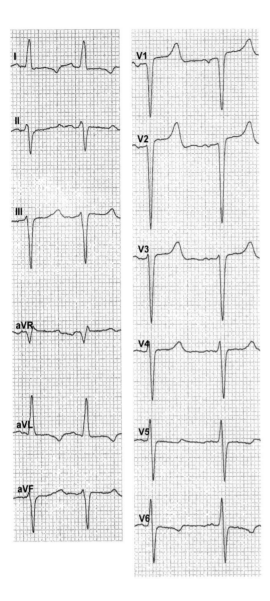

ECG 5.8

71y/m. LVH in LAFB. The index $S_{III} + (R + S)_{maximal\ precordial}$ ≥ 30 mm (Gertsch et al [17]) is positive: $S_{III} = 12$ mm; R + S in $V_2 = 21$ mm; Sum = 33 mm. All other voltage indices (e.g. R_{aVL}, $R_I + S_{III}$, Cornell and Sokolow) are negative.

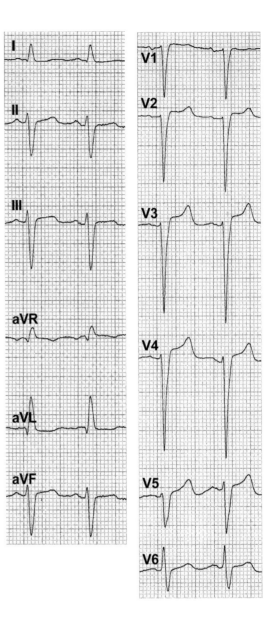

ECG 5.9

77y/m. LVH in LAFB. *Positive indices*: Gertsch et al (36 mm), Cornell (32 mm). *Negative indices*: R_{aVL}, $R_I + S_{III}$, Sokolow.

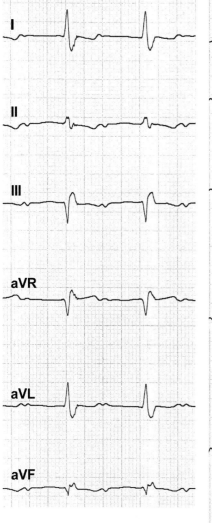

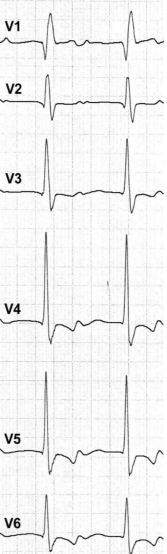

ECG 5.10

57y/m. LVH in RBBB. Hypertensive and coronary heart disease. Besides sinus rhythm with an extreme AV block 1° and a pathologic Q wave in V_1/V_2, the great R wave amplitudes in leads V_4/V_5 in the presence of RBBB suggest LVH. T negativity in V_4 to V_6 due to LV overload and/or ischemia.

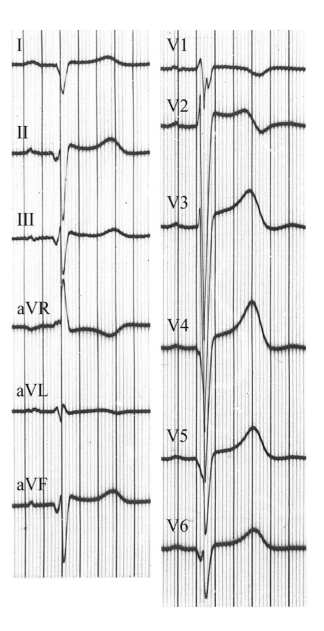

ECG 5.11a
Short Story/Case Report 1. 22y/m. HOCM. ECG (50 mm/sec): sinus rhythm. Striking QRS vector in the limb and precordial leads. ÂQRS$_F$ about − 130°, with a positive QRS complex only in lead aVR. Giant S waves in V$_2$/V$_3$. QS complexes in leads I, II, V$_4$ to V$_6$, as in extensive lateral myocardial infarction (however positive discordant T waves).

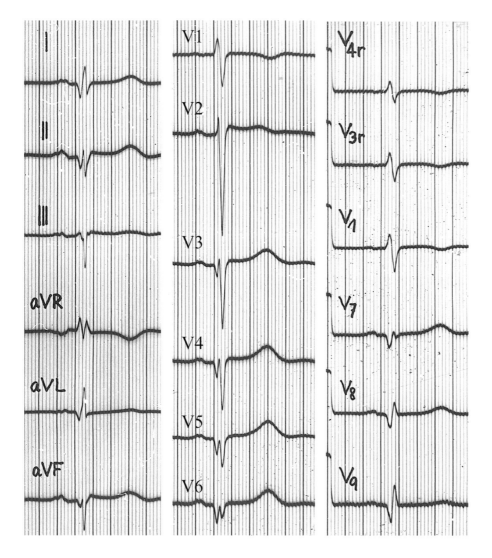

ECG 5.11b

Short Story/Case Report 1. 27y/f. HOCM. ECG (50 mm/sec): sinus rhythm. Striking QRS vector in the limb and precordial leads. ÅQRS$_F$ about - 100°. QS complexes in leads V$_5$/V$_6$, prominent Q waves in leads I, II, aVL, aVF and V$_3$/V$_4$ and in the posterior leads V$_7$ to V$_9$. The QRS vector and the Q waves are very similar to those in ECG 5.11a.

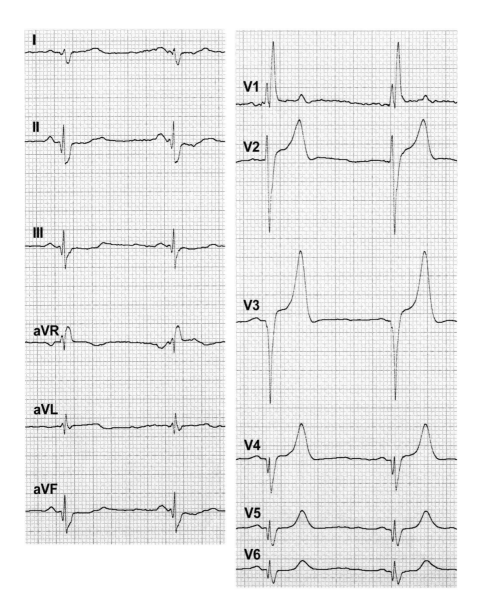

ECG 5.12

28y/m. 'Typical' pattern in HOCM. QS in V$_3$, pathologic Q waves in V$_4$ to V$_6$ and in I, II, aVF and III (as manifestation of at least abnormal septal activation). ECG 18 months after alcohol ablation, unchanged besides new RBBB. LV gradient reduced from 48(116) mmHg to 10(19) mmHg (with amylnitrate).

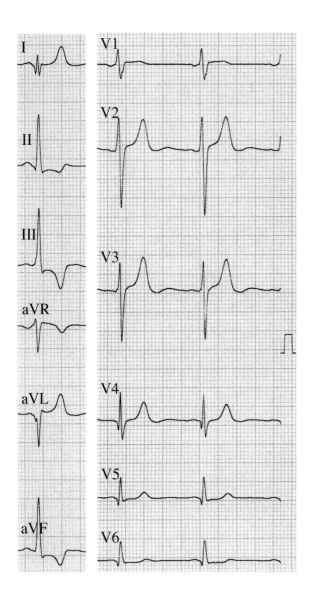

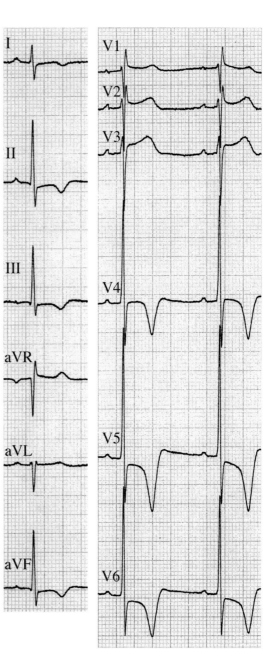

ECG 5.13
25y/m. HOCM. QS in aVL, slightly prominent Q in I and V_4 to V_6 (half calibration of the precordial leads). Striking ST depression and negative T waves in II/aVF/III. Echo/Doppler: gradient 33 mmHg at rest, 70 mmHg with amylnitrate.

ECG 5.14
39y/m. Apical hypertrophy. High R amplitude with significant ST depression and 'giant' negative T waves in V_4 to V_6. Incomplete RBBB. Echo: LV mass 270 g/m^2.

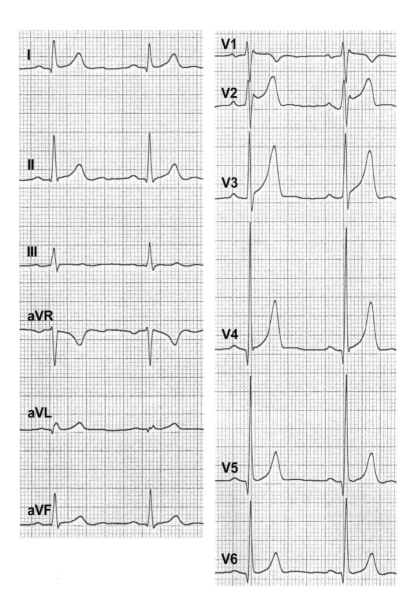

ECG 5.15
64y/m. Mild aortic valve incompetence. Typical pattern of 'diastolic overload'. Relatively deep Q waves and tall, narrow R waves, slight ST elevation and positive, high and peaked T waves in V_3 to V_6. The pattern is probably also due to low rate sinus rhythm.

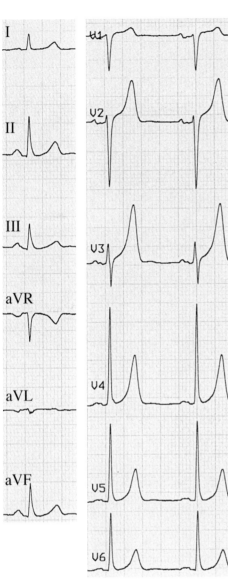

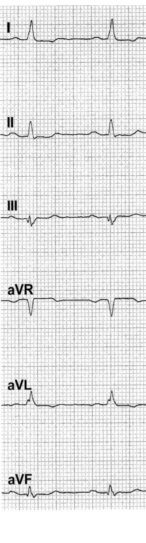

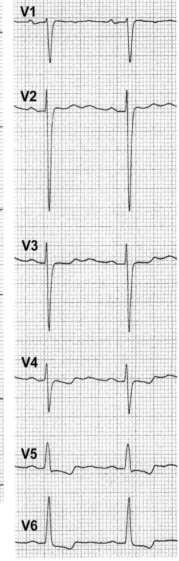

ECG 5.16

Short Story/Case Report 2. ECG: there is minimal ST elevation in V5 and V6 combined with relatively high and symmetroid T waves.

ECG 5.17

77y/m. LVH with LV dilatation. There is clockwise rotation in the precordial leads, R in V6 is significantly higher than R in V5. All voltage criteria are negative. LVH can be assumed by deep S wave in V2.

Chapter 6
Right Ventricular Hypertrophy

At a Glance

Right ventricular hypertrophy (RVH) is only detectable in the ECG if the normally thin wall of the right ventricle develops hypertrophy up to a grade that more or less balances the left ventricular mass. This alteration always takes time, generally months or years.

Excessive RVH (with a right ventricular mass at least as great as the left ventricular mass) can be reliably diagnosed. In moderate RVH, the ECG manifestations allow only some suspicion of the presence of RVH. It is much rarer than left ventricular hypertrophy and is encountered in congenital heart diseases in its extensive form.

ECG

Lead V_1 is the most proximal to the anteriorly positioned right ventricle and therefore shows exclusively the *direct* and specific alterations of RVH, demonstrating the augmented RV vectors, directed anteriorly and to the right. Thus, lead V_1 represents the *key lead for RVH*, in the absence of incomplete or complete right bundle-branch block. The special right-precordial leads V_{3R} to V_{6R} are not used for the diagnosis or exclusion of RVH, but for the detection of RV infarction in the presence of inferior myocardial infarction.

1   ECG Conditions for RVH

RVH may be present in three conditions:

i.   without RV conduction disturbance
ii. with incomplete right bundle-branch block (iRBBB)
iii. with complete right bundle-branch block (RBBB).

Frontal *QRS right-axis deviation* ($\mathring{A}QRS_F \geq 90°$) is often present. Additional *ST depression* and especially *T inversion* in leads V_1 to V_2/V_3 favor the diagnosis of RVH in conditions (i) and (ii), but not in (iii).

1.1   RVH without RV Conduction Disturbance

The ECG is characterized by a single positive QRS deflection that is a *pure R wave in lead V_1* (ECGs 6.1–6.3). This condition is encountered in pulmonary valve stenosis (which can also be associated with iRBBB), severe RVH in congenital heart diseases with *Eisenmenger* syndrome, and in some cases of mitral stenosis and severe cor pulmonale. In general there is associated frontal QRS right-axis deviation.

If some well-defined conditions are excluded, such as true posterior myocardial infarction and one type of pre-excitation, an R complex in V_1 is very specific for RVH.

A *qR complex in lead V_1* is also a reliable sign of RVH (ECG 6.4). The Q wave is due to RVH and RV (and right atrial!) dilatation and not due to anteroseptal necrosis. A qR complex is occasionally found in severe acute pulmonary embolism in this case due to RV and right atrial *dilatation*.

An *RS complex in lead V_1* with a ratio R : S of more than 1 : 1 (ECG 6.5) favors the presence of RVH, but is less reliable. This statement is also valid for an *R wave* > 7 mm in V_1 or an *S wave* < 2 mm in V_1, always in the case of an RS complex.

1.2   RVH with iRBBB (QRS Duration Normal)

An rSr' complex in V_1 with an r' that is *smaller* than the initial R wave is rarely associated with RVH and is rather common in healthy young persons (ECG 6.6). If the r' is evidently *greater* than the initial R wave, RVH is present in about 40% of cases. On one hand, this rSr' type (r' > r) is typical of patients with 'atrial septal defect of the secundum type' (90% have this anomaly), generally with asymmetric, negative T waves in V_1 to V_3 (ECG 6.7) and may also be found in chronic pulmonary embolism, valvular pulmonary stenosis, and occasionally in cases of mitral stenosis. On the other hand, the pattern may occasionally represent an *intermediate* state between iRBBB and RBBB. The etiology in this case is manifold and includes fibrosis of the right bundle branch or coronary heart disease. However it should be emphasized that an rSr' type with r' > r can occur in normal individuals and is not unusual in people with funnel chest.

1.3 RVH with RBBB (QRS Duration > 0.12 sec)

For RBBB with or without RVH, the typical pattern is an *rsR' complex in lead V_1*. In some cases the S wave is lacking because of projections and only a single broad and notched R wave is present. RVH can only be diagnosed or suspected if the amplitude of R' exceeds 12 mm and/or the QRS duration is > 0.14 sec, caused by an atypically broad and often notched R' wave. An associated QRS right-axis deviation is almost obligatory (ECG 6.8). The T wave is always negative in lead V_1, in many cases also in V_2 to V_4, with and without RVH. The classical pattern of associated right atrial hypertrophy/enlargement, the 'p pulmonale', can only be detected in patients with cor pulmonale 'parenchymale' – that is, due to obstructive lung disease.

Statistically RBBB is much more frequent in patients *without* RVH than in patients with RVH, with a ratio of about 20 : 1.

It is generally advisable to correlate the ECG with the clinical findings, especially in borderline 'ECG RVH' and using the echocardiogram as a direct and better diagnostic method.

The Full Picture

The ECG diagnosis of RVH is limited because the condition must be extensive in order to outweigh a normal or even hypertrophic left ventricle. Some ECG criteria are highly specific for severe RVH.

In cases with supposed RVH, an echocardiogram is imperative.

2 Etiology and Prevalence

Extensive RVH is observed in patients with congenital heart diseases such as tetralogy of Fallot, valvular pulmonary stenosis, and the advanced stages of anomalies with left-to-right shunt complicated by the Eisenmenger reaction. In acquired heart diseases such as cor pulmonale and mitral stenosis, and in 'secondary' RVH following left heart failure, the RVH is generally moderate. Due to the limitations of the ECG in these cases, the echocardiogram is preferable. RVH can be quantified to a certain degree and RV function is measurable using this method.

RVH is about 10–20 times rarer than left ventricular hypertrophy. Reliable epidemiological data is lacking.

ECG Special

3 Vectors in RVH

The normal human ventricular ECG is a *levogram*. This means that the thickness of the wall of the left ventricle (10–12 mm) far exceeds that of the right (2–3 mm). Similarly, in normal conditions, the left ventricular mass (115 g/m² body surface in males and 95 g/m² in females) is evidently greater than the RV mass (about 20 g/m² body surface). Thus, the *LV vectors* are normally responsible for the *QRS complex*. In the frontal leads, the QRS axis is variable, whereas in the precordial leads there is a negative deflection (S wave) in leads V_1 to V_3 (with a small initial R wave due to septal activation) and a positive deflection (R wave) in leads V_4 to V_6 (with a small 'septal' Q wave). The opposite small RV vectors, directed anteriorly and to the right are completely canceled ('swallowed') by the dominating great LV vectors. It is obvious that a slight-to-moderate degree of RVH is not detectable in the ECG. ECG changes can only be observed if the RV muscle mass reaches more than about half of the left ventricular muscle mass. In anatomic studies, and also echocardiographically, RVH is diagnosed if the wall thickness exceeds 5 mm without ventricular dilatation, and 4 mm with associated RV dilatation [1]. Expressed in weight, RVH is also defined as a RV weight of more than 70 g (about 40 g/m^2) [2]. If RV weight exceeds about 30% of the left ventricle, the expression 'relative RVH' is used.

RVH enhances the amplitude of the main RV vector as well as the duration of the RV depolarization, without broadening the QRS complex, except in the presence of an RBBB pattern.

The typical changes are observed in lead V_1, due to its proximity to the right ventricle. Moreover, the RV vectors are magnified by the 'proximity effect'. V_1 is the only lead to reflect directly the increased RV vectors directed not only anteriorly but also to the right.

The most characteristic sign for RVH is a *qR complex in lead V_1* (highly specific but relatively rare; ECG 6.4) or a *single tall R wave in lead V_1* (ECGs 6.1–6.3). The Q wave is a consequence of the abnormal septal vector, which is directed more posteriorly than to the right, caused by hypertrophy of the right part of the interventricular septum. In some cases, lead V_1 reflects endocardial RV potentials (RV potentials registered by a 'pseudo-epicardial' lead upon a dilated right atrium) [3]. This means that an alteration of the ventricular depolarization may express – exceptionally and indirectly – an atrial abnormality! In this case a Q wave (QR complex in lead V_1) indicates excessive right atrial dilatation (Chapter 14 Differential Diagnosis of Pathologic Q Waves).

4   RVH in the ECG

4.1   Single R Wave, QR Complex or RS Complex in Lead V_1

The more severe the RVH, the greater is the amplitude of the R wave in V_1, with or without Q wave. Therefore, the highest R waves are seen in heart diseases with a severe elevation of systolic RV pressure lasting for many years, e.g. in congenital heart diseases in patients with *Eisenmenger* syndrome on one hand (ECG 6.9) and in severe *pulmonary valve stenosis* on the other hand (see section 5, differential diagnosis).

A single tall R wave in V_1 is quite rare in patients with pulmonary hypertension of other origin, such as severe mitral stenosis or cor pulmonale. In these conditions the R wave has an amplitude of only 2–4 mm (ECG 6.10), or shows an RS complex, or in other cases an incomplete or complete right bundle-branch block.

An R/S ratio in lead V_1 > 1 is due to RVH in about 60% of cases. Again, a concomitant frontal QRS right-axis deviation supports the diagnosis. Roman et al [4] demonstrated in a anatomic-electrocardiographic study of 118 hearts that the criteria of $R_{V_1} + S_{V_5}$ or S_{V_6} > 10.5 mm (Sokolow-Lyon index for *RVH*) and S_{V_5} or S_{V_6} > 7.0 mm are of little value for the detection of RVH.

4.2   Incomplete Right Bundle-Branch Block

If the r' is greater than the initial R wave, RV hypertrophy or dilatation – or both – *may* be the cause, especially if negative asymmetric T waves in leads V_2/V_3 and a right frontal QRS-axis deviation are present. In other cases this rsr' configuration is an intermediate stage between incomplete right bundle-branch block (iRBBB) and complete RBBB.

Based on vectorcardiographic criteria, Chou et al [5] found a sensitivity of 66% in 97 selected patients with atrial septal defect, mitral stenosis and chronic obstructive lung disease. The specificity was not tested. In a large study of 819 autopsies, Flowers and Horan [6] reported insufficient sensitivity of about 10% but excellent specificity of 87%–100% for most of the mentioned ECG criteria for RVH. However, these publications are based on selected patient cohorts. In daily practice about 50% of the rSr' patterns with r' > r in lead V_1 are found in healthy, especially younger, individuals. iRBBB with r' < r represents a normal variant in most cases.

4.3   Complete Right Bundle-Branch Block

RBBB is encountered more often without RVH than in combination with RVH (relation about 20 : 1). RVH is present:

i.   if the R' is higher than 12 mm
ii. if the QRS duration is equal to or greater than 0.14 sec, due to a strikingly broad R' wave
iii. if there is frontal QRS axis deviation.

An rsR' type or negativity of the T wave up to leads V_3 or V_4 is not a reliable sign for RVH, without associated QRS right-axis deviation.

4.4 S_I/S_{II}/S_{III} Type

This configuration is seen more often as a normal variant than in RV hypertrophy or dilatation. In the latter cases, the S waves are generally deeper than the R waves, and the S wave is deeper in lead II than in lead III. ECG 6.11 shows S_I/S_{II}/S_{III} type in a young individual with a normal heart.

4.5 Rare Type of RVH

A very rare ECG pattern in RVH is characterized by an *rS type in all precordial leads* (ECG 6.12). The R waves are sometimes so small that extensive anterolateral infarction cannot be excluded. However, the T waves are generally positive in all leads and infarction can be excluded by other clinical findings. A concomitant right-axis deviation or a $S_I/S_{II}/S_{III}$ type supports the diagnosis of RVH. The electrophysiologic mechanism of this rS pattern is not completely clear. An extreme rotation of the heart is assumed, eventually associated with a special RV conduction disturbance, with RV vectors pointing more backwards than forwards.

4.6 P Wave Alterations

It is surprising that alterations of the p wave rarely provide additional information in suspected RVH based on QRS alterations. A classical 'p pulmonale' (tall p waves in the inferior leads, negative p wave in lead aVL) is only detectable in patients with 'cor pulmonale' due to chronic obstructive lung disease (ECG 6.13). In younger patients with severe asthma or heavy nicotine abuse, QRS right-axis deviation and a pattern of p pulmonale may be present without RVH. In these cases the precordial leads are generally normal.

In patients with severe RVH due to pulmonary hypertension on the basis of severely increased precapillary pulmonary arterial resistance (e.g. in Eisenmenger syndrome, in chronic pulmonary embolism, in pulmonary hypertension after intake of aminorectic drugs [7]), a special pattern of right atrial overload may be seen, called 'p pulmonale vasculare' by some authors. The orientation of the frontal p vector is less oriented to the right than in 'p pulmonale parenchymale'. *Consequently the amplitude of the p wave is greater in lead I than in lead III.* In lead V_1 or/and V_2 the p waves are generally peaked (ECG 6.14).

5 Differential Diagnosis of Possible Signs of RVH

5.1 Frontal QRS Right-Axis Deviation

An isolated right-axis deviation (that is without possible signs for RVH in lead V_1) may be seen in the following conditions:

i.   Normal children: in newborns the axis is more than + 110° in > 90%, after 4 weeks the axis is about + 90° or more [8].

ii. Young adults: in 2%–3% of 20–30-year-olds [9].

iii. Chronic bronchoobstructive lung disease without RVH.

iv. After left pneumectomy.

v.   Isolated left posterior fascicular block (extremely rare *without* combination with inferior myocardial infarction) with a QRS axis of + 90° to + 120°; in left posterior fascicular block *with* inferior infarction, the QRS axis is about + 60° (Chapter 9 Fascicular Blocks).

vi. Extensive anterolateral infarction: pathologic Q waves and T wave abnormalities in the anterolateral leads (and often in I and aVL) make this diagnosis easy.

vii. Unknown and inexplicable origin (rare).

5.2 qR Type in Lead V_1

i.   Extreme rotation of the heart, leading to projection of left ventricular vectors on lead V_1 (e.g. in cases after left pneumectomy).

ii. In right atrial and RV *dilatation* (in about 10% of cases of acute massive pulmonary embolism).

iii. A Q wave in combination with RBBB is due to anteroseptal infarction, if pathologic Q waves are also present in adjacent leads (V_2 to V_3 (V_4)).

5.3 Tall R Wave and RS Complex in Lead V_1

i.   In children a tall R wave in V_1 is frequent up to the age of 8 years, it occurs in 20% of those aged 8–12 years, and in 10% of 12–16-year-olds [9]. An R/S ratio of > 1 in lead V_1 is rare in healthy adults (about 1%), whereas an R/S ratio > 1 in lead V_2 is found in 10% [10].

ii. An RS complex or a single R wave in V_1 and V_2 (V_3) is typical for *true posterior infarction*. The diagnosis is supported by pathologic Q waves or QS complexes in leads V_7 to V_9 (Chapter 13 Myocardial Infarction).

iii. *Pre-excitation* (former type A) may lead to a tall R wave. The correct diagnosis is easy based on the shortened PQ interval and the delta wave.

iv. In rare cases a single R or an RS complex in V_1 may be observed in pulmonary emphysema (without RVH) or in cases of displacement of the heart by surgical removal of the left lung, in left pneumothorax, in great pleural effusions, in kyphoscoliosis and in cachectic patients (possibly due to the 'proximity effect' in this case).

In all conditions with possible RVH signs in lead V_1 an associated frontal QRS right-axis deviation strongly favors the diagnosis of RVH, whereas an isolated QRS right-axis deviation is unspecific.

Tall R waves (up to 10 mm) in V_1 are also seen in two rare congenital heart diseases, namely in *single ventricle* and in *transposition of the great arteries* (also *after* operative correction by the 'Mustard operation' or 'atrial switch').

5.4 Incomplete Right Bundle-Branch Block

An r' wave smaller than the initial R wave is seen in many normal, especially young, individuals, overall in 7% [11]. An r' wave that is evidently greater than the R wave is more common in normal individuals than was assumed in older publications. This rSr' type may also be an intermediate state between incomplete RBBB and complete RBBB.

5.5 Complete Right Bundle-Branch Block

The differentiation between RBBB with right-axis deviation and RVH (ECG 6.15) and RBBB associated with left posterior fascicular block (ECG 6.16) is not easy. In typical cases of this type of bifascicular block, a delayed intrinsic deflection of the inferolateral portion of the left ventricle can be observed in lead V_6. A terminal slurring of the R wave reduces the duration of the S wave (ECG 6.16).

5.6 $S_I/S_{II}/S_{III}$ Type

As mentioned before, this ECG pattern is rarely found in RVH and RV dilatation and more frequently represents a normal variant without any other abnormality. It may be accompanied by thoracic deformations.

6 Systolic and Diastolic Overload

The old concept of Cabrera and Monroy [12] distinguishes between systolic RV overload (characterized by an R or RS complex in lead V_1) and diastolic RV overload (characterized by iRBBB). This concept has lost its clinical importance but may be of some interest in some selected patients. However, newer studies have revealed the unreliability of this statement [13]. Furthermore, Gurtner et al [14] found an iRBBB in > 90% of 24 patients with moderate-to-severe pulmonary hypertension due to the intake of the aminorectic drug aminorex

fumarate (a typical condition of systolic overload). The ECGs in these cases were very similar to those studied by Gertsch et al [15] in 203 patients with atrial septal defect of the secundum type (a typical condition of diastolic overload).

7 Effect of Systolic Pressure in the Right Ventricle and Pulmonary Artery on the ECG

A reliable correlation has been confirmed only in excessive elevation of the systolic pressure in the right ventricle, in pulmonary stenosis and in congenital heart disease with Eisenmenger syndrome. A single R wave > 20 mm in lead V_1 indicates a systolic pressure of > 100 mmHg in the right ventricle [16]. In moderately elevated systolic pressure the relation is much less reliable [17]. However, the higher the pressure is, the higher the quotient R/S in lead V_1 is. In general, severe pulmonary hypertension, or a very high RV systolic pressure in pulmonary stenosis, results in a single R or qR complex in V_1, whereas a moderately elevated systolic pressure leads to an RS complex or an rSr' configuration in V_1. In atrial septal defects, the rare patterns of a qR or an rSr's' generally indicate a higher pulmonary arterial pressure than in the presence of the usual rSr' pattern [17].

References

1. Walker IC, Helm RA, Scott RC. Right ventricular hypertrophy: I. Correlation of isolated right ventricular hypertrophy at autopsy with the electrocardiographic findings. Circulation 1955;11:215
2. Bove KE, Rowlands DT, Scott RC. Observations on the assessment of cardiac hypertrophy utilizing a chamber partition technique. Circulation 1966;33:558
3. Sokolow M, Lyon TP. The ventricular complex in right ventricular hypertrophy as obtained by unipolar precordial and limb leads. Am Heart J 1949;38:273
4. Roman GT Jr, Walsh TJ, Massie E. Right ventricular hypertrophy: Correlation of electrocardiographic and anatomic findings. Am J Cardiol 1961;7:481
5. Chou TC, Masangkay MP, Young R, et al. Simple quantitative vectorcardiographic criteria for the diagnosis of right ventricular hypertrophy. Circulation 1973;48:1262
6. Flowers NC, Horan LG. Hypertrophy and infarction: Subtle signs of right ventricular enlargement and their relative importance. In: Schlant RC, Hurst JW (eds): Advances in Electrocardiography. New York: Grune & Stratton, 1972
7. Gurtner HP. Pulmonary hypertension, 'plexogenic pulmonary arteriopathy' and the appetite depressant drug aminorex: post or propter. Bull Eur Physiopathol Resp 1979;15:897

8. Barboza ET, Brandenburg RO, Swan HJC. Atrial septal defect: The electrocardiogram and its hemodynamic correlation in 100 proved cases. Am J Cardiol 1958;2:698

9. James FW, Kaplan S. The normal electrocardiogram in the infant and child. Cardiovasc Clin 1973;5:295

10. Hiss RG, Lamb LE, Allen MF. Electrocardiographic findings in 67 375 asymtomatic subjects: X. Normal values. Am J Cardiol 1960;6:200

11. Ziegler RF. Electrocardiographic studies in normal infants and children. Springfield, IL: Charles C Thomas, 1951

12. Cabrera E, Monroy JR. Systolic and diastolic loading of the heart: II. Electrocardiographic data. Am Heart J 1952;43:669

13. Silver AM, Siderides LE, Antomius NA. The right precordial leads in congenital heart diseases manifesting right ventricular preponderance. Am J Cardiol 1959;3:713

14. Gurtner HP, Gertsch M, Salzmann C, et al. Häufen sich die primär vasculären Formen des chronischen Cor pulmonale? Schweiz med Wschr 1968;98:1579–94

15. Gertsch M, Kaufmann M, Althaus U. Zur Circumclusion des Ostium-secundum-Defektes. Schweiz med Wschr 1973;103:281

16. Cayler GG, Ongley F, Nadas AF. Relation of systolic pressure in the right ventricle to the electrocardiogram: A study of patients with pulmonary stenosis and intact ventricular septum. N Engl J Med 1958;258:979

17. Burch GE, De Pasquale NP. Electrocardiography in the diagnosis of congenital heart disease. Philadelphia: Lea & Febiger 1967, p 322

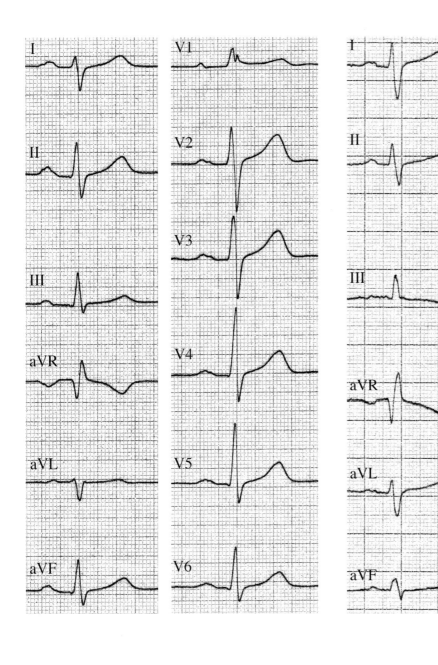
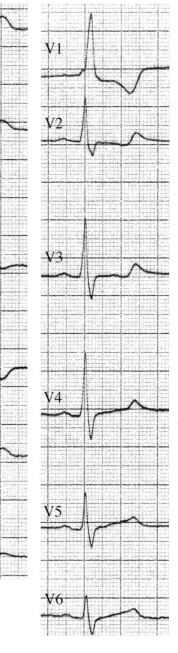

ECG 6.1

29y/m. Severe pulmonary valve stenosis (gradient 40 mmHg at rest, 100 mmHg during exercise with 120 Watt). ECG (paper speed 50 mm/sec): ÅQRS$_F$ + 130°. Single R wave (5 mm) with preterminal slurring in V$_1$. S$_I$/S$_{II}$/S$_{III}$ type.

ECG 6.2

19y/m. Severe pulmonary valve stenosis (gradient 90 mmHg). ECG (paper speed 50 mm/sec): ÅQRS$_F$ + 120°. Tall single R wave (15 mm), ST depression and negative T wave in V$_1$. R > S in V$_2$.

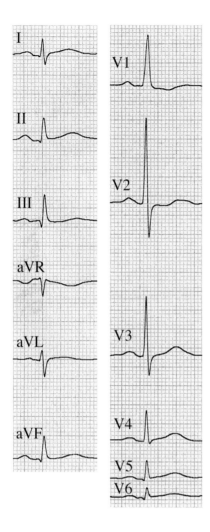

ECG 6.3

10 days/f. Severe pulmonary valve stenosis (gradient 60 mmHg). ECG (paper speed 50 mm/sec): ÅQRS$_F$ + 80°. Tall single R wave (13 mm) in V$_1$, R > S$_{V2(V3)}$, minimal ST depression in V$_1$/V$_2$.

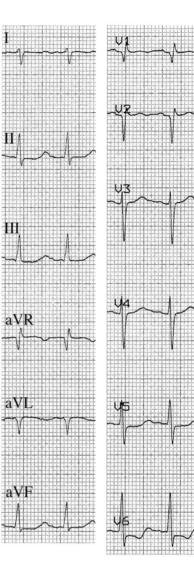

ECG 6.4

43y/f. Severe mitral stenosis with tricuspid regurgitation. Mitral valve replacement and tricuspid De Vega plastique 2 years before. ECG: sinus rhythm 116/min. P duration > 200 msec. The first peak of the p wave is partially hidden within the T wave. AV block 1°. ÅQRS$_F$ + 115°. Qr in V$_1$ and V$_2$. Alteration of the repolarization. Coronary and LV angiography: normal.

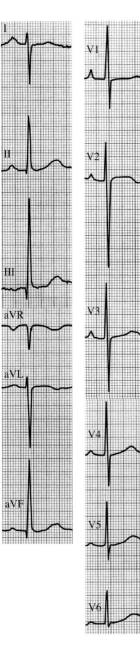

ECG 6.5
2y/m. Tetralogy of Fallot, unoperated. ECG (50 mm/sec): QRS right-axis deviation. R > S in lead V_1.

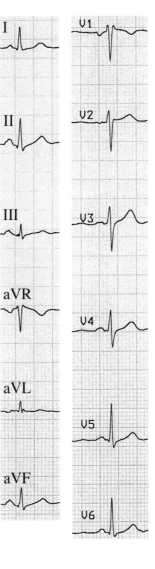

ECG 6.6
51 y/f. Normal heart. ECG: iRBBB with r' < r, as a normal variant.

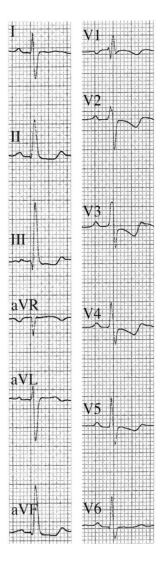

ECG 6.7
49y/f. Atrial septal defect of the secundum type (ASD II), left to right shunt > 60%. Pulmonary artery pressure normal. ECG: ÅQRS$_F$ + 105°. iRBBB with r' > r, T negative up to lead V_5.

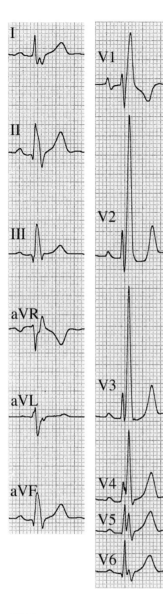

ECG 6.8

26y/m. Tetralogy of Fallot operated 10 years before. ECG: ÂQRS_F (of the first 60 msec) + 75°. Direct pattern of RBBB in V_1 up to V_5 (V_6), with giant amplitude of R' in V_2/V_3 corresponding to persisting severe RVH confirmed with echocardiogram.

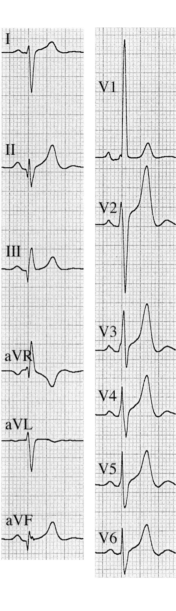

ECG 6.9

27y/m. Huge ventricular septal defect with early Eisenmenger reaction at the age of 2 years. ECG: QRS right-axis deviation. Single R wave (30 mm) in V_1. Positive T wave in all precordial leads.

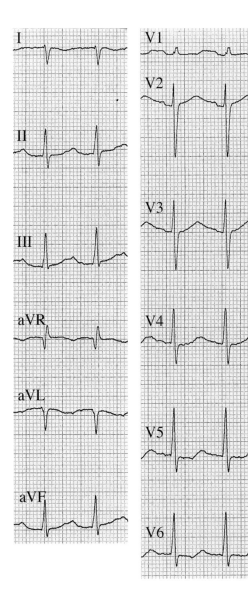

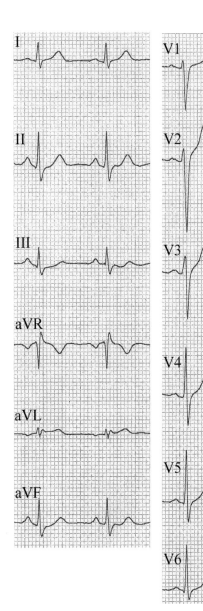

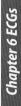

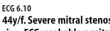

ECG 6.10
44y/f. Severe mitral stenosis with pulmonary hypertension. ECG: probable p mitrale (T–P fusion). ÅQRS$_F$ about + 110°. Single R wave in V$_1$ (2 mm).

ECG 6.11
27y/m. Normal heart. S$_I$/S$_{II}$/S$_{III}$ type.

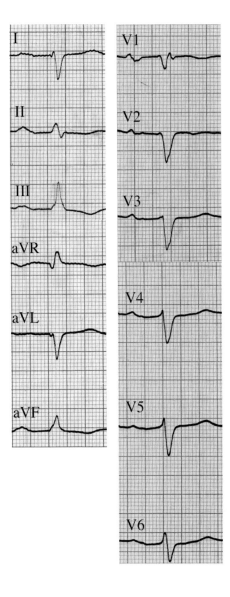

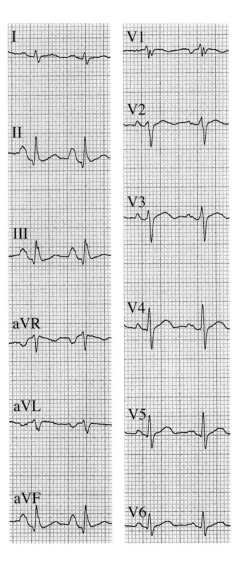

ECG 6.12

73y/f. Chronic obstructive pulmonary disease with global respiratory failure. Hypertension and pulmonary arterial hypertension. RV heart failure. ECG (50 mm/sec): sinus rhythm. ÂQRS_F about + 130°. rS complex in all precordial leads. Thorax x-rays: Cor bovinum. No echo. This rare pattern may also be seen in smaller hearts.

ECG 6.13

63y/m. Severe obstructive pulmonary disease. ECG: P wave high in II, aVF and III, negative in aVL. So-called 'p pulmonale parenchymale'.

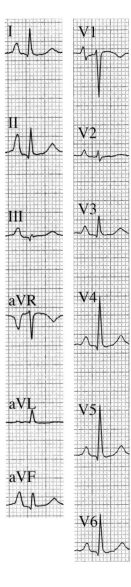

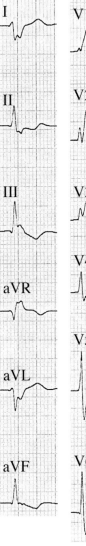

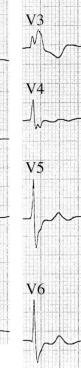

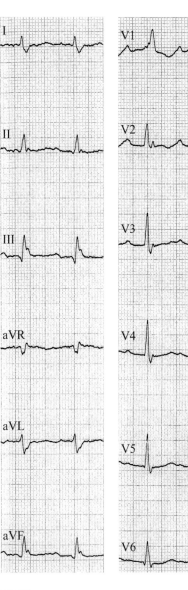

ECG 6.14

48y/f. Severe primary pulmonary hypertension (systemic pressure in the pulmonary artery). ECG: Giant p wave in II (4 mm) and aVF. P amplitude in I greater than in III. Peaked p wave in V_1 and V_2 (V_3 to V_6). So-called 'p pulmonale vasculare'.
$ÅQRS_F + 30°(!)$.

ECG 6.15

70y/f. Right and left heart failure, probably due to chronic pulmonary embolism and arterial hypertension. ECG: atrial fibrillation, f waves not visible. $ÅQRS_F$ (first 60 msec) $+ 75°$. Complete RBBB with single notched broad R wave in V_1. Note: *Broad S wave in V_6*. Echocardiogram: extensive RVH, mild LVH. Marked reduction of RV ejection fraction and left ventricular EF.

ECG 6.16

72y/m. Surgical problem. No pulmonary disease. No history of coronary heart disease or hypertension (Lenègre disease?). No syncope hitherto.
Echocardiogram: normal left ventricular function. ECG: RBBB + LPFB + AV block 1° (= incomplete trifascicular block). RBBB with notched broad R wave in V_1. Frontal vertical axis of the first 60 msec of QRS. Note *slurred R downstroke* with consequently *smaller S wave in lead V_6*. The notching/slurring in leads III/aVF are very probably due to RBBB and not due to left posterior fascicular block.

Chapter 7
Biventricular Hypertrophy

At a Glance

The reliable detection of biventricular hypertrophy (BVH) is done with the echocardiogram. With the ECG the diagnosis can only be made if excessive right ventricular hypertrophy (RVH) outweighs left ventricular hypertrophy (LVH).

ECG

For decades the following 'classical' ECG configurations have been proposed for the diagnosis of BVH:

i. $S_{V1} + R_{V5(or\ V6)} > 35$ mm (positive Sokolov index), combined with a vertical frontal QRS axis ($\mathring{A}QRS_F > + 90°$). The index can only be used in patients over 30 years; it has an acceptable specificity of 70%–80% but an extremely low sensitivity.

ii. $S_{V6} \geq 7$ mm (without RBBB); this sign is also seen in isolated RVH.

iii. Probably the best sign for BVH is the *combination of some typical RVH patterns with left atrial enlargement* (p duration $\geq$ 120 msec):
   a) $S/R \geq 1$ in V_5/V_6 + left atrial enlargement
   b) $S_{V6} \geq 7$ mm + left atrial enlargement (ECG 7.1)
   c) $\mathring{A}QRS_F > + 90°$ + left atrial enlargement (in the presence of right bundle-branch block (RBBB) the frontal QRS axis is determined on the basis of the first 60 msec of QRS).

These three criteria have a good specificity but a very low sensitivity.

In suspected cases of BVH an echocardiogram and other diagnostic tests, such as heart catheterization and investigations for lung diseases, are necessary to identify the disease, or diseases, that lead to BVH.

The Full Picture

Most ECG indices for isolated *left* ventricular hypertrophy have a high specificity but a low sensitivity and are applicable only to individuals over 40 years. Isolated *right* ventricular hypertrophy is more difficult to diagnose in the ECG because the RV vectors are counterbalanced by LV vectors. It is obvious that in *biventricular* hypertrophy the mutual influence of the RV and LV vectors, pointing in opposite directions, is fundamentally important and inhibits a reliable diagnosis in many (or most?)

cases. RVH must be excessive to influence an ECG that is primarily dominated by LVH.

ECG Special

In contrast to the electrocardiographic detection of LVH, where new ECG indices are still being described, publications about ECG or vectorcardiographic diagnosis of BVH have much declined. This proves that for *diagnosis* and *grading*

BVH, the ECG has definitively been replaced by the echocardiogram and other imaging methods.

1 Usual ECG Signs for BVH

The most recent study by Jain et al [1] in 1999 investigated the ECGs of 69 patients with BVH, based on two-dimensional echocardiographic results. In only 17 of 69 patients (25%) could BVH be identified by ECG signs; in 25 (36%) LVH was diagnosed; in 14 (20%) RVH was diagnosed; and in 13 (19%) neither LVH nor RVH was diagnosed.

The most frequent sign for BVH was $S_{V5/V6} > 7$ mm (10 patients). A 'Katz-Wachtel sign' (see section 2.2) was seen in four patients.

In a necropsy study of 323 patients with ventricular hypertrophy, Murphy et al [2] found with the three criteria for BVH listed above (S/R ≥ 1 in V_5/V_6; $S_{V6} \geq 7$ mm; $ÅQRS_F > + 90°$, all combined with left atrial enlargement) a high specificity of 94% and a very low sensitivity of 20% for BVH.

2 Other ECG Signs for BVH

Occasionally other ECG patterns are seen in BVH.

2.1 Shallow S_{V1}, Deep S_{V2}

ECGs 7.2 and 7.3 show an overall high QRS voltage in V_2 to V_6, suggesting LVH. Only the S wave in lead V_1 is small ('shallow'), with an amplitude < 4 mm, due to partial canceling of a deep S wave (caused by LVH) by opposite vectors produced by additional RVH. The difference between the small S in V_1 and the deep S in V_2 (≥ 12 mm) is striking.

2.2 Katz-Wachtel Sign

The original description by Katz and Wachtel [3] refers to a huge biphasic QRS complex (RS or QR) in the leads II, III or I,

found in children with different congenital heart diseases. Later a 'precordial Katz-Wachtel index', $(R + S)_{V3} \geq 40$ mm, was proposed for detecting BVH in children (ECG 7.4).

2.3 Special QRS Pattern in Right Bundle-Branch Block

Complete right bundle-branch block (RBBB) (also without RVH) reduces the R amplitude in leads V_5/V_6. In ECG 7.5 the high R waves in V_5 (V_6), in the presence of RBBB favor the presence of LVH. The duration of QRS is 160 msec, with a large R' typical for RVH. Moreover, an rsR' complex is present up to lead V_3, an unusual finding in LVH without associated RVH. The p wave is not only prolonged (140 msec), typical for left atrial enlargement, but also peaked in V_1/V_2, suggesting right atrial enlargement. Indeed this 72-year-old patient suffered from hypertensive heart disease and from severe pulmonary hypertension for 6 years, due to chronic pulmonary embolism. The echocardiogram/Doppler revealed dilatation of the right atrium and ventricle. The calculated systolic pulmonary artery pressure was 82 mmHg, the mass of the dilated left ventricle 182 g/m^2. In several other cases with similar clinical findings, only ECG signs for RVH, or LVH, or no signs of ventricular hypertrophy were observed.

References

1. Jain AM, Chandna H, Silber EN, et al. Electrocardiographic patterns of patients with echocardiographically determined biventricular hypertrophy. J Electrocardiol 1999;32:269–173
2. Murphy ML, Thenabadre PN, de Soyza N, et al. Reevaluation of electrocardiographic criteria for left, right and combined ventricular hypertrophy. Am J Cardiol 1984;53:1140–7
3. Katz LN, Wachtel H. The diphasic QRS type of electrocardiogram in congenital heart disease. Am Heart J 1937;13:202–6

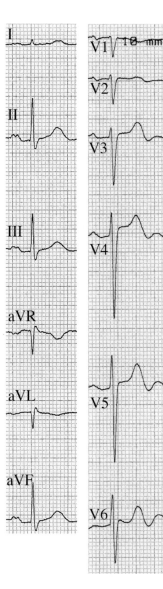

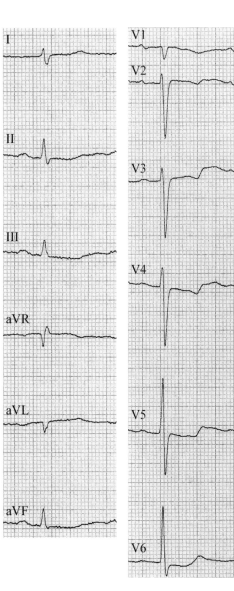

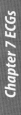

ECG 7.1
83y/f. $S_{V6} > 7$ mm plus left atrial
enlargement. Combined aortic valve
disease, severe mitral regurgitation.
ECG: sinus rhythm. P duration
120 msec: S in V_6 10 mm. The rS configuration in V_1 to V_6 suggests RV
and/or LV dilatation. Echo: hypertrophic and dilated RV and LV.
Dilated atria. Thoracic x-rays: cor
bovinum.

ECG 7.2
67y/f. 'Shallow S_{V1}/deep S_{V2}'. Combined rheumatic valve disease, mitral
valve reconstruction 14 years ago, biventricular heart failure. ECG: sinus
rhythm(!), P duration 160 msec. $ÅQRS_F + 110°$ strongly favors RVH. The relative deep S wave in lead V_2 (in the presence of a shallow S wave in V_1) and
the relative high R waves in V_5/V_6 suggest LVH. The repolarization is consistent with hypokalemia. Potassium (K^+) 3.1 mmol/l. Echo/Doppler: severe LV
and RV hypertrophy and dilatation, severely impaired function of both
ventricles. Left and right atria dilated. Moderate mitral stenosis, severe
mitral and tricuspid regurgitation.

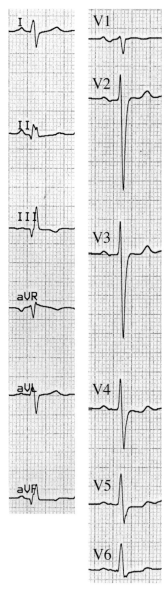

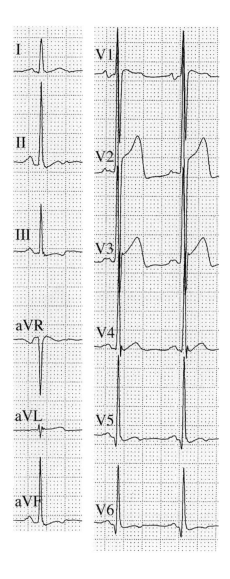

ECG 7.3
73y/m. 'Shallow S$_{V1}$/deep S$_{V2}$'.
Combined aortic and mitral valve
disease. Sinus rhythm, p duration
120 msec. ÂQRS$_F$ + 110°.
S$_{V1}$ = 3.5 mm, S$_{V2}$ = 14 mm.
Negative T waves in V$_1$ to V$_4$.
Echo: BVH and dilatation.

ECG 7.4
27y/m. 'Katz-Wachtel sign', false positive.
Hypertrophic left ventricular cardiomyopathy,
asthenic habitus. ECG: (R + S)$_{V2}$ = 60 mm.
R + S$_{V3}$ = 32 mm. No S wave in V$_6$. Echo: LV mass
182 g/m$_2$. RV normal.

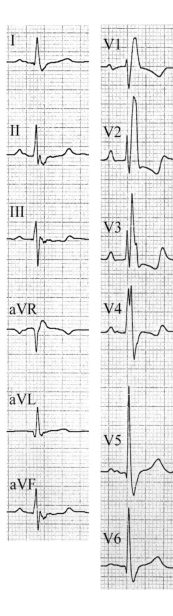

ECG 7.5
72y/m. BVH and RBBB. For clinical diagnoses and explanation of the ECG see text.

Chapter 8
Pulmonary Embolism

At a Glance

Acute pulmonary embolism (acPE), limited to the first 48 hours of the disease, is a very dangerous situation with considerable mortality, often because of misdiagnosis. It is therefore necessary to establish the diagnosis and to begin therapy *within the shortest possible time.* The fastest and most reliable methods are the echocardiogram and helical (spiral) computerized tomography (CT), combined with plasma D-dimer measurement. With this approach (diagnostic accuracy in about 95%) pulmonary artery angiography can be avoided in most cases. A positive result of lower-limb venous compression ultrasonography is useful for the diagnosis, especially in *subacute* PE (subacPE) with symptoms lasting for more than 48 h. A lung scan is only diagnostic in about 50%, but is helpful for diagnosis of subsegmental embolization. The ECG is unreliable for the diagnosis of acPE, yet it may reveal the first hint of right ventricular overload.

ECG

In acPE the *acute* rise of pulmonary artery resistance and pulmonary arterial pressure leads to *dilatation* (not to hypertrophy) of the *right ventricle* (RV) and often of the right atrium. As a consequence, a number of ECG alterations may be present.

1 ECG Alterations
1.1 Alterations of QRS

i. Shift of the frontal QRS axis ($\mathring{A}QRS_F$) to the *right,* often with a S_I/Q_{III} (condition $S_I \geq 1.5$ mm; $Q_{III} \geq 1.5$ mm) or S_I/rSr'_{III}.
ii. Rotation of the heart in its horizontal axis (also provoked by right ventricular (RV) dilatation), leading to *clockwise* displacement of the transition zone (QRS clockwise rota-

tion) in the precordial leads. If QRS counterclockwise rotation is encountered, it is due to pre-existing RV hypertrophy or due to other reasons.
iii. RV conduction disturbance: *incomplete* (or, rarely, complete) right bundle-branch block (iRBBB), with rSr' complex (or rsR' complex in complete RBBB) in lead V_1. A QR complex (Qr) in lead V_1 is seen in about 10%, especially in massive pulmonary embolism (> 80% obstruction of the pulmonary arteries).

1.2 Alterations of Repolarization

i. T negativity in III *and* aVF
ii. T negativity in V_2/V_3, also without incomplete RBBB or RBBB
iii. ST depression in leads V_1 to V_3, or ST elevation in leads V_1 and III
iv. ST or T alterations in the left precordial leads (rare).

1.3 Rhythm Disturbances

Sinus tachycardia is by far the most frequent ECG abnormality in acPE, occurring in 70%–80%. Atrial flutter occurs in 5%–10%, whereas atrial fibrillation is rare.

1.4 Alterations of the P Wave

Relatively high and peaked p waves may be seen in some leads, especially in II and V_2. The definition of this alteration (also described as 'p pulmonale vasculare') is a conundrum and so is its prevalence. The classical 'p pulmonale' ('p pulmonale parenchymale' with an amplitude ≥ 2.5 mm in lead II, and purely negative in aVL) is seen only exceptionally. Possible ECG signs in acPE are listed in Table 8.1.

Table 8.1
Possible ECG signs in acute pulmonary embolism

	Prevalence*
Sinus tachycardia (rate ≥ 100/min)	70%
Sinus rhythm (rate ≥ 90%)	80%
S_I/Q_{III} type or S_I/rSr'_{III} type	40%
S_I/Q_{III} or S_I/rSr'_{III} + *negative* T in III and aVF	25%
Incomplete right bundle-branch block (rSr' or QR in V_1) 40%	7%(!)–60%
QRS clockwise rotation in precordial leads	35%
$ÅQRS_F$ shift to the right up to ≥ + 60° at the age > 30 years	30%
T negativity in leads V_2 and V_3	30%
Right atrial enlargement (atypical 'p pulmonale')	10%?
Atrial flutter	5%
Complete right bundle-branch block	3%

*For more details and results from the literature see Table 8.2.

It should be emphasized that eventual ECG signs due to acPE are *transitory* (reversible) in successfully treated patients. The *combination* of several different ECG signs of ventricular overload are helpful (although still insufficient) for the diagnosis of acPE. ECGs 8.1–8.6 were registered in patients with severely symptomatic massive acPE at admission to the emergency unit of our hospital during the winter of 2001. AcPE was proven by helical CT (and echocardiogram).

Only three patients showed five current ECG signs of RV overload, three showed only one to three signs. Only three patients suffered from sinus tachycardia, however five had sinus rates of > 90/min. Five patients recovered with thrombolysis; one young woman (the patient in ECG 8.6) admitted 2 weeks after giving birth, died despite thrombolysis and surgical thrombectomy.

Some general comments apply to the findings in ECGs 8.1–8.6:

a) all patients were women, but the female/male ratio in acPE is about 3:2
b) all patients suffered from massive life-threatening acPE with corresponding symptoms (tachypnea, severe dyspnea at rest, hemoptysis in four cases) and clinical findings (pre-shock, distended jugular veins, fast heart rate in five patients, cyanosis in four).

These examples and the literature support the general opinion that the ECG is *unreliable* for the diagnosis of acPE, due to its modest specificity and low sensitivity. Therefore, the ECG should not be used as a diagnostic method. In too many patients pre-existing ECG alterations may be (falsely) suggestive for acPE and, much worse, the ECG may lack any sign of RV overload even in patients with massive acPE. Moreover, it is often impossible to differentiate between 'signs of RV overload' and normal variants (Chapter 3 The Normal ECG and its Normal Variants).

2 Value of ECG in Suspected Acute PE

If the ECG is unreliable for the diagnosis of PE, then where, if indeed anywhere, is its place in suspected acPE?

2.1 Differentiation of AMI from Acute PE

As every physician knows, the diagnosis of acPE based on symptoms (and anamnestic findings) is not always easy to make. Often acute myocardial infarction (AMI) has to be excluded. In inferior AMI a striking ST elevation is generally seen in leads III, aVF and II. An older inferior infarction shows not only pathologic Q waves in III and aVF, but also a Q (q) wave in II. In contrast, a Q (q) wave in lead II is *extremely rare* in acute RV overload. AMI of other localizations may be detected by the usual criteria.

2.2 Analysis of Heart Rhythm and Conduction Disturbances

Only with the ECG can arrhythmias and conduction disturbances be diagnosed reliably.

2.3 ECG Signs of Acute RV Overload

In the presence of ECG signs suggesting acute RV overload, the possibility of acute PE (or subacute PE if symptoms last more than 48 h) should be considered. Patients with acute PE, especially those with the subacute form, may have a history that is a conundrum, with puzzling symptoms. We have seen many patients where multiple ECG signs of RV overload gave the first clue for the diagnosis of pulmonary embolism. This happened more often in subacute than in acute PE. It should also be mentioned that only a few hospitals worldwide have access at all times to spiral CT or to experienced specialists in echo/Doppler. Under these circumstances, the ECG may be helpful for the diagnosis of acPE, in combination with the history, symptoms, and other clinical findings.

2.4 Control of Clinical Evolution

Is the ECG useful for controlling clinical evolution? The regression of ECG signs of RV overload (if present in acute or subacute PE) may be a useful bystander sign for a favorable clinical follow-up. However there is no strict time correlation between the objective findings (e.g. in the echo) and the ECG. ECG alterations may regress sooner or persist longer than expected.

2.5 Subacute and Chronic repetitive PE

As suggested above, the ECG is more useful in patients with subacute PE (after 48 h), although not with sufficient diagnostic accuracy. In chronic *repetitive* PE, RV *hypertrophy* develops.

The Full Picture

ECG Special

3 Prevalence of ECG Signs Suggesting PE

The value of the S_I/Q_{III} type (or $S_I/Q_{III}/T_{III}$ type) was first recognized by McGinn and White [1] in 1935 and is therefore called McGinn-White type. This accounts for about 30% of cases. In some cases a small r wave precedes the negative deflection in lead III. Thus a S_I/rsr'_{III} type is present. Rarely, the negative deflection in III is lacking. In this case an S_I/R_{III} type may reflect acute RV overload. A QR type in lead V_1, instead of the more common rSr' type, was described by Weber and Phillips [2] who found this sign in 10 out of 60 patients with acute PE. A QR configuration (in most cases a Qr) in lead V_1 is an ominous sign and generally occurs in massive and *life-threatening* acPE with extensive *right ventricular and atrial enlargement.*

Early publications, such as that by Cutforth and Oram [3] from 1958, revealed an astonishingly high number of ECG signs suggesting RV overload in patients with acute (and subacute) PE, especially in cases which had a lethal outcome. In later studies the contribution of the ECG to the diagnosis of acPE was considered modest. Stein et al [4] studied 90 patients with massive or submassive acPE documented by pulmonary artery angiography, and found the most frequent sign was T negativity in the precordial and limb leads (42%), but an RBBB or iRBBB, a right-axis deviation, or an S_I/Q_{III} type in only 6%–12%. The authors noticed that after recovery the T alterations persisted markedly longer than the QRS abnormalities. Szucs et al [5] used a similar cohort of 50 patients and found a frontal QRS right axis shift in 15% and an iRBBB in 8%. Sutton et al [6] detected in 35 patients with massive acPE an RBBB in

26% and an S_I/Q_{III} type in 52%, combined with T inversion in 26%. By far the most frequent ECG abnormality in all studies was *sinus tachycardia*, in 70%–90% (partially defined as a sinus rhythm at a rate of > 90/min).

The prevalence of the different ECG alterations possible in acPE varies *greatly* in the published studies (Table 8.2). The reasons probably stem from the relatively small cohorts of patients studied, the differences in grade of PE, the use of dif-

Table 8.2
Prevalence of possible ECG signs in acute pulmonary embolism

	Our experience	Literature
Sinus tachycardia (rate ≥ 100/min)	70%	70%–90%
Sinus rhythm (rate ≥ 90/min)	80%	70%–90%
S_I/Q_{III} type or S_I/rSr'_{III} type	40%	10%(!)–60%
S_I/Q_{III} or S_I/rSr'_{III} plus T negativity in III and aVF	25%	11%–40%
Incomplete right bundle-branch block (rSr' or Qr in V_1)	40%	7%(!)–60%
QRS clockwise rotation in precordial leads	35%	13%–40%
ÅQRS$_F$ shift to the right up to ≥ + 60° (age > 30 years)	30%	15%–50%
T negativity in leads V_2 and V_3	30%	10%–40%
Right atrial enlargement (p pulmonale)	5%?	2%–20%(!)
Atrial flutter	5%	2%–30%(!)
ST depression (> 1 mm) in V_1 to V_3 *or* ST elevation (> 1 mm) in V_1 or III	? 10%	–
Peripheral low voltage	5%	–
Complete right bundle-branch block	3%	–
Atrial fibrillation		2%–3%
Isolated T negativity in left precordial leads	1%–2%	–

ferent 'gold standards', and because of mixed patient groups of those with acute and subacute PE.

A completely normal ECG (besides sinus tachycardia) in acute PE is not rare. Differentiating between *pathologic* and *normal* is often impossible, because most direct and indirect ECG signs of acute *RV overload* are also seen in normal individuals. Sometimes other misleading signs, including sinus bradycardia, isolated left precordial ST/T abnormalities, or AV block 1°, may arise as the only ECG manifestations of acute PE. Moreover, in pre-existing ECG abnormalities, like those seen in severe left ventricular hypertrophy, bundle-branch block, and myocardial infarction, signs of RV overload are only exceptionally detectable.

Overall, the incidence of ECG signs of RV overload depends more on the extent of pulmonary artery occlusion than on the sum of ECG registrations. In massive acute PE *multiple* signs of acute RV overload may be observed (ECGs 8.1, 8.2 and 8.6).

4   ECG Signs and Grade of Acute PE

Two recent publications deal with the relation between ECG signs and severity of acute PE. Kucher et al [7] found in 70 acute PE patients (confirmed by echo/Doppler and proved by spiral CT) a *QR (Qr) complex in lead V_1* (n=12) correlated best with RV pressure overload and high pulmonary artery occlusion rate (> 80%), with a specificity of 100% and sensitivity of 28%. Furthermore, ST elevation in V_1 and T negativity in V_2/V_3 were good predictors of massive acute PE. Daniel et al [8] established an ECG point-scoring system with 22 ECG signs and a maximum possible score of 21 points. T negativity in V_1 to V_4 scored highest with 4 points. A score of $\geq$ 10 was interpreted as highly suggestive for severe pulmonary hypertension by PE. These results can be improved by some modifications, in the opinion of Daniel et al. In our opinion, the rather complex method leads to useful bystander ECG results in less urgent cases. In other patients with acute PE there is no place (and no time) for any point-score index, whether it refers to the ECG or to the echo (see Short Story/Case Report 1).

5   Practical Procedures in Suspected Acute PE

Fortunately, the prognosis of even massive acute (and subacute) PE has improved considerably in many hospitals over the last few years, due to time-saving diagnostic methods (echocardiogram, D-dimer, and helical CT) and early therapy (especially thrombolysis). The following list summarizes the standard emergency procedures:

i.   history (chronic disease, recent operation, long journey in car or airplane)
ii. symptoms (tachypnea, dyspnea at rest, hemoptysis)
iii. clinical examination (heart rate, blood pressure, inspection of jugular veins, and auscultation of the lung)
iv. routine laboratory exams including D-dimer
v.   echo/Doppler and ECG
vi. in case of 'positive echo' (and positive D-dimer) give immediate therapy with thrombolytic agents
vii. spiral CT (if available) to prove and quantify pulmonary artery obstruction, with a back-up reanimation team. When spiral CT is negative, a lung scan may detect subsegementary PE; when spiral CT is positive, transfer the patient to the intensive care unit.

The Short Story/Case Report illustrates how in dramatic cases of suspected acute PE there may not even be time to implement these standard emergency procedures.

Short Story/Case Report 1

In October 2000 a 61-year-old man was admitted to the emergency department of our hospital because of sudden onset of severe dyspnea and syncope 3 h before. Rapid clinical examination revealed a life-threatening condition as shown by shock (systolic blood pressure 70/40 mmHg, heart rate 135/min), breathing frequency of 50/min, and cyanosis and thick neck veins. The patient was not able to give further information. Emergency transthoracic echocardiography revealed severe RV and RA dilatation. The LV showed subnormal contraction. The ECG (ECG 8.7) was interpreted as suspicious for acute RV overload. However, the lack of Q in III and a QR complex in V_1 as well as a QS complex in V_2, together with slight ST elevation, caused some confusion (anteroseptal AMI?). Fifteen minutes after admission, echocardiographically confirmed electromechanical dissociation (EMD) occurred, and vigorous cardiopulmonary resuscitation (CPR) was performed immediately. At the same time, two intravenous bolus injections of 15 mg alteplase were given, followed by infusion of 70 mg within 60 min, while CPR was continued. Spontaneous carotid pulses were observed 25 min later, and the patient's hemodynamics recovered with support from catecholamines. Emergency spiral CT revealed more than 80% occlusion of the proximal pulmonary arteries. The patient was transferred to the intensive care unit. Three hours after successful

CPR and thrombolysis, the patient developed hemorrhagic shock due to liver and spleen rupture as a consequence of prolonged mechanical chest compression, and abdominal blood pooling due to severely impaired RV function. After emergency splenectomy and liver revision, the patient's hemodynamics stabilized 14 h after admission. Ten days after successful treatment of acute central PE there were no signs of RV overload as shown by normalization of the echocardiogram and the ECG.

In conclusion, the patient was saved because of typical clinical symptoms and echo (and ECG) findings that were strongly suggesting massive acute PE, and because resuscitation and rapid thrombolysis were applied quickly. The patient was also lucky to survive a severe complication. The origin of the disease that caused development (without symptoms) of deep lower-limb vein thrombosis remained unclear. Retrospective detailed analysis of the admission ECG revealed, besides sinus tachycardia, at least six signs of acute RV overload (ECG 8.7). The QR and QS complexes in V_1/V_2 (together with slight ST elevation) proved to be ominous signs of extreme RV and RA dilatation and were not due to anteroseptal AMI.

6 ECG in Subacute PE

As mentioned previously, the ECG is unreliable and may be misleading in the diagnosis of acute PE (PE that is diagnosed within 48 h of the onset of symptoms). However, only about half of patients enter the hospital with severe acute symptoms, within 48 h of the beginning of symptoms, or die suddenly (postmortem diagnosis). The other half are hospitalized with relevant symptoms days or even weeks after the first symptoms, and these are only connected with PE retrospectively.

It also seems reasonable, therefore, to consider the value of ECGs in diagnosis of subacute PE. In a recent publication, Sreeram et al [9] investigated 49 patients with proven PE (aged 44–88 years) with acute or aggravated symptoms (dyspnea, chest pain, palpitations, collapse requiring resuscitation). Of these patients, 13 showed symptoms for < 3 h and up to 48 h (acute PE), and 36 showed symptoms for 2–7 days (subacute PE). If three ECG signs out of seven suggesting acute RV overload were present, PE was correctly presumed in 37 patients (78%). The seven signs are:

i.   incomplete or complete RBBB, often with ST elevation in V_1
ii. S wave in I and aVL > 1.5 mm

iii. shift of the transition zone to V_5
iv. Q waves in III and aVF, but *not* in II
v.   frontal QRS right-axis deviation or intermediate axis
vi. peripheral QRS low voltage (a 'new' sign suggested by Sreeram et al [9] present in 21%!)
vii. T wave inversion in III and aVF, or in V_1 to V_4.

Twelve patients had normal ECGs at admission, but serial ECGs revealed diagnostic signs in three. Yet in this situation the ECG was definitively less valuable than the echo/Doppler that showed increased end-diastolic RV dimension, increased RV systolic pressure, and tricuspid valve regurgitation in 100% of the patients, at admission. In a prospective study with 246 patients suspected of having PE (49 of them with definitive PE), Rodger et al [10] could not confirm the results of Sreeram et al [9]. The diagnosis was made or excluded by ventilation perfusion scans. Out of 28 studied ECG signs, only incomplete RBBB and 'tachycardia' were statistically more frequent in patients with PE than in patients without PE. The great discrepancy between the results of the studies by Sreeram [9] and Rodger [10] may be explained by a) different severity of the disease (probably less in the Rodger cohort); b) different stages of PE; and c) different 'gold standards' (echo/Doppler versus ventilation perfusion scan). Moreover, it is striking that in the Rodger publication, the prevalence of a 'late R' in lead aVR (quite a common pattern in normal ECGs and in patients with PE) was zero.

In summary, the ECG may be slightly more helpful for diagnosis (suspicion) of subacute PE than it is for acute PE. However, in suspected subacute PE, the use of echo/Doppler is indispensable as a fast, reliable and cheap method.

7 Historical Perspective

Let us not underestimate the 'old' clinical physicians. In 1966, the aforementioned Weber and Phillips [2] investigated 60 patients with massive acute PE, and diagnosed 37 cases on clinical findings only. They found a QR complex in lead V_1 in 10 patients (16.6%). In 2003, Kucher et al [7] studied 71 patients with acute PE, controlled by echo/Doppler and D-dimer, and proved by spiral CT. They described the same ECG sign, a QR (Qr) complex in V_1, in 14 patients (19.7%). Thus, the results elaborated by the two groups are nearly identical, clearly showing that these 'old' physicians were able to reliably diagnose massive acute PE without the benefits of a modern armamentarium. And, by the way, Weber and Phillips [2] reported an astonishingly high incidence of (intermittent) atrial flutter (30%), and sinus tachycardia in only 48%.

References

1. McGinn S, White PD. Acute cor pulmonale resulting from pulmonary embolism. Its clinical recognition. J Am Med Assoc 1935;104:1473–80
2. Weber DM, Phillips JH Jr. A re-evaluation of electrocardiographic changes accompanying acute pulmonary embolism. Am J Med Sci 1966;251:381–98
3. Cutforth RH, Oram S. The electrocardiogram in pulmonary embolism. Br Heart J 1958;20:41–60
4. Stein PD, Dalen JE, McIntyre KM, et al. The electrocardiogram in acute pulmonary embolism. Prog Cardiovasc Dis 1975;17:247–57
5. Szucs MM, Brooks HL, Grossman W, et al. Diagnostic sensitivity of laboratory findings in acute pulmonary embolism. Ann Intern Med 1971;74:161–6
6. Sutton GC, Honey M, Gibson RV. Clinical diagnosis of acute massive pulmonary embolism. Lancet 1969;1(7589):271–3
7. Kucher N, Walpoth N, Wustmann K, et al. QR in V1—an ECG sign associated with right ventricular strain and adverse clinical outcome in acute pulmonary embolism. Europ Heart J 2003, in press
8. Daniel KR, Courtney DM, Kline JA. Assessment of cardiac stress from massive pulmonary embolism with 12-lead ECG. Chest 2000;120:474–81
9. Sreeram N, Cheriex EC, Smeets JL, Gorgels AP, Wellens HJJ. Value of the 12-lead electrocardiogram at hospital admission in the diagnosis of pulmonary embolism. Am J Cardiol 1994;73:298–303
10. Rodger M, Makropoulos D, Turek M, et al. Diagnostic value of the electrocardiogram in suspected pulmonary embolism. Am J Cardiol 2000;86:807–9

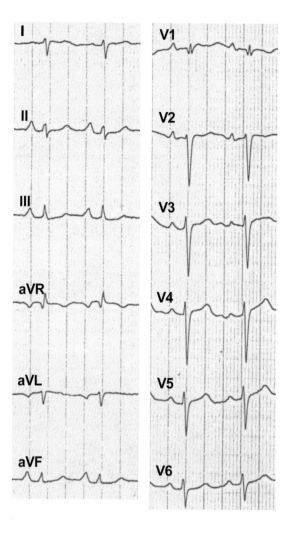

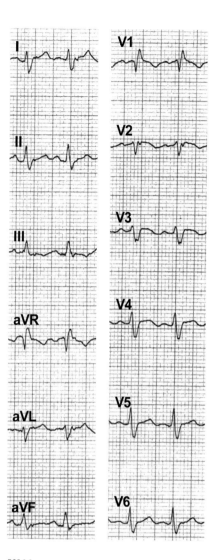

ECG 8.1

53 y/f. Sinus rhythm, rate 93/min. Peaked p waves inferiorly and in V_1/V_3 (rare finding). $\mathring{A}QRS_F + 140°$, peripheral QRS low voltage. S_I, but no Q_{III}. iRBBB. Excessive clockwise rotation in the precordial leads, rS up to V_6. No negative T waves in the right or other precordial leads >>> 5 possible signs of acute RV overload.

ECG 8.2

69 y/f. Sinus tachycardia 126/min, normal p. $\mathring{A}QRS_F +140°$, near QRS low voltage. S_I, but no Q_{III}. iRBBB. Marked clockwise rotation. Negative T waves up to V_4 >>> 5 signs.

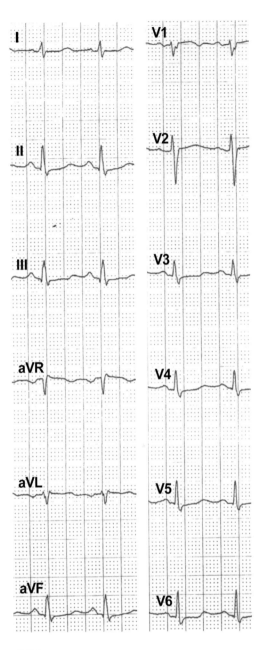

ECG 8.3
43 y/f. Sinus rhythm, 92/min, normal p. ÅQRS$_F$ +80°.
S$_I$/Q$_{III}$ type. Pseudo-iRBBB. No clockwise rotation, no T
negativity in precordial leads >>> 2 signs.

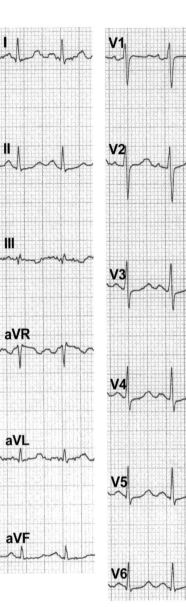

ECG 8.4
45 y/f. Sinus tachycardia 126/min. Peaked p
waves in V$_2$. ÅQRS$_F$ +40°. Discreet S$_I$/rsr′$_{III}$ type.
Near QRS low voltage. No clockwise rotation. No
T negativity >>> 3 signs.

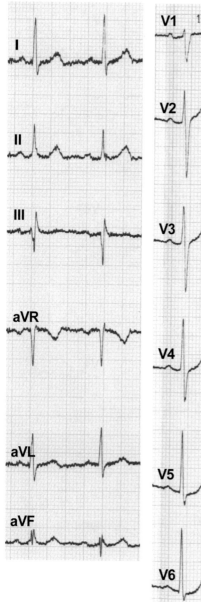
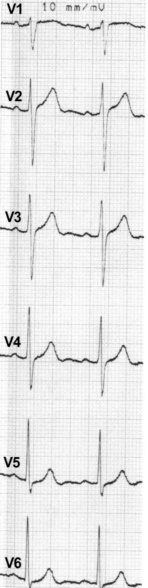

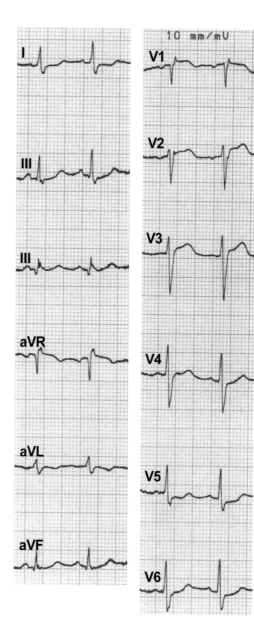

ECG 8.5

53 y/f. SR 79/min, normal p. ÅQRS$_F$ about +40°. S$_I$/rSr'$_{III}$ type. Slight clockwise rotation. No T negativity >>> 1 sign.

ECG 8.6

34 y/f. Sinus tachycardia 104/min, negative p wave in V$_1$ as a sign of left atrial overload. ÅQRS$_F$ +75°. S$_I$/Q$_{III}$ type. iRBBB with Qr in V$_1$. Clockwise rotation. Slight ST elevation in V$_1$ (and V$_2$/V$_3$). ST depression in V$_5$/V$_6$. No negative T waves >>> 5 signs.

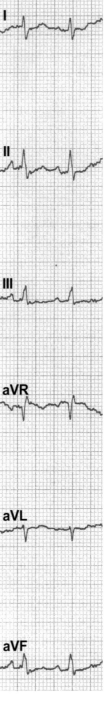
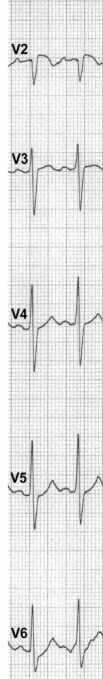

ECG 8.7
Short Story/Case Report 1. 60 y/m. ECG: sinus tachycardia, 120/min. Peaked p waves in II/aVF. ÅQRS$_F$ + 100°. S$_I$/Rs$_{III}$ type (in this case equivalent to S$_I$/Q$_{III}$ type, due to extreme rotation of the heart). Qr complex in V$_1$ (and QS complex in V$_2$). Clockwise rotation in precordial leads. ST elevation of 0.5–1.0 mm in V$_1$/V$_2$. T negativity in V$_2$ >>> at least 7 signs.

Chapter 9
Fascicular Blocks

At a Glance

The concept of fascicular blocks is based on the predominantly *trifascicular* infrahisarian ventricular conduction system, the *right bundle branch* on one side, and the *left anterior* and *left posterior fascicle* (forming the left bundle branch) on the other. The expression 'fascicular block' is a synonym of the older expression 'hemiblock'. In some patients fascicular blocks progress to bifascicular/bilateral blocks and then to complete atrioventricular (AV) block. Thus they represent potential precursors of complete infrahissian AV block, which is generally associated with syncope and increased mortality.

Etiology and Prevalence

Left anterior fascicular block (LAFB) and left posterior fascicular block (LPFB) are both left (mono-)fascicular blocks but differ very much in their prevalence, their etiology, and their correct diagnosis. The etiology is manifold, including left ventricular hypertrophy, coronary heart disease (CHD) with or without myocardial infarction (MI), fibrosis of the infrahisarian conduction system (*Lenègre* disease), and others.

In a general population LAFB does not generally develop before the age of 40 years; it is found in 4%–6% at 60 years, and up to 10% at 80 years. Occasionally, LAFB completely masks an inferior or anterior infarction.

LPFB is very rare in middle-aged patients of medical and cardiology departments (0.15% and 0.3% respectively) and is even rarer in a general population. However, the diagnosis is important because LPFB is combined with inferior MI in over 90% of patients. In inferior MI, LPFB is found in 6% of patients and often masks the classical infarction signs.

ECG

If we assume a mean normal QRS duration of 0.09 sec, the QRS duration in LAFB and in LPFB is prolonged to 0.10–0.11 sec, without left ventricular hypertrophy.

1 Left Anterior Fascicular Block

LAFB is easy to diagnose (ECGs 9.1–9.3). The *first* main characteristic of LAFB is a *QRS left-axis deviation* in the frontal leads, with a frontal QRS axis (ÅQRS_F) between $-30°$ and $-90°$. A small q wave in I and aVL may be present. In leads I and aVL a slurred R downstroke is often found. The T wave is positive and asymmetric in the inferior leads III, aVF, and II, negative in aVR and variable in I and aVL (positive, flat, negative).

The *second* main characteristic of LAFB (often forgotten in the literature) is a *smooth* or *absent transition zone of QRS* in the horizontal leads with an *RS* configuration in all precordial leads. Generally there is an rS complex (R smaller than S) in V_1 to V_6. In some cases R and S have about the same amplitude in V_2/V_3 and/or V_4 to V_6, and very rarely R is higher than S in V_2/V_3. The T wave is positive and asymmetric in V_1 to V_6.

2 Left Posterior Fascicular Block

LPFB is difficult to diagnose because only minor alterations may allow the differentiation from a normal variant with vertical ÅQRS_F.

LPFB is commonly associated with inferior infarction and, in this condition, is characterized by a frontal QRS axis between $+50°$ and $+80°$, by a q wave of variable duration in III and aVF, and variable T waves in the same leads. Generally there is a slurred R downstroke in leads III and aVF. The alterations in the precordial leads are minimal but they do have diagnostic value. In most cases we also find a slurred R downstroke in V_6, there is no s wave or only a minimal s wave in this lead.

LPFB masks the pattern of old inferior infarction *partially* or *completely*.

The difference is obvious between the ECG patterns of an old inferior MI without LPFB and an old inferior MI associated with LPFB. Instead of the typical loss of QRS vectors resulting in *pathologic Q waves* ($\geq$ 0.04 sec) or *QS waves* in leads III and aVF (II), often with negative and symmetric T waves (ECG 9.4), we find tall R waves in these leads with small or only slightly enlarged or absent Q waves, combined with negative, flat, or positive T waves (ECGs 9.5 and 9.6).

The extremely rare LPFB without inferior infarction shows the pattern mentioned above with small q waves and even greater R waves in the inferior leads, leading to $\mathring{A}QRS_F$ between + 80° and + 120°.

The pattern of LPFB (also in its common combination with inferior infarction) may easily be *confounded* by other conditions with an $\mathring{A}QRS_F$ between + 50° and + 80° (or even + 120°), for example in a *normal* ECG in young individuals (especially with asthenic habitus) (ECG 9.7), or *right ventricular hypertrophy* (RVH) or *extensive anterior (anterolateral) infarction*. All these conditions represent exclusion criteria for the diagnosis of LPFB. For correct diagnosis, the QRS duration, the fine alterations described above, and a history of (inferior) MI must be considered. In cases of doubt an inferior infarction can be confirmed or excluded by echocardiography.

The Full Picture

The concept of left (and right!) fascicular blocks was described in 1917 by Rothberger and Winterberg [1] in a fascinating publication of 63 pages, based on animal experiments. The typical ECG patterns were demonstrated in the limb leads only, because the precordial leads were introduced by Wilson only in 1944. However, their publication [1] from Vienna was forgotten, and for decades fascicular block-like patterns were interpreted as 'peri-infarction blocks'. Moreover, the clinical significance of these intraventricular conduction disturbances was not known at that time. In 1956 Grant [2] described a conduction block in the superior division of the left bundle branch as a cause of left-axis deviation, and in 1968 Rosenbaum et al reintroduced the concept of fascicular blocks in his famous book *Los Hemibloqueos*, published in English 2 years later [3]. At about the same time, fascicular blocks and bilateral/bifascicular blocks were recognized as potential precursors of acquired complete atrioventricular blocks, and cardiac pacemakers as adequate therapy were available. Thus the exact identification of fascicular blocks represents one of the most important progresses in electrocardiography in recent decades.

3 Intraventricular Conduction System Anatomy

In around 50% of dog hearts, as well as human hearts, the intraventricular conduction system is trifascicular, consisting of the right bundle branch and the left anterior and left posterior fascicle (Figure 9.1a). In the remaining 50% an additional medial fascicle is found in the left ventricle (Figure 9.1b), and more rarely multiple fascicles are found (Figure 9.1c). Therefore, the expression 'fascicular block' seems more adequate than the expression 'hemiblock'. These variations may also explain the diagnostic difficulties experienced in some cases.

The left posterior fascicle is the most voluminous one, and which leaves the His bundle first and separately. Thereafter, the His bundle is divided into the right bundle branch and into the left anterior fascicle (or into two or more fascicles). In general, in diseases of the intraventricular conduction system, the fascicles are affected in their most proximal parts within the surrounding tissue of the end of the His bundle. To a certain degree this explains why the somewhat isolated left posterior fascicle is more resistant to diseases than the other fascicles. Additionally, the posterior fascicle has a dual supply of blood from the left and right coronary arteries [4].

4 Etiology of Fascicular Blocks

4.1 Etiology of LAFB

Early epidemiological studies of middle-aged patients with left-axis deviation or later studies about LAFB, suggest that

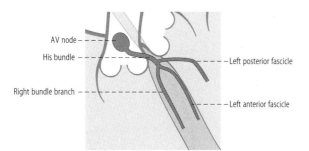

Figure 9.1a
Trifascicular ventricular conduction system

AV node
His bundle
Right bundle branch
Left posterior fascicle
Left anterior fascicle

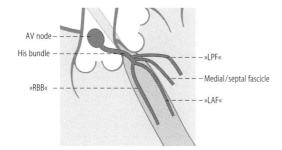

Figure 9.1b
Quadrifascicular ventricular conduction system

AV node
His bundle
»RBB«
»LPF«
Medial/septal fascicle
»LAF«

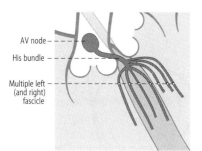

Figure 9.1c
Plurifascicular ventricular conduction system

AV node
His bundle
Multiple left (and right) fascicle

40%–60% of these patients suffer from, in order: CHD, hypertensive heart disease, or diabetes [5–7]. Patients with fibrosis of the intraventricular conduction system without CHD, known as Lenègre disease [8], are responsible for another 10%–20%, and are not included in this number. Chronic CHD is found in about 30% of LAFB cases. However, in acute MI, isolated LAFB appears extremely rarely. Of 480 patients with acute myocar-

dial infarction, LAFB developed in only one patient; in 19 patients LAFB was pre-existing [9]. Rare conditions for the development of LAFB are dilating cardiomyopathy, myocarditis, collagenous and neuromuscular disease, and hyperkalemia [6,7]. Intermittent LAFB during coronary angiography is very rare. After heart valve operations, especially aortic valve replacement, isolated fascicular blocks are extremely rare, while bilateral bifascicular blocks and complete AV blocks are seen in 2%–4%. During operations, unintentional damage may occur to the His bundle, or to the fascicles that run down the His bundle very close to each other. The very rare pattern of left-axis deviation in acute pulmonary embolism probably does not always correspond to true LAFB. It may be explained by *right* anterior fascicular block (see section 7.3 below). The common pattern of left-axis deviation in endocardial cushion defects, especially atrial septal defects of the 'ostium primum' type ('ASD I') and AV canal defects, are not due to true conduction blocks but due to anomalies of the conduction system (interruption or absence of the left anterior fascicle). In these cases a slurred R downstroke in leads I and aVL, often seen in LAFB, is never observed. Also in some congenital heart diseases, such as tricuspid atresia, single ventricle and corrected transposition, left-axis deviation is rarely detected. In childhood (or later) congenital left-axis deviation may be present without congenital heart disease [10], perhaps caused by a minimal endocardial cushion defect involving only the left anterior fascicle. Some cardiologists call this an 'electric ASD I'.

4.2   Etiology of LPFB

Isolated LPFB is associated with inferior myocardial infarction in most cases. Other very rare etiologies such as Lenègre disease, hypertension, aortic valve disease, cardiomyopathy, aortic dissection type A, angiography of the right coronary artery, and others, have been described, mostly in case reports (see 6.2 Special Remarks).

ECG Special ————————————————

5   Left Anterior Fascicular Block

5.1   Vectors and the ECG

In conduction blocks within the left anterior fascicle, a part of the septum and the inferoposterior left ventricular wall are activated first, over the posterior fascicle, thus leading to a vector pointing inferiorly (>>> small r wave in the inferior limb leads). An abrupt change of the direction of the vector occurs very early, about 20 msec after the beginning of QRS. This is due to a *great vector* produced by excitation along the myocardium of the lateral and high lateral wall, directed *upwards and to the left*. This great vector completely masks the vectors pointing inferiorly during activation of the inferior wall. In the ECG we find a frontal QRS left-axis deviation with a deep S wave and an rS type in the leads III, aVF, and II. The vectorcardiogram shows a counterclockwise QRS loop in the frontal plane (Figure 9.2a). The delayed activation of the lateral wall of the left ventricle leads to a broadening of QRS by 15–20 msec and often to a slurred R downstroke in leads I and aVL. In the horizontal plane the QRS vector loop (also counterclockwise) shows many variations and may be oriented more or less anteriorly (at the beginning), to the left and backwards (middle to late vectors), and to the right (last vectors) (Figure 9.2b). This explains the RS complex with its varying amplitudes of the R and S waves in the different precordial leads. A frequent pattern is an rS complex in all precordial leads. Often the R and S wave have about the same amplitude in the lateral leads (ECG 9.8).

5.2   Variants

In general, LAFB is characterized by an rS complex in all horizontal leads. In some cases, with or without left ventricular hypertrophy, the R wave may be tall and more or less equal to the S wave in lead V_2 (ECG 9.9). In other cases (in about 10%) a small q wave is found in leads V_2 and V_3 [11], as shown in ECG 9.10. This may be due to a short initial orientation of the QRS vector backwards (mimicking anteroseptal infarction) or due to real anteroseptal infarction. Other documented cases prove that on rare occasions LAFB may completely *mask* anteroseptal, anterior or inferior infarctions. In the latter case, the LAFB pattern predominates the frontal leads – there is an rS wave in III and aVF, with positive asymmetric T waves.

Left ventricular hypertrophy associated with LAFB does not produce q waves in the lateral leads V_5 and V_6 (for the diagnosis of left ventricular hypertrophy in LAFB see Chapter 5). It is believed that left ventricular hypertrophy itself may result in left-axis deviation, without LAFB (ECG 9.11). In these cases we find distinct q waves and tall R waves in V_5 and V_6. The diagnosis of LAFB with borderline left-axis deviation or of incomplete LAFB is arbitrary.

Overall LAFB is responsible for about 85% of left-axis deviations. The most important differential diagnosis is old inferior MI, showing broad Q waves or a QS complex in III and aVF,

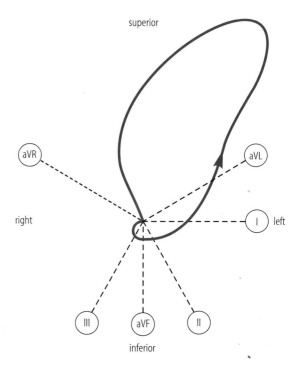

Figure 9.2a
Frontal QRS vector loop in left anterior fascicular block (LAFB)

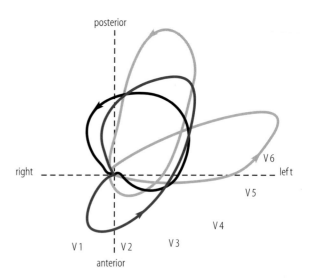

Figure 9.2b
Horizontal QRS vector loop in left anterior fascicular block (LAFB)

in many cases associated with negative and symmetric T waves. Those may also be flat or positive in older infarctions, positive also as a result of mirror image, due to left ventricular overload.

5.3 Prognosis

The prognosis of isolated LAFB is generally good, in consideration of the underlying cardiac disease. LAFB develops to a bilateral block or even complete AV block (Chapter 11 Bilateral Blocks) only in a small percentage and this process generally lasts decades. In exceptional cases LAFB (as isolated RBBB or LBBB) may be combined with syncope. Histopathologic studies [12,13] have shown that severe damage of the intraventricular conduction system may be found in the presence of only minor conduction disturbances in the ECG.

Short Story/Case Report 1

In 1984 a 46-year-old man had two sudden episodes of syncope, one of 10 sec duration and one of about 30 sec, on the second occasion with a fracture of his right hand. He was transferred from the orthopedic to the neurologic station. Clinical and laboratory findings were normal, as was an electroencephalogram. The cardiology consultant found a sinus rhythm and LAFB at rest. The echocardiogram was normal; the exercise test revealed excellent work capacity, without other ECG abnormalities. As there were no risk factors for CHD, coronary angiography was not performed. The patient was dismissed and an ambulatory ECG was proposed. Ten days later, on a train returning from work, the patient suddenly died. In the autopsy no cause of sudden death could be found macroscopically. The coronary arteries were normal. However, extensive histopathologic examination of the intraventricular conduction system revealed extensive fibrosis of the proximal portions of the right bundle branch, the left anterior, and also the left posterior fascicle (Lenègre disease). It was assumed that the patient died during his third Morgagni-Adams-Stokes attack, due to complete AV block and ventricular asystole, possibly with consecutive ventricular fibrillation.

To conclude: the cardiologist was not aware of the possible discrepancy between the ECG and histopathologic findings. Unfortunately, he *neglected* the history typical for arrhythmogenic syncope. An ambulatory ECG should have been performed and an electrophysiologic study made during hospitalization, and implantation of a pacemaker should have been discussed. Pacemaker implantation would have been more appropriate in this case than for asymptomatic patients with borderline sick sinus syndrome diagnosed in the ECG.

6 Left Posterior Fascicular Block

6.1 Vectors and the ECG

If the conduction is blocked in the posterior fascicle, a portion of the septum is activated first, over the anterior fascicle. The abnormal and relatively early activation of the inferior wall on a broad front results in a great vector directed inferiorly, dominating the vectors directed superiorly (activation of the high lateral wall), thus determining the ECG pattern with a frontal QRS axis of + 80° to + 120° (in the usual combination with inferior infarction about + 60°), with a small q wave and a tall R wave in the leads III, aVF, and II. The vectorcardiogram shows a clockwise QRS loop. The delayed activation of the inferior wall often results in a *slurred R downstroke in the inferior leads III and aVF*. LPFB produces little alteration in the horizontal leads, however, of diagnostic importance. A *slurred R downstroke* and an *absent s wave in* V_6 (found in about 80% of the cases) often confirms the diagnosis (ECGs 9.5 and 9.6).

6.2 Special Remarks: ÅQRS$_F$, ECG Patterns and Etiology

Here are a few facts and reflections about the discrepancies in the literature in respect to ÅQRS$_F$, ECG pattern, and etiology.

In the literature, the opinions about LPFB are rather controversial and even confusing. The main reason is probably that most publications date from 1968 to 1975 and lack comparison with left ventricular angiography and coronary arteriography. In older papers a mean frontal QRS axis of + 90° to + 120°, and even to + 180° is described as typical. However, a mean QRS axis of + 70° is also discussed as possible in complete and incomplete LPFB, or in LPFB combined with inferior infarction. Medrano et al [14] insist on the diagnostic importance of a slurred R downstroke in the inferior leads III and aVF, and V_6, without an s wave in this lead. Unless these *morphologic signs* are observed, the pattern of LPFB may be easily confounded with normal variants.

Some examples of 'LPFB' published in the literature [15] represent normal variants in younger people. It is generally accepted that an age of less than 30–40 years, asthenic habitus, RVH, or extensive anterior/lateral infarction are exclusion criteria for the diagnosis of LPFB, because a shift of the frontal QRS axis to the right is common. However, in all these conditions the 'fine' alterations of real LPFB, associated with inferior MI, are lacking.

More recently the pattern of LPFB in inferior MI has been qualified as 'peri-infarction block' [16]. Indeed, some patterns of intraventricular conduction disturbances in MI, such as rSr' type in leads V_2 to V_6 in anterior infarction [17], may be called 'peri-infarction block', as they are today. However, in such a 'peri-infarction block' there is never a great QRS vector directed opposite to the infarcted area. Thus a tall R wave, associated with inferior MI, can only be explained by an important conduction disturbance – in this case a block of the left posterior fascicle.

Many *etiologies* for LPFB have been described, mainly concerning a few or single cases. CHD is the most frequent cause. Overall, by far the largest number of LPFB patterns (documented with ECGs) that have been published are *associated with inferior MI* [18]. Very rare causes (without inferior infarction) include fibrosis of the left posterior fascicle (Lenègre disease), hypertension, aortic valve disease, cardiomyopathy, aortic dissection, and other conditions [3,11,13,18,19]. Transient LPFB sometimes occurs, though rarely, during exercise testing and angina [20].

One more recent clinical study about LPFB dates from 1993 [18]. It compares the ECG with left ventricular angiographic and coronary angiographic findings. In a retrospective 1-year study, 9 of 163 patients (5.5%) with old inferior (or inferoposterior) infarction showed LPFB. In a prospective 1-year study of patients in departments of cardiology and internal medicine, LPFB was detected in 6 of 2502 ECGs (0.24%). In 5 of those 6 patients an invasive study was performed, revealing inferior infarction; the sixth patient had an inferior aneurysm of the left ventricle in the echocardiogram. Thus all 15 patients with LPFB had an inferior infarction. In a 1-year period no other etiology could be found. There was severe two-to-three-vessel CHD in 12 of 14 patients undergoing invasive studies, and 9 (64%) underwent coronary bypass grafting (mean 3.2 grafts). The pattern of inferior infarction was partially or completely masked by the LPFB in all cases; the correct diagnosis was made only once, before hospitalization. The authors concluded that LPFB is mostly found in patients with inferior infarction (in some cases with additional anterior infarction) and is generally associated with severe CHD, therefore requiring invasive investigation to evaluate coronary revascularization. Based on an extensive study of the published literature on LPFB (including the published ECG patterns of LPFB), the authors did not find valuable arguments against the concept that LPFB is mostly encountered in patients with inferior infarction. In this study the mean frontal QRS vector was about + 60°, varying from + 50° to + 80°.

Explaining the different ÅQRS$_F$ in LPFB without inferior MI and in LPFB with inferior MI, is not difficult. There is a link between the apparent discrepancies in the older and newer literature. There is no doubt that LPFB *without* inferior infarction generally produces a mean frontal QRS vector between + 80° and + 120°. However, this condition is very rare. It is also obvious that some previously published ECGs and vectorcardiographic patterns of so-called LPFB, especially in younger people without heart disease and with normal QRS duration [15], represent normal variants. LPFB combined with inferior infarction results in a minor shift of the frontal QRS vector to the right. Some loss of vectors directed inferiorly, caused by necrosis, produces a q wave in III and aVF that is generally deeper and somewhat broader (but < 40 msec) than the q wave in LPFB without inferior infarction, thus reducing the shift of the QRS to the right and resulting in a mean QRS vector of about + 60°.

6.3 Prognosis

Because the diagnosis of LPFB is not easy, the prognosis primarily depends on the treating physician… In cases of doubt the patient history and risk factors for CHD should be evaluated and an echocardiogram performed. Coronary angiography is mandatory in suspected infarction to evaluate revascularization. The prognosis then depends on left ventricular function and the feasibility of coronary bypassing.

In the evolution of monofascicular over bifascicular to trifascicular block and complete AV block, the left posterior fascicle plays the part of 'joker'. Due to its special conditions (thick fascicle with early and separate division from the His bundle; double blood supply), the left posterior fascicle is the most resistant portion of the intraventricular conduction system (Chapter 11 Bilateral Blocks). There is a lack of publications about the risk for patients with isolated LPFB (with or without inferior infarction) of developing complete AV block. Because there must be some risk, these patients should be controlled.

7 Very Rare Patterns of Fascicular Blocks

7.1 LAFB plus LPFB

In very rare cases the combination of LAFB and LPFB may be suspected. ECG 9.12 shows an example in which a medial fascicle is responsible for left ventricular activation.

7.2 Left Septal Fascicular Blocks

Until now it has not been possible to identify the ECG pattern of the block in the medial (septal) fascicle, in a convincing manner [21].

7.3 Right Fascicular Blocks

Funnily enough, the right ventricular conduction system in both dog and human hearts is divided into two (or three) fascicles. Right ventricular fascicular blocks have been extensively studied by Rothberger and Winterberg 1917 [1], by Uhley and Rivkin 1961 [22], and by Medrano and De Micheli 1975 [23]. Interestingly right anterior fascicular blocks may occasionally result in left-axis deviation, similar to LAFB, without the pattern of incomplete RBBB in lead V_1. This might be one explanation for the rare cases of left-axis deviation in acute PE. Otherwise, right ventricular fascicular blocks do not seem to have clinical importance.

References

1. Rothberger CI, Winterberg H. Experimentelle Beiträge zur Kenntnis der Reizleitungsstörungen in den Kammern des Säugetierherzens. Zeitschr ges exper Med 1917;5:264
2. Grant RP. Left-axis deviation. An electrocardiographic–pathologic correlation study. Circulation 1956;14;233
3. Rosenbaum MB, Elizari MV, Lazzari JO. The hemiblocks. New concepts of intraventricular conduction based on human anatomical, physiological and clinical studies. Oldsmar, FL: Tampa Tracings, 1970
4. Frink RJ, James TN. Normal blood supply to the human His bundle and proximal bundle branches. Circulation 1973;47:8–18
5. Eliot RS, Millhon WA, Millhon J. The clinical significance of uncomplicated marked left-axis deviation in men without known disease. Am J Cardiol 1963;12:767
6. Ostrander LD. Left-axis deviation: Prevalence, associated conditions and prognosis. An epidemiologic study. Ann Intern Med 1971;75:23–8
7. Corne RA, Beamish RE, Rollwagen RL. Significance of left anterior hemiblock. Br Heart J 1978;40:552–7
8. Lenègre J. Les blocs auriculoventriculaires complets chroniques. Etudes des causes et des lesions à propos de 37 cas. Mal cardiovasc 1962;3:311
9. Scheinman M, Brenman B. Clinical and anatomic implications of intraventricular conduction blocks in acute myocardial infarction. Circulation 1972;46:753–60
10. Gup AM, Granklin RB, Hill HE. The vectorcardiogram in children with left-axis deviation. Am Heart J 1965;69:619
11. Gertsch M, Bernoulli D. Fascicular block patterns – observations on differential diagnosis. In: Lüderitz B (ed). Cardiac Pacing. Diagnostic and Therapeutic Tools. Heidelberg: Springer 1976, pp 111–8
12. Rossi L. Sistema di conduzione trifascicolare ed emiblocchi di branca sinistra. G Ital Cardiol 1971;1:55–62
13. Demoulin JC, Kulbertus HE. Histopathologic correlates of left posterior fascicular block. Am J Cardiol 1979;44:1083–8
14. Medrano GA, Brenes C, De Micheli A, Sodi-Pallares D. Clinical electrocardiographic and vectorcardiographic diagnosis of left posterior subdivision block, isolated or associated with RBBB. Am Heart J 1972;84:727–37
15. Lopes VM, Miguel JM, dos Reis DD, et al. Left-posterior hemiblock. Clinical and vectorcardiographic study of twenty cases. J Electrocardiol 1974;7:197–214
16. Braunwald E. Heart Disease. A Textbook of Cardiovascular Medicine, fifth edn. Philadelphia: WB Saunders Company 1997, p 133
17. Varriale P, Chryssos BE. The RSR' complex not related to right bundle branch block: Diagnostic value as a sign of myocardial infarction scar. Am Heart J 1992;123:369–76
18. Godat FJ, Gertsch M. Isolated left posterior fascicular block: A reliable marker for inferior myocardial infarction and associated severe coronary artery disease. Clin Cardiol 1993;16:220–4
19. Scott RC, Manitsas GT, Kim OJ, et al. Left posterior hemiblock – A new diagnostic sign in dissecting aneurysm? J Electrocardiol 1971;4:261–6
20. Madias JE, Knez P. Transient left posterior hemiblock during myocardial ischemia – eliciting exercise treadmill testing: a report of a case and a critical analysis of the literature. J Electrocardiol 1999;32:57–64
21. Sanches PCR, Moffa PJ, Sosa E, et al. Electrical, endocardial mapping of 5 patients with typical ECG of left middle fascicular Block. J Electrocardiol 2001;34:323
22. Uhley HN, Rivkin LM. Electrocardiographic patterns following interruption of main and peripheral branches of the canine right bundle of His. Am J Cardiol 1961;7:810
23. Medrano GA, De Micheli A. Contribucion experimental al diagnostico de los bloquéos fasciculares derechos. Arch Inst Card Mex 1975;45:704–19

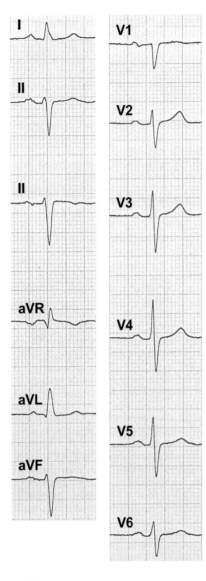

ECG 9.1
74 y/m. Typical LAFB. ÅQRS$_F$ - 75°, slurred R downstroke in I/aVL, and 'smooth' transition zone in precordial leads.

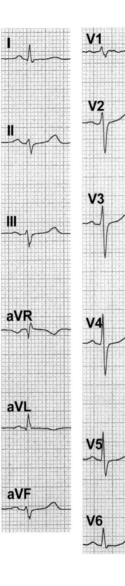

ECG 9.2
54 y/m. Typical LAFB. ÅQRS$_F$ - 60°, mirror image of slurred R downstroke in III, and 'smooth' transition zone in precordial leads.

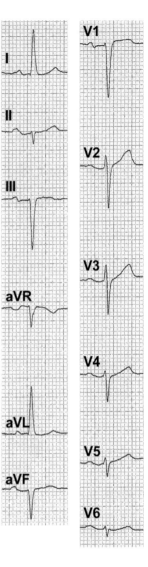

ECG 9.3
80 y/f. LAFB without apparent slurring (a frequent pattern). ÅQRS$_F$ about - 40°. Absent transition zone in the horizontal leads, with extreme clockwise rotation.

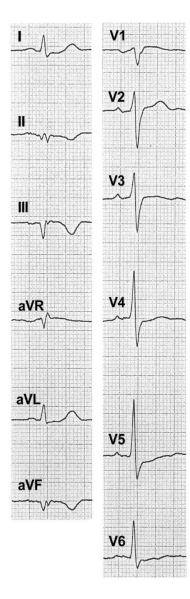

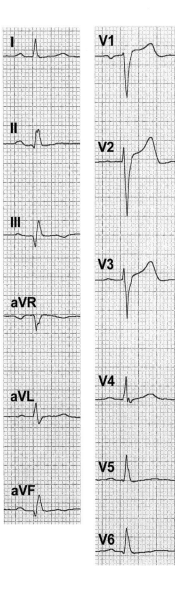

ECG 9.4
73 y/m. Old inferior MI without LPFB. ÂQRS$_F$ - 50°. Q > 0.04 sec in III, aVF (II) and symmetric negative T waves in the same leads.

ECG 9.5
68 y/m. LPFB, partly masking old inferior MI. ÂQRS$_F$ + 55°. Q wave < 0.04 sec in III, aVF. Slurred R downstroke in II (III/aVF) and V$_6$/V$_5$. Negative T wave in III. Note the absence of S wave in V$_6$ (and V$_5$). Coro: closed right coronary artery, inferior aneurism, ejection fraction 42%. Moreover, 60% stenosis of LAD and 70% stenosis of CX.

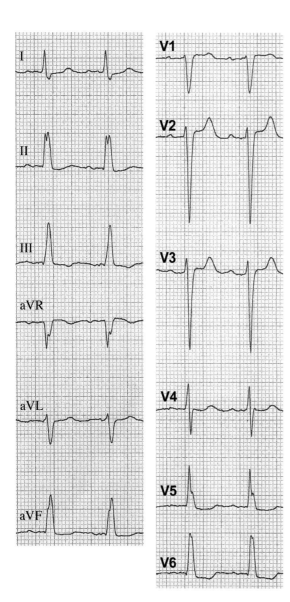

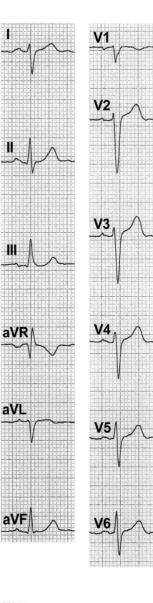

ECG 9.6

72 y/f. LPFB, completely masking old inferior MI. Left atrial enlargement. ÂQRS$_F$ + 80°. Slurred R downstroke in V$_5$ and as mirror image in aVR. Tall and broad R waves in II, aVF and III. Only minimal Q waves in the same leads. Coro: closed right coronary artery, inferior akinesia, ejection fraction 50%. Also 80% stenosis of CX.

ECG 9.7

32 y/m. No apparent heart disease, weight 115 kg. Unexplained right-axis deviation. ÂQRS$_F$ about + 130°. No signs for LPFB (see also broad S wave in V$_6$ and small S wave in aVF). This pattern is much more frequent in asthenic young people.

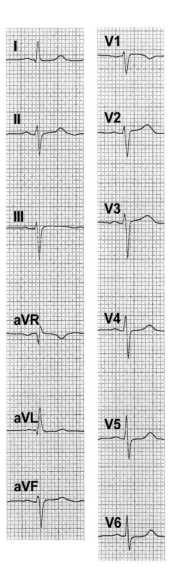

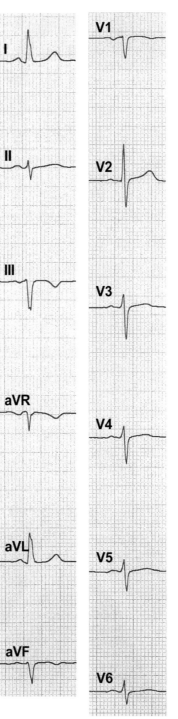

ECG 9.8
53 y/f. LAFB. ÅQRS$_F$ - 50°. Only minimal
terminal R slurring in aVL. Horizontal
leads: rS type in V$_1$ to V$_4$, R=S in V$_5$/V$_6$.

ECG 9.9
66 y/f. LAFB. ÅQRS$_F$ - 45°. Slurred R
downstroke in I/aVL. Tall R wave in
V$_2$ as a variant of LAFB.

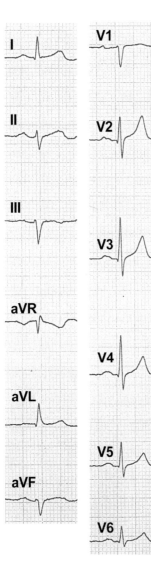

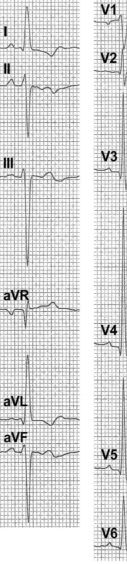

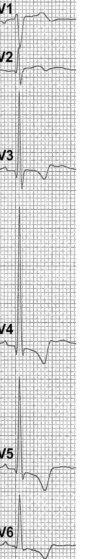

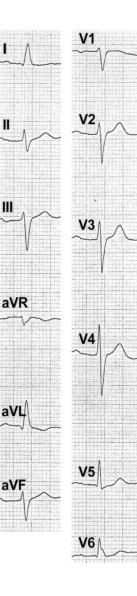

ECG 9.10
52 y/m. Variant of LAFB, with small Q waves in leads V_2 and V_3 (V_4). Differential diagnosis: old anteroseptal MI.

ECG 9.11
53 y/m. Severe aortic valve disease. Left-axis deviation without LAFB. ÂQRS$_F$ - 50°. Horizontal plane: QRS counterclockwise rotation. Significant q waves in V_2 to V_6. Evident left ventricular hypertrophy with strain pattern.

ECG 9.12
67 y/m. Possible LAFB + LPFB. ÂQRS$_F$ - 40°. Slurred R downstroke in I, aVL *and* V_6.

Chapter 10
Bundle-Branch Blocks (Complete and Incomplete)

At a Glance

Bundle-branch blocks (BBB) are the most common ECG patterns of *aberration* of the ventricular conduction, in the presence of a supraventricular rhythm, mostly sinus rhythm. This means that the electric impulse is not conducted over both bundle branches at the same time but is blocked in one bundle branch. Consequently, one ventricle is activated with delay, through the interventricular septum.

Other types of aberration in the ventricles are fascicular blocks (including bifascicular and/or bilateral blocks) and pre-excitation in individuals with an accessory pathway.

Differentiating between complete *right* bundle-branch block (RBBB) and complete *left* bundle-branch block (LBBB) is almost as important for a physician as it is for a driver to differentiate between right-hand drive and left-hand drive cars.

The prevalence of RBBB depends predominantly on age and on the presence or absence of coronary heart disease. Overall it seems that RBBB is more frequent than LBBB. The etiologies for both blocks include hypertension, coronary heart disease, degenerative disease of the intraventricular conduction system (Lenègre disease), and heart valve replacement.

ECG

The normal human ECG is a 'levogram' due to the important muscle mass of the left ventricle (LV) compared to that of the right (RV), at a ratio of 8 : 1. Thus, the great LV vectors outweigh the small RV vectors. In the 12-lead ECG we generally do not see anything of right ventricular excitation, but there are two exceptions: right ventricular hypertrophy (see Chapter 6 Right Ventricular Hypertrophy) and RBBB.

The expression 'conduction block' may be misleading. Often there is no real conduction block but an extensive slowing of the conduction; in the ECG the block may be incomplete, or complete. In complete blocks an extreme reduction of the conduction velocity may be the reason for the pattern of bundle-branch block.

The block may be reversible: after a heart operation, after recovery from myocardial infarction, pulmonary embolism (RBBB), or infectious heart disease, and in some cases after thoracic trauma (RBBB) or by treatment of arterial hypertension (mostly LBBB).

1 Complete Right Bundle-Branch Block

RBBB and LBBB are characterized by a *broad QRS complex* and a special *QRS configuration*. QRS duration in LBBB is generally longer than in RBBB. Without concomitant ventricular hypertrophy, QRS in RBBB measures 0.12 sec (0.12–0.14 sec) and in LBBB 0.14 sec (0.14–0.16 sec).

In RBBB, right ventricular excitation is especially well detectable, because the right ventricle is activated *after* the left. The activation of the left and the right ventricles can be seen separately. The QRS vector in RBBB is similar to that of normal ventricular activation, with exception of the last part. The initial and middle vectors are only slightly altered, whereas the delayed excitation of the right ventricle produces a great vector oriented to the right. There are only *two leads* in the 12-lead standard ECG that explore rightward-oriented vectors *directly*, that is by a *positive deflection*: V_1 and aVR (up to a certain degree also lead III). For RBBB a *terminal broad R wave* is characteristic in these leads (ECGs 10.1 and 10.2). In *lead V_1* the classical pattern is an *rsR' complex* with a R' of great amplitude, about 5–16 mm. In some cases a *simple broad* but *always notched* R complex is present, due to projections (ECG 10.3). In uncomplicated RBBB, a qR type in V_1 is quite rare and RVH must be excluded in this case. The positive terminal R wave in aVR and often also in III confirms the diagnosis of RBBB. The absence of a terminal R wave in aVR excludes RBBB, and other conditions for a single R wave in lead V_1 – such as pre-excitation or posterior myocardial infarction – must be considered.

In RBBB, the leads I, aVL and V_5/V_6 (as mirror-image leads for the delayed right ventricular activation) show broad terminal S waves with an amplitude of 1–6 mm.

2 Incomplete Right Bundle-Branch Block

Incomplete RBBB (iRBBB) is characterized by a normal broad *rSr' complex* in lead V_1, always with a terminal R wave in lead aVR. The r' wave in V_1 may be smaller, equal or greater than the initial r wave. The pattern is quite common (up to 5%) and is considered as a normal variant in most cases (ECGs 10.4 and 10.5). An r' wave in V_1 significantly broader than the initial r wave may be caused by right ventricular hypertrophy or enlargement, especially if the T waves are negative in V_2 and V_3 (ECG 10.6).

3 Complete Left Bundle-Branch Block

In the complete form of LBBB, QRS measures at least 0.12 sec, in most cases ≥ 0.14 sec, also without left ventricular hypertrophy (LVH). In contrast to RBBB, in LBBB the QRS complex is extremely deformed, because the great septal and LV vectors are directed from *the right to the left* (and upwards or downwards, and backwards) producing a unique and somewhat bizarre QRS complex. The QRS pattern in the horizontal leads is strikingly uniform, with a broad rS complex in V_1 to V_4 (in < 20% of cases with a QS complex) and an *abrupt change* to a positive deflection in V_5 and V_6 with a broad, notched (or not notched) or bifid R wave, *without* a Q wave (ECG 10.7). Occasionally, this abrupt change can be observed between lead V_3 and V_4, or between V_5 and V_6.

In the frontal leads, the QRS axis often points to the left and upwards (left-axis deviation). We find a broad R wave (without Q wave) in I and aVL, and in the inferior leads III and aVF generally an rS complex, and rarely a QS complex (as occasionally in V_1 to V_4), that may be confounded with an infarction pattern. However, in LBBB the QRS is broad and the T wave is discordant and asymmetric (ECG 10.8) – and not (as usual) concordant and symmetric as in myocardial infarction.

4 Incomplete Left Bundle-Branch Block

The pattern of iLBBB is relatively rare. Its definition is a QRS duration of about 0.12 sec and the typical behavior of the LBBB pattern in V_1 to V_6, with a sudden change from a negative QRS deflection in V_4 to a positive one in V_5 (ECG 10.9). Most so-called iLBBB, without an abrupt change of QRS polarity between V_4 and V_5, are simple patterns of LVH with prolonged QRS. In cases of doubt, iLBBB may be classified as LBBB.

The Full Picture

The heart has its own special system for conduction of the electric impulse. If the function of this system is disturbed, nature looks 'automatically' for another way to conduct it. In the case of LBBB the left ventricle is activated from the right ventricle, over the septum, bypassing the normal conduction system – in this case the left bundle branch. If this did not happen, the left ventricle would stand still and death would occur. Correspondingly, in RBBB the right ventricle would stand still without activation over the septum. Thus the electrical conduction in bundle-branch block is an example of the wonderful reserve mechanisms of nature.

5 Etiology and Prevalence

Common etiologies are hypertension, coronary heart disease (especially myocardial infarction), degenerative disease of the ventricular conduction system (Lenègre disease) in middle-age and the elderly, thoracic trauma, heart operation (especially aortic valve replacement and closure of ventricular septum defect), and inflammatory and other diseases [1–5]. If bundle-branch block is found in individuals with an otherwise normal heart [6], fibrosis of the ventricular conduction system is assumed. The prevalence of bundle-branch blocks depends on the studied population and therefore differs considerably in the literature. Gertsch et al [7] studied 5000 ambulatory patients from a cardiac institute, and found RBBB in 1.62% and LBBB in 0.74%. Out of 7073 patients referred for exercise treadmill testing with thallium imaging, Hesse et al [8] found an RBBB in 3% and an LBBB in 2%. In the Tecumseh study by Ostrander et al, the prevalence of bundle-branch block was 2.4% [9]. Eriksson et al [10] reported, in a general male population, a rise of bundle-branch block from 1% to 17% between the ages of 50 years and 80 years.

All publications report an increase of bundle-branch blocks with aging and a higher prevalence of RBBB compared to LBBB. The last observation is astonishing, because the diseases of the left heart are far more frequent than those of the right. The reasons are speculative. The fact that the right bundle is supplied by branches of the right *and* left coronary arteries, and may be blocked by disease of both coronary arteries, may play a role. A *new* bundle-branch block in association with acute myocardial infarction was observed in about 2%–6% [11,12].

ECG Special _____

6 Complete Right Bundle-Branch Block

6.1 QRS Vectors

The schemes of ventricular vectors in Figures 10.1 and 10.2 are somewhat simplified but correlate well with the ECG. In Figure 10.1 normal ventricular vectors are shown. It is obvious that the vectors in RBBB (Figure 10.2) are quite similar to the normal vectors. In RBBB a portion of the interventricular septum and the whole free wall of the left ventricle, including its inferior and high lateral segments, are normally activated through the left bundle branch. The right bundle branch being blocked, the electric impulse automatically breaks through the interventricular septum from the left to the right, at about 80 msec before the left ventricle is completely activated. This produces an abnormal vector 1. The vector has the same direction as the normal septal vector but a relatively great magnitude and long duration. This has two consequences. First, the septal vector is enhanced, visible (by the proximity effect) only in the precordial leads V_2 and V_3, as a higher initial R wave that may mimic the mirror image of true posterior infarction. With leads V_7 to V_9 true posterior infarction can be confirmed or excluded. Second, and more important, the vector 1 (as also the vector 3) reduces to a certain extent the main LV vector (vector

2), which means the amplitude of the R waves in V_4 to V_6. The mirror-image deflections – the S waves in the anteroseptal leads – are extremely reduced (by the proximity effect). This makes the ECG diagnosis of LVH even more difficult than under normal conditions. However, a higher R voltage than normal in leads $V_4/V_5/V_6$ (about ≥ 15 mm) renders LVH probable at an age of ≥ 40 years (ECG 10.10).

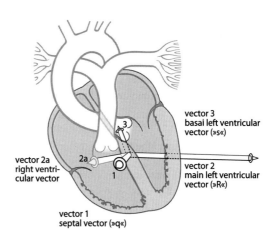

Figure 10.1
Scheme of the ventricular vectors in normal conduction

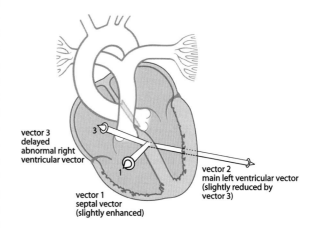

Figure 10.2
Scheme of the ventricular vectors in right bundle-branch block

The vector 3 originates from the delayed activation of the RV, on a broad front, partially neglecting the specific conduction system. Consequently, this vector again has great amplitude and long duration. In lead V_1 the terminal R (R') wave is astonishingly high in respect to the thin wall of the right ventricle. This can be explained by the 'proximity effect'. In the mirror-image leads (e.g. I, aVL, V_5/V_6) the corresponding S waves are as broad but of smaller amplitude than the R' wave in V_1, because the proximity effect is lacking.

Generally the rSR' is only seen in V_1. From V_2 to V_6 the mirror image of the delayed right ventricular activation is seen as negative terminal deflection. In some cases the delay in right ventricular activation (with or without T-wave negativity) is visible in lead V_2 or even up to V_4 (ECG 10.11). In these cases, right ventricular hypertrophy must be excluded. Without right ventricular hypertrophy, this pattern is difficult to explain with the vector theory. This is an example of the limits of the vectorial approach.

6.2   Repolarization Vectors

In RBBB the ST and T vectors of the right ventricle are more or less pointing in the opposite direction of the R' – that is to the left, upwards and slightly backwards. In the ECG we find a minimal ST depression in V_1 and III (and aVF) and a negative and asymmetric T wave in the same leads. At *exercise,* the T wave becomes negative in more precordial leads, up to lead V_4, rarely to V_5. This should not be misinterpreted as ischemic response.

6.3   Determination of Frontal QRS Axis in RBBB

In the ECG without RBBB, the frontal QRS axis (ÅQRS_F) reflects the frontal QRS axis of the LV vectors. In the presence of RBBB, only the first 60–70 msec of the QRS complex correspond to the LV vectors. Thus we determine the frontal QRS axis in RBBB by regarding only the first *60 or 70 msec* of QRS. After some practice this is possible with a precision of about 20°. But even accurate measuring is not completely precise, because this 'LV axis' is slightly shifted to the right by the influence of vector 1 of RBBB. Generally the axis is between - 30° and + 90°. In right-axis deviation (formerly called classical type RBBB) RVH or an additional left posterior fascicular block (LPFB) must be excluded. In left-axis deviation (formerly called Wilson type RBBB) an additional left anterior fascicular block (LAFB) has to be considered. Not every RBBB with left-axis deviation (of the first 60 msec of QRS) corresponds to a bilateral block of the type RBBB + LAFB. If there is no decrease in S width in lead I and especially lead aVL (where the S wave is often completely lacking in the presence of additional LAFB), isolated RBBB with left-axis deviation can be assumed (ECG 10.12).

6.4   Myocardial Infarction in RBBB

In RBBB the pattern of acute and old myocardial infarction can be recognized almost as well as without RBBB, in contrast to infarctions with LBBB (Chapter 13 Myocardial Infarction).

6.5   Right Ventricular Hypertrophy in RBBB

Differentiation between RBBB with and without right ventricular hypertrophy is not as easy as one might think (Chapter 6 Right Ventricular Hypertrophy).

7   Incomplete Right Bundle-Branch Block

iRBBB is defined as delayed intrinsic deflection in right ventricular activation exceeding about 35 msec, producing an rSr' complex in lead V_1 and some times in III, without prolonging QRS duration.

In the past two different types have been distinguished. Type A has a r' that is smaller (in duration and often amplitude) than r. Type A was interpreted as a harmless normal variant. Type B, with a r' greater than r, was thought to be combined with right ventricular hypertrophy (ECGs 10.5 and 10.6). This opinion can be partially abandoned. If a greater and unselected cohort with type A or type B is compared, there is no statistical difference. That means that type B may also be a normal variant, and type A (more rarely) may be combined with right ventricular hypertrophy. In selected patients suffering from diastolic or systolic right ventricular overload (in patients with atrial septal defects or chronic pulmonary embolism) the type B will be much more frequent, however. It is also evident that iRBBB with a negative T wave, not only in V_1 but also in V_2 and V_3, is a better marker of right ventricular disease than the type of iRBBB. Chronic systolic and diastolic overload cannot be distinguished, neither by characteristics of QRS (both show a broad r' in V_1) nor by the repolarization (both have negative T waves in V_2 to V_3 that are generally asymmetric) (Chapter 6 Right Ventricular Hypertrophy).

The Mexican school of electrocardiography has its own nomenclature for the types of patterns of RBBB, based on the degree of conduction slowing:

a. first degree: former type A of iRBBB, with r' smaller than r
b. second degree: former type B of iRBBB, with r' greater than r
c. third degree: complete right bundle-branch block (RBBB).

These definitions may be useful to a certain extent for a general population that is growing older today and subject to hypertensive, coronary and degenerative heart diseases.

In the presence of iRBBB the ECG should always be interpreted in context with the patient history and the clinical findings.

Short Story/Case Report 1

In May 1978 the specialist for infectious diseases was called to a very obese 64-year-old woman who had had an operation on both knees 4 days before, and who had been on heparin (underdosed). She suffered from moderate dyspnea at rest, with hyperventilation; her pulse rate had increased from 90 to 130/min within 2 h and her blood pressure decreased from 170/100 to 120/90 mmHg. At the same time her body temperature had risen from normal to 39 °C. Blood cultures were ordered. Occasionally, the preoperative and new ECGs were shown to an 'ECG specialist' (who was not an experienced clinical cardiologist). The first ECG revealed signs of LV hypertrophy and overload; the second showed, besides the fast sinus rate, only one minimal difference: a notch in the ascending branch of the S wave in V_1, a very incomplete RBBB. Based on this sign, and without so much as a glance at the patient, the ECG specialist made the diagnosis of acute pulmonary embolism. Consecutive investigations included blood gases (pO_2 48; pCO_2 22) and urgent lung scintigraphy that showed complete obstruction of the left pulmonary artery. With anticoagulation the patient recovered within 3 days clinically and the scintigram was normalized after 3 months. The fever was probably caused by an acute infection of the urinary tract.

In conclusion, the correct diagnosis was (fortunately) made by the detection of a very silly ECG sign that could have been an innocent alteration. In fact, acute pulmonary embolism was possible, likely even, from the very beginning, on the basis of the patient history and clinical findings. Acute pulmonary embolism should never be diagnosed on the ECG alone (Chapter 8 Pulmonary Embolism).

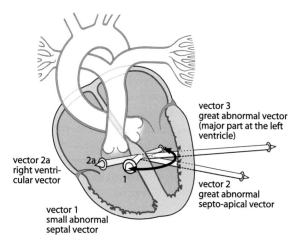
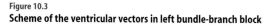

Figure 10.3
Scheme of the ventricular vectors in left bundle-branch block

8 Complete Left Bundle-Branch Block

8.1 QRS Vectors

In contrast to RBBB, where almost only the end of the QRS complex is altered, LBBB provokes a substantial deformation of the QRS. In the presence of a blocked left bundle branch the right ventricle is activated through the right bundle branch as normal. The early penetration of the electrical impulse through the left part of the interventricular septum from *the right to the left* and slightly anteriorly (in most cases this means with rS in lead V_1 to V_4) produces a small vector 1 (Figure 10.3). The great abnormal vector 2, pointing mainly to the left, corresponds to a delayed excitation of the whole septum. As in normal ventricular conduction, the relatively small right ventricular vector 2a is completely absorbed. Also the delayed and magnified vector 3, that corresponds to the activation of the great muscle mass of the left ventricle, is directed to the left. Thus in LBBB the two great vectors 2 and 3 are directed to the left, backwards and slightly superiorly or inferiorly. The consequence is an extremely uniform pattern in the horizontal plane. Whereas in leads V_1 to V_4 we find a broad rS complex (in < 20% of cases a broad QS complex), there is an abrupt change between V_4 and V_5 from completely negative to completely positive deflections. In leads V_5 and V_6 we observe a broad and sometimes notched or bifid R wave, without a Q wave (ECG 10.7). A sudden change from negative to positive QRS may also be seen from lead V_3 to lead V_4 (ECG 10.13,

ECG 10.14) or from lead V_5 to lead V_6, especially in (left and/or right) ventricular dilatation (ECG 10.8). In uncomplicated LBBB there are no 'notches' or 'slurrings' in leads V_1 to V_4, and the small R wave is generally slightly increasing from V_1 to V_4. It is important to memorize these typical patterns, e.g. for the differentiation of *typical* ECG patterns of *myocardial infarction* in LBBB (Chapter 13 Myocardial Infarction), and the differentiation of *supraventricular tachycardias* with LBBB aberration from *ventricular* tachycardias (Chapters 23 AV Junctional Tachycardias and 26 Ventricular Tachycardias). In the frontal plane the most common pattern is a broad R wave in I and aVL and a broad rS, and occasionally a broad QS complex in the inferior leads.

8.2 Repolarization Vectors

Corresponding to the abnormal QRS vectors in LBBB the ST and T vectors are also strongly altered, pointing to the opposite direction of QRS vectors, namely to the right, forward and inferiorly. ST and T is therefore always opposite to the QRS deflection. The ST segment may be elevated in V_2 and V_3 (V_4) up to 3–4 mm, without hypertrophy or ischemia. In V_5 and V_6 ST depression generally does not exceed 1–2 mm. The T wave is also discordant to the QRS and asymmetric. In some cases we find in I, aVL, V_5 and V_6 biphasic (negative/positive) or positive T waves, instead of the usual negative T waves. The former concept – that this behavior of the T wave corresponds to ischemia – has not been confirmed.

8.3 Determination of Frontal QRS Axis in LBBB

In contrast to RBBB, the separate activation of the ventricles is not visible. Thus we determine the QRS axis as usual, considering the whole QRS complex. However, this axis is not the true QRS axis that would be present without LBBB. Generally LBBB provokes a substantial left-axis deviation of the QRS axis (ECG 10.8), but also other QRS axes are seen (ECGs 10.7 and 10.13).

8.4 Myocardial Infarction in LBBB

LBBB masks typical myocardial infarction in more than 70% of cases (see Chapter 13 Myocardial Infarction).

8.5 Left Ventricular Hypertrophy in LBBB

Based on the uniformity of the QRS vectors of LBBB in the horizontal plane, the detection of LVH (ECG 10.14) seems to be easier than in the ECG without conduction disturbance (Chapter 5 Left Ventricular Hypertrophy).

8.6 Incomplete Left Bundle-Branch Block

If we accept the definition of iLBBB, that the ECG pattern should reveal the same characteristics as LBBB with the exception of a slightly prolonged QRS duration of about 0.12 sec (ECG 10.9), iLBBB is rarely encountered (let us remember that in LBBB QRS generally measures $\geq$ 0.14 sec). If we argue that we are not able to differentiate in the ECG between real conduction block and extensive conduction slowing, it is probable that in iLBBB a portion of the left ventricle is activated with delay over the left bundle branch but the main portion from the right to the left, by the abnormal activation of the septum [13,14]. Furthermore, in some cases of typical (complete) LBBB we cannot exclude the possibility of a small segment of the left ventricle being activated over the left bundle branch, and almost the whole muscle of the left ventricle being activated by the mechanism described above. In practice we use the difference of QRS duration for the distinction between iLBBB and LBBB.

9 Special Aspects of Bundle-Branch Blocks

9.1 Rate-Dependent Bundle-Branch Block

Due to the longer refractory period of the right bundle, compared to that of the left bundle, rate-dependent RBBB occurs more often than LBBB. RBBB aberration is not rare at the beginning of a supraventricular tachycardia, for some beats; LBBB aberration is rarer in this condition (Chapter 23 AV Junctional Tachycardias). Bundle-branch block may also be triggered by bradycardia [15]. For new onset bundle-branch block during exercise see Chapter 27 Exercise ECG.

9.2 Alternating, Intermittent and Reversible BBB

At the beginning of the development of bundle-branch block, occasionally alternating or intermittent bundle-branch block (ECG 10.15) may be observed [16,17].

Reversible bundle-branch block may be observed after heart operation, after recovery from myocardial infarction, after pulmonary embolism (RBBB) or infectious heart diseases, in some cases after thoracic trauma (RBBB) or by treatment of arterial hypertension (mostly LBBB). This is one hint more for the functional component in bundle-branch block and other conduction blocks.

9.3   Difference of QRS and QT Duration in RBBB and LBBB

QRS duration is longer in LBBB than in RBBB. This is based on the fact that the abnormal conduction through the septum lasts longer from the right to the left than from the left to the right. The reason is not completely clear. Some findings argue for an 'electrical barrier' that exists only in the septal activation from the right to the left [18]. More evident is the reason for the larger vector 3 in LBBB, compared to vector 3 in RBBB. It takes more time to activate the greater muscle mass of the left ventricle than that of the right. Consequently, also the QT time in LBBB lasts about 20 msec longer than the QT time in RBBB, that means about 30–40 msec longer than in normal ventricular conduction.

10   Prognosis

Principally, the prognosis of bundle-branch block depends on the underlying disease. In the absence of heart disease, the prognosis is generally good. However, a certain percentage of patients with bundle-branch block, especially with LBBB, develop cardiac disease after years, mostly coronary artery disease. In the Reykjavik study [19,20], the Tecumseh study [9] and the Framingham study [21] bundle-branch block was not connected with an increased mortality, in the absence of coronary heart disease. In the study by Eriksson et al [10] in older men there was no significant relation to coronary heart disease or mortality. However, the patients with bundle-branch block were prone to greater left ventricular volume and to developing heart failure. In bundle-branch block appearing during acute myocardial infarction the prognosis is different. Melgarejo-Moreno et al [22] and Newby et al [23] found that new and permanent bundle-branch block was an independent predictor of increased mortality. Hod et al [24] found that in patients with acute inferior infarction the subgroup of those with bundle-branch block (5%, in 79% RBBB) had significantly increased mortality at 1 year, 5 years and 10 years. Finally, a more recent study by Hesse et al [8], with a huge cohort of 5290 men and 1783 women, confirmed some old results and revealed some new ones. RBBB was more frequent overall than LBBB; RBBB was more frequent in men and LBBB was more frequent in women. Women and men with bundle-branch block had more abnormalities in stress thallium images and were more likely to have coronary heart disease. After a follow-up of 6 years, LBBB and RBBB were associated with increased mortality.

References

1. Haft JI, Herman MV, Gorlin R. Left bundle-branch block: etiologic, hemodynamic and ventriculographic considerations. Circulation 1971;43:279–87
2. Lenègre J. Contribution à l'étude de bloc de branche. Paris: IB Bailliere et Fils 1958
3. Lev M, Unger PN, Rosen KM, et al. The anatomic substrate of complete left bundle-branch block. Circulation 1974;50:479–86
4. Kulbertus HE, Cojne JJ, Hallidoe-Smith KA. Conduction disturbances before and after surgical closure of ventricular septal defect. Am Heart J 1969;77:123
5. Zimmermann R. Intraventrikuläre und atrioventrikuläre Reizleitungsstörungen nach Herzoperationen. Inauguraldissertation. University of Bern 1979
6. Rotman M, Triebwasser JH. A clinical and follow-up study of right and left bundle-branch block. Circulation 1975;51:477–84
7. Gertsch M, Medrano GA, De Micheli A. Schenkelblock, bilateraler bifaszikulärer und bilateraler trifaszikulärer Schenkelblock. Schweiz med Wschr 1974;104:1623–7
8. Hesse B, Diaz LA, Snader CE, et al. Complete bundle-branch block as an independent predictor of all-course mortality: report of 7073 patients referred for nuclear exercise testing. Am J Med 2001;110:253–9
9. Ostrander LD, Brandt RL, Kjelsberg MO, Epstein FH. Electrocardiographic findings among the adult population of a total natural community, Tecumseh, Michigan. Circulation 1965;31:888–98
10. Eriksson P, Hansson P-O, Eriksson H, Dellborg M. Bundle-branch block in a general male population. The study of men born in 1913. Circulation 1998;98:2494–500
11. Nimetz AA, Shubrocks SJ, Hutter AM, et al. The significance of bundle-branch block during acute myocardial infarction. Am Heart J 1975;90:439–44
12. Scheidt S, Killip T. Bundle-branch block complicating acute myocardial infarction. J Amer Med Assoc 1972;222:919–24
13. Sodi Pallares D, Estandia A, Soberson J, et al. Left intraventricular potential of the human heart: II. Criteria for diagnosis of incomplete left bundle-branch block. Am Heart J 1950;40:655
14. Schamroth L, Bradlow BA. Incomplete left bundle-branch block. Brit Heart J 1964;26:285
15. Massumi RA. Bradycardia-dependent bundle-branch block: A critique and proposed criteria. Circulation 1968;38:1066
16. Krikler DM, Lefevre D. Intermittent left bundle-branch block without obvious heart disease. Lancet 1970;1:498–500
17. Swiryn S, Abben R, Denes P, Rosen KM. Electrocardiographic determinants of axis during left bundle-branch block; Study in patients with intermittent left bundle-branch block. Am J Cardiol 1980;46:53–8
18. Medrano GA, De Micheli A. Is the concept of 'jumping wave' still valid? Arch Inst Cardiol Mex 2000;70;19–29
19. Hardarson A, Arnarson T, Eliasdon JG, et al. Left bundle-branch block: prevalence, incidence, follow up and outcome. Europ Heart J 1987;8:1075–9

20. Thrainsdottir I, Hardarson T, Thorgeirsson G, et al. Epidemiology of right bundle-branch block and its association with cardiovascular morbidity. The Reykjavic study. Europ Heart J 1993;14,1590–6
21. Kreger BE, Anderson KM, Kannel WB. Prevalence of intraventricular block in the general population; the Framingham study. Am Heart J 1989;117:903–10
22. Melgarejo-Moreno A, Galcera-Tomas J, Garcia-Alberola A, et al. Incidence, clinical characteristics and prognostic significance of right bundle-branch block in acute myocardial infarction: a study in the thrombolytic era. Circulation 1997;96:1139–44
23. Newby KH, Pisano E, Krucoff MW, et al. Incidence and clinical relevance of the occurrence of bundle-branch block in patients treated with thrombolytic therapy. Circulation 1996;94:2424–8
24. Hod H, Goldbourt U, Behar S. Bundle-branch block in acute Q wave inferior wall myocardial infarction. A high risk subgroup of inferior myocardial infarction patients. The SPRINT study group. Secondary Prevention Reinfarction Israeli Nifedipine Trial. European Heart J 1995;4:471–7

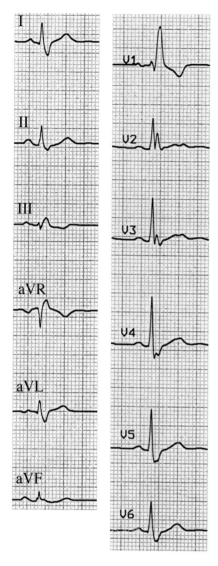

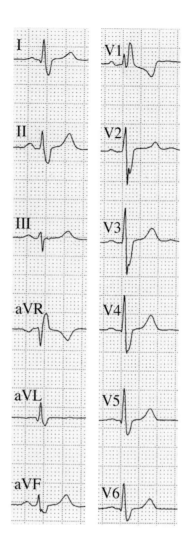

ECG 10.1
59y/m. RBBB with the typical rsR' in V$_1$, and an Rsr' configuration in V$_2$/V$_3$. Coronary artery disease (one-vessel disease), normal left ventricular function.

ECG 10.2
33y/m. RBBB with the typical RSR' (rsR') configuration only in V$_1$. Normal heart.

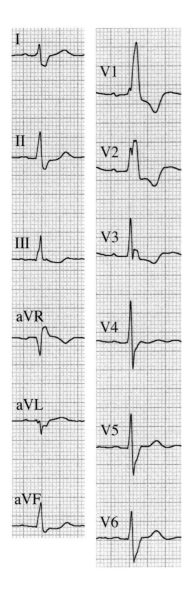

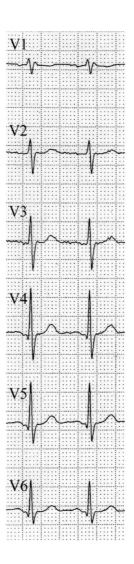

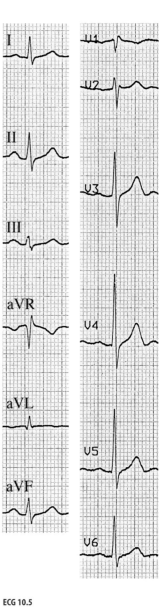

ECG 10.3
58y/f. RBBB without an rsR′ complex in V₁, but with a notched broad R wave in V₁/V₂ and an Rsr′ complex in V₃. Hypertension, normal heart.

ECG 10.4
31y/m. Incomplete RBBB with r > r′ in V₁. Normal heart.

ECG 10.5
62y/m. Incomplete RBBB with r < r′ in V₁ and V₂. Slight LVH.

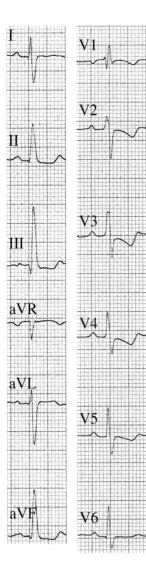

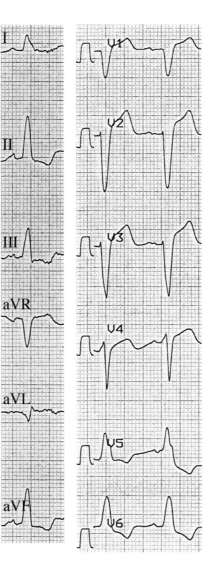

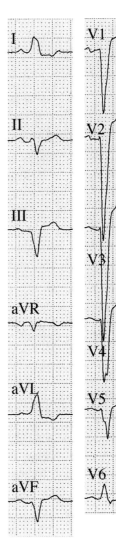

ECG 10.6
49y/f. Incomplete RBBB with r < r′ in V₁ and T negativity in V₂ up to V₅! Atrial septal defect with left to right shunt > 60%.

ECG 10.7
49y/f. LBBB, QRS duration 0.14 sec (half calibration in precordial leads). Sudden change of QRS polarity from V₄ to V₅. Hypertension, LVH, pulmonary emphysema. Normal coronary arteries.

ECG 10.8
54y/m. LBBB, QRS 0.14 sec. Change of QRS polarity between V₅ and V₆, with Rs in V₆. *QS in III*. Dilating cardiomyopathy of the left ventricle. No significant coronary artery stenosis.

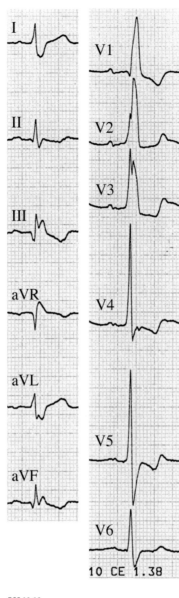

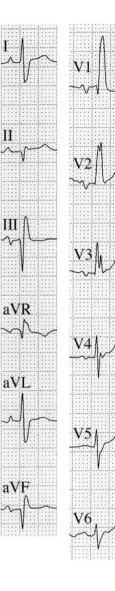

ECG 10.9
72y/f. Incomplete LBBB (QRS 126 msec!). Change of QRS polarity between lead V_4 and lead V_5. Hypertension, LVH.

ECG 10.10
63y/m. RBBB plus LVH. High R waves in V_4 and V_5 (up to 26 mm). Relatively broad Q wave in III/aVF. Alteration of the repolarization also in left precordial leads. Moderate to severe aortic regurgitation. Normal coronary arteries.

ECG 10.11
47y/f. RBBB with visible right ventricular activation delay up to V_4. Height 172 cm, weight 45 kg. No RVH, small heart.

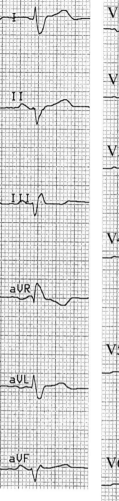

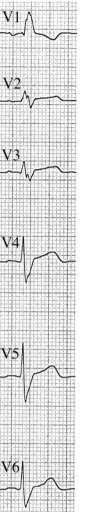

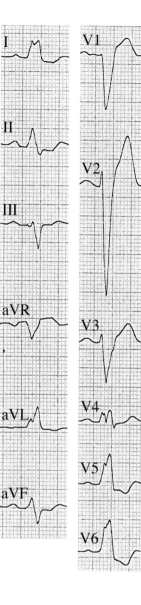

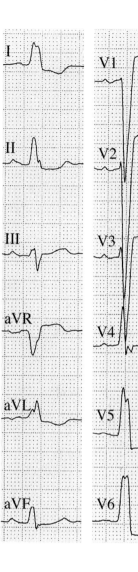

ECG 10.12
69y/m. RBBB with left axis deviation of the first 60 msec of QRS. No signs for additional left anterior fascicular block (note the broad S wave in aVL). Left atrial enlargement (p duration 0.13 sec). Hypertension.

ECG 10.13
72y/m. LBBB (QRS 0.13 sec). Sudden change of QRS polarity between V_3 and V_4. Slight LVH.

ECG 10.14
67y/f. LBBB with a frontal axis about + 40°. Hypertension, coronary artery disease. 90% stenosis of left anterior descending coronary artery, normal left ventricular EF.

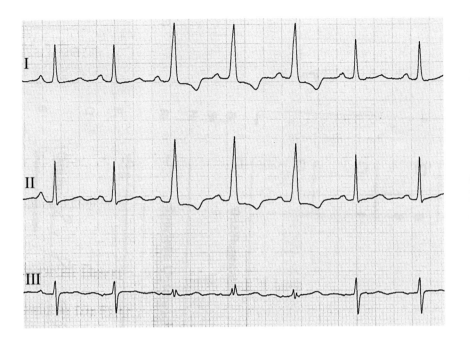

ECG 10.15
Intermittent incomplete LBBB.

Chapter 11
Bilateral Bifascicular (Bundle-Branch) Blocks

At a Glance

Bilateral bifascicular blocks, also called bilateral bundle-branch blocks, include complete right bundle-branch block (RBBB) combined with either left anterior fascicular block (LAFB) or left posterior fascicular block (LPFB).

The prevalence of the combination RBBB + LAFB in hospital patients is 0.5%–1%, the combination RBBB + LPFB is at least 20 times rarer. The etiologies of these conduction block patterns are the same as for isolated fascicular blocks: coronary heart disease (CHD) and cardiomyopathies of other origins, Lenègre disease, hypertensive heart disease, heart valve operations, and rare conditions.

Bilateral bifascicular blocks are clinically important because they represent potential precursors of complete infra-Hissian atrioventricular (AV) block.

ECG

1 RBBB + LAFB

This type of bilateral bifascicular block (Figure 11.1) is relatively *frequent*. The delayed excitation of the right ventricle (RBBB) and of high lateral portions of the left ventricle alter the QRS vector loop in the frontal and horizontal planes. The ECG is characterized by:

i. QRS duration > 0.12 sec
ii. typical RBBB pattern in lead V_1 with an rsR' complex (sometimes with a pure broad and slurred R wave, or a qR complex). The S wave in V_6 is broad (mirror image of lead V_1)
iii. frontal left-axis deviation of the first 0.06 sec of the QRS. Often small Q waves in aVL and I; rS complex in III/aVF/II with positive T waves

iv. clockwise rotation of left ventricular QRS vector in the precordial leads, mostly with an rS complex and (in most cases) without a Q wave in leads V_5/V_6.

A slurred R downstroke in leads I and aVL – due to a visible delayed intrinsicoid deflection – is not compulsory. Therefore the ECG pattern in the limb leads may differ considerably (either with broad or absent S waves in leads aVL and I), whereas the QRS configuration in the horizontal plane is quite uniform. ECGs 11.1–11.6 demonstrate the different patterns in the limb leads.

In general the S wave in leads I and especially aVL are smaller than the S wave in lead V_6 (ECGs 11.1 and 11.2). Often the S waves in I and especially aVL are missed, thus imitating an LBBB pattern in the limb leads (ECGs 11.3 and 11.4). In many cases there is no distinct slurred R downstroke and occasionally the S waves are only moderately or minimally diminished in leads I and aVL. In such cases it may be impossible to distinguish the pattern of RBBB + LAFB from that of isolated RBBB with left-axis deviation on the basis of a single ECG. In

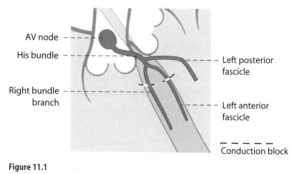

AV node

His bundle

Right bundle branch

Left posterior fascicle

Left anterior fascicle

- - - - Conduction block

Figure 11.1
Bilateral block of the type RBBB + LAFB

ECG 11.5, with obvious frontal left-axis deviation, nobody can reliably confirm or exclude additional LAFB. On one hand the broad S waves in aVL and I and the rSR' type in III (and aVF), with negative T waves, favor isolated RBBB. On the other hand, the absence of a Q wave in V_5/V_6 is quite rare in isolated RBBB and is extremely frequent in RBBB + LAFB.

ECG 11.6 illustrates this rare finding in RBBB + LAFB – a preserved Q wave in leads V_6/V_5 (and V_4). ECG 11.7 shows RBBB with minor frontal QRS left-axis deviation, probably *without* associated LAFB.

2   RBBB + LPFB

This type of bilateral bifascicular block is *rare* (Figure 11.2). The typical RBBB pattern in lead V_1 is combined with a vertical axis of the first 0.06 sec of the QRS complex in the frontal plane. The delayed activation of the inferior left ventricular (LV) portions generally leads to a visible delayed intrinsicoid deflection, a slurred R downstroke in leads aVF and III, and also in lead V_6 (V_5). The S wave in this lateral (inferolateral) lead is generally smaller than usual. The Q wave in leads V_5 and V_6 is preserved (ECG 11.8).

As in isolated LPFB, the diagnosis of RBBB + LPFB should not be made in clinical conditions that may also lead to a vertical frontal axis of the LV vector; these conditions include: age < 40 years, right ventricular hypertrophy (RVH), lung diseases such as pulmonary emphysema, asthenic habitus and, of course, lateral infarction. As for isolated LPFB, RBBB + LPFB generally masks an old myocardial infarction (MI), reducing the Q wave in the inferior leads (ECG 11.9) or even masking it.

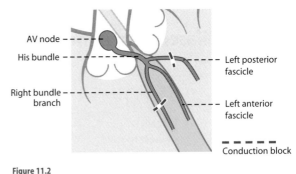

Figure 11.2
Bilateral block of the type RBBB + LPFB

3   Prognosis

Bilateral bifascicular blocks represent potential precursors of a complete AV block (AV block 3°). The progression of RBBB + LAFB to AV block 3° is generally slow (about 4% per year), whereas a RBBB + LPFB is more often an immediate precursor of AV block 3°. However the indication for pacemaker implantation depends also on clinical findings and symptoms such as dizziness, presyncope, or syncope. A Holter ECG may help to discover episodes of AV block 2° or 3° in patients with unclear symptoms. In selected cases, the duration of the HV interval is measured. For detailed indications for permanent pacing see The Full Picture.

The Full Picture

Based on the concept of the trifascicular (or quadrifascicular) *ventricular conduction system* that consists of the right bundle branch and the two (or three) left fascicles, we prefer the term 'bilateral bifascicular block'. However, the term 'bilateral bundle-branch block' is *identical* and is used more frequently.

4   Etiology

Similarly to isolated fascicular blocks, bilateral fascicular blocks are generally due to coronary artery disease (CAD), primary fibrosis of the ventricular conduction system, hypertensive heart disease, and iatrogenic lesions during heart surgery, approximately in this order. In many cases the etiology can only be presumed. The definitive etiology can only be detected by pathologic–anatomical examinations. This may be one of the reasons why the prevalence of etiology varies considerably in the literature. However, most publications deal with the combination RBBB + LAFB. Information about RBBB + LPFB is very rare. In 40%–60% of people CAD is responsible for chronic bilateral bifascicular block [1,2] and is seen in acute MI

(AMI) in 4%–7% [2–4], usually RBBB + LAFB in anterior AMI (the right bundle branch and the left anterior fascicle are both supplied by septal branches of the left anterior descending artery (LAD). In 1964 Lenègre first described a 'sclerodegenerative process' of the ventricular conduction system, responsible for bilateral bundle-branch block and complete AV block in the absence of CAD [5]. Of 61 cases with bilateral bundle-branch block or complete AV block, postmortem examination revealed CAD in 32 (28 with MI) (52%), and 'primary' fibrosis of the ventricular conduction system (in the right bundle branch and in the left fascicles) in 19 cases (31%). In these last cases, no other cause could be detected, especially no coronary artery pathology [5].

The prevalence of hypertensive heart disease in patients with a bilateral fascicular block, mostly RBBB + LAFB, is about 20%. RBBB + LAFB occurs also during heart operations, in 11% of corrections of Fallot, in 6% of closures of ventricular septal defects [6], in a low percentage of aortic valve replacements, and occasionally in mitral or tricuspid valve replacements [7–9]. In these instances a bilateral block is due to direct damage to the conduction fascicles. A unifascicular block may pre-exist. A bilateral block after coronary bypass is very rare. In an early publication [10] the prevalence reached 3.5% and was due to inadverted ischemia.

Other rare etiologies include non-coronary cardiomyopathy [11], aortic valve disease [12], Lev disease in older patients (sclerosis and calcification of the left heart skeleton) [13], congenital heart disease [14], heart transplantation [15], and hyperkalemia [16].

In practice it is often not possible to determine the etiology if the patient has neither proven CAD, nor has he had a heart operation.

i. an LBBB-like pattern (ECGs 11.3 and 11.4)
ii. a slurred R wave downstroke in leads aVL and I, with smaller S waves (ECGs 11.1, 11.2 and 11.6)
iii. only minimally increased duration of the R wave in aVL/I, with practically normal broad S waves (ECG 11.5). In these cases, the pattern is hardly to distinguish from that of isolated RBBB. Both RBBB and LAFB decrease the amplitude of the R wave in leads V_4 to V_6. Consequently, we find an rS complex in these leads, in most cases without a Q wave.

6 Differential Diagnosis of RBBB + LPFB

Most cases with RBBB and a vertical axis of the first 0.06 sec of the QRS complex are due to pulmonary diseases with emphysema and/or RV hypertrophy and are also seen in young people and in asthenic individuals. ECG 11.11 shows RBBB in a young asthenic patient. The rare pattern of RBBB + LPFB can only be reliably diagnosed in a single ECG on the basis of a slurred R downstroke in lead V_6 (V_5) in expense of the RBBB-induced S wave (ECGs 11.8 and 11. 9). Serial ECGs may be very helpful. In the presence of RBBB an abrupt rightward change of the frontal LV QRS vectors (the first 0.06 sec) indicates additional LPFB, in the absence of acute pulmonary diseases.

7 Differential Diagnosis of RBBB + LAFB + LPFB *Without* Complete AV Block

In this very rare condition, the ventricular conduction is only guaranteed by a medial (septal) left fascicle (Figure 11.3). The very rare pattern is characterized by the common pattern of RBBB (rsR' in V_1) and the behavior of the intrinsicoid deflection of LAFB *and* LPFB. Therefore we can observe a slurred R

ECG Special

5 Differential Diagnosis of RBBB + LAFB

The pattern of RBBB in V_1 (rsR' or broad notched R wave) is not altered by LAFB or by LPFB.

In RBBB + LAFB, the pre-existing QRS axis, the caliber of the left anterior fascicle, incomplete block in the anterior fascicle, and the presence or absence of a distinct medial fascicle, may all influence the QRS configuration, making the diagnosis difficult. While a left-axis deviation of the first 0.07 sec of QRS is compulsory, the influence of LAFB on the frontal QRS loop is very variable. The three different patterns are:

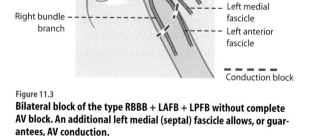

Figure 11.3
Bilateral block of the type RBBB + LAFB + LPFB without complete AV block. An additional left medial (septal) fascicle allows, or guarantees, AV conduction.

downstroke in leads I and aVL (caused by LAFB) *and* V_6 (caused by LPFB), with small S waves in these leads. The total frontal QRS axis in this pattern is about – 30° (ECG 11.10). Astonishingly, the PQ interval may be normal.

This pattern represents an *immediate* precursor of complete AV block and should therefore be recognized. Because there is no striking frontal right- or left-axis deviation, the pattern is sometimes misinterpreted as uncomplicated RBBB (ECG 11.10 with a QRS axis (first 0.06 sec) of + 75°).

Short Story/Case Report 1

In 1984, a 73-year-old patient was admitted to hospital because of three episodes of syncope during the previous week (one complicated by fracture of his right arm). There was a history of hypertension. The ECG (ECG 11.10) was interpreted as sinus rhythm, normal PQ interval, and complete RBBB. An additional remark was made: no sign of associated LAFB (absent left-axis deviation). Based on his history the patient was monitored. He suffered another period of loss of consciousness due to intermittent complete AV block with ventricular asystoly. A pacemaker was implanted. After operation, two ECGs revealed sinus rhythm with the pattern of RBBB + LAFB + LPFB. In later control ECGs, constant complete AV block was diagnosed (without PM funtion).

In conclusion: the pattern should have been recognized immediately. At least the patient was put on the ECG monitor because of his history of syncope.

8   Prognosis

The progression of RBBB + LAFB to AV block 3° is generally slower in patients with Lenègre disease and with unknown etiology than in patients where there is an association with chronic CAD. A prolonged His-ventricle (HV) interval probably enhances the development to AV block 3°. However, a prolonged HV interval is not always helpful for predicting the prognosis [17]. Overall a yearly progression of about 3% [18] to 7% [1] is estimated. In the setting of AMI, AV block 3° develops much more frequently (in up to 43% of patients) and is associated with a high mortality rate of about 50% [19]. In general the cause of death is progressive heart failure due to extensive infarction.

For the combination RBBB + LPFB a much higher rate of developing AV block 3° has been described, from 8%–60% within 1–2 years [1,20].

9   Indications for Pacemaker Implantation

The indications for permanent pacing in chronic bi- and trifascicular block are listed in the ACC/AHA Guidelines [21]. It is obvious that all symptomatic patients (with syncope or presyncope) should receive a pacemaker urgently. In asymptomatic patients the problem is not definitively resolved. It is generally acknowledged that the presence of both patterns of bilateral bundle-branch block at different times in the same patient represents an indication for pacing. In patients with a *bilateral bifascicular block* associated with *infra-His AV block 1° (or 2°)* – called 'incomplete trifascicular block' – a pacemaker should be implanted, also in asymptomatic patients. This intervention is valuable also for patients with *LBBB* with infra-His AV block 1° (and 2°). In the presence of *RBBB + LAFB* without AV block 1° or 2°, close control of the patient is sensible. However, the younger the patient, the greater is the possibility of developing AV block 3°. External conditions, for instance if the patient is employed as a driver, will influence the decision for a prophylactic pacemaker implantation.

In the presence of *RBBB + LPFB* we usually implant a pacemaker. The rare pattern of *RBBB + LAFB + LPFB without* AV block 3° [22,23] requires urgent pacemaker implantation. We have seen this rare pattern only in symptomatic patients immediately before or after pacemaker implantation, often alternating with the pattern of complete AV block.

References

1. Scanlon PJ, Pryor R, Blount SG. Right bundle-branch block associated with left superior or inferior intraventricular block: Clinical setting, prognosis and relation to complete heart block. Circulation 1970;42:1123–33
2. Col JJ, Weinberg SL. The incidence and mortality of intraventricular conduction defects in acute myocardial infarction. Am J Cardiol 1972;29:344–50
3. Nimetz AA, Shubrooks SJ, Hutter AM, et al. The significance of bundle-branch block during acute myocardial infarction. Am Heart J 1975;90:439–44
4. Waugh RA, Wagner GS, Haney TL, et al. Immediate and remote prognostic significance of fascicular block during acute myocardial infarction. Circulation 1973;47:765–75
5. Lenègre J. Etiology and pathology of bilateral bundle-branch block in relation to complete heart block. Progr Cardiovasc Dis 1964;6:409–44
6. Downing JW, Kaplan S, Bove KE. Postsurgical left anterior hemiblock and right bundle branch block. Br Heart J 1972;34:263–70

7. Zimmermann R, Gertsch M. Intraventricular and atrioventricular conduction disturbances after cardiac heart surgery. Abstract. 20th European Heart Congress, Amsterdam 1972

8. Lehmann G, Deisenhofer I, Zrenner B, Schmitt C. Recurrent symptomatic bilateral bundle-branch block in a 74-year-old patient with prosthetic aortic valve: a description of a case and review of the literature. Int J Cardiol 1999;71:283–6

9. Aravindakshan V, Elizari MV, Rosenbaum MB. Right bundle-branch block and left anterior fascicular block (left anterior hemiblock) following tricuspid valve replacement. Z Kreislaufforsch 1970;59:895–902

10. Zeldis SM, Morganroth J, Horowitz LN. Fascicular conduction disturbances after coronary bypass surgery. Am J Cardiol 1978;41:860–4

11. Watt TB, Pruitt RD. Character, cause and consequence of combined left-axis deviation and right bundle-branch block in human electrocardiograms. Am Heart J 1969;77:460–5

12. Thompson R, Mitchell A, Ahmed M, et al. Conduction defects in aortic valve disease. Am Heart J 1979;98:3–10

13. Lev M. Anatomic basis for atrioventricular block. Am J Med 1964;37:742

14. Shaher RM. Left ventricular preponderance and left-axis deviation in congenital heart disease. Br Heart J 1963;25:726

15. Chou Te-C. Electrocardiography in Clinical Practice, fourth edn. Philadelphia: WB Saunders 1996, p 592

16. Bashour T, Hsu I, Gorfinkel HJ, et al. Atrioventricular and intraventricular conduction in hyperkalemia. Am J Cardiol 1975;35:199–203

17. Dhingra RC, Palileo E, Strasberg B, et al. Significance of the HV interval in 517 patients with chronic bifascicular block. Circulation 1981;64:1265–71

18. Suravicz B. Prognosis of patients with chronic bifascicular block. Circulation 1979;60:40–2

19. Scanlon PJ, Pryor R, Blount SG. Right bundle-branch block associated with left superior or inferior intraventricular block associated with acute myocardial infarction. Circulation 1970;42:1135–42

20. Rosenbaum MB. The hemiblocks: diagnostic criteria and clinical significance. Mod Concepts Cardiovasc Dis 1970;39:141–6

21. ACC/AHA. Guidelines for Implantation of Cardiac Pacemakers and Antiarrhythmia Devices. J Am Coll Cardiol 1998;37:1175–209

22. Medrano GA, Brenes C, De Micheli A, Sodi Pallares D. El bloquéo de la subdivision anterior y posterior de la rama izquierda del Haz de His (bloqéo bifascicular) y su asociacion con bloquéo de la rama derecha (bloquéo trifascicular). Estudio electrocardiografico experimental y clinica. Arch Inst Cardiol Mex 1969;39:672–87

23. Gertsch M. Die linksfaszikulären Blockierungen. Diagnostik, Bedeutung und therapeutische Konsequenzen. Bull schweiz Akad med Wiss 1975;31:59–78

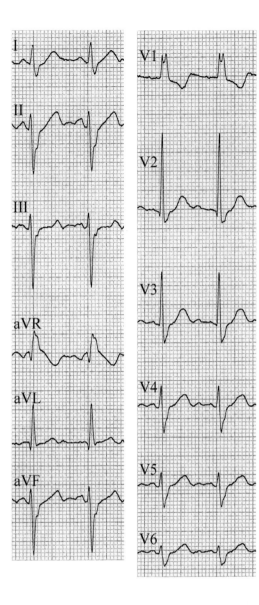

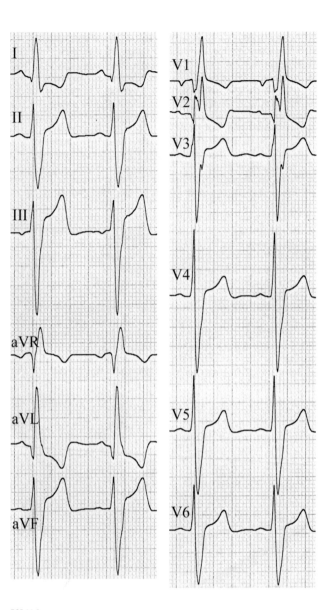

ECG 11.1

73 y/f. Hypertension. ECG: RBBB with single and notched R in V₁. QRS left-axis deviation in limb leads. Relative broad S in I but very small s in aVL. Atypical qR in V₂ (due to a 'variant' of LAFB). Typical rS complexes in V₅/V₆.

ECG 11.2

40 y/f. Aortic valve replacement for severe aortic valve incompetence. Surgically induced bilateral block. ECG: bilateral block. RBBB with rsR′ in V₁. QRS left-axis deviation in limb leads. Relative small s wave in I, absent s wave in aVL. rS complex in V₅/V₆, without a q wave. The great LV vectors are due to LV hypertrophy. Echo: LV mass 260g/m².

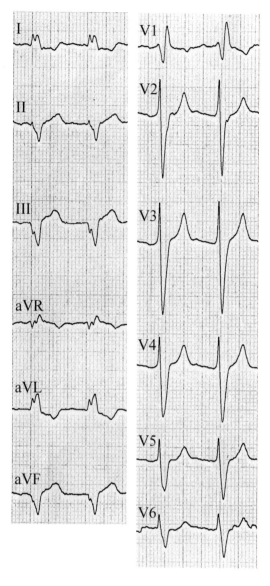

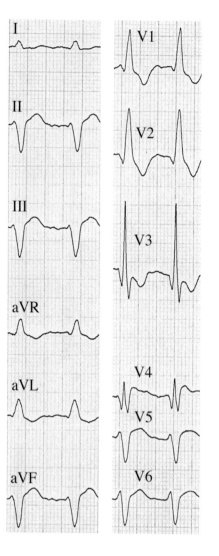

ECG 11.3

68 y/m. Old inferior MI. ECG: bilateral block. RBBB with rsR' in V$_1$. Frontal QRS left-axis deviation. QS in III/aVF, due to old MI. Minimal s wave in I, absent s wave in aVL, with broad notched QRS. The ECG pattern in the limb leads imitates LBBB. Clockwise rotation of LV vector in precordial leads. Absent Q wave in V$_6$.

ECG 11.4

59 y/f. 2-day-old anterior MI. ECG: bilateral block. RBBB with qR in V$_1$. Frontal QRS left-axis deviation. Absent s waves and broad R waves in aVL/I. Again the pattern in the limb leads imitates LBBB. In leads V$_5$/V$_6$ rS complex. Note that the pathologic q waves in (V$_1$) V$_2$ to V$_4$ and the ST elevation in V$_4$ are due to anterior MI. Atrial fibrillation.

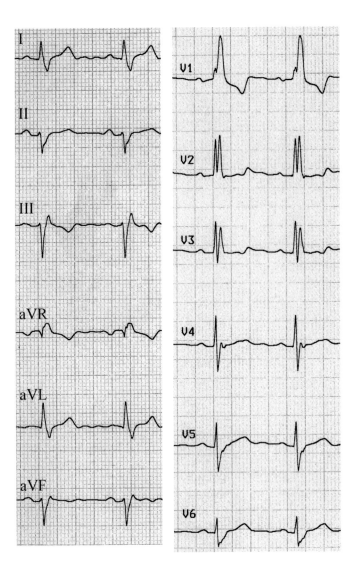

ECG 11.5
**67 y/m. No history for CHD. Echo within normal limits.
ECG: RBBB with or without associated LAFB (see text
section ECG).**

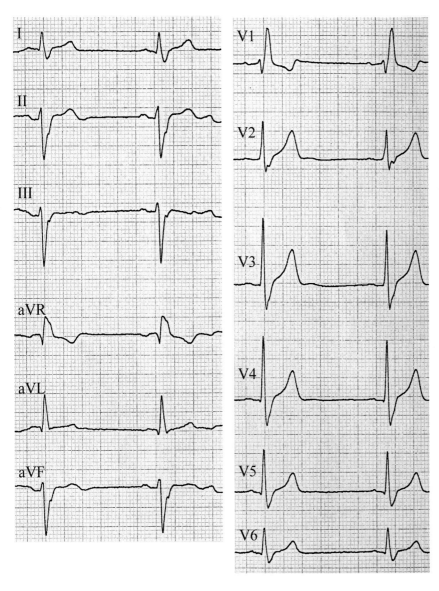

ECG 11.6

50 y/m. Hypertension. Echo: LV mass at upper normal limit. ECG: bilateral block with q waves in leads V$_4$ to V$_6$. RBBB with rsR' in V$_1$. Frontal left-axis deviation. Relative broad S wave in I, but small s wave in aVL. Small q waves in leads V$_4$ to V$_6$.

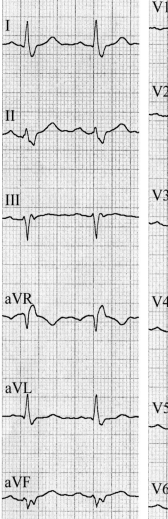
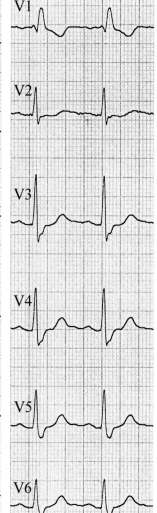

ECG 11.7 ▲

64 y/m. No history for CHD. ECG: probably isolated RBBB, with rsR' in V$_1$. Borderline QRS frontal left-axis deviation (first 0.07 sec about - 30°). Broad S waves in I and aVL. Rs complex in V$_5$/V$_6$.

ECG 11.8 ▶

72 y/m. Surgical problem. No pulmonary disease. No history of CHD or hypertension (Lenègre disease?). No syncope hitherto. Echo: normal LV function. ECG: RBBB + LPFB + AV block 1° (incomplete trifascicular block). RBBB with notched R wave in V$_1$. Frontal vertical axis of the first 60 msec of QRS. Slurred R downstroke with consequent smaller s wave in lead V$_6$. The notching/slurring in leads III/aVF are probably due to RBBB and not due to LPFB. Follow-up: in an ambulatory ECG two episodes of AV block 2:1. The patient received a pacemaker and developed complete AV block 4 months later.

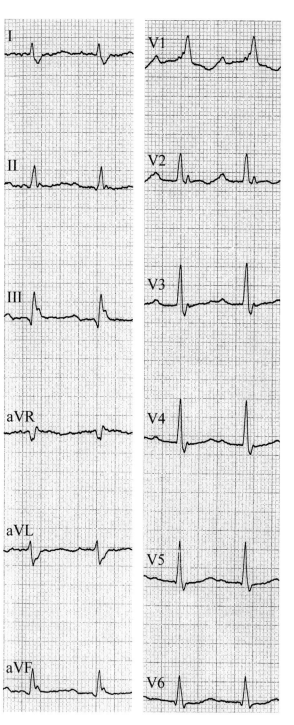

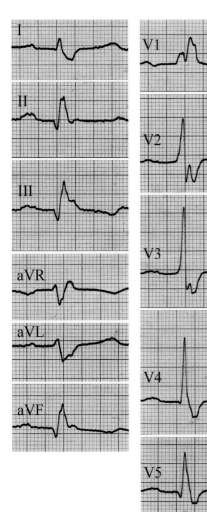

ECG 11.9

72 y/m. 1-year-old inferoposterior (lateral) MI. ECG (50 mm/sec!): RBBB + LPFB. RBBB with notched R wave in V$_1$. *Note* **the broad first portion of the R wave, and the tall R waves in V$_2$/V$_3$, caused by posterior MI. Frontal vertical axis of the first 0.06 sec of QRS. The fine** *first* **slurring of the R downstroke in III and aVF is caused by LPFB. Also slurred R downstroke in V$_5$/V$_6$, with reduction of S duration.** *Note* **that the S wave gets smaller from V$_2$ to V$_6$ (not** *broader* **as in isolated RBBB). The q waves in III/aVF/V$_6$ are somewhat striking, but do not exceed 25 msec (paper speed 50 mm/sec).**

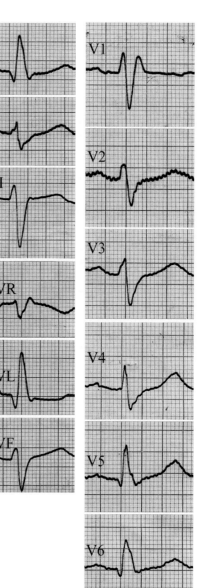

ECG 11.10
73 y/m. Short Story/Case Report 1. ECG (50 mm/sec!): RBBB + LAFB + LPFB, without complete AV block. RBBB with rSr' in V$_1$ (rsR' in another ECG of the same patient, not shown here). Frontal axis of the first 0.06 sec of QRS about - 30°. Slurred R downstroke in leads I/aVL *and* V$_5$/V$_6$, with consecutive reduction of s wave duration. The PQ interval is not prolonged.

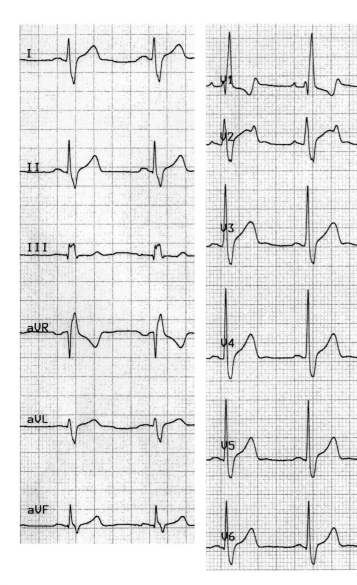

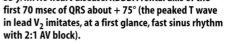

ECG 11.11
33 y/m. No heart disease. RBBB. Frontal axis of the first 70 msec of QRS about + 75° (the peaked T wave in lead V$_2$ imitates, at a first glance, fast sinus rhythm with 2:1 AV block).

Chapter 12
Atrioventricular Block and Atrioventricular Dissociation

At a Glance

Atrioventricular (AV) block is not only linked to some important electropathophysiologic mechanisms such as conduction slowing and escape rhythm, but also to typical ECG patterns such as Wenckebach period or Mobitz block, and to other potential precursors of complete AV block such as fascicular blocks and their combinations. All in all, AV block in its various degrees is of great clinical importance.

Principally a 'conduction block' represents a prolongation of conduction time and not necessarily an absolute and fixed conduction block. Therefore, any conduction block (bundle-branch, fascicular, sinoatrial, or AV block) may be a variable condition, which may be reversible under some circumstances.

AV dissociation represents a complex term and its significance depends on several conditions.

ECG

1 Anatomic Localization of AV Block

This is illustrated in Figure 12.1. Anatomically, AV block is localized:

i.   either within the AV node or in the upper part of the His bundle (a *supra-His* block)
ii. or it is localized within the infra-hissian fascicles of the right and left ventricle (right bundle branch, left anterior and posterior (and 'medial') fascicle) or within the lower part of the His bundle where it spreads into the fascicles (an *infra-His* block).

2 Degrees of AV Block

AV block is divided into three categories:

i.   in AV block 1° every atrial impulse is conducted to the ventricles, with a prolonged PQ interval
ii. in AV block 2° (subdivided into three different types) there is a *change* of conduction and complete AV block of the atrial impulses
iii. in AV block 3° (complete AV block) *all* atrial impulses are AV blocked. The actions of the atria and the ventricles occur absolutely independently from each other. If no (AV nodal or ventricular) escape rhythm arises, ventricular *asystole* occurs.

2.1 AV block 1°

Defined by PQ interval > 0.20 sec (ECG 12.1). Isolated AV block 1° does not represent a block but a prolonged AV conduction; it is mostly harmless, generally showing little or no progression over years or decades. It is also found in healthy individuals or may be due to digitalis and other drugs.

The prolongation of the AV conduction generally occurs in the AV node ('supra-His').

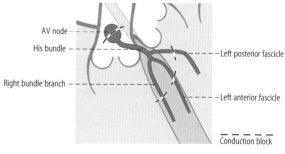

Figure 12.1
Anatomical localization of AV block. Supra-His versus infra-His

2.2 AV block 2°

2.2.1 AV block 2° Type Wenckebach

This type is characterized by an increasing PQ interval, *up to one* completely AV blocked atrial impulse, resulting in a short ventricular pause (ECG 12.2). This behavior is often repetitive. This 'Wenckebach period' generally includes three to four atrial impulses (p waves). Like AV block 1°, AV block 2° type Wenckebach (Figure 12.1) occurs *within* the AV node (supra-His) and is harmless in most cases. It may progress to complete AV block in inferior acute myocardial infarction and digitalis excess.

2.2.2 AV block 2° Type Mobitz

This type is characterized by *intermittent* and *sudden* complete AV block of one (or more) atrial impulses, often without an escape beat or escape rhythm for one or more cycles. There is *no increase* of the (often normal) PQ interval before the ventricular pause. In the conducted beats, a bundle-branch block or a bilateral bundle-branch block is present in most cases (ECG 12.3). AV block 2° of the Mobitz type represents an immediate precursor of chronic complete AV block and is therefore dangerous. ECGs 12.4 and 12.5 illustrate that in Mobitz block an escape rhythm may fail for some seconds or longer.

The block occurs *distal* to the His bundle in most cases (infra-His, Figure 12.1). Patients with Mobitz block (and preexisting bundle-branch block) have often had or will soon suffer from syncope. Thus, a true Mobitz block is a clear indication for a pacemaker (as distinct from 'pseudo-Mobitz' as discussed in section 5.2.2a The Full Picture).

2.2.3 AV block 2° Type Advanced

This type is also called 'high degree'. Both terms are somewhat misleading because this type of AV block 2° is generally far removed from complete AV block, in contrast to the Mobitz type.

As for the Wenckebach type, there is a *periodic change* between conducted and completely AV blocked atrial impulses. The block occurs in the manner of a 2 : 1 or 3 : 1 AV block (up to about 8 : 1, especially in atrial flutter) usually with a constant and normal PQ interval (ECG 12.6). In AV block 2 : 1 every second atrial impulse is completely AV blocked and one impulse is conducted. In AV block 3 : 1 two of three atrial impulses are completely AV blocked and one impulse is conducted, and so on.

In general AV block 2° of the advanced type is localized *supra-His*; the conducted beats do not show a bundle-branch

block. Progression to complete AV block is uncommon in cases without bundle-branch block (exceptions are inferior acute myocardial infarction, digitalis excess, and certain rare conditions). The significance of the block type usually depends on the rate of atrial rhythm and the number of AV blocked beats. A sinus rhythm at a rate of 90/min and a 3 : 1 AV block result in a ventricular bradycardia of 30/min and impaired hemodynamics. In cases with bundle-branch block (ECG 12.7) the progression to complete AV block is more frequent. In atrial flutter the usual 2 : 1 AV block is beneficial, inhibiting an excessive ventricular rate. A 2 : 1 AV block can also be interpreted as the *shortest possible* Wenckebach period. In some cases of atrial flutter, the interval between the flutter waves and the QRS complex may be irregular, due to superimposed Wenckebach phenomena.

2.3 Complete AV Block

This occurs when the conduction between atria and ventricles is completely blocked. The atria follow an atrial rhythm (mostly sinus rhythm) and the ventricles, completely independently, follow an AV nodal or ventricular escape rhythm. If the escape rhythm does not arise, *ventricular asystole* occurs. The symptoms depend on the duration of asystole. An asystole lasting 3–6 sec leads to dizziness and presyncope; an asystole of > 6 sec leads to syncope. In patients with preexisting impairment of cerebral circulation, an asystole of 3–4 sec may provoke a syncope.

A syncope due to *cardiac arrhythmia* is called a Morgagni-Adams-Stokes attack (MAS attack). If asystole lasts more than about 4–7 min, irreversible organic damage results (especially cerebral). Longer ventricular asystole leads to death, sometimes provoked by secondary ventricular fibrillation.

2.4 Types of Complete AV Block

As mentioned before, there are *two* types of complete AV block, which differ in evolution, etiology, and clinical significance.

2.4.1 Infra-His Complete AV Block

This AV block is localized *distal* to the His bundle (infra-His), within the ventricular fascicles and bundles respectively (Figure 12.1). Thus, fascicular blocks, bundle-branch blocks and bilateral bundle-branch blocks represent 'precursors' of infra-His complete AV block (Figure 12.2). The transition from AV block 2° to complete AV block often occurs as the *Mobitz* type.

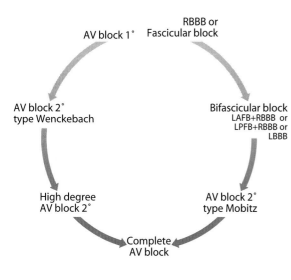

Figure 12.2
Common development to complete supra-His AV block (left side) and to complete infra-His AV block (right side)

The rate of the ventricular escape rhythm is low at 10–45/min, generally about 40/min (ECG 12.8) and is not increased during exercise. Thus, hemodynamics are moderately to severely impaired. Moreover, the ventricular *escape rhythm* is not reliable in many cases and episodes of asystole are frequent.

The etiology is predominantly coronary artery disease (CAD) and idiopathic fibrosis of the infra-His conduction system (Morbus Lenègre). Infra-His complete AV block is more frequent than supra-His complete AV block and is generally irreversible.

2.4.2 Supra-His Complete AV Block

This AV block is localized *proximal* to the His bundle (supra-His) in the region of the AV node (Figure 12.1). The precursors of supra-His complete AV block are AV block 1° and two types of AV block 2°, namely the Wenckebach and *advanced* types (Figure 12.2; ECG 12.9). Because the AV junctional escape rhythm is often reliable and the rate is 45–65/min, episodes of asystole are quite rare and hemodynamics are only modestly impaired. At exercise, the rate of the escape rhythm may be accelerated up to 100/min or more. Supra-His complete AV block is most frequently encountered in inferior acute myocardial infarction (AMI) (ECG 12.10), in about 8% of people with this condition. In > 90% of these, complete AV block is

reversible within hours, days or a week. A temporary pacemaker may be needed. AV block is also reversible in digitalis intoxication (after digitalis withdrawal), usually after several days. Other rare etiologies of supra-His block include congenital heart disease (with irreversible block) and infections of the heart.

Today there is a general agreement that, principally, *every* patient with chronic complete AV block of infra-His or supra-His localization should be treated with a pacemaker.

3 AV Dissociation

The term 'AV dissociation' is used on one hand as a *general* term and on the other as a *special* term. The general term includes complete AV block and the special types of AV dissociation. The *special* term is only applied to the three special forms of AV dissociation. The so-called 'AV dissociation in ventricular tachycardia' (corresponding to functional complete AV block) is discussed in section 6.1.3 in The Full Picture.

In the three special forms of AV dissociation the AV conduction system is *not* affected by a disease. Because impulse formation occurs in two centers (one in the sinus node, the other in the AV junction) almost concurrently, each impulse only penetrates the AV conduction system. Complete conduction is inhibited by the other impulse, arriving from the opposite site. Thus, only a *secondary, functional* AV block is present. The ventricles follow an AV junctional center, whereas the atria are activated by the sinus node. However, in contrast to complete AV block, there is a strong *temporal* connection between the two centers.

The subdivision into three types is more or less arbitrary. All three forms of special AV dissociation are basically characterized by the same ECG pattern. The p waves are 'wandering' through the QRS complexes, sometimes appearing immediately before or after the QRS, and often hidden within the QRS (ECGs 12.11 and 12.12). The rate of the AV junction rhythm and the sinus rate only differ in small limits; over a longer episode the rate of the two centers is the same. In contrast, in *complete* AV block, the p waves are 'wandering' through full heart cycles, due to the higher rate of the sinus impulses compared to the rate of the independent AV junctional or ventricular escape rhythm.

3.1 Three Types of AV Dissociation

3.1.1 AV Dissociation with Accrochage

The AV dissociation occurs only for some beats.

3.1.2 Isorhythmic AV Dissociation

The AV dissociation lasts for minutes, and very occasionally for hours.

3.1.3 AV Dissociation with Interference

Otherwise known as 'interference AV dissociation', the AV dissociation is interrupted from time to time by conducted sinus beats – so-called 'ventricular captures'.

The special forms of AV dissociation are mostly seen in healthy individuals, especially during sleep, and in athletes, and are harmless in these cases. In patients after recent heart operations or other interventions, AV dissociation may occasionally provoke a fall of blood pressure, due to the atrial contraction against the closed tricuspid valve. The rarest type, AV dissociation with interference, is occasionally observed in organic heart disease and/or digitalis intoxication.

The Full Picture

Even experienced ECG readers may have trouble differentiating between complete AV block and AV dissociation.

4 Nomenclature and its Implications

4.1 Differences Between Complete AV Block and AV Dissociation

There is some confusion about the term 'AV dissociation' in general, and in respect to AV block. The reason is based on the fact that the term AV dissociation is used both as a *general* term and as a *special* term. Table 12.1 illustrates this clearly. As a general term, AV dissociation includes complete AV block and the three special forms of AV dissociation. For the description of these three forms, AV dissociation is used as special term. It is essential to understand that AV dissociation in complete AV block, and AV dissociation in the three forms of special AV dissociation are completely different, with respect to their pathophysiology, their manifestation in the ECG, and their clinical significance.

Table 12.1
AV dissociation as a 'general' term and as a 'special' term

AV dissociation	
Complete AV block	Three types of special AV dissociation:
	1. AV dissociation with accrochage
	2. Isorhythmic AV dissociation
	3. AV dissociation with interference

4.2 Pathophysiology and the ECG

In complete AV block, AV dissociation is complete. There is absolutely no connection between the atrial (mostly sinus) rhythm and the slower escape rhythm that originates from the AV junction or from one of the ventricles. The connection between the atria and the ventricles is interrupted by organic lesions and generally remains *irreversible* (exceptions include inferior AMI and digitalis intoxication).

The three forms of special AV dissociation (details are given in section 6.1) represent functional, intermittent and *reversible* arrhythmias. In general there is also complete AV dissociation, but the two impulse centers – one in the sinus node and the other in the AV junction – are in close temporal connection. The mechanism of the phenomenon is not completely understood. Several mechanisms have been discussed, such as the relative discharge of the dominant and subsidiary pacemaker, baroreceptor reflex mechanisms, the chronotropic response to sinoatrial stretch, and the responsiveness of the sinus node to accelerating forces [1]. Based on the older concept, AV dissociation depends on the *electrotonus* – the electric field in the body – which is produced by the electrical activity of the heart. Electric discharge of the sinus node induces, over the electrotonus, the discharge of the AV junction region, *without* using the AV conduction system. Similarly, by electrotonus, electrical discharge of the AV junction induces discharge of the sinus node. The transmission of the electrical signal by the electrotonus occurs much more rapidly than, under normal conditions, the conduction of the electric impulse over the conduction system. Thus, there is a strong time connection between the two pacemakers, and their rates differ only within narrow limits. This explains why in all three special forms of AV dissociation the p waves are 'dancing' around the QRS complexes, appearing sometimes immediately before or after the QRS, or hidden within the QRS. In special AV dissociation, AV conduction is principally preserved. However, the normal AV conduction pathway *cannot* be used, because the sinus node and the AV junction center discharge at about the same time, so that each stimulus inhibits the conduction of the other, antegradely or retrogradely. This behavior is called '*functional* complete AV block due to AV dissociation'. The atria are stimulated by the sinus node, the ventricles by the AV junction center.

In complete AV block, the p waves, with their higher rate, 'wander' through the heart cycles. In special AV dissociation, the p waves are always in close proximity of the QRS complex, or are hidden within the QRS. The sinus rhythm and the AV junction rhythm have the same rate per minute.

Last but not least, AV dissociation occurs only in bradycardia, mostly in sinus bradycardia or sinus rhythm at a rate up to 75/min. One exception is AV dissociation in ventricular tachycardia – a special condition discussed in section 6.1.3 below.

4.3 Clinical Significance

Complete AV block is a severe conduction disturbance with hemodynamic and often life-threatening consequences. The clinical significance of *special* AV dissociation is based on the underlying rhythm disorder (mostly sinus bradycardia) and the basic heart disease (usually absent). It is generally a *harmless, intermittent* phenomenon that occurs mainly in *normal* individuals. Special AV dissociation is rarely associated with manifestations of the sick sinus syndrome, such as sinoatrial (SA) block or intermittent sinus arrest. Only in this combination can AV dissociation, as a secondary phenomenon, induce severe hemodynamic complications or syncope. In postoperative patients, AV dissociation occasionally provokes a fall in blood pressure and may require atrial pacing. The rarest form, 'AV dissociation with interference', may be associated with severe heart disease or digitalis intoxication.

ECG Special

5 Atrioventricular Block

AV block is divided into three degrees, in AV block 1°, in AV block 2° with its three types and in AV block 3° (complete AV block).

5.1 AV Block 1°

In AV block 1° the PQ time (PQ interval) is > 0.20 sec. Although there is some relation to sinus rate (longer PQ interval in bradycardia, shorter PQ interval in tachycardia), this definition is used for all rates, in practice. AV block 1° does not provoke an arrhythmia (of course) and generally has no influence on hemodynamics. In rare cases, the PQ interval may reach 0.7 sec. AV block is usually harmless and has a good prognosis. Mymin et al [2] conducted a 30-year follow-up study of 3983 healthy members of the Royal Canadian Air Force; they found 52 individuals (at the beginning) and 124 (at the end) with AV block 1°, about 70% with a PQ interval of < 0.23 sec. Only two individuals showed progression to AV block 2°. AV block 1° is found in about 6% of healthy people, also in athletes, and in some cases may be induced by drugs such as digitalis, verapamil, or beta-blockers.

5.1.1 Hemodynamics in AV Block 1°

Recently it has been stated that AV block 1° may considerably impair cardiac output. Indeed, Barold [3] produced an article entitled: 'Indications for permanent cardiac pacing in first-degree AV block: class I, II or III?' Indeed, a double-chamber pacemaker, with a relatively short AV interval, may improve cardiac output in selected patients, especially in those with mitral incompetence and moderate heart failure. However, pacemaker implantation for isolated AV block 1° remains a rare procedure. Temporary AV sequential pacing is occasionally used during the first days after heart operations because of AV rhythm with retrograde atrial activation or isorhythmic AV dissociation, conditions that may really impair cardiac output and arterial pressure.

5.2 AV block 2°

In AV block 1° *every* atrial impulse is conducted to the ventricles; in complete AV block (AV block 3°) *no* impulses are conducted from the atria to the ventricles. AV block 2° is characterized by the *change* between AV-conducted and AV-blocked atrial impulses.

The three types differ:

i.   in the mode of conducted/nonconducted beats
ii. in the anatomic localization of the block (with overlaps) and
iii. in clinical significance and prognosis.

5.2.1 AV Block 2° Type Wenckebach

This type is characterized by an increasing PQ interval (increasing AV block 1°), up to a single completely AV blocked supraventricular impulse, resulting in a single ventricular pause (ECG 12.2). The same mechanism (Wenckebach period) is repeated one or more times. The first beat of the period often already shows some prolongation of the PQ time (AV block 1°). The increment of the increasing PQ time gets shorter in *typical* Wenckebach, and therefore the R–R interval decreases, up to the ventricular pause. In *atypical* Wenckebach (which in fact occurs in about 50% of cases), the increment of PQ prolongation remains constant, or it increases. Here the R–R interval remains constant or increases.

In more than 90% of Wenckebach type blocks, the AV block 2° is localized supra-His, which means *proximal* to the His bundle or in the *upper* part of the His bundle, mostly in the AV node. Wenckebach block is harmless in nearly all cases and can be found in healthy young people, especially in athletes (under enhanced vagal tone), and during the night. Progression to complete AV block is seen in association with inferior AMI and digitalis intoxication, and sometimes in hyperthyreosis, sarcoidosis, and in infections like borreliosis.

5.2.1a Infra-His AV Block 2° Type Wenckebach

This condition is rare [4].

5.2.1b Atypical Forms of AV Block 2° Type Wenckebach

'Wenckebach behavior' is only typical in about 50% of cases, with an increasingly prolonged PQ interval, up to the pause; decreasing increment of PQ prolongation, with the consequence of decreasing R–R intervals in the conducted beats.

Atypical forms:

i.   The PQ interval does not increase before the pause (equal to Mobitz block). However, the PQ interval in the first beat *after* the ventricular pause is *shorter* (ECG 12.13). Usually the conducted beats show AV block 1° and the QRS are small (in contrast to Mobitz block). In a Holter ECG of such a patient we often also find 'typical Wenckebach behavior'.

If the conducted beats show a wide QRS (bundle-branch block), Mobitz block cannot be excluded. Thus the first QRS after the pause can be interpreted as a (ventricular) escape beat, although this is a rare condition in Mobitz block. In cases of doubt, differentiating between (harmless) atypical Wenckebach and (dangerous) Mobitz should be based on electrophysiologic study, always taking into consideration the clinical findings.

ii. The increment of the PQ prolongation is *increasing*. Consequently, the R–R interval increases also. This type may be harmless or may indicate some higher degree of AV block 2°.
iii. In rare cases, the Wenckebach period is interrupted by a *supraventricular* (AV junctional) escape beat during the expected ventricular pause or before restart of the next period (ECG 12.14). The Wenckebach period thus remains incomplete.

5.2.2 AV Block 2° Type Mobitz

This type is characterized by a sudden and unexpected complete block of AV conduction, for one or more heart cycles, *without* previous increasing prolongation of the PQ interval. In the conducted beats AV block 1° is often lacking. Mobitz type of AV block 2° is localized very proximally within the three (or four, or more) ventricular *fascicles* (right bundle branch + left anterior fascicle + left posterior fascicle (+ left 'medial' fascicle)), generally within the lower part of the His bundle. The block is called *infra-His*. Usually the nonblocked beats show a bundle-branch block or bilateral bundle-branch block, as indicators for a disease of the infra-hissian conduction system (ECGs 12.3–12.5). The Mobitz type is dangerous because it represents an immediate precursor of *permanent complete* AV block. Moreover, Mobitz type represents an unstable condition because at the 'beginning' of complete AV block, episodes of conducted beats and complete AV block may change abruptly. This initial phase of complete AV block is especially dangerous because the escape rhythm is even less reliable than in chronic complete AV block.

In conclusion, a typical Mobitz block represents an indication for a pacemaker. In practice, the transition from bifascicular or incomplete trifascicular block into complete AV block can only rarely be documented by an ECG.

5.2.2a Pseudo-Mobitz Block

As mentioned before, one form of 'atypical Wenckebach' (constant PQ interval before the pause and shorter PQ interval after) may be misinterpreted as Mobitz block. An ECG pattern formally identical to that of Mobitz block occurs in the intensive care unit, especially in the early postoperative period. The phenomenon is due to enhanced vagal tone and *always* coincides with a decrease in sinus rate [5], a condition that is not seen in true Mobitz. Moreover pseudo-Mobitz occurs supra-His. Therefore the conducted beats show a narrow (normal) QRS complex.

Pseudo-Mobitz episodes are not infrequently encountered in patients of any age during the first days after an operation (ECG 12.15). The AV block is supra-His, often without AV junction escape beats. In general there is a strong correlation with incidences such as vomiting or maneuvers that enhance vagal tone. Most often the episodes of ventricular asystole are asymptomatic (the ventricular asystole lasting only a few seconds), and during normal rhythm we find no bundle-branch block or fascicular block.

These pseudo-Mobitz episodes disappear after atropine therapy, or spontaneously, and do not need a pacemaker.

5.2.3 AV Block 2° Type Advanced (High Degree)

This type of AV block 2° is characterized by periodical change of AV conduction and complete AV block. In most cases we find a constant 2 : 1 AV block, that means that one supraventricular impulse is *alternately* conducted and completely AV blocked. AV blocks of 3 : 1 or 4 : 1 or higher (e.g. 6 : 1) are also possible. The advanced type is localized proximal to the His bundle more often than it is localized distally. The conducted beats may show AV block 1° or they may not.

It is now generally acknowledged that the advanced type may show Wenckebach behavior or Mobitz behavior. Wenckebach behavior is the more common, where there is no tendency to develop complete AV block. The 2 : 1 AV block may be interpreted as the shortest possible Wenckebach period: the PQ time of the second supraventricular atrial impulse (in this short Wenckebach period of only two beats) greatly increases for one beat so that one ventricular beat is missed. In atrial flutter the 2 : 1 degree (or higher) of AV block inhibits an excessively high ventricular rate and is therefore beneficial in this case.

The more rare Mobitz behavior may lead suddenly to longer episodes of complete AV block or to chronic complete AV block with the danger of ventricular asystole.

In some cases with changing 2 : 1 and 3 : 1 (or 4 : 1) AV blocks, the interval between the p wave or the flutter wave and the following QRS complex is variable. This is due to a superimposed Wenckebach phenomenon, resulting in the *combination* of AV block 2° advanced type with AV block Wenckebach type. ECG 12.16 shows an example of a patient with atrial flutter. This illustrates that these two types of block generally belong close together.

The combination of AV block 2° advanced type *with* AV block Mobitz type is less common and occurs only rarely in cases with AV block 2° advanced type with 'Mobitz behavior' (mentioned above). ECGs 12.17a–b show examples of this, with pre-existing bilateral bundle-branch block.

Note that in some publications, AV block 2° of advanced type is mixed up with (or incorporated into) AV block 2° of the Mobitz type.

5.2.3a Pseudo 2 : 1 AV Block

Sometimes an alteration of the T wave, that mimics a p wave, may suggest an AV block 2:1, at a first glance (ECG 12.18). A careful analysis of the ECG allows the correct diagnosis.

5.3 AV Block 3°

AV block 3° and complete AV block are *identical* and represent a severe conduction disturbance, in which the conduction from the atrial stimulus to the ventricles is completely interrupted. The atria follow an atrial, mostly sinusal rhythm, but the ventricles (completely *independent* from the atrial rhythm) follow an AV nodal or ventricular escape rhythm at a *lower* rate. The site of the block may be at anatomically different levels (Figure 12.1).

The site may be located proximal to the His bundle (supra-His), in the AV junction region. In this form, the escape rhythm (with a rate of 45–60/min) is localized just *distal* to the blocked area, in the *lower* part of the AV junction.

The other localization is distal to the His bundle (infra-His) and is due to the combination of conduction blocks in all three intraventricular fascicles: right bundle branch + left anterior fascicle + left posterior fascicle. The escape rhythm arises distal to the blocked fascicles, in a more *peripheral* part of a fascicle, in the right or left *ventricle*. The rate of the ventricular escape rhythm is markedly *lower* than that of an AV junction rhythm, generally about 40/min; in some patients the rate is down to 20/min or lower.

Short Story/Case Report 1

In 1980 a 72-year-old patient came on foot to our department of cardiology. The author met him at reception, where he was sitting on a stool. He told the author that he had had vertigo for several days and near syncope on the way to the hospital. The author felt his wrist for a pulse but found none...finally there was a beat...and after 4 seconds there was another...after 4 seconds another...and so on. The rate was about 15/min. The ECG revealed complete AV block with a ventricular escape rhythm of 16/min. The patient was informed about the possibility of therapy with a pacemaker and he agreed to immediate implantation. During the intervention he complained several times about vertigo that regularly disappeared with coughing. Each cough produced a beautiful spike of the arterial pressure (ECG 12.19 with simultaneous arterial pressure). After the implantation of a ventricular inhibited pacemaker the patient was enthusiastic about his pulse rate of 70/min and insisted on going home on foot, as it was only a 20–minute walk. He argued that he had walked to the hospital with a heart rate of 16 beats/min, and walking home with a rate of 70/min would be much easier. Furthermore, he wanted to surprise his wife with the pacemaker. A young colleague followed him home (unnoticed). During the next week the patient came to the hospital twice for pacemaker and wound control, walking each time of course.

Complete AV block is clinically important and often dangerous for two reasons:

i. If the rate of the escape rhythm is very low, hemodynamic consequences may lead to symptoms such as impaired work capacity, general malaise, or heart failure. This is especially true for a *ventricular* escape rhythm (in infra-His block) that has a primary low rate and does not respond to sympathetic stimulation.

ii. If the escape rhythm does not emerge, or shows intermittent failures, ventricular *asystole* occurs. Asystole for a few seconds may be without symptoms or may lead to dizziness or presyncope. Asystole lasting more than 5–7 sec leads to loss of consciousness and the patient suffers from a Morgagni-Adams-Stokes attack [6–8]. Again an *infra-His* block is far more dangerous than a supra-His block, because a ventricular escape rhythm is not as reliable as an AV junctional escape rhythm. Thus, ventricular asystole occurs much more frequently in complete AV block that is localized distal to the His bundle. Ventricular asystole may last for minutes and leads to death caused by persistent asystole or secondary ventricular fibrillation. Moreover, infra-His AV block is generally a chronic disorder, whereas supra-His block is often reversible (as in the case of inferior AMI or in treated digitalis intoxication).

5.3.1 Simultaneous Supra-His AV Block and Bundle-Branch Block

Occasionally complete supra-His AV block is combined with a bundle-branch block. In these cases a ventricular escape rhythm can be excluded on the basis of a rate of about 60/min (AV junctional escape rhythm) and the typical pattern of bundle branch aberration. ECGs 12.20 and 12.21 show two examples.

5.3.2 AV Blocked Atrial Premature Beats

This arrhythmia is especially encountered in Holter ECGs. If an atrial premature beat occurs very early and falls into the refractory period of AV conduction, it is completely AV blocked. In the ECG the p wave is visible as a 'notch' at the end of the T wave, or is hidden within the apex of the T wave, which is peaked in this case (ECG 12.22). The next sinus beat occurs after the usual postextrasystolic pause. The arrhythmia may be misinterpreted as an SA block, especially in cases of bigeminy. In ECG 12.23 the p waves are clearly detectable, however.

Short Story/Case Report 2

During a check-up in 1992 a 48-year-old woman told us that she had received a pacemaker implant 3 years before, in another hospital, because of two episodes of presyncope and a sick sinus syndrome. She mentioned palpitations occurring during the night especially. The ventricular inhibited pacemaker was programmed at 50/min and not pacing at rest (sinus rhythm 68/min). The exercise test was normal; echo/Doppler showed no abnormality. The Holter ECG revealed six AV blocked atrial premature beats with a consecutive ventricular pause, interrupted by one ventricular pacemaker beat. Two of these episodes were registered as discomfort by the patient. Her previous doctor kindly sent us the ECG from 1988 before pacemaker implantation. This showed some AV blocked atrial premature beats, twice in bigeminy (ECG 12.24) during six cycles; the arrhythmia had been misdiagnosed as SA block and therefore a pacemaker was implanted. We programmed the device to a rate of 30/min and the patient remained without palpitations or other symptoms. Retrospectively, the episodes of presyncope were interpreted as vagovasal during a bowel infection.

5.3.3 Development of Complete AV Block
(Also see Chapter 11 Bilateral Blocks.)

The evolution from precursors to complete AV block differs in the supra-His type and in the infra-His type (Figure 12.2).

Supra-His AV block progresses from AV block 1°, over AV block 2° Wenckebach type and over AV block 2° advanced type to complete AV block. The conduction disturbance occurs in the AV node. His bundle derivations show prolongation of the AH interval or a block between the atrium and the His region. In completely blocked beats the potential of the His bundle is lacking, because the stimulus is blocked *above* the His bundle. The ventricular escape rhythm is localized in the lower part of the AV junction and shows a normal QRS duration. If complete AV block is reversible the regression occurs in reverse order, from complete block to AV block 2° advanced type/Wenckebach type, to AV block 1°, often with final normalization of the PQ interval.

In contrast, in *Infra-His* block the first precursor is a monofascicular block: right bundle-branch block (RBBB) or left anterior fascicular block (LAFB) which develops to bifascicular (bilateral) block, mostly RBBB + LAFB or left bundle-branch block (LBBB). In this context LBBB is understood as 'unilateral bifascicular block' (LAFB + LPFB). Isolated left posterior fascicular block (LPFB) is very rare and is mostly associated with inferior infarction. The combination of RBBB + LPFB is also very rare.

Bifascicular block may be combined with additional AV block 1°, or 2° of advanced type (and very rarely with Wenckebach type). This combination is called *incomplete trifascicular block*. In this case, the prolongation of the AV time occurs within all three ventricular fascicles. In two fascicles the conduction is completely blocked and in the third fascicle there is an AV block 1° or 2° of advanced type. The His bundle derivations show a prolonged HV interval or a block distal to the His bundle. Thus the potential of the His bundle is always detectable. However, in bifascicular blocks, the PQ interval (and the HV interval) is often normal, also immediately before the development of complete AV block. In these cases, episodes of AV block 2° *Mobitz* type may occur. In Mobitz block, the conduction in the third fascicle is also completely blocked, for one or more heart cycles, inducing complete AV block. As a matter of fact – and by definition – any progression of a bifascicular block with a normal PQ time to complete AV block is based on the Mobitz phenomenon. Of all three types of AV block 2° Mobitz type is by far nearest to complete AV block. If typical Mobitz block (with unilateral or bilateral bundle-branch block during the conducted beats) is detected in an ECG, pacemaker implantation is indicated, in *most* cases.

The escape rhythm in infra-His complete AV block arises in the conduction tissue distal to the blocks, in the right or left ventricle, showing wide QRS complexes (generally QRS > 0.14 sec). The ventricular rate is low at 40/min or less.

Infra-His block is a progressive disease and complete infra-His block is never completely reversible. As mentioned before, in some patients a fluctuation between complete AV block and sinus rhythm with bilateral bundle-branch block (with or without AV block 1° or 2°) may be observed. This represents an unstable and dangerous situation because an escape rhythm is very unreliable in these cases.

The His bundle itself may be damaged during open-heart surgery, producing complete 'intra-His block'. Such a block may be reversible.

5.3.4 Etiology and Clinical Significance of Complete AV Block

5.3.4a *Supra-His*

A supra-His block is mostly encountered in inferior AMI, where it occurs in 8% [9,10] and generally persists for hours or days. It is reversible in more than 90%. Some patients need a provisional pacemaker. If complete block is irreversible a permanent pacemaker is necessary. Occasionally supra-His block is seen in digitalis intoxication [11] (Chapter 30 Digitalis Intoxication). It is also reversible after digitalis withdrawal, within days up to a week. Other rare etiologies include sarcoidosis [12,13] and infections like borreliosis [14,15], and congenital AV block [16]. More recently, special attention has been drawn to young patients with congenital supra-His complete AV block *without* other heart disease. In this subgroup the incidence of severe complications, death included, has been underestimated [17–19]. Therefore, these patients should also receive pacemakers [17,18]. Overall, in patients with permanent pacemakers implanted for complete AV block, supra-His block accounts for only about 10%.

5.3.4b *Infra-His*

Infra-His block is predominantly due to coronary heart disease (CHD) and 'fibrosis' of the infra-His conduction system (Morbus Lenègre). Rare etiologies include congenitally corrected transposition of the great arteries [20] and 'absent His bundle' [16]. For details of the variety of etiologies see Chapter 9 Fascicular Blocks.

In patients with permanent pacemakers implanted for complete AV block, infra-His block is present in 90%, a fact which clearly shows the clinical significance of this type of block. The older literature reveals a mortality rate of about 50% within 6–12 months in patients with untreated complete infra-His block.

5.3.5 His Bundle Derivations

The intracardiac derivations of the His bundle potential, first described by Puech et al in 1970 [21], have definitively made it easier to distinguish supra-His from infra-His conduction disturbances, and – at least as importantly – the differences between ventricular tachycardia and supraventricular tachycardia (SVT) with aberration. For some years, the indication for pacemaker implantation in bilateral bundle-branch block was guided by the behavior of the HV interval [22]. A prolonged HV interval was thought to be combined with a faster progression to AV block 3°. Later publications have questioned this opinion to a certain extent [23]. Today the His bundle potential is still recorded during every invasive electrophysiologic study, for many purposes. However, in practice it plays a minor role in the selection of patients for pacemaker implantation; today it is based more on the conventional ECG, Holter registration, and the symptoms.

5.3.6 ECG and Anatomical Lesions

In a series of anatomical investigations Rossi [24] showed that there is no strong correlation between the severity of (especially) infra-His conduction disturbances and the severity of anatomical damage. Relatively small and localized lesions may interrupt AV conduction completely, whereas in more severe and diffuse lesions AV conduction may be preserved or only mildly impaired.

5.3.7 Therapeutic Conclusions

It is generally accepted that all patients with *chronic* complete AV block should be treated with a permanent pacemaker, irrespective of the site of the block (infra-His or supra-His). *Why* then are there so many discussions about AV block? Recognizing the *precursors* of complete AV block allows risk stratification. Incomplete *supra*-His block does not generally develop to complete AV block. Yet there are exceptions:

i. inferior AMI
ii. digitalis intoxication (should not be overlooked in elderly patients with unperceived renal insufficiency)
iii. some cases with AV block 2° advanced type with Mobitz behavior.

In contrast, incomplete *infra*-His blocks have a long-term tendency to progress to complete AV block. The recognition of fascicular block, bilateral block and AV block 2° Mobitz type allows adequate treatment of symptomatic patients with a pacemaker *before* chronic complete AV block has developed. In practice, intermittent episodes of complete AV block can only be manifested with an ECG in about half of patients with presyncope or syncope. Bilateral bundle-branch block or Mobitz block associated with typical symptoms are sufficient for pacemaker implantation. For the differences between LAFB + RBBB and LPFB + RBBB in respect to development of AV block 3° see Chapter 11 Bilateral Blocks.

6 Special AV Dissociation

Knowledge about the existence and the mechanism of special AV dissociation is far more important than differentiation between the three different types, which are defined in a more or less arbitrary manner. In fact, they mainly differ in relation to the duration of the arrhythmia and to the presence or absence of intermittently conducted sinusal beats, along the normal AV conduction system. If not combined with SA block or intermittent sinus arrest, AV dissociation generally arises in *sinus bradycardia*, a condition in which the rate of the sinus rhythm approaches the inherent rate of the AV junctional center. Special AV dissociation between sinus bradycardia and a ventricular center is extremely rare.

Generally, three types of AV dissociation are distinguished:

i. Type 1: AV dissociation with accrochage; in this type AV dissociation occurs only for some beats.
ii. Type 2: AV dissociation with synchronization; AV dissociation is present for minutes or hours, very occasionally for days. There is no clear distinction between the two types. However in both types, the arrhythmia disappears and sinus rhythm arises after exercise (ECGs 12.25a–b) and often after a sympathomimetic drug or atropine, if the sinus rate clearly exceeds the rate of the AV center.
iii. Type 3: AV dissociation with interference (interference dissociation); this type is characterized by intermittent conduction of a sinus beat, a ventricular capture. Again, the definition is not convincing because capture beats are also observed in type 1 with accrochage. In older publications, interference dissociation has been attributed to digitalis intoxication and/or severe heart disease. In fact this type also occurs in healthy individuals.

6.1 Special Conditions in AV Dissociation

6.1.1 AV Dissociation in a Postextrasystolic Beat

AV dissociation in the beat following a (mostly ventricular) premature beat is a common feature, seen especially in Holter

ECGs. In the ECG the p wave appears immediately before the QRS complex or is hidden within the QRS. The sinusal stimulus is not conducted, the QRS is induced by a *postextrasystolic AV junctional* escape beat. Thus, this AV dissociation for one beat is due neither to a common form of special AV dissociation nor to AV block, but to almost simultaneous discharge of the sinus node (a normal discharge, however relatively late, after the premature beat) and the AV junction (escape beat after the long postextrasystolic pause).

6.1.2 Ventriculophasic Sinus Arrhythmia

In complete AV block with a 'physiologic' or 'artificial' (pacemaker-induced) escape rhythm and a regular sinus rhythm of the atria, the discharge of the sinus node is influenced for a short period by the ventricular excitation, *without* retrograde AV conduction. If the p wave occurs within about 150 msec after a QRS, it appears anticipated by 20–50 msec. It is assumed that this phenomenon, like ventriculophasic modulation of atrioventricular nodal conduction, is induced by baroreceptor-mediated phasic changes in vagal tone [25]. The arrhythmia is interesting but has no clinical importance.

6.1.3 AV Dissociation in Ventricular Tachycardia

The term 'AV dissociation' is not used here in the sense of one of the 'special forms' of AV dissociation but in the sense of a *functional* complete AV block, due to the tachycardic action of the ventricles and to retrograde, concealed (and incomplete) conduction in the AV node. In special conditions, the AV node is not refractory for a very short time and a sinusal impulse may reach and activate the ventricles. This is called 'ventricular capture' (by the sinus impulse) or 'Dressler beat'. A *fusion beat* is produced by simultaneous activation of the ventricles by the sinusal impulse and the ventricular center. Both phenomena prove the ventricular origin of a wide QRS complex tachycardia. It is useful to know that in about 40% of ventricular tachycardias there is permanent 1 : 1 retrograde atrial activation (Chapter 26 Ventricular Tachycardias).

References

1. Patel A, Pumill R, Goldman D, Damato AN. Isorhythmic atrioventricular dissociation revisited. Am Heart J 1992;124:823–9
2. Mymin D, Mathewson FA, Tate RB, Manfreda J. The natural history of primary first-degree atrioventricular heart block. N Engl J Med 1986;315:1183–7
3. Barold SS. Indications for permanent cardiac pacing in first-degree AV block: class I, II, or III? (editorial). PACE 1996;29:747–51
4. Puech P, Wainwright RJ. Clinical electrophysiology of atrioventricular block. Cardiol Clin 1983;1:209–24
5. Barold SS, Hayes DL. Second-degree atrioventricular block: a reappraisal. Mayo Clin Proc 2001;76:44–57
6. Morgagni JB. De Sedibus et Causis Morborum, second edn. Patavii, sumpt. Remondini, Venice 1761
7. Adams R. Cases of diseases of the heart, accompanied with pathological observations. Dublin Hosp Rep 1827;4:353
8. Stokes W. Observations on some cases of permanently slow pulse. Dublin J Med Sci 1846;2:73
9. Simon AB, Steinke WE, Curry JJ. Atrioventricular block in acute myocardial infarction. Chest 1972;62:156–61
10. Norris RM. Heart block in posterior and anterior myocardial infarction. Br Heart J 1969;31:352–6
11. Ma G, Brady WJ, Pollack M, Chan TC. Electrocardiographic manifestations: digitalis toxicity. J Emerg Med 2001;20:145–52
12. Fleming HA. Sarcoid heart disease and complete heart block. Sarcoidosis 1986;3:78
13. Ford PG, Jorizzo JL, Hitchkock MG. Previously undiagnosed sarcoidosis in a patient presenting with leonine facies and complete heart block. Arch Dermatol 2000;136:712–4
14. Nagi KS, Joshi R, Thakur RK. Cardiac manifestations of Lime disease: a review. Can J Cardiol 1996;12:503–6
15. McAlister HF, Klementowicz PT, Andrews C, et al. Lyme carditis: an important cause of reversible heart block. Ann Intern Med 1989;110:339–45
16. James TN. Congenital disorders of cardiac rhythm and conduction. J Cardiovasc Electrophysiol 1993;4:702–18
17. Michaelsson M, Jonzon A, Riesenfeld T. Isolated congenital complete atrioventricular block in adult life. A prospective study. Circulation 1995;92:442–9
18. Friedman RA. Congenital AV block. Pace me now or pace me later? Circulation 1995;92:283–5
19. Michaelsson M, Riesenfeld T, Jonzon A. Natural history of congenital complete atrioventricular block. Pacing Clin Electrophysiol 1997;20:2098–101
20. Connelly MS, Liu PP, Williams WG, et al. Congenitally corrected transposition of the great arteries in the adult: functional status and complications. J Am Coll Cardiol 1996;27:1238–43
21. Puech P, Grolleau R, Latour H, et al. Recording of electric activity of His bundle in spontaneous AV blocks. Arch Mal Coeur Vaiss 1970;63:784–809
22. Haft JI. The His bundle electrogram. Circulation 1973;47:897–911
23. Phibbs B, Friedman HS, Graboys TB, Lown B, et al. Indications for pacing in the treatment of bradyarrhythmias. Report of an independent study group. J Am Med Assoc 1984;252:1307–11
24. Rossi L. Trifascicular conduction system and left branch hemiblock. Anatomical and histopathological considerations. G Ital Cardiol 1971;1:55–62
25. Skanes AC, Tang AS. Ventriculophasic modulation of atrioventricular nodal conduction in humans. Circulation 1998;97:2245–51

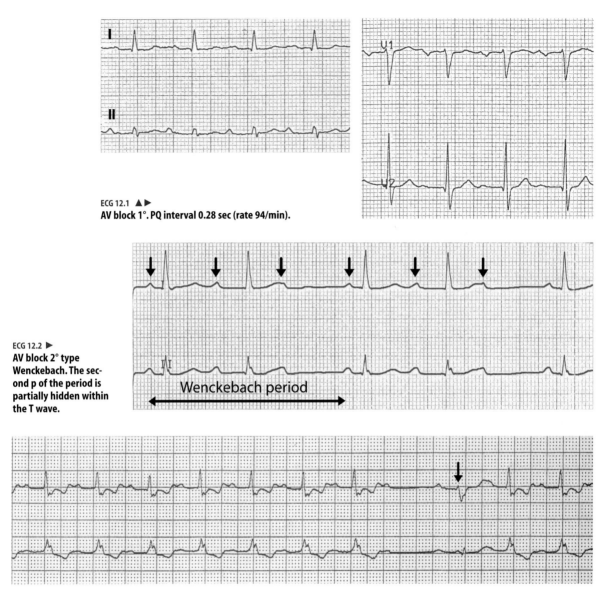

ECG 12.1 ▲ ▶
AV block 1°. PQ interval 0.28 sec (rate 94/min).

ECG 12.2 ▶
AV block 2° type Wenckebach. The second p of the period is partially hidden within the T wave.

Wenckebach period

ECG 12.3
Sinus rhythm, rate 95/min. AV block 1° (PQ 0.2 sec) and RBBB. The eighth p wave, without preceding increase of PQ interval, is completely AV blocked: AV block 2° Mobitz type. Probably the ninth p is also AV blocked and the following QRS (↓) represents a ventricular escape beat (PQ before this beat 260 msec).

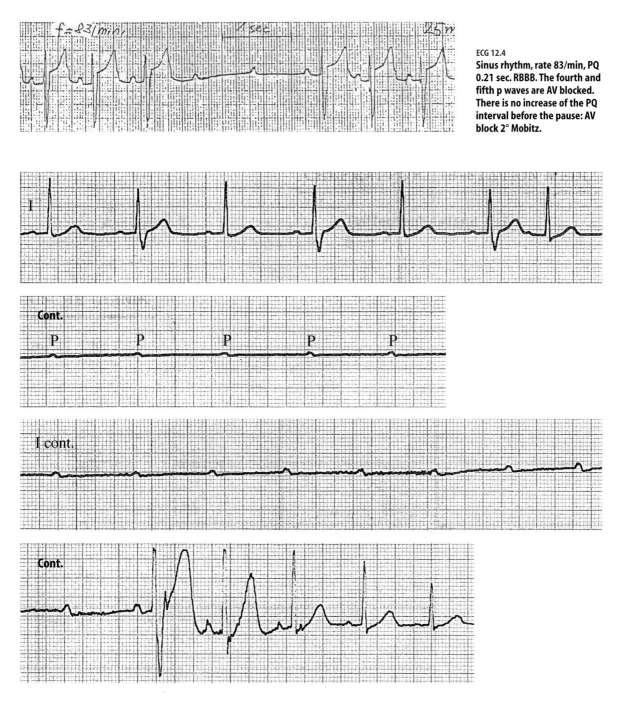

ECG 12.4
Sinus rhythm, rate 83/min, PQ 0.21 sec. RBBB. The fourth and fifth p waves are AV blocked. There is no increase of the PQ interval before the pause: AV block 2° Mobitz.

ECG 12.5
Continuous monitor stripe, showing Mobitz block. Sinus rhythm, rate 62/min. PQ 0.2 sec. Alternating RBBB. After an atrial premature beat 15 consecutive p waves are AV blocked, resulting in ventricular asystole of 13 sec. After one ventricular escape beat, sinus rhythm continues. Note: the rate of the nonconducted p waves gradually increases, due to sympathetic stimulation. The two first T waves after the pause are artificially altered.

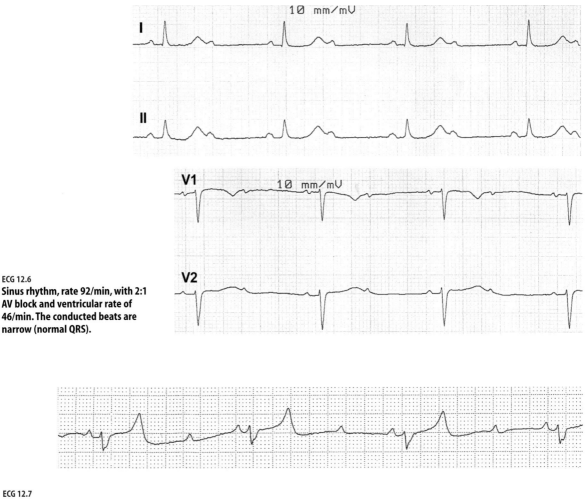

ECG 12.6
Sinus rhythm, rate 92/min, with 2:1 AV block and ventricular rate of 46/min. The conducted beats are narrow (normal QRS).

ECG 12.7
Sinus rhythm, rate 108/min, PQ normal in conducted beats. RBBB. AV block 2° 3 : 1, ventricular rate 36/min. One p wave is hidden within the apex of the T wave. The ECG changed between 2 : 1, 3 : 1 and complete AV block within minutes (not shown).

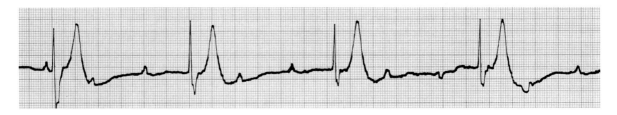

ECG 12.8
Sinus rhythm (of the atria), rate 75/min. Complete AV block with wide QRS, rate of ventricular escape rhythm 25/min.

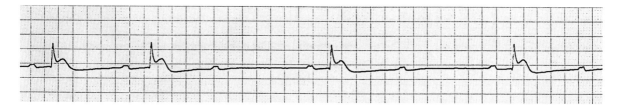

ECG 12.9
Patient with acute inferior infarction. ECG: AV block 2° Wenckebach progressing to AV block 2° 2 : 1, with a ventricular rate of 23/min.

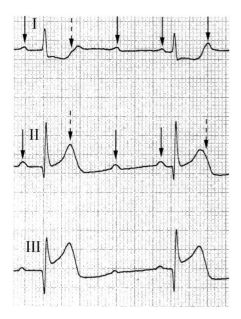

ECG 12.10
Complete AV block in acute inferior infarction (leads I, II, III). Sinus rhythm of the atria, rate 120/min (arrows: p waves). AV junctional escape rhythm, rate 44/min.

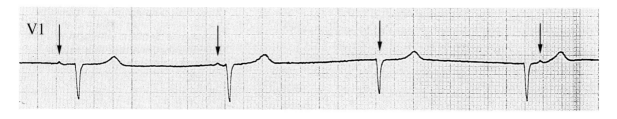

ECG 12.11
Bradycardic AV dissociation 'with accrochage', rate about 37/min. The first beat is a sinus beat, the PQ time of the second p wave is shortened, the third p is hidden within the QRS complex, the last p wave appears shortly after QRS. The 3 last QRS are AV junctional beats.

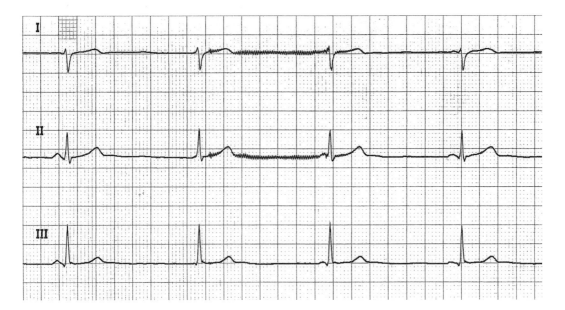

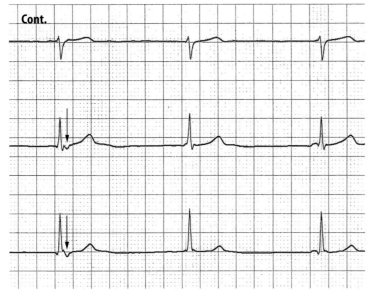

ECG 12.12
Isorhythmic AV dissociation, rate 46/min. The p waves appear shortly before or after QRS, or are hidden in the QRS. In one beat there is probably VA conduction (arrow). Note: no atrial impulse is conducted – too short a PQ interval!

ECG 12.13
'Atypical' Wenckebach. The PQ interval is constantly 0.28 sec. After the pause the PQ time is 0.25 sec for one beat.

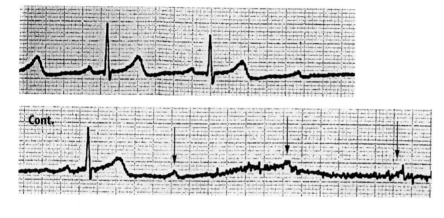

ECG 12.14
'Interrupted Wenckebach period'. Before the Wenckebach period restarts, an AV junction escape beat arises (third and sixth QRS complex).

Cont.

ECG 12.15
47 y/f. Several episodes of pseudo-Mobitz and ventricular asystole up to 4.5 sec, during the first 36 h after removal of the gall-bladder, while in the intensive care unit. Condition: nausea or vomiting. Rhythm strip: sinus bradycardia 53/min, normal QRS duration. Sudden 2:1 AV block for one cycle, then complete AV block without ventricular escape rhythm. The arrhythmias disappeared spontaneously, together with episodes of nausea. Holter ECG was normal. Like comparable cases, the patient had no cardiac complaints in the next years.

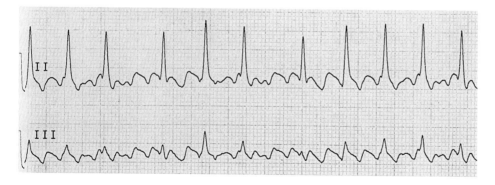

II

III

ECG 12.16
64 y/m. CAD. Paroxysmal atrial flutter. ECG: atrial flutter with irregular AV conduction. The distance between the flutter waves and the QRS complexes varies constantly. Explanation: 2:1 AV block with superimposed Wenckebach phenomenon.

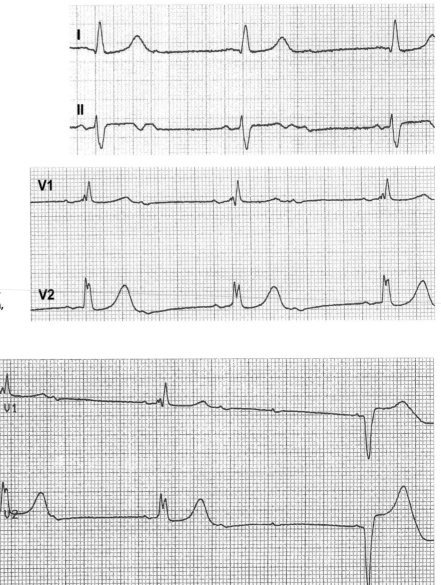

ECG 12.17a
86 y/f. CAD. Several episodes of syncope. AV block 2° 2 : 1. Sinus rhythm, rate 74/min, with RBBB and LAFB.

ECG 12.17b
Same patient. Irregular sinus node activity (additional SA block). The second QRS (and probably also the first beat, p missed) is conducted. Then two p waves are AV blocked. The last beat is a ventricular escape beat > > > progression to complete AV block.

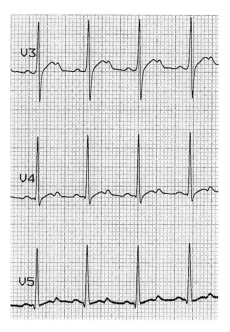

ECG 12.18

42 y/m. Guillain-Barré syndrome. Leads V₃ to V₅. ECG mimicking 2 : 1 AV block. At a first glance, an unspecific alteration of the repolarization mimics 2 : 1 AV block. However in other leads no second p wave is detectable (not shown), and the distance from p to pseudo-p is longer than the one from pseudo-p to p.

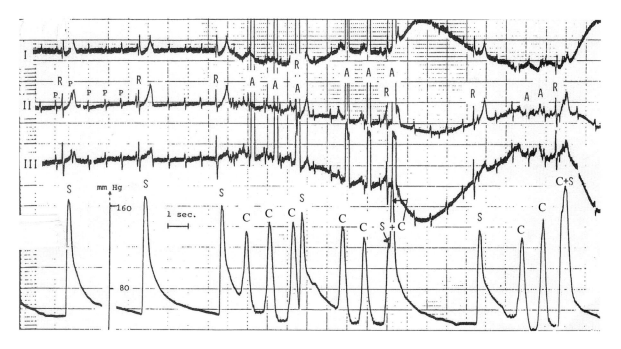

ECG 12.19

Short Story/Case Report 1. ECG leads I, II and III written with 10 mm/sec. Complete AV block with an atrial rate of 66/min and a ventricular rate (see R) of 16/min. Lower curve: arterial pressure. Note: coughing (C) induces impressive systolic pressure waves (and artifacts in the ECG (A)). S = systolic pressure induced by ventricular escape rhythm. C + S = summation of S and coughing.

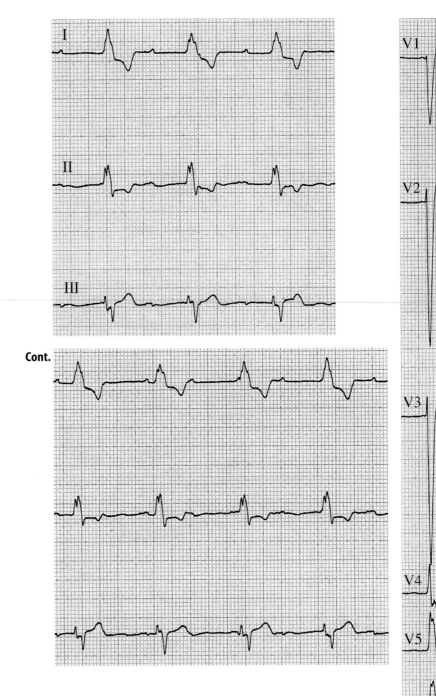

ECG 12.20

Complete AV block supra-His + LBBB aberration. Complete AV block with AV junction escape rhythm, rate 66/min. A ventricular escape rhythm can be excluded by the relatively high rate and the typical LBBB aberration pattern (leads V_1 to V_6).

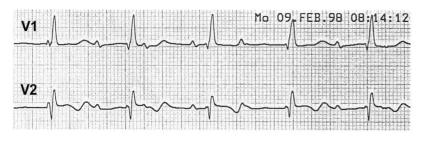

Mo 09 FEB.98 08:14:12

ECG 12.21
Complete AV block supra-His + RBBB aberration. Complete AV block with AV junction escape rhythm (rate 70/min) and RBBB aberration (see the typical rsR' configuration in V_1 and V_2).

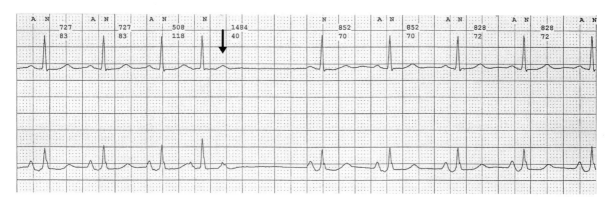

ECG 12.22
AV blocked atrial premature beat. The fourth complex is an atrial premature beat, the fifth p is AV blocked (scarcely visible in the upper Holter stripe; easily detectable in lower stripe).

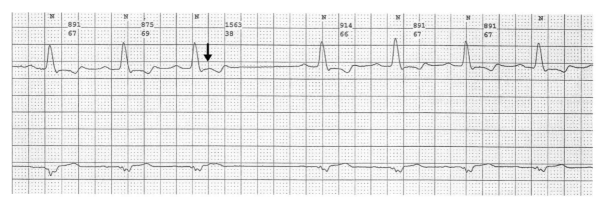

ECG 12.23
AV blocked atrial premature beat. An AV blocked p is visible, only with care, within the T wave of the third cycle, before the pause.

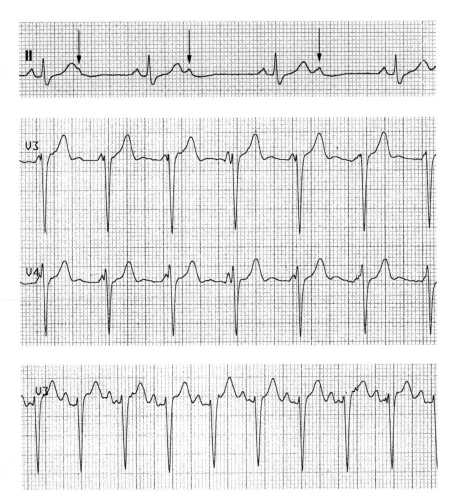

ECG 12.24
Short Story/Case Report 2. AV blocked atrial PBs in bigeminy, resulting in bradycardia of 47/min. The first blocked p wave is partially hidden within the T wave.

ECG 12.25a
56 y/m. AV dissociation at rest (rate 84/min).

ECG 12.25b
Same patient. Sinus tachycardia at exercise with 7 MET.

Chapter 13
Myocardial Infarction

At a Glance

Besides cardiac arrhythmias, myocardial infarction (MI) represents the most important subject in electrocardiography, due to the high prevalence and severity of the disease.

About 40%–50% of acute and old MIs can be recognized in the ECG by *typical* ST elevation and/or pathologic Q waves, many cases with combined infarctions or with right bundle-branch block (RBBB) included. Another 20% of MIs are detectable by *complex* ECG patterns (with bundle-branch block or fascicular blocks) and by *special* ECG patterns (e.g. the so-called 'non-Q-wave infarction' or new nonsignificant Q waves).

After the introduction of urgent percutaneous transluminal coronary angioplasty (PTCA) and fibrinolysis, the accurate diagnosis of acute MI has become more important than ever. It is therefore also necessary to recognize atypical infarction patterns and to consider the differential diagnosis of the Q wave, of the ST elevation, and of the T wave.

Etiology

More than 90% of MIs are due to atheromatous coronary arteries with consecutive thrombosis, the latter often provoked by plaque rupture. Coronary artery spasm seems to contribute to necrosis in many cases. MI may also occur as a bystander disease in conditions such as aortic dissection, connective tissue disease, cardiac trauma, tumors, cocaine abuse among others. Congenital MI (due to coronary artery anomalies) is extremely rare.

ECG

About 70% of MIs are recognizable in the ECG, based on well-defined criteria. About 30% of acute and old MIs are not recognizable in the ECG. The reasons are:

i.   small infarctions
ii. infarctions associated with left bundle-branch block (LBBB)
iii. multiple infarctions, where one infarction pattern masks the other
iv. and last, but not least, because the ECG is an *indirect method*.

It is therefore astonishing that so many MIs can be recognized in the ECG, in many cases with reliable determination of localization and stage. Often the *clinical evolution* of MI can be observed, corresponding also (like pericarditis) to an *evolution of ECG alterations*.

1   ST Vectors, Q Vectors and T Vectors

Thanks to an electropathophysiologic rule – or perhaps to a gift from God – the infarction pattern at any stage appears in the direct detecting leads, irrespective *of the pre-existing QRS configuration*, whether it is a qR complex, an rS complex, or another QRS complex. This fact very much simplifies the diagnosis of 'classical' acute and old MI.

The *injury (lesion) ST vector* points to the region of infarction, resulting in *ST elevation* (Figure 13.1a).

The *necrosis QRS vector* points in the opposite direction to the infarcted area, producing a *pathologic Q wave or QS wave* (Figure 13.1b).

Similarly, the so-called *ischemia vector* (in 'chronic ischemia') points away from the infarction zone, resulting in *negative and symmetric T waves* (Figure 13.1c). For definition of the different grades of ischemia see Chapter 1 Theoretical Basics.

2 Stages of Myocardial Infarction

Principally there are four different approaches for the description of the stage of MI (acute/subacute/old), concerning different aspects:

i. the electropathophysiologic evolution *or*
ii. the international nomenclature *or*
iii. the histopathologic evolution *or*
iv. the clinical findings and the general clinical experience.

This is a source of general confusion, because the four different approaches do not coincide in time evolution (details about the different nomenclatures for the stages are given in the section The Full Picture and in Figure 13.4).

Regarding the electrophysiologic evolution, three stages can be distinguished, each one characterized by typical alterations of repolarization and depolarization:

2.1 Acute Stage

Marked ST elevation (generally > 3 mm, up to 12 mm). This represents a *transmural lesion* (transmural injury).

2.2 Subacute Stage

Moderate ST elevation plus *Q waves or QS waves*. This represents *minor injury* and *necrosis*. The T wave is generally negative and symmetric, representing *ischemia*.

2.3 Old (Chronic) Stage

'Classical' *Q waves* (duration ≥ 0.04 sec) or *QS waves*, with isoelectric ST segment. A Q wave or QS wave due to infarction represents *necrosis*. The T wave remains negative or has normalized.

Note: For the description of the ECG examples in this book, the *international nomenclature* (that does not distinguish between acute and subacute MI) is used. However, where it is convenient and possible, the effective age of infarction is mentioned (in hours, days, months, and years).

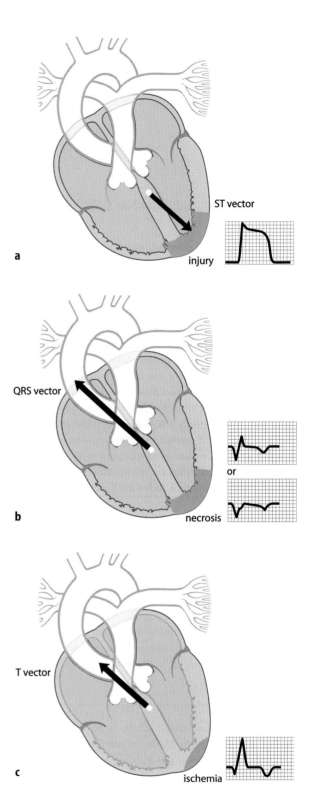

Figure 13.1 ▶
ST vector, QRS vector and T vector in myocardial infarction
a. **ST injury vector**
b. **QRS vector in necrosis**
c. **T ischemia vector**

3 Localization of Q-Wave Infarction

According to its localization, the infarction pattern manifests itself in different leads. If one considers the three-dimensional exploration of the cardiac vectors by the 12 standard ECG leads, it is easy to determine the localization. The direct ('optical') *correlation between the localization of infarction and the exploring leads* is schematically demonstrated in Figures 13.2a–13.2f, as well as the *most frequent localizations of* coronary artery obstruction, for each infarction localization. Figure 13.3 shows the nomenclature for the coronary arteries and branches.

3.1 Anteroseptal Infarction

See Figure 13.2a. As the leads V_2 and V_3 are placed over the interventricular septum (and V_4 over the apex), anteroseptal infarction will produce the typical pattern in these leads (plus in V_1), according to the infarction stage.

ECG 13.1a (ECG 13.1b after thrombolysis), ECG 13.2 and ECG 13.3 show an acute MI; ECG 13.4 is an old anteroseptal infarction involving the apex. Leads I and aVL are not influenced, because they explore anterolateral regions of the left ventricle.

3.2 Extensive Anterior (Anterolateral) Infarction

See Figure 13.2b. Anterolateral infarction includes infarction of the septum, the apex and lateral portions of the left ventricle (LV). Therefore, the infarction pattern is seen not only in the leads (V_1) V_2 to V_4 but also in lead V_5 and often V_6. In this infarction type the pattern is also detected by leads I and aVL (in the latter when the high lateral portion of the LV is involved). ECG 13.5, ECG 13.6a, ECG 13.6b and ECG 13.7 are examples of acute extensive anterior (anterolateral) MI; ECGs 13.8 and 13.9 are examples of old anterolateral infarction.

3.3 Lateral Infarction (Isolated MI of the Lateral Wall)

See Figure 13.2c. This infarction is rare in its isolated form. As the leads V_5 and V_6 directly explore the lateral wall, the typical pattern is seen in these leads. Depending on the infarct size the typical signs may also be present in leads I and aVL. In *high lateral infarction* the best direct (and sometimes the only) exploring lead is lead *aVL*. Therefore, this MI type can easily be overlooked.

ECG 13.10 shows acute high lateral and posterior MI, with ST elevation only in lead aVL and extensive 'mirror images' in other leads. ECG 13.11 shows a 4-day-old high lateral MI with a pathologic Q wave in aVL and symmetric negative T waves also in V5/V6 (in these leads there are no pathologic Q waves).

3.4 Inferior Infarction

See Figure 13.2d. According to Einthoven's triangle, the leads III (at + 120°), aVF (at + 90°) and II (at + 60°) directly reflect inferiorly oriented vectors. The pattern of inferior infarction will therefore be detected in these leads. In practice, the alterations are best seen in leads aVF and III, less distinctly in lead II. However, a Q wave also in lead II favors the diagnosis of inferior infarction, whereas in pulmonary embolism a Q wave in II is lacking.

ECGs 13.12 and 13.13 show acute inferior MI. In a substantial number of cases, acute inferior MI is associated with a 'right ventricular infarction' (see 3.6 below). ECGs 13.14 and 13.15 show an old inferior MI.

3.5 Posterior ('True' Posterior) Infarction

See Figure 13.2e. For one special reason this infarction pattern is difficult to understand. According to the definition of pathologic Q waves, and with reference only to the 12 standard ECG leads, the pattern is not a Q-wave infarction. We only see the *mirror image* of the original pattern in some of these leads. The additional posterior leads V_7, V_8 and V_9 provide the direct infarction pattern. The mirror image is seen in the anterior (anteroseptal) leads V_2 and V_3 (and sometimes V_1), consisting of an *ST depression* (instead of an ST elevation) and/or *a great and broad R wave* (instead of a broad Q wave), depending on infarction stage. In the absence of pathologic Q waves and/or ST elevation in the 12 standard leads, the possibility of infarction is often not considered. Thus, in the presence of the following alterations in *leads V_1 to V_3* the diagnosis of posterior infarction should always be confirmed or excluded with the help of leads V_7 to V_9:

i. single R wave and/or an Rs complex, with an R duration of ≥ 0.04 sec
ii. isolated ST depression
iii. combination of (i) and (ii).

ECGs 13.16 and 13.17 show acute posterior MI. ECG 13.18 reflects an old posterior MI.

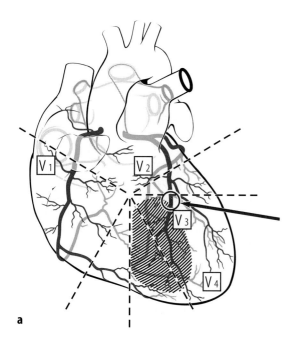

a

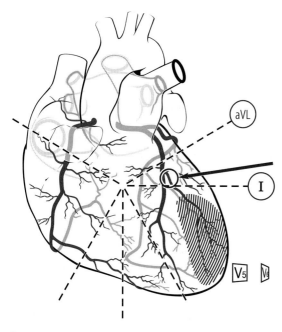

c

b

d

Figure 13.2a–d
Correlation between localization of infarction and occlusion of coronary artery (arrow), and exploring ECG leads
a. Anteroseptal infarction

b. Extensive anterior infarction (anterolateral infarction)
c. Isolated lateral infarction
d. Inferior infarction

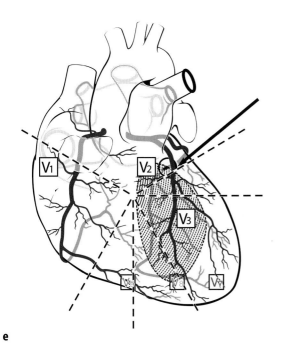

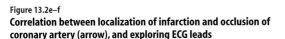

e

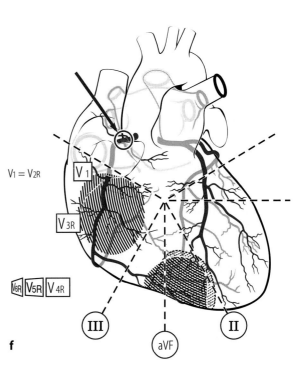

f

Figure 13.2e–f
Correlation between localization of infarction and occlusion of coronary artery (arrow), and exploring ECG leads

e. Posterior infarction
f. Right ventricular 'infarction' (combined to inferior infarction)

An Rs complex with a relatively high and broad R wave (≥ 0.40 sec) in leads V_1 to V_3 is not rare in healthy – especially young – individuals, whereas an isolated ST depression in these leads does not exist in an otherwise normal ECG, and consequently suggests acute posterior MI. In doubtful cases and in combination with clinical signs, an echocardiogram or even a coronary angiography should be considered.

3.6 Right Ventricular Infarction

See Figure 13.2f. An isolated right ventricular infarction is extremely rare. However, an *acute inferior infarction* (and no other infarction type) is combined with an *acute right ventricular (RV) infarction* in a strikingly high percentage of cases of about 40%, generally in cases with proximal occlusion of the right coronary artery. In contrast to posterior infarction, right ventricular infarction does not produce a mirror image in any of the standard leads. The direct infarction pattern is only detectable with the additional *right ventricular leads V_3R, V_4R, V_5R and sometimes V_6R*. Acute inferior MI combined to acute

right ventricular 'infarction' is frequently associated with atrioventricular (AV) block of all degrees (ECG 13.19a).

ECGs 13.19b–19c and ECG 13.20 show 'right ventricular infarction' in acute inferior MI.

As a strong rule, the right ventricular leads V_3R to V_6R *must* be applied as soon as possible in every patient with an acute inferior infarction. The medical treatment differs in the presence of right ventricular infarction. Moreover, the typical ECG signs for right ventricular infarction disappear in 50% of cases, 48 h after the first symptoms. One week after right (and inferior or left) ventricular infarction, the typical signs of right ventricular infarction are often no longer detectable in the ECG and right ventricular contraction has generally normalized. This proves that 'RV infarction' is not a real infarction but represents a severe but reversible ischemia of the right ventricle, corresponding to *hibernating myocardium*. However, the term 'RV infarction' is still in general use.

By far the best – often life-saving – therapeutic intervention of acute inferior MI with right ventricular infarction is *immediate PTCA*. The second best is thrombolysis.

171

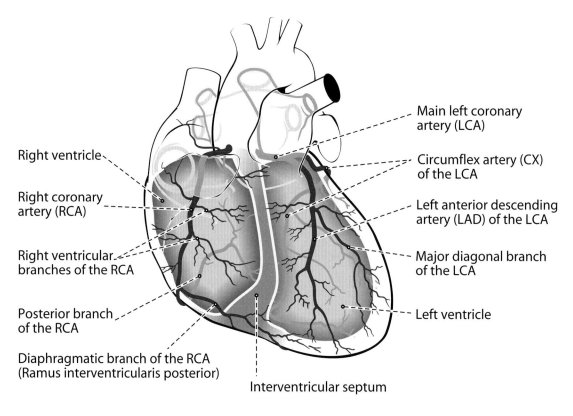

Figure 13.3
Anatomy of the coronary arteries

4 Differential Diagnosis of 'Classical' Infarction Patterns (Pathologic Q waves, ST Elevation, Abnormal T Waves)

See Table 13.1. The differential diagnosis of formally *pathologic Q waves* is extensive and includes, for example, hypertrophic obstructive cardiomyopathy, pulmonary embolism, normal variants (Q_{III}!) and as an artifact in false poling of the limb leads (discussed extensively in Chapter 14 Differential Diagnosis of Pathologic Q Waves).

ST elevation is seen in pericarditis (ST < 3 mm, concave, *without* development of pathologic Q waves), as a mirror image of ST depression due to left ventricular (LV) overload or left bundle-branch block, in 'early repolarization', in the Brugada syndrome, and in other conditions. ST elevation with an amplitude of several millimeters may also be present as

normal variant in leads V_2 and V_3 (ECG 13.21). In *Prinzmetal angina* the elevated ST segment returns (with or without chest pain) to the isoelectric line, generally within a few minutes, up to 20 min. Often episodes of reversible ST elevation can only be detected in an ambulatory ECG. Of course those patients need further evaluation (with coronary angiography), because significant coronary artery stenosis is common.

The so-called *non-Q-wave infarction pattern* is characterized by *negative symmetric T waves* (about 2–7 mm) in several precordial leads, and in I, II and/or aVL (ECG 13.22), or in leads III and aVF. The differential diagnosis of negative and symmetric T waves is *extensive* and includes *ischemia without necrosis,* subacute or chronic pericarditis, the so-called 'syndrome X' and many other conditions (Table 13.1).

Tall, positive and symmetric or symmetroid T waves are not only seen occasionally in the very early (peracute) stage of MI but also in hyperkalemia and in normal patients with sinus bradycardia (in leads V_2/V_3).

To summarize: for the diagnosis of MI, it is extremely important to consider the history, the symptoms, and the clinical findings and, in suspected acute or subacute infarction, the laboratory findings such as creatin kinase (CK), myocardial-bound CK (CK-MB), troponin, and myoglobin. The presence of several risk factors for coronary heart disease augments considerably the probability of infarction of all stages (Bayes theorem).

5 Complex Infarction Patterns

The term 'complex infarction patterns' is used for infarction in combination with the classical *intraventricular conduction disturbances:* left bundle-branch block (LBBB), right bundle-branch block (RBBB), left anterior fascicular block (LAFB), left posterior fascicular block (LPFB), and bilateral blocks.

An *old* infarction associated with *LBBB* is diagnosable with reliability in the presence of certain criteria (high specificity) such as:

i.   Q wave in at least two of the leads I, aVL, V_5, V_6
ii. regression of R wave amplitude from V_1 to V_4
iii. notching of the S wave in V_3 to V_5, the 'Cabrera sign'.

However, in the *absence* of these signs, an old MI cannot be excluded (low sensitivity). An *acute* myocardial infarction *with*

LBBB may be suspected or even diagnosed by the unusual behavior of repolarization, for example ST elevation instead of LBBB-related ST depression (details of MI and LBBB are covered in the ECG Special section below).

In contrast, an *old* infarction in RBBB is generally easy to identify in inferior and anterior localization. Identical pathologic Q waves are present (as without RBBB) because necrosis influences the first about 40–60 msec of the QRS complex, whereas RBBB produces alterations of the last 50–60 msec of QRS (ECG 13.23). Paradoxically, an *acute* MI in *RBBB* is sometimes overlooked. However, the diagnosis may be suspected (as in LBBB) on the basis of unusual ST alterations that are not related to RBBB.

LAFB may imitate or mask an old anteroseptal infarction, or mask an inferior infarction. The latter condition is very rare. Extensive anterior infarction is detectable in spite of LAFB.

LPFB represents a special condition. In practice, this rare conduction disturbance occurs only (more accurately in 95% of cases) in inferior MI, often completely masking the infarction. The LPFB pattern is similar to a normal ECG, the typical alterations are subtle. ECG 13.24 shows LPFB completely masking an old inferior MI, ECG 13.25 provides a similar pattern in a young healthy individual. In patients at the age > 40 years, with an $\text{Å}QRS_F$ of about + 60°, and with or without suspicious Q waves in leads III and aVF, the diagnosis of inferior infarc-

Table 13.1
Differential diagnosis of acute and old myocardial infarction in the ECG

Acute infarction	Old infarction	Classical non-Q infarction
ST ↑ without Q	Pathologic Q, isoelectric ST	T inversion only
Prinzmetal angina	Normal variants: 'Q_{III}'; QS in V_2/V_3	Ischemia without infarction
Early repolarization	LVH: 'Q_{III}'	Ventricular overload
Pericarditis	False poling	Normal variants
Mirror image of LV overload	Pre-excitation (WPW)	Syndrome X
Rare conditions such as Brugada syndrome	LBBB	Pericarditis (stage 3 and 4)
Pneumothorax	HOCM	Myocarditis
	Situs inversus	Anemia
	Other rare conditions*	Pancreatitis
		Funnel chest
		Upright position
		Drugs
		Many other conditions**

HOCM, hypertrophic obstructive cardiomyopathy; LBBB, left bundle-branch block; LVH, left ventricular hypertrophy; WPW, Wolff-Parkinson-White syndrome.
*   Discussed in Chapter 14 Differential Diagnosis of Pathologic Q waves.
** Discussed in Chapter 17 Alterations of Repolarization.

tion with LPFB should be considered – especially in patients with risk factors for coronary heart disease. For details about LPFB see the section 6 in Chapter 9 Fascicular Blocks.

6   Special Infarction Patterns

Principally, the *special patterns* of MI are identical to *non-Q-wave infarctions*. Note that this definition is based on the absence of a broad Q wave, with a duration of ≥ 0.04 sec. Therefore MI patterns with a Q wave < 0.04 sec are included in the 'non-Q wave' patterns.

The special infarction patterns include:

i.   Patterns *without* Q waves: a) symmetric negative T waves (classical non-Q-wave infarction); b) ST depression > 3 mm.
ii.   Patterns with *reduction* of R wave amplitude and *with* Q waves in the classical leads (for instance in aVF and III, in inferior infarction) with a duration of < 0.04 sec.
iii. *New and/or small* Q waves (< 0.04 sec) in leads where they should not be present.
iv.   An RSR' pattern in leads I and aVL and/or in $\geq$ two precordial leads V_2 to V_6.

In the conditions (ii–iv) the presence of symmetric negative T waves in the respective leads may be helpful for diagnosis.

The so-called *non-Q-wave* infarction pattern represents the most important and most frequent special pattern. It is charac-terized (also in the acute stage!) by *symmetric, negative T waves* in leads V_1 to V_5 (V_6) and often I and aVL by normal or only slightly reduced R waves (ECG 13.26). A non-Q-wave infarction pattern in leads III and aVF is rare. In the acute stage, ST may be minimally elevated, with above-convex configuration. The infarction may be *transmural* or *nontransmural.*

In patients with non-Q-wave infarction, a Q-wave infarction occurs in about 30% in the following 6 months. Therefore, early coronary angiography is mandatory in order to confirm the diagnosis, with performance of PTCA or coronary artery bypass grafting (CABG) if necessary.

Sometimes we find a 'mixture' of non-Q-wave infarction and Q-wave infarction. The predominating typical deep and symmetric and negative T waves are associated with patholog-ic Q waves in one or more leads (ECG 13.27). This pattern is by definition a Q wave MI. In ECG 13.28 a late ventricular prema-ture beat (VPB) reveals pathologic Q waves in the precordial leads – but this is not a reliable sign. The morphology of VPBs may also imitate a Q-wave MI.

Conclusion

The general rule is that only a well-instructed ECG reader (who is also a good clinician) should interpret ECGs and arrhyth-mias; this rule is especially valid when applied to cases of sus-pected MI.

The Full Picture

It is not sufficient for an ECG reader only to be able to identify a classical *Q-wave pattern* of old inferior or anterior myocar-dial infarction (MI). Patients are not interested whether their MI can be detected in the ECG at first glance or whether it is difficult to diagnose (e.g. in the case of mirror image of infarc-tion signs, or in the presence of intraventricular conduction defects). What is your opinion? If a close relative or a friend had an infarction that was difficult to detect in the ECG, would you accept the fact that the ECG reader responsible would not be able to make, or even suppose, the correct diagnosis and therefore introduce an adequate therapy? Or would you be happy if this patient were to undergo fibrinolysis or urgent coronary angiography on the basis of an innocent thoracic pain and ST elevation corresponding to a normal variant of the ECG (such as an ST elevation of 2–3 mm in leads V_2/V_3)? Worse still is the fact that an undiagnosed acute MI often has severe consequences and leads to death in many people.

7.1   Arteriosclerotic Coronary Artery Disease (Common)

MI generally develops in patients with atheromatous coronary arteries. The pathogenic mechanisms have been discussed by Fischer et al [1] and Gutstein and Fuster [2].

Coronary artery spasm is the mechanism for vasospastic or Prinzmetal angina [3]. This coronary spasm represents an important coexisting pathophysiologic factor in the evolution of MI [4,5]. Risk factors include contraceptives and nicotine (especially in combination), and cocaine. Coronary spasm and late resolution of thrombotic material are the most probable causes of infarction in patients with normal coronary arteries. This is true in most cases also for acute MI during pregnancy or within the first three months after delivery, a rare but often misdiagnosed event, with a high mortality of 20%–38%(!). In these women, generally aged 30 to 40 years, dissection of coronary arteries has also been described [17]. ECGs 13.29, 13.30a–b and 13.31 show cases of spasm-induced reversible ST elevations. If the spasm affects the right coronary artery (RCA), intermittent atrioventricular (AV) block 2° or 3° may be observed.

7.2   Congenital Coronary Artery Disease (Rare)

Coronary artery fistula is an abnormal connection between a normal coronary artery and the right heart or the pulmonary artery, often producing a typical systolodiastolic murmur. The consequences, due to left-to-right shunt and coronary steal effect, are heart failure, anginal pain, and very occasionally infarction that appears after the age of 20 years.

The origin of the left coronary artery from the pulmonary artery (Bland-White-Garland syndrome [6]) is a special entity with a worse prognosis, and which leads to MI in the newborn, arrhythmias, and sudden death. An extraordinary case of a patient who has reached adult age is presented.

Short Story/Case Report 1

In 1976 a 41-year-old woman without cardiac history who drove daily to work suffered syncope and was clinically investigated. The heart was slightly enlarged and moderate mitral incompetence was diagnosed with a systolic 2/6 murmur over the apex. The abnormal Q waves in the precordial leads were misinterpreted as septal ventricular hypertrophy (that ECG was unfortunately lost); the syncope was misdiagnosed as vagovasal. Some months later, while shopping, the patient had another severe syncope with cardiac and respiratory standstill. She was immediately reanimated by a cardiac pediatrician just passing by, and hospitalized, where the ventricular fibrillation was treated by external shock. Coronary angiography revealed an abnormal origin of the left coronary artery from the pulmonary artery, a great akinetic zone anterolaterally, and a reduced LV ejection fraction of 40%. On operation, the abnormal left coronary artery was closed at its origin from the pulmonary artery and an aortocoronary venous bypass was connected to the left coronary artery. Some months later the woman returned to work with improved LV function (50%), and only mild mitral incompetence. In the ECG, R waves appeared in the precordial leads (ECG unfortunately lost). Fourteen years later the patient was still well, without cardiac failure (although she has now been lost from control).

Abnormal passage of the left or right coronary artery between the aorta and the pulmonary artery/right ventricle is due to aberrant origin of the coronary artery from the contralateral aortic sinus. MI and sudden death may occur [7].

Coronary artery anomalies in various forms may be associated with *congenital* heart diseases [8,9].

Myocardial bridging, leading to narrowing of the proximal or middle part of the left anterior descending coronary artery (LAD) (rarely of circumflexa [CX]) may induce angina, and exceptionally infarction [10]. In children with hypertrophic cardiomyopathy it may represent a risk factor for sudden death [11].

7.3   Other Conditions of Coronary Artery Disease (Rare)

All of the following conditions are very rare compared to the common cause of coronary heart disease (atheromatous alterations of the coronary arteries and consecutive thrombosis).

Diseases of the *aorta* include dissection, Takayasu arteritis, and syphilis. Dissection of the aorta type A provokes MI in some cases, due to dissection of a coronary artery or to obstruction by hematoma. In a study of 89 patients, Hirata et al [12] found acute ST–T changes in more than 50% of type A dissection and in 20% of type B dissection. The authors attribute the ECG abnormalities to involvement of the ostial coronary artery, shock from tamponade, and pre-existing coronary artery disease. The other conditions mentioned are extremely rare.

Another rare condition is *coronary embolism*, in patients with bacterial endocarditis, prosthetic valves, left atrial myxoma, mural thrombus in LV aneurysm, or in severe dilating cardiomyopathy.

MI *during or shortly after* therapeutic interventions are encountered in coronary artery bypass grafting (CABG) and percutaneous transluminal coronary angioplasty (PTCA). Infarction in patients with CABG is more frequent than expected and varies between 10% and 20% [13,14]. Only in rare cases does a great infarction occur.

Short Story/Case Report 2

[With the kind permission of the patient.]

A 59-year-old man (whose last name is Frischherz, meaning 'fresh heart'), suffered from angina due to severe three-vessel coronary disease, with a normal LV ejection fraction (EF) of 72%. Mild valvular aortic stenosis was present. The ECG (13.32a) showed a probable LV hypertrophy with some alteration of the repolarization. In September 1990 a quintuple aortocoronary bypass operation was performed. Immediately afterwards, ST elevation in the inferior and lateral leads was observed, but on immediate reoperation no abnormalities of the grafts could be detected. However, a great inferolateral infarction occurred with atypical ECG signs (ECG 13.32b) and a reduction of EF to 45%. During the following years, progressive heart failure developed due to rapid progression of aortic stenosis with an aortic valve-opening area of 0.9 cm^2 and a severe diffuse progression of coronary artery disease, with at least four of the five grafts open, on coronary angiography. The EF was 25% in 1997. During the winter of 1997–98 end-stage heart failure developed and in May 1998, heart transplantation was performed. Besides intermittent renal failure, the course was uneventful; 4 years after the operation, everyone is happy for Mr Frischherz – with his fresh heart and near-normal ECG (ECG 13.32c).

Rossiter et al [15] found, in combined valvular and coronary bypass surgery, an incidence of perioperative infarction of 21% in aortic valve replacement plus CABG, and of 5% in mitral valve replacement plus CABG, respectively. Improvements in surgical techniques have considerably lowered mortality and perioperative infarction rates [16]. Furthermore, the technique of aortocoronary bypass without using extracorporal circulation shortens operation times and may minimize the incidence of perioperative infarction.

The incidence of acute infarction *during* or shortly *after* PTCA is much lower at about 1.6% [18]. Patients undergoing PTCA have generally milder coronary artery disease [CAD] and a better LV function than patients who need bypass surgery. Moreover, the interventional cardiologist can immediately visualize an obstruction or spasm and prevent infarction by a prompt reintervention.

Cocaine has become one of the most frequent causes of acute MI in young people in some countries. If taken intravenously, cocaine leads to vasoconstriction and arterial hypertension within minutes; if sniffed, this happens within an hour. Coronary artery spasm may enhance thrombus formation *and* plaque rupture. An unusual progression of coronary artery disease was observed in some patients. Acute MI (generally occurring within 1 h after cocaine intake) was observed with normal or stenotic coronary arteries [19,20].

Other *rare causes* of MI are connective tissue diseases (lupus erythematodes, periarteritis nodosa, rheumatoid arthritis), amyloidosis, neurologic disorders (Friedreich ataxia, progressive muscular dystrophy), penetrating and nonpenetrating cardiac trauma, primary and metastatic heart tumor, homocystinuria, and contraceptives (especially in combination with nicotine). Some cases are described after carbon monoxide poisoning and after honeybee stings [21]. Cerebral hemorrhage and severe shock may lead to subendocardial infarction [22].

ECG Special

8 Nomenclature of Infarction Stages

As mentioned in the previous section, there are four different approaches for describing the stages of MI *that do not coincide in time evolution* and which cause some confusion. Each approach considers different aspects of MI (Figure 13.4).

8.1 Electropathophysiologic Evolution

This ECG description considers the *electropathophysiologic evolution* of MI. The acute stage (only ST elevation) lasts for some hours, the subacute stage (ST elevation plus pathologic Q or QS waves) lasts several days (up to 1 week), followed by the chronic stage (only pathologic Q/QS, without ST elevation). Thus, a 5-day-old infarct cannot be distinguished from one that

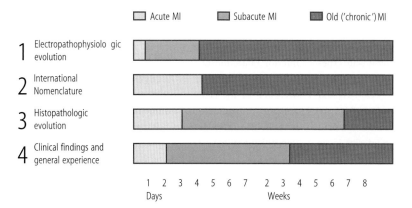

Acute MI   Subacute MI   Old ('chronic') MI

1 Electropathophysiologic evolution

2 International Nomenclature

3 Histopathologic evolution

4 Clinical findings and general experience

1 2 3 4 5 6 7   2 3 4 5 6 7 8
Days   Weeks

is several years old on the basis of the ECG alone. The behavior of the T wave is not reliable.

8.2 International Terminology

ECG descriptions can follow *international terminology*. This nomenclature *does not* distinguish between the acute and subacute stages (in the sense of the electropathophysiologic description mentioned above). Every infarction stage with ST elevation – without or with pathologic Q/QS – is described as 'acute'. The term 'subacute' is used when the ST segment has returned to the isoelectric line. Consequently, the subacute stage cannot be distinguished from the old stage on the basis of the ECG alone. T alterations may or may not help to distinguish between the two.

8.3 Histopathologic Evolution

This is a description of infarct stage based on *histopathologic evolution*, without taking ECG alterations into consideration. The acute stage lasts for days. The subacute stage lasts about 6 weeks, up to *histopathologic healing* of infarction (fibrotic scar). Thereafter the infarction is described as old.

8.4 Clinical Findings and Practical Experience

Estimation of infarction stages may rely on *clinical findings* and *practical experience*. The acute stage lasts for a few days and the subacute stage for 2–3 weeks. After this time, the patient is usually allowed to work again. It is accepted, howev-

er, that great operative interventions should only be performed 6 weeks after the onset of MI (after healing of the infarction). Figure 13.4 illustrates the four different approaches for the stages of MI *in relation to time*. It must be mentioned that the ECG stage of infarction varies considerably depending on *individual evolution* and on *therapy*. Fibrinolysis or emergency PTCA generally shortens the acute stage.

As mentioned before, this book uses *international nomenclature* for the description in the ECG examples. However, this approach does not distinguish between subacute and acute infarction (as the *electrophysiologic* nomenclature does).

The acute *and* subacute stages are summarized under the term 'acute stage' and are characterized by ST elevation, without or with Q waves. In order to avoid confusion, we give – where possible – the real age of infarction in hours, days, weeks, months or years.

9 Combination of Infarction Patterns

We distinguish between the combination of infarction of two (or three) adjacent myocardial areas, and the combination of infarction of separated or opposite areas.

9.1 Infarction of Adjacent Areas

The five locations of left ventricular MI mentioned in the previous section are arbitrary. An adjacent area is often also involved by the infarction. In fact, *anterolateral* MI is a combination of two *adjacent* infarcted areas, one anteroseptal and the other anterolateral. Another common combination is *posterolateral* MI.

In some cases of posterior MI, lateral involvement may be present but difficult to identify. If the R wave diminishes from lead V_4 to V_6, together with augmentation of the Q wave from V_4 to V_6, there is partial involvement of the lateral wall, especially if the T wave in V_6 (and V_5) is negative (ECG 13.33).

Inferoposterior MI is a common combination (ECG 13.34 and 13.35). *Inferolateral* (ECG 13.36) and *inferoposterolateral* MI are also not rare. In the inferoposterior combination, we may find a Q or QS or a minimal initial R wave in the inferior leads (ECGs 13.37–13.39). In all these cases, the diagnosis is made by the presence of typical alterations in the corresponding leads. Often one localization is dominant, and at the other location the alterations are only borderline (ECG 13.40). Generally, this type of combined localization, such as inferoposterior and inferoposterolateral, is caused by *one* occluded great coronary branch of the left coronary artery (mostly CX) or an occluded dominating right coronary artery.

9.2 Infarction of Separate or Opposite Localization

The typical 'double infarction' affecting two *separate* areas of the left ventricle is the combination of *anteroseptal and inferior* MI. Again, the ECG diagnosis is made by alterations in the different corresponding leads (ECGs 13.41–13.44). In this type of MI, occlusion of the right coronary artery, also of a branch of the left coronary artery, can be assumed.

In relatively rare cases, MI patterns of opposite localization may *mask* each other (ECG 13.45). In these patients severely impaired LV function is often erroneously attributed to 'dilating cardiomyopathy of unknown etiology', whereas in fact severe coronary artery disease with multiple infarcts is present. Differentiation may also be difficult in the echocardiogram. Also, in combined *posterior* and *anteroseptal* (or anteroapical) infarction the diagnosis is difficult or impossible, because the ECG alterations of the two infarcts cancel themselves out partially or completely. Sometimes the diagnosis can be suspected (in the context of clinical findings) on the basis of relatively tall R waves in leads V_1 to V_3, preceded by a Q wave (ECG 13.59, with additional RBBB).

ECG 13.46 demonstrates that ECG diagnosis of MI is sometimes very difficult, for several reasons. This ECG of a patient 2 days after CABG suggests, at first glance, acute anterior MI (see leads V_5 and V_6, where the elevated ST segment arises directly from the R wave). However, a frontal ST vector of +75° and other signs favor the diagnosis of acute pericarditis.

Further coronary angiography revealed open grafts; LV function was unchanged.

Another type of combined MI of separate areas is acute inferior infarction of the *left ventricle* associated with acute infarction of the *right* (ECG 13.47), mostly due to proximal occlusion of the right coronary artery. This combination is much more frequent than assumed 10 years ago, and is found in 30%–50%(!) of patients with acute inferior MI [23–25]. Recognizing right ventricular infarction (with the help of leads V_3R to V_6R) is essential for therapeutic reasons. Vasodilators must be avoided and fluid (over-)restitution must be guaranteed. Severe complications such as AV block, repetitive ventricular fibrillation, and shock, are more frequent than in other types of acute MI. While the in-hospital mortality of this combination of infarctions is excessive (about 16%) *without* early coronary artery reperfusion in the acute stage, long-term survival is equal to patients with inferior infarction *without* RV infarction. The explanation is simple: in most cases RV 'infarction' is *not* an infarction but corresponds to *hibernating myocardium*. In fact, after 48 h, in > 50% of cases, not only have ST elevation but also pathologic Q waves in the right precordial leads disappeared. The reasons for recovery are thought to be a minor oxygen requirement by the thin wall of the right ventricle, direct perfusion (by venous blood!), and special collateral conditions (ischemic precondition) [25]. In-hospital mortality has *dramatically decreased* by early reperfusion of the right coronary artery, thus enabling prompt recovery of hibernating right ventricular myocardium (and partially also of inferior LV myocardium). Out of 40 successfully reperfused patients with early PTCA by Bowers et al [25], 39 patients (98%) survived without right ventricular failure, after 1 month. However, these excellent results can only be expected in modern hospitals, with invasive cardiologic equipment.

10 Complex Infarction Patterns

The term 'complex infarction pattern' is used for MI *associated with* bundle-branch blocks (RBBB and LBBB), fascicular blocks, and bilateral blocks. Bundle-branch block due to acute MI considerably increases mortality, also in inferior infarction [26].

10.1 Infarction Associated with Right Bundle-Branch Block

The pathologic Q wave of *old* MI is equally detectable in the presence of as in the absence of RBBB, because the initial depolarization of the left ventricle is not, or is only modestly, influenced by RBBB. Only the enhancement of the septal vector may lead to tall primary R waves in leads V_2 and V_3, that may be misdiagnosed as (a mirror image of) posterior MI. ECGs 13.48–13.52 show different localizations of MI; ECG 13.53 shows the combination of old anteroseptal and inferior infarction.

Acute MI can be easily diagnosed in many cases. In the case of acute anteroseptal infarction the ST elevation in leads V_1 to V_3 may be at least partially canceled by the ST depression caused by RBBB. However, distinct ST elevations (and Q waves) in leads V_1/V_2 often indicate clearly acute anteroseptal infarction (ECGs 13.54 and 13.55). The corresponding alterations in the inferior leads allow the diagnosis of acute inferior MI. ECG 13.56a–b (RBBB occurring with latency) and ECGs 13.57–13.59 show several localizations of acute MI associated with RBBB.

In practice, the MI pattern in the presence of RBBB is sometimes overlooked, because the eye of the observer is impressed by the RBBB pattern, often meaning that no further consideration is given to the Q waves and the behavior of the ST segment.

10.2 Infarction Associated with Left Bundle-Branch Block

In the presence of LBBB the diagnosis of an *old* MI is often difficult or impossible. This can be explained by two facts. First, LBBB produces abnormal QRS vectors pointing mainly from the right to the left, and more or less backwards and upwards, thus severely deforming the QRS pattern. These abnormal QRS vectors prevent the appearance of a typical necrosis pattern. Second, a QS complex due to LBBB may mimic an infarction.

An rS complex (sometimes with a very small initial R wave) is common in leads V_1 to V_4 and should not be interpreted as anteroseptal/anterior MI. A QS complex in V_1 to V_3 or V_4 is found in LBBB with or without MI. Similarly a QS complex in leads III and aVF may imitate an inferior infarction or be caused by it. In both cases, the T waves are generally positive and asymmetric.

ECG signs suggesting old MI in the presence of LBBB are presented in Table 13.2.

i.   A *qR complex* (with a Q wave generally < 0.04 sec) in at least two of the leads I, aVL, V_5, V_6 is specific in about 90% of old anterior MI in the presence of LBBB. The sensitivity is low.

ii. An *rsR' complex* in leads I (aVL) and in some precordial leads generally indicates extensive old anterior MI. Low sensitivity.

iii. Decreasing *R wave amplitude* from (V_1) V_2 to V_4 is typical for old anterior MI (theoretically with involvement of the posterior septum). Low sensitivity.

iv. The Cabrera sign (notched/slurred S wave upstroke in leads V_3 to V_5 [27]) indicates old anterior MI in 60%–90%. Low sensitivity.

The four ECG patterns (i–iv) have an acceptable to excellent specificity but a very low sensitivity. In the presence of more than three of the mentioned signs, the infarct size is generally medium to extensive, because the LBBB pattern can only be altered substantially by a massive loss of LV vectors.

v.   A *Q wave* (generally ≥ 0.03 sec) in leads III and aVF may indicate inferior MI. However, Q waves or even a QS con-

Table 13.2
Specificity and sensitivity of ECG signs suggesting old myocardial infarction in LBBB

	Specificity(%)*	Sensitivity(%)*
Q wave (mostly < 0.04 sec) in ≥ two of leads I, aVL, V_5, V_6	80–100	5–20
rsR' in ≥ two of leads I, aVL, V_5, V_6	80–100	8–24
Decreasing of R wave from V_1 (V_2) to V_4	70–90	5–30
Notched S wave upstroke (Cabrera sign) in V_3 to V_5	60–90	8–32
Q in III and aVF (without left-axis deviation)	30–70	30?
Notched R wave upstroke in leads I, aVL, V_5, V_6 (Chapman sign)	22–62	20–26
Notched R wave in ≥ two inferior leads	34–74	10–32
Multiple notching in (> four?) limb and precordial leads	?	?
QS in leads V_1 to V_4	about 50	20–40

*Values based on the literature.

figuration may be present in these leads in left-axis deviation, without MI.

vi. *Chapman* sign: notched/slurred R wave upstroke in leads I, aVL (and V_5 or V_6), indicating anterior MI. Unreliable.

vii. *Notched R wave* in inferior leads, a possible sign for inferior MI.

viii. Multiple *notching/slurring of QRS* in several leads, seen especially in anterior MI.

ix. A *QS complex* in V_1 to V_4 is occasionally seen without MI. In the combination with (anterior) MI, other signs such as the Cabrera sign or a Q wave in $\geq$ two of the leads I, aVL, V_5, V_6 are often present.

The signs (v–ix) have an insufficient sensitivity and a low specificity.

In the study by Hands et al [28], 24 of 35 patients with LBBB had old and/or acute MI, 12 had no MI. The author found an excellent specificity of 90%–100%, combined with a low sensitivity of 5%–30%, for the following signs:

i. Q wave in $\geq$ 2 of leads I, aVL, V_5, V_6
ii. R wave regression V_1 to V_4
iii. late notching of S wave in V_3 to V_5 (Cabrera sign)
iv. notched R wave in $\geq$ 2 of inferior leads
v. Q wave in III (left-axis deviation excluded)
vi. QS in V_1 to V_4.

The value of the results is limited by the very small number of patients, who, additionally, had old and/or acute MI. Weiner et al [29] showed the superiority of the vectorcardiogram over the ECG, with specificities of 85.7% and 80.9%, and sensitivities of 71.8% and 53.1%, respectively. Wackers [30] emphasizes the importance of *serial* ECGs for the diagnosis of acute and old MI in the presence of LBBB.

ECGs 13.60–13.64 show patterns of old MI in LBBB. The reader will notice that in some ECGs *several* signs suggesting MI are present.

It should be mentioned that all these patterns (with the exception of i. Q waves in I, aVL, V_5/V_6) may also be seen in noncoronary heart diseases where there is a severely damaged left ventricle, especially in severe hypertrophic and dilated LV cardiomyopathy. However, coronary heart disease is by far the most common cause for these 'abnormal' LBBB patterns.

In *acute* MI the diagnosis is also difficult. Depending on the different leads, ST elevation in acute infarction is either partially *canceled* by ST depression caused by LBBB, or ST elevation is *superimposed* to ST elevation caused by LBBB.

Consequently, *acute infarction* in the presence of LBBB may be diagnosed and localized in the presence of the following signs [31]:

i. ST depression (mirror image of ST elevation posteriorly) in leads V_2/V_3: acute posterior MI.

ii. ST elevation in leads where LBBB alone would induce ST depression (examples: ST elevation in leads I and/or leads aVL, V_4 to V_6: acute anterior MI; ST elevation in leads III, aVF (II): acute inferior MI (ECG 13.65)).

iii. Striking ST elevation in leads V_2 to V_3 > 5 mm: acute anterior infarction (ECG 13.66a–b).

Based on these criteria, acute anterior or inferior MI may be diagnosed in many cases if the ECG is registered within the first hours after the event. A recent publication by Madias et al [32] suggests – and our own experience also supports this – that in 124 patients with LBBB out of 4193 patients with acute MI, ST elevation in V2/V3 is somewhat less specific (especially in severe LVH) than the ST alterations mentioned in (i) and (ii) above.

10.2.1 Infarction in Pacemaker Patients

In a few pacemaker recipients, the electrode is implanted epicardially on the left ventricle. The QRS complex therefore shows an atypical RBBB pattern. Consecutively, the pattern of acute and old MI generally can be recognized.

In most patients, the electrode is implanted intravenously in the right ventricle, with a consecutive *atypical* LBBB pattern. Depending on the localization of the tip of the electrode, we find different QRS axes in the frontal plane. However, a single broad R wave in leads I and aVL and a QS type in III, aVF and II are most common. In contrast to the usual LBBB, we mostly miss a positive QRS deflection in V_5 and V_6, thus imitating a loss of QRS vectors. In lead V_1 a completely atypical pattern with a Qr complex (without MI) may be encountered. Overall the diagnosis of acute and old MI in the presence of right ventricular pacing is often very difficult or impossible (ECG 13.67). In extensive anterior MI the LBBB pattern may show significant notching.

10.3 Infarction in Left Anterior Fascicular Block

Left anterior fascicular block (LAFB) may mask or in rare cases imitate an *old* infarction [33,34]. The typical Q or QS complexes and the common negative T waves in inferior infarction are completely masked by LAFB. However the association of LAFB with inferior infarction is very rare.

Occasionally, anterior infarctions of moderate size are also masked by LAFB. Generally, anteroseptal/apical and extensive anterior infarctions are detectable (ECGs 13.68–13.72). A variant of LAFB (in 5%–10%) with a small Q wave (QRS complex) in leads V_2 (and V_3) imitates a small anteroseptal necrosis [33,34]. The diagnosis of *acute* infarction is generally not compromised (ECGs 13.73–13.75b (follow-up)). Coronary angiographic findings in patients with or without LAFB are not significantly different [35].

10.4 Infarction in Left Posterior Fascicular Block

LPFB represents a special condition (Chapter 9 Fascicular Blocks). On one hand, > 6% of old inferior infarctions are combined with LPFB. On the other hand, LPFB is associated in > 90% to an old inferior MI [36]. Therefore, the LPFB pattern itself allows the diagnosis of old inferior MI, in most cases, although LPFB masks the common pattern of inferior MI partially or completely. ECGs 13.76 and 13.77 show typical examples of LPFB where the extensive inferior MI is masked. ECG 13.78 shows LPFB with old inferior MI and acute anteroseptal MI.

The presence of LPFB indicates not only inferior MI in most cases, but generally also severe two-to-three coronary vessel disease [36], representing a valid indication for coronary angiography. Considering the facts mentioned above, it is important to know the *exact* and *fine* diagnostic ECG criteria of LPFB (Chapter 9 Fascicular Blocks). In a patient older than 40 years without RV hypertrophy, and a frontal QRS vector of about + 60°, with preterminal slurring of the R wave in leads III and/or V_6, the presence of LPFB should be considered (regardless of the presence or absence of Q waves in the inferior leads). In doubtful cases an echocardiogram or a coronary angiography are decisive for the diagnosis.

10.5 Infarction in Bilateral Block

10.5.1 Infarction in RBBB + LAFB

In this *common* type of bilateral block, the ECG pattern is predominantly determined by LAFB, with the exception of leads V_1 (V_2). Consequently, inferior and small anterior infarctions may be masked. However, in many cases anterior MI is detectable by pathologic Q waves, often combined with reduction of R amplitude and/or notched QRS in the adjacent leads

(ECGs 13.79–13.81). Equally, a non-Q wave MI can be suspected (ECG 13.82). In our experience, LAFB partially impairs the development of T negativity in the precordial leads.

10.5.2 Infarction in RBBB + LPFB

As isolated LPFB, also LPFP in combination with RBBB, generally masks partially or completely an old inferior MI. The diagnosis can only be assumed in the presence of suspicious Q waves in the inferior leads. This is not the case in ECG 13.83. The differential diagnosis of this *rare* type of bilateral block, with or without inferior infarction, is RBBB associated with right ventricular hypertrophy (Chapter 11 Bilateral Blocks).

11 Special Infarction Patterns

The special infarction patterns may be divided into the following types:

i.   the 'classical' non-Q-wave infarction (with negative symmetric T waves);
ii. infarction with ST depression > 3 mm;
iii. infarction with 'nonsignificant' Q waves (< 0.04 sec) at *usual* localization;
iv. infarction with 'non-significant' Q waves (< 0.04 sec) at *unusual* localization (often associated with 'notching of QRS');
v.   infarction with RSR' type in precordial (and limb) leads;
vi. infarction with pure reduction of R wave amplitude (often combined with 'notching' of QRS);
vii. atrial infarction (a special condition of special infarction patterns).

11.1 The So-Called Non-Q-Wave Infarction

Although there are other types of non-Q-wave infarction, this term is generally reserved for the 'so-called' non-Q-wave infarction that is characterized by extensive and relatively deep negative (symmetric) T waves in the precordial leads (V_1) V_2 to V_5 (V_6) and often also in leads I (II) and aVL. Inferior non-Q-wave infarction (with symmetric negative T waves in III and aVF) is rarer. The pattern is seen in the acute stage of infarction and may last for weeks or even months. The R amplitude is often *slightly reduced* compared to a previous ECG. In the acute stage a moderate (1–2 mm) convex-upward ST elevation or ST depression may be seen (ECG 13.84).

Based on an early experimental study of Prinzmetal et al [37] non-Q-wave infarction was generally accepted to be nontransmural. Many years later this concept was questioned by other authors: a non-Q-wave infarction may be *transmural* or *non-transmural*. Interestingly, Prinzmetal himself revoked his own hypothesis 3 years after the first publication [38]. This type of non-Q-wave infarction is by far the *most frequent* of all unusual infarction patterns. De Zwaan et al [39] observed *negative symmetric* and also *biphasic terminally negative T waves* in the precordial leads V_2 to V_4 (V_5) in 180 (of 1260) patients with unstable angina, due to severe stenosis of the proximal left anterior descending coronary artery (LAD). Most of these patients had systolic and diastolic wall contraction abnormalities, which were interpreted by the authors as stunning myocardium rather than as infarction.

The following story describes an extraordinary evolution of non-Q-wave infarction after surgical revascularization.

Short Story/Case Report 3

In 1984, a 42-year-old man was admitted for heart catheterization with the clinical diagnosis of severe aortic valve stenosis and symptomatic non-Q-wave infarction. The ECG showed LV hypertrophy and deep symmetric T waves anterolaterally (ECG 13.85a). Both diagnoses were confirmed. Besides a gradient of 70 mmHg at the aortic valve, severe stenosis of the left anterior descending coronary artery, with a huge aneurysm of the anterior wall of the left ventricle, was found (ejection fraction 45%). Aortic valve replacement and CABG to the left anterior descending coronary artery were performed. Three weeks after operation the patient complained of atypical chest pain. Technetium/thallium scintigraphy revealed no ischemia and – to everyone's surprise – normalized LV function. The aneurysm was therefore not due to a fibrotic scar but to hibernating myocardium. Twenty years after operation the patient remains well; the ECG showed regression of LVH and slight alteration of the repolarization (ECG 13.85b).

To conclude, surgical (or interventional) revascularization may lead, in favorable cases, to striking recovery of LV function, due to recovery of hibernating myocardium. This phenomenon was first described by Chatterjee et al [40] in patients after CABG, and may occur also in patients with a Q-wave infarction.

Differential diagnosis: there is a vast range of diseases to be differentiated from non-Q-wave infarction, such as late-stage pericarditis, cerebral hemorrhage, severe anemia/shock, the so-called syndrome X [41], and acute pancreatitis (see Table 13.1). The knowledge of the *other types of special infarction patterns* is also impor-

tant. Some ECG patterns have been recognized better only in recent decades, with increasing number of coronary angiography. These ECGs reflect the real infarct size even less than Q-wave patterns. Many patients with unusual infarction patterns need further investigation and all should be followed and treated as patients with 'usual' infarction patterns. Most of the ECG examples shown below were observed within an 8-month period in our 1000-bed university hospital. Thus, these patterns are not as rare as one might believe. Most infarctions were confirmed by coronary and LV angiography.

11.2 Infarction with ST depression ≥ 3 mm

This type is defined as ST depression of ≥ 3 mm in at least one precordial lead, at rest (generally V_3 to V_5); it is relatively rare (ECG 13.86).

11.3 Infarction with 'Nonsignificant' Q Waves at Usual Localization

Short Story/Case Report 4

In March 2000 a 54-year-old colleague told the author about a slight 'pulling' pain localized to the region of the left great pectoral muscle, that had occurred for a week since exercising with dumb-bells. He had also some general malaise. He denied having risk factors for coronary heart disease. His blood pressure was 170/100 mmHg at rest. The ECG revealed an 'unusual' infarction pattern with an inferoposterior localization, without significant Q waves in the inferior leads, but with suspect symmetrical negative T waves in these leads (ECG 13.87a). The family doctor instantly faxed the ECG made at a check-up 3 years before, which was completely normal (ECG 13.87b). The stress test revealed an excellent work capacity (rate of 160/min at 17 MET (maximal exercise test). However, the strange 'muscular' pain could be reproduced. Heart enzymes were normal. Coronary angiography performed the next day showed a complete proximal obstruction of a great circumflex artery with some collateralization, LV angiography showed a minor circumscript hypokinesia inferoposteriorly, with a normal EF of 70%. The other coronary arteries were normal. Recanalization and stenting was performed, with a good result. With a repeat of the exercise test the following day, no pain occurred. Risk factors such as moderate hypertension, hypercholesterinemia, and moderate adiposity were treated. Surprisingly the 'special' ECG pattern unveiled the infarction better than LV angiography in this case.

ECG 13.88a shows an atypical pattern of old inferior MI (without pathologic Q waves) and notched QRS in the limb leads and in V_6 (possible lateral involvement). Five months later the ECG (ECG 13.88b) revealed a typical pattern of inferior Q-wave MI.

11.4 Infarction with 'Nonsignificant' Q Waves at Unusual Localization

This infarction pattern is often associated with some reduction of R amplitude and a notched QRS complex. Also, symmetrical negative T waves may support the diagnosis (ECGs 13.89–13.91).

11.5 Infarction with RSR' Type in Precordial (and Inferior) Leads

ECGs 13.92–13.95 demonstrate cases with this 'unusual' infarction pattern. Of course an incomplete RBBB must be excluded (rSr' in V_1, terminal R wave in aVR).

The MI pattern with rsR' in I and/or aVL, and V_6 or V_5/V_6 is *especially important*, because it is often associated with an extensive anterolateral infarction with consecutively severely reduced LV function (ECGs 13.96–13.99).

The predominance of a severe two-to-three-vessel coronary disease and hypokinetic and akinetic zones at different locations sustain the suspicion that some of those MI patterns are provoked by pattern superposition of two or more MIs from opposite localization.

Varriale and Chryssos [42] described 26 patients with documented old MI, admitted within 2.5 years (11 women, 15 men, average age 66 years), with an RSR' pattern in V3 to V6 (13 pat.), in II/aVF/III (9 pat.) and in both anterior and inferior leads (4 pat.). The QRS duration was 0.11–0.16 sec (-0.18 sec); RBBB and LBBB were excluded by vectorcardiography. An RSR' type was observed in one lead in 11 patients and in ≥ two leads in the other 16 patients. Additional pathologic Q waves were present in 12 patients. The RSR' type was generally associated with severely impaired LV function (10% to 58%, average 26.3%) with heart failure in 18 of 26 patients. Ten patients died during the follow-up period of 3 years.

Incidentally, similar infarction patterns were described by Grant in 1957 [43], called *peri-infarction block* at that time. As some peri-infarction block patterns were later recognized as left fascicular blocks (hemiblocks), this term was abandoned. However, the RSR' pattern corresponding to an old MI principally represents a peri-infarction block, due to a terminal conduction delay of fractionated viable myocardial tissue around the infarction scar [42].

In our opinion, an isolated RSR' type in the inferior leads may be misleading and may correspond to a normal variant, for instance an incomplete RBBB. Notched QRS in other leads or pathologic negative T waves favor the diagnosis of old MI, as do pathologic Q waves in other leads. The RSR' (rsR') pattern may also be observed in leads I, aVL and/or V_5/V_6, in MI patterns in the presence of LBBB (see section 10.2 above).

11.6 Infarction with Pure or Predominant Reduction of R Wave Amplitude

The diagnosis of MI in this condition is very often uncertain or impossible. However, in some cases, especially with notched QRS, MI can be suspected (ECGs 13.100 and 13.101).

In summary, the 'special' infarction patterns described in points 11.3–11.5 above represent *typically atypical*(!) infarction patterns for an experienced ECG reader, who compares the ECG with angiographic findings. As a matter of fact, many ECG readers have no experience in invasive cardiology and worse, some invasive cardiologists are not interested enough in electrocardiology.

On one hand, formally *evident* pathologic Q waves, so-called significant ST elevation and negative (also symmetric) T waves, found in normal individuals, are due to artifacts (false poling of the limb leads) or other conditions and diseases far removed from MI. On the other hand, there are ECG patterns with *minor* special alterations that allow the probable and sometimes definitive diagnosis of MI. It is evident that a comparison with a previous ECG is very helpful in these cases.

Remember that not every infarction pattern is as typical as that shown in ECG 13.102, with a pattern of acute MI involving more or less all walls of the left ventricle (and probably also the right).

To conclude with the ECG examples: ECG 13.103 shows a *classical non-infarction pattern*(!) – a completely normal ECG. However the patient suffered from mild angina during exercise and had a borderline exercise test. The coronary angiogram revealed an occluded LAD, with good collateralization from the right coronary artery and CX. LV ejection fraction was 75%. An attempt to reopen the LAD failed and the patient was controlled with drug therapy. – Let us remember that a normal ECG at rest does not exclude a severe CHD.

11.7 Atrial Infarction

The pattern of *atrial infarction* represents a special condition of special infarctions, because the atrial muscle is involved. The real prevalence of atrial infarction is not known. Gardin and Singer [44] found it in 1%, whereas in a book on auricular electrocardiograms by Zimmerman et al [45] an incidence of 17% is indicated. The reason for this discrepancy is probably a different use of the common criteria, which are: a) Elevation of the segment between the end of the p wave and the beginning of the QRS complex ('PQ elevation'), the most reliable sign in the opinion of Gardin and Singer; b) Depression of that segment; and c) Notched p waves. It is also obvious that the criteria are rather vague. Atrial infarction may be responsible for atrial arrhythmias, but is not clinically important overall. Moreover, some published ECGs of 'atrial infarction' are more representative of innocent atrial repolarization, or even atrial arrhythmias, but not infarction (see ECG (B) on page 1346 of ref [44] where atrial flutter is present). *PQ depression* in acute MI is more often combined with infarction-related pericarditis than with atrial infarction. Nagahama et al [46] observed in 304 patients with acute anterior MI that PQ depression (present in only a minority of the patients with additional pericarditis) is associated with greater infarct size and with a significantly higher hospital mortality rate.

12 Differential Diagnosis of 'Classical' Q-wave Infarction Patterns

The differential diagnosis of the 'classical' infarction patterns is given in Table 13.1. Regarding *acute MI* versus *acute pericarditis* it can generally be said that in acute MI the elevated ST segment arises from the R wave, whereas in acute pericarditis the elevated ST segment arises from the S wave. On one hand, however, the ST segment may arise from the S wave in the precordial leads V_1 to V_3 (with pre-existing deep S waves), also in acute MI. On the other hand, the ST segment may arise from the R wave in leads V_5/V_6 in acute pericarditis, if there is no pre-existing S wave.

The differential diagnosis of the *pathologic Q waves* is extensively discussed in Chapter 14. Acute pericarditis is diagnosed in most cases by the behavior of the frontal ST vector, that is between + 30° and + 70° (see chapter 15 Acute and Chronic Pericarditis).

13 Localization of Infarction and Localization of Coronary Occlusion

The correlation between the infarction location and the site of coronary lesion is not reliable because of anatomical variations of the coronary arteries (e.g. dominance of one vessel or one great branch), the extent of collateral vessels (culprit or bystander stenosis), the position of the heart and other conditions. However, some correlation between the localization of the infarct and the site of occlusion of coronary vessels is quite common (Figures 13.2a–f). Also the usual ECG terms for infarct site are not precise. For practical use it is still convenient, however, to use the traditional terms 'inferior MI', 'posterior MI', 'anteroseptal MI', 'extensive anterior MI', and so on.

14 Estimation of Infarct Size

In only about 60% of *old* Q-wave infarction can the size be estimated reasonably, by application of the rule: *the more leads that show a Q wave, and the greater the size of the Q waves (QS), the greater the infarcted area is (and vice-versa).* This is especially valid for anterior infarction. However, in about 40% of cases the relation is not found. For example, an ECG with QS waves in V_1 to V_4 and a Qr complex in V_5 may also correspond to a circumscript apicoseptal aneurysm with modest reduction of LV ejection fraction. In contrast, a big anterolateral infarction with a severely impaired LV function may only show a QS complex in leads V_1 to V_3, without pathologic Q waves in the other precordial leads or in I and aVL. The reasons for this discrepancy are not known. However, the limitations of the ECG, as an indirect method, are demonstrated once more.

As LV function is very important for heart performance and prognosis, the infarct size should not be estimated on the basis of ECG alterations but should be measured by a direct method (e.g. the echocardiogram).

In a pattern of *acute* infarction, the definitive extent of necrosis cannot be predicted in most cases. Generally, more leads show signs of injury (ST elevation) than leads revealing signs of necrosis thereafter (Q/QS waves). The definitive infarct size depends on many variables. The behavior of the lesion section around the central necrosis is favorably influenced by collaterals, and negatively affected by apposition of additional thrombotic material in the coronary artery. Infarct size may be reduced by early PTCA and thrombolysis.

Question: If the ECG is unreliable at defining the size and precise localization of MI, then why should the 'exact' description of the infarction type be necessary? (Not a bad question...)

Answer: A detailed analysis of the ECG sharpens the interpreter's eye for detection of atypical or minor alterations of clinical importance (e.g. posterior infarction, 'complex' and 'special' infarction patterns).

Acute infarction

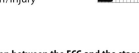

- ischemia
- lesion/injury

Figure 13.5a
Acute infarction: correlation between the ECG and the stage of myocardial ischemia. Monophasic ST deformation/'transmural' lesion=lesion/injury

Subacute infarction

- »necrosis«
- ischemia
- lesion/injury

Figure 13.5b
Subacute infarction: correlation between the ECG and the stage of myocardial ischemia (ST elevation=lesion, pathologic Q wave=necrosis, negative T wave=ischemia)

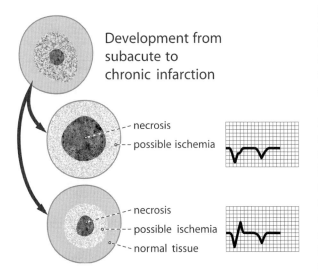

Development from subacute to chronic infarction

- necrosis
- possible ischemia

- necrosis
- possible ischemia
- normal tissue

Figure 13.5c
Evolution of subacute infarction to chronic infarction

15 Electropathophysiology

The description of the infarction stages related to the electropathophysiologic evolution corresponds quite well with the real myocardial damage.

15.1 Acute Stage

Thrombotic occlusion of a coronary artery leads to ischemia, with a central zone of major ischemia (lesion/injury). The ECG shows transmural lesion or a so-called 'monophasic deformation'; the R wave, the ST segment, and the T wave are incorporated into a *single positive deflection* (Figure 13.5a).

15.2 Subacute Stage

Necrosis develops in the central zone; in the ECG a *Q wave* appears. The necrotic zone is surrounded by a lesion zone (minor ST elevation in the ECG), that is itself surrounded by an ischemic zone, with T negativity beginning in the ECG (Figure 13.5b).

15.3 Old (Chronic) Stage

The lesion (or injury) zone is of great importance for the evolution of infarction. Figure 13.5c shows two possibilities of the evolution from subacute to old/chronic infarction: either (rarely) the whole lesion zone develops to necrosis, thus increasing infarct size (Figure 13.5c, short arrow), and we find broad Q or QS waves in the ECG; or (frequently) the lesion zone recovers partially, thus limiting the infarct size (Figure 13.5c, long arrow), and we find less broad Q waves in the ECG. In old infarction the ST segment has returned to the isoelectric line and the T wave is generally symmetric and negative. Often the T wave normalizes after weeks or months.

Transmural lesion is a potentially reversible stage. Complete recovery occurs regularly in Prinzmetal angina due to reversible spasm of a coronary artery branch. In MI regression of the lesion to ischemia or to normal myocardium is enhanced by collaterals and therapeutic procedures such as fibrinolysis or PTCA. This phenomenon is called recovery of 'hibernating myocardium': A zone, formerly unable to contract, regains its vitality. Indeed, even portions of extremely ischemic myocardium (characterized in the ECG by a part of the pathologic Q wave) may recover. This explains the general observation that the size and duration of Q waves decrease during the first weeks or months after an acute infarction. A *pathologic Q wave, in its strict sense,* represents *nondepolarizable* myocardium, and *not* necrosis. Consequently, in very rare cases, Q waves may be completely reversible. Necrosis is *never* reversible, by definition.

It must be emphasized that the comments about the correlation between infarct size and QRS configuration are 'didactic'. In practice there is sometimes a good correlation, but in many cases the correlation is bad or even lacking. This is true also for non-Q-wave infarction.

16 Complications of Acute MI

A brief overview of this subject seems appropriate for a book on ECGs.

16.1 Arrhythmias and Conduction Defects

Arrhythmias represent the *most frequent direct complications* of acute MI, including ventricular premature beats (VPBs), monomorphic ventricular tachycardia (VT) and ventricular fibrillation, AV blocks of all degrees, and ventricular tachycardia (VT) of the type torsade de pointes, in some cases.

In inferior infarction, especially in combination with RV infarction, complete AV block of suprahissian localization develops in about 12% and generally regresses spontaneously over AV block 2° and 1° to normal AV conduction within days. Definitive pacing is rarely required. Complete infrahissian AV block is rare, it indicates severe damage of the left ventricle and is seen in extensive anterior infarction. The appearance of a new RBBB, LBBB or bilateral block in the course of acute infarction is observed in 0.5%–8% [26, 28–30, 48, 49]; RBBB occurs more frequently than LBBB. A new LAFB is remarkably rare, occurring in < 5% of cases. Scheinman and Brenman [49] found 20 cases of LAFB in 480 patients with acute MI, but in 19 cases LAFB was pre-existant. In the publication by Bosch et al [35], the number of LAFB due to acute MI (out of 28 cases of LAFB in 141 patients) was not clearly determined.

16.2 Nonarrhythmic Complications

Ventricular aneurysm is quite frequent in anterior infarctions. A study in 80 patients indicates that persisting ST elevation of more than 1 mm in > three anterolateral leads, in anterior Q-wave infarctions, represents a reliable sign for aneurysm [47]. In our experience, in many aneurysms of the anterior LV wall, ST elevation is missed. For unknown reasons (perhaps due to the absence of the 'proximity effect' in the limb leads) inferior aneurysm is only exceptionally detectable by persisting ST elevation in leads aVF, III (and II).

For *rupture of the LV free wall* and for ventricular *septal perforation* there are no reliable ECG signs.

In some cases a 'second' ST elevation may announce imminent wall rupture [50]. ST elevation in lead aVL in the ECG at admission (within 6 h of the onset of chest pain) may be a predictor of free-wall rupture [51]. However, the correlation is quite poor. In the series by Yoshino et al [51] only four of the seven patients with free-wall rupture had an ST elevation in aVL > 0.1 mV, compared to 51 patients *without* rupture but with the same ECG alteration.

Thus, the common *nonarrhythmic complications* of MI, including shock, acute mitral regurgitation due to rupture of subvalvular tissue and ventricular septal defect, are diagnosed on the basis of typical clinical findings [52,53] and with the help of echo/Doppler, the Swan-Ganz catheter (determination of right heart oxygen saturation in the case of septal perforation), or with conventional heart catheterization.

For further information about the ECG in myocardial infarction (and unstable angina) see the recently published book by Wellens et al [54].

References

1. Fischer A, Gutstein DE, Fuster V. Thrombosis and coagulation abnormalities in the acute coronary syndromes. Cardiol Clin 1999;17:283–94
2. Gutstein DE, Fuster V. Pathophysiologic and clinical significance of atherosclerotic plaque rupture. Cardiovasc Res 1999;41:323–33
3. Prinzmetal M, Kennamer R, Corday E, et al. Angina pectoris. I. A variant form of angina pectoris. Am J Med 1959;27:375–88
4. Maseri A. Coronary vasoconstriction: visible and invisible. N Engl J Med 1991;325:1579–80
5. Yasue H, Ogawa H, Okumura K. Coronary artery spasm in the genesis of myocardial ischemia. Am J Cardiol 1989;63:29E–32E
6. Bland EF, White PD, Garland J. Congenital anomalies of the coronary arteries: report of an unusual case associated with cardiac hypertrophy. Am Heart J 1933;8:787
7. Liberthson RR, Dinsmore RE, Fallow JT. Aberrant coronary artery origin from the aorta. Report of 18 patients, review of literature and delineation of natural history and management, Circulation 1979;59:748–54
8. Felmeden D, Singh SP, Lip GY. Anomalous coronary arteries of aortic origin. Int J Clin Pract 2000;54:390–4
9. Johnston TA, Dyer K, Armstrong BA, Bengur AR. Anomalous origin of the left coronary artery in tetralogy of Fallot associated with abnormal mitral valve pathology. Pediatr Cardiol 1999;20:438–40
10. Tauth J, Sullebarger T. MI associated with myocardial bridging: case history and review of the literature. Catheter Cardiovasc Diagn 1997;40:364–7
11. Yetman AT, McCrindle BW, MacDonald C, et al. Myocardial bridging in children with hypertrophic cardiomyopathy – a risk factor for sudden death. New Engl J Med 1999;341:288–90
12. Hirata K, Kyushima M, Asoto H. Electrocardiographic abnormalities in patients with acute aortic dissection. Am J Cardiol 1995;76:1207–12
13. Bonchek LI: How should we manage suspected perioperative infarction after coronary bypass surgery? Am J Cardiol 2001;87:761–2
14. Brasch AV, Khan SS, Denton TA, et al. Twenty-years follow-up of patients with new perioperative Q waves after coronary artery bypass grafting. Am J Cardiol 2000;86:677–9
15. Rossiter SJ, Hultgren HN, Kosek JC, et al. Myocardial damage

in combined valvular and coronary bypass surgery. Circulation 1975;52(Suppl 2):119–25

16. Nunley DL, Grunkemeier GL, Starr A. Aortic valve replacement with coronary bypass grafting. Significant determinants of ten-year survival. J Thor Cadiovasc Surg 1983;85:705–11

17. Roth A, Elkayam U. Acute myocardial infarction associated with pregnancy. Ann Intern Med 1996;125:751–62

18. Lincoff AM, Popma JJ, Ellis SG, et al. Abrupt vessel closure complicating coronary angioplasty. Clinical, angiographic and therapeutic profile. J Am Coll Cardiol 1992;19:926–35

19. Mittleman MA, Mintzer D, Maclure M, et al. Triggering of MI by cocaine. Circulation 1999;99:2737–41

20. Hollander JE. The management of cocaine-associated MI. N Engl Med 1995;333:1237–41

21. Sanghvi S, Vyas V, Hakim A, et al. Reversible transmural inferior wall ischemia after honeybee sting. Indian Heart J 1997;49:79–80

22. Harries AD. Subarachnoid heamorrhage and the electrocardiogram – a review. Postgrad Med J 1981;57:293–6

23. Zehender M, Kasper W, Kauder E, et al. Right ventricular infarction as an independent predictor of prognosis after acute inferior MI. N Engl J Med 1993;328:981–8

24. Wellens HJJ. Editorial: Right ventricular infarction. N Engl J Med 1993;38:1036–8

25. Bowers TR, O'Neill WW, Grines C, et al. Effect of reperfusion on biventricular function and survival after right ventricular infarction. N Engl J Med 1998;338:933–40

26. Hod D, Goldbourt U, Behar S. Bundle-branch block in acute Q wave inferior wall MI. A high risk subgroup of inferior MI patients. The SPRINT study group (Secondary Prevention Reinfarction Israeli Nifedipine Trial). Eur Heart J 1995;16:471–7

27. Cabrera E, Friedland C. LA onda de activacion ventricular en el bloquéo de rama izquierda con infarto: un nuevo signo electrocardiografico. Arch Inst Cardiol Mex 1953;23:441–60

28. Hands ME, Cook EF, Stone PH, et al. The LIS Study Group. Electrocardiographic diagnosis of MI in the presence of complete left bundle-branch block. Am Heart J 1988;116:23–31

29. Weiner R, Makam S, Gooch AS. Identification of MI in the presence of left bundle-branch block: correlation of electrocardiography, vectorcardiography, and angiography. Am Osteopath Assoc 1983;83:119–24

30. Wackers FJ. The diagnosis of MI in the presence of left bundle-branch block. Cardiol Clin 1987;5:393–401

31. Sgarbossa EB, Pinski SL, Barbagelata A, et al. Electrocardiographic diagnosis of evolving acute MI in the presence of left bundle-branch block. N Engl J Med 1996;334:481–7

32. Madias JE, Sinha A, Asthiani R, et al. A critique of the new ST-segment criteria for the diagnosis of acute MI in patients with left-bundle-branch block. Clin Cardiol 2001;24:652–5

33. Rosenbaum MB, Elizari MV, Lazzari JO. The hemiblocks. Oldsmar, FL: Tampa Tracings 1970

34. Gertsch M, Bernoulli D. Fascicular block patterns – Observations on differential diagnosis. In: B Lüderitz (ed) Cardiac pacing. Berlin: Springer Verlag 1976, pp 111–18

35. Bosch X, Theroux P, Roy D, et al. Coronary angiographic significance of left anterior fascicular block during acute MI. J Am Coll Cardiol 1985;5:9–15

36. Godat FJ, Gertsch M. Isolated left posterior fascicular block: a reliable marker for inferior MI and associated severe coronary artery disease. Clin Cardiol 1993;16:220–6

37. Prinzmetal M, Shaw CM, Maxwell MH Jr, et al. Studies on the mechanism of ventricular activity. The depolarization complex in pure subendocardial infarction – role of the subendocardial region in the normal electrocardiogram. Am J Med 1954;16:469–88

38. Pipberger H, Schwartz L, Massumi RA, Weiner SM, Prinzmetal M. Studies on the mechanism of ventricular activity. XXI. The origin of the depolarization complex with clinical applications. Am Heart J 1957;54:511–29

39. De Zwaan C, Bär FW, Jannsen JHA, et al. Angiographic and clinical characteristics of patients with unstable angina showing an ECG pattern indicating critical narrowing of the proximal LAD coronary artery. Am Heart J 1989;117:657–65

40. Chatterjee K, Swan HJ, Parmley WW, et al. Depression of left ventricular function due to acute myocardial ischemia and its reversal after aortocoronary saphenous-vein bypass. N Engl J Med 1972;286;1117–22

41. Maseri A, Crea F, Cianflone D. Myocardial ischemia caused by distal coronary vasoconstriction. Am J Cardiol 1992;70:1602–5

42. Varriale P, Chryssos BE. The RSR' complex not related to right bundle-branch block: Diagnostic value as a sign of MI scar. Am Heart J 1992;123:369–76

43. Grant RP. Clinical electrocardiography. New York: McGraw Hill 1957, pp 176–181

44. Gardin JM, Singer DH. Atrial infarction. Importance, diagnosis, and localization. Arch Intern Med 1981;141:1345–8

45. Zimmerman HA, Bersano E, Dicosky C. The auricular electrocardiogram. Springfield, IL: Charles C Thomas, 1968

46. Nagahama Y, Sugiura T, Takehana K, et al. Clinical significance of ST segment depression in acute Q wave anterior wall MI. J Am Coll Cardiol 1994;23:885–90

47. Dubnow MH, Burchell HB, Titus JL. Postinfarction ventricular aneurysm. A clinicomorphologic and electrocardiographic study of 80 cases. Am Heart J 1965;70:753–60

48. Okabe M, Fukuda K, Nakashima Y, et al. A quantitative histopathological study of right bundle-branch block complicating acute anteroseptal MI. Br Heart J 1991;65:317–21

49. Scheinman M, Brenman BA. Clinical and anatomic implications of intraventricular blocks in acute MI. Circulation 1972; 46:753–60

50. Hurst JW. Abnormalities of the S–T segment – Part II. Clin Cardiol 1997;20:595–600

51. Yoshino H, Yotsukura M, Yano K, et al. Cardiac rupture and admission electrocardiography in acute anterior MI: implication of ST elevation in aVL. J Electrocardiol 2000;33:49–54

52. Prieta A, Eisenberg J, Thakur RK. Nonarrhythmic complications of acute MI. Emerg Clin Med North Am 2001;19:397–415

53. Mixon TA, Tak T, Lawrence ME. Cardiac tamponade complicating MI in the era of thrombolytics and platelet IIb/IIIa: case report and literature review. Am J Geriatr Cardiol 2001;10:133–8

54. Wellens HJJ, Gorgels AM, Dovendans PA. The ECG in acute myocardial infarction and unstable angina. Kluwer Academic Publishers. Boston/Dordrecht/London 2002

Note for all texts to the ECGs: Coro indicates LV angiography plus coronary angiography. PTCA may be with or without stenting (in recent years, additional stenting has been performed in about 75% of cases).

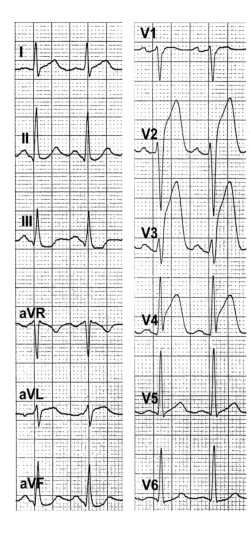

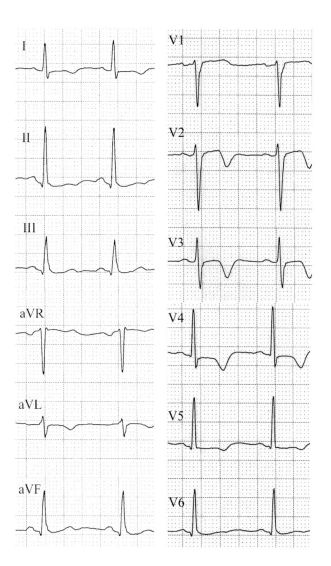

ECG 13.1a
64y/m. Acute 2-hour-old anteroseptal MI. ECG: ST elevation of up to 10 mm in most leads arising from the S waves! No pathologic Q wave. Echo: ejection fraction 65%, anteroapical hypokinesia.

ECG 13.1b
Same patient. ECG 4 hours later, after thrombolysis: ST segment normal, T negative in I, aVL and V_2 to V_4 (V_5). No pathologic Q waves. No coro.

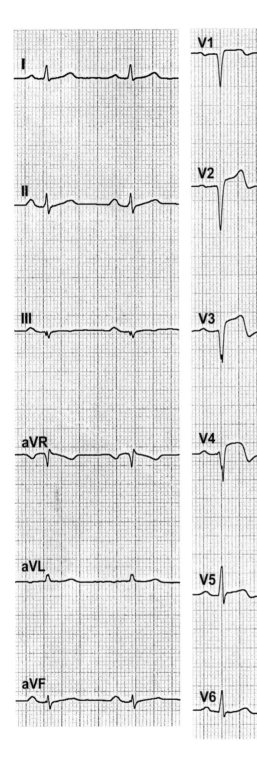

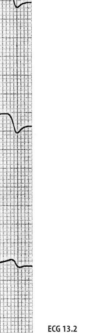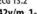

ECG 13.2

42y/m. 1-day-old acute anteroseptal MI. ECG: combination of QS in V$_1$/V$_2$ and minimal R wave in V$_3$/V$_4$ (with notching) with ST elevation in (V$_1$) V$_2$ to V$_5$, and terminally negative T wave in V$_3$/V$_4$. Coro: 99% stenosis of LAD and first diagonal branch. Apical hypokinesia, EF 70%. PTCA.

189

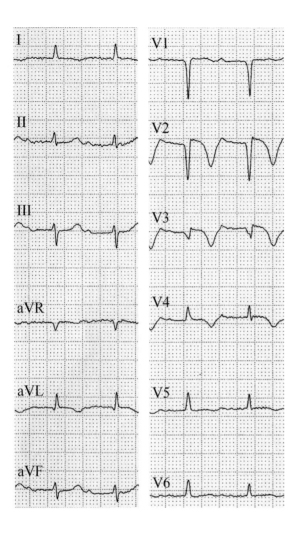

ECG 13.3
94y/m. 2-day-old acute anteroseptal MI. ECG: Qr in V_2/V_3 (notching in V_4), with slight ST elevation. Negative and symmetric T waves in V_2 to V_4 and aVL. No coro (note the age!).

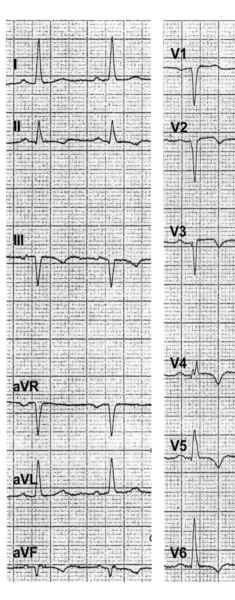

ECG 13.4
63y/m. 1-year-old anteroseptal MI. ECG: QS in V_2, Qr in V_3, notched QRS in V_4 (V_3). Minimal ST elevation in anteroseptal leads. Negative symmetric T waves in V_2 to V_6 and inferior limb leads. Coro: 50% LAD stenosis (spontaneous recanalizaton of LAD). Anteroseptal akinesia. LV EF 60%.

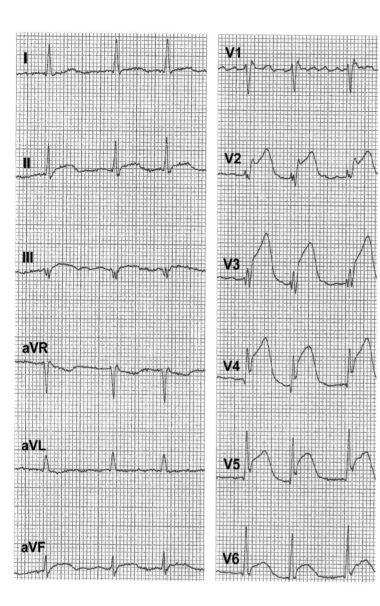

ECG 13.5

64y/m. Acute 1-hour-old acute extensive anterior MI. ECG: atrial fibrillation (incomplete RBBB). ST elevation up to 7 mm in leads V_2 to V_6, in V_2/V_3 arising from the S wave, and tall/broad T waves. Notched QRS in V_2/V_3. No pathologic Q waves. Coro: Occlusion of LAD. Anteroapical hypokinesia, EF50%. PTCA.

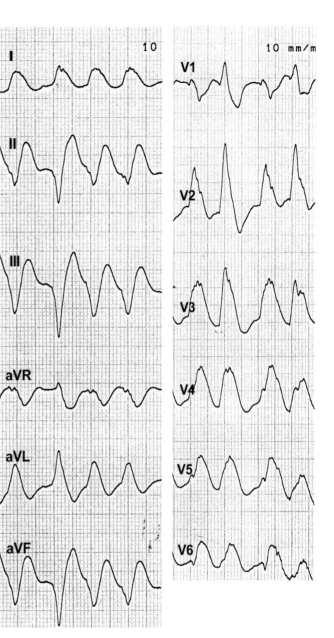

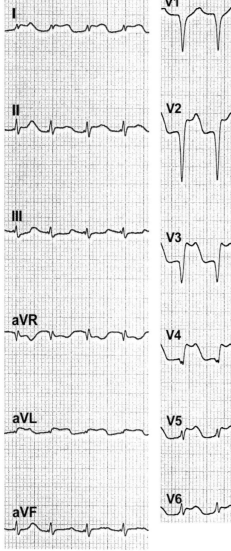

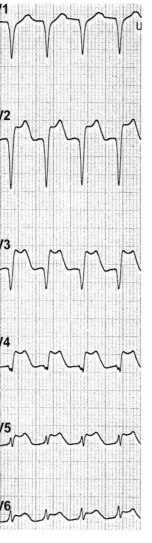

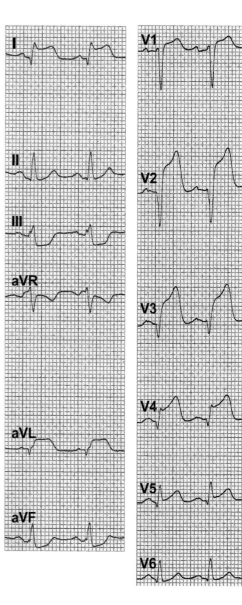

ECG 13.6b

Same patient. ECG 35 min later: probable atrial flutter type II with 1 : 2 AV conduction, ventricular rate 149/min. Peripheral low voltage. QS waves in leads V_1 to V_3, pathalogic Q in V_4. ST segment elevation up to 4 mm in I, II, aVL, V_2 to V_6. Coro: 20 mm long 60% proximal stenosis of LAD. Anterolateral hypokinesia, EF 58%. Interpretation: spontaneous recanalization of LAD. PTCA.

ECG 13.7

36y/m. Acute 3-hour-old extensive anterolateral MI. ECG: sinus tachycardia. QS (minimal r) in V_2/V_3, relatively deep and broad Q in V_4, I and aVL. ST elevation up to 5 mm in the corresponding leads. Coro: occlusion of the middle LAD. Anterolateral hypokinesia to akinesia, EF 40%. PTCA.

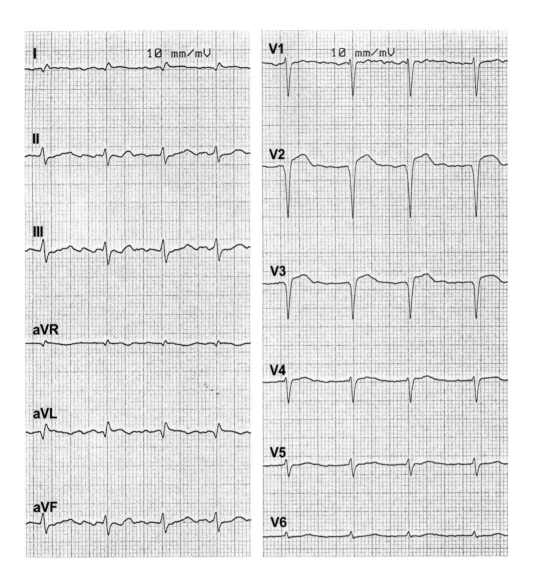

ECG 13.8

66y/m. 4-week-old 'acute' anterolateral MI. ECG: atrial fibrillation. QS complex in leads V_2 to V_3 and pathologic Q waves in I and aVL. Reduction of R amplitude in V_4 to V_6. Slight ST elevation in leads V_2 to V_3 (V_4, I, aVL). Coro: 90% stenosis of LAD and CX. Anterolateral akinesia, diffuse hypokinesia, EF 28%. PTCA of LAD and CX.

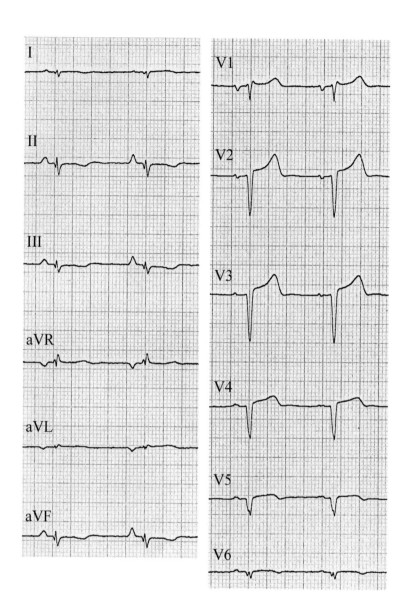

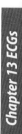

ECG 13.9

63y/m. 15-year-old anterolateral MI with aneurysm. ECG: QS in leads V_2 to V_6. Peripheral low voltage. Nonsignificant Q waves in I, II, aVF and III, rsr' in aVL. Slight ST elevation in (V_1) V_2 to V_5. Negative T waves in inferior leads (asymmetric), and in V_6 (symmetric). Echo: extensive anterolateral aneurysm, EF 45%.

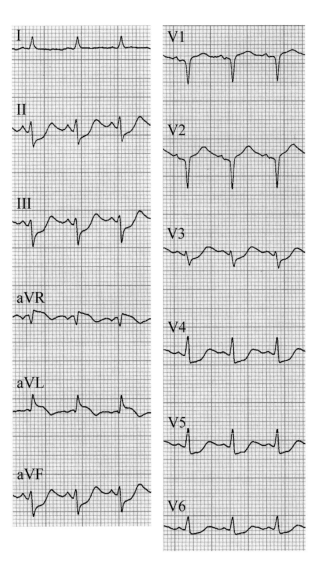

ECG 13.10

78y/f. Acute 2-day-old high lateral/posterior MI due to peri-interventional dissection of RCX. 8-month-old anteroseptal MI. ECG: sinus tachycardia. LAFB. ST elevation only in aVL (and aVR), with 'mirror image' ST depression in II, aVF, III and V_3 to V_6. QT interval prolonged. The old anteroseptal MI can be suspected by QS in V_1/V_2. Coro: closed LAD, intermittently closed CX. EF 60%.

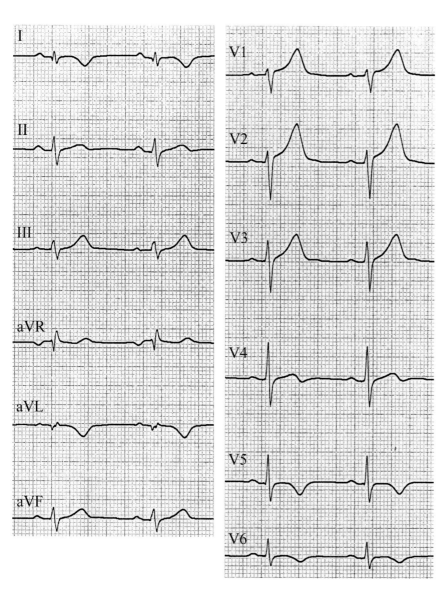

ECG 13.11
72y/m. Old high lateral MI. ECG: Qr in aVL, with symmetric T waves in aVL, I, V$_5$/V$_6$.

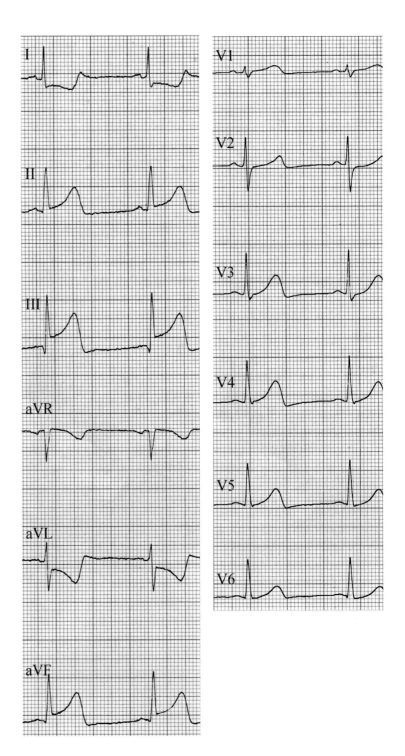

ECG 13.12
63y/f. Acute inferior infarction, chest pain since 2 hours. ECG: ST elevation in III/aVF(II), ST depression in I/aVL as mirror image. Coro: 90% RCA stenosis. EF 62%. PTCA.

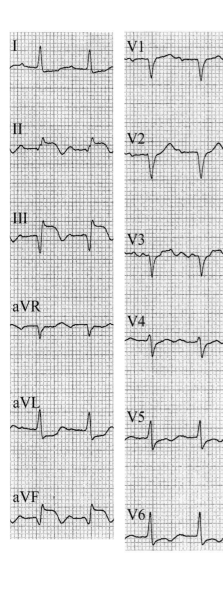

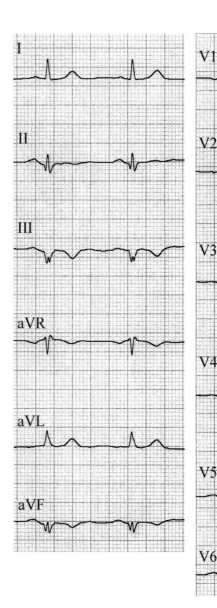

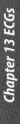

ECG 13.13

72y/f. Acute 24-hour-old inferior (and old anteroseptal?) MI. ECG: AV block 1°. Pathologic Q waves, ST elevation and T wave inversion in leads II, aVF and III. Poor R progression in V$_2$ to V$_4$. Negative T waves in V$_5$ to V$_6$. Coro: three-vessel disease, closed RCA and LAD. Inferior and anterior hypokinesia, EF 45%.

ECG 13.14

67y/m. Old inferior MI. ECG: nonsignificant Q in II and aVF (with reduction of R wave), QS in III. Negative symmetric T waves in III and aVF. Broad R waves in V$_1$ to V$_3$ might indicate posterior involvement. Coro: three-vessel disease, inferior hypokinesia, EF normal.

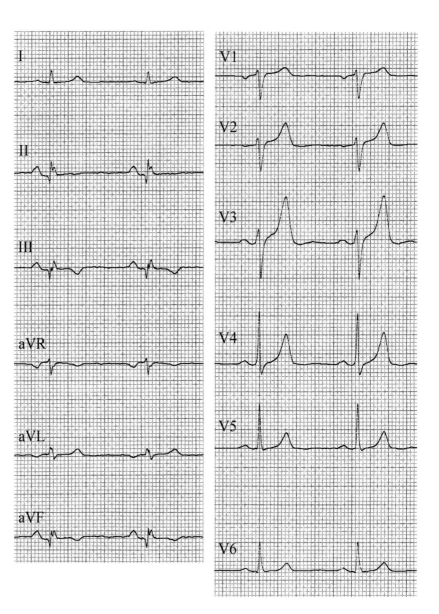

ECG 13.15
59y/m. 3-year-old inferior MI. ECG: Q in inferior leads with T inversion in III and aVF. Notched QRS in inferior and other leads. Coro: > 50% stenosis of RCA and LAD. EF 45%.

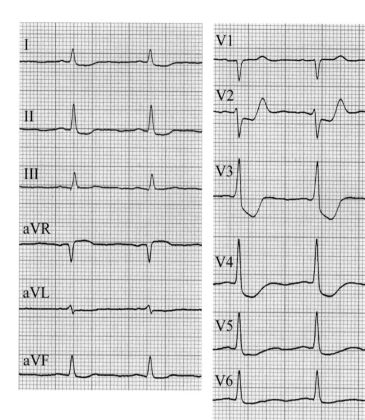

ECG 13.16

60y/m. Acute 6-hour-old posterior MI. ECG (half calibration): enormous ST depression (mirror image of posterior ST elevation) especially in V_2 to V_6. High and broad R in V_3. Coro: three-vessel disease with occlusion of the dominating RCX. EF 36%.

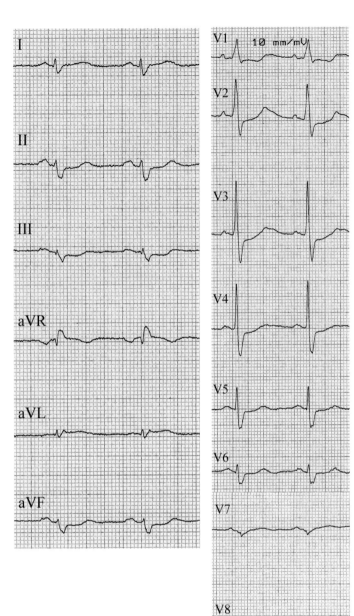

ECG 13.17

74y/m. Acute 5-day-old posterior MI. ECG: tall and broad R wave in V_1 and $V_2(V_3)$, slight ST depression in V_1 to V_5, both corresponding to mirror image of alterations in the posterior leads. See: QS in V_7/V_8, Qr in V_9.

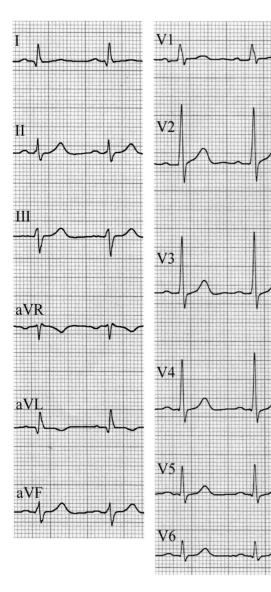

ECG 13.18

69y/m. 6-year-old posterior MI (and 9-month-old lateral MI). ECG: tall and broad R wave in V_1 and V_2. Slightly enlarged Q waves in I and aVL, R wave reduction in leads V_5/V_6 due to lateral MI. Coro: three-vessel disease with occluded LAD(!) and 70% stenosis of RCX. Inferior, posterior and lateral hypokinesia. LV EF 55%.

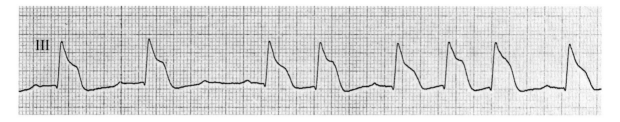

ECG 13.19a ▲
47y/m. Acute 12-hour-old inferior MI with RV involvement. Rhythm strip. SR, AV block 2° (Wenckebach and 'high degree').

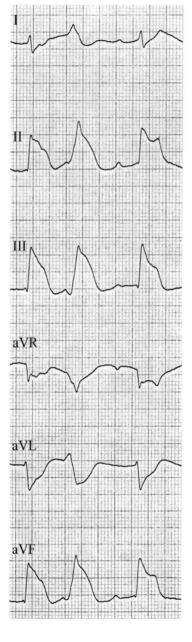

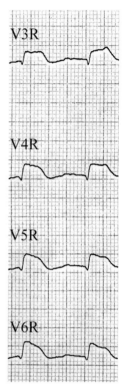

ECG 13.19c ▲
Same patient. Right precordial leads: monophasic deformation in II, aVF and III. Small q wave and extensive ST elevation in right precordial leads V$_3$R to V$_6$R. The patient refused any intervention and died 3 days later by cardiogenic shock. Probably dominating RCA.

ECG 13.19b ▶
Same patient. Limb leads: bizarre ST elevation ('monophasic deformation')

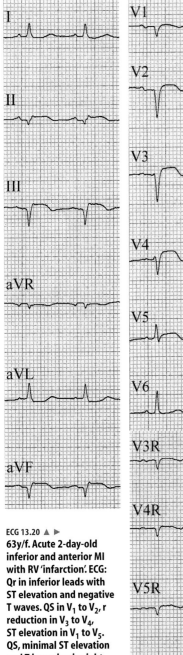
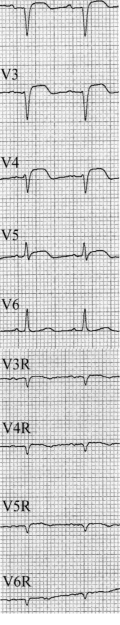

ECG 13.20 ▲ ▶
63y/f. Acute 2-day-old inferior and anterior MI with RV 'infarction'. ECG: Qr in inferior leads with ST elevation and negative T waves. QS in V_1 to V_2, r reduction in V_3 to V_4, ST elevation in V_1 to V_5. QS, minimal ST elevation and T inversion in right precordial leads V_3R to V_6R.

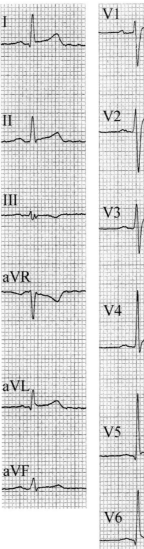
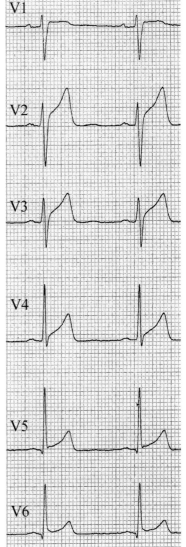
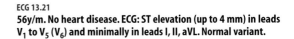

ECG 13.21
56y/m. No heart disease. ECG: ST elevation (up to 4 mm) in leads V_1 to V_5 (V_6) and minimally in leads I, II, aVL. Normal variant.

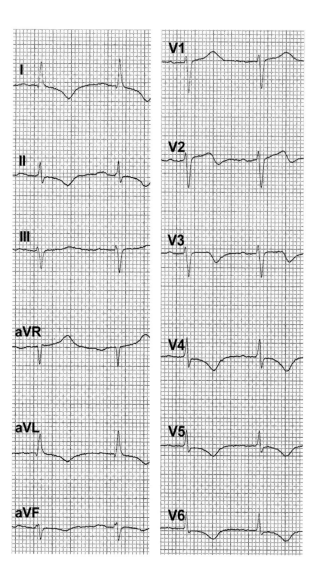

ECG 13.22

72y/f. 2-day-old non-Q-wave MI. ECG: SR, AV block 1°. Symmetric negative T wave in leads I, II, aVL (aVF) and V$_3$ to V$_6$. No significant Q waves, but slightly reduced R waves in V$_4$ to V$_6$. Coro: 60% stenosis of LAD, anterolateral akinesia, EF 40%. Interpretation: spontaneous recanalization of LAD. PTCA.

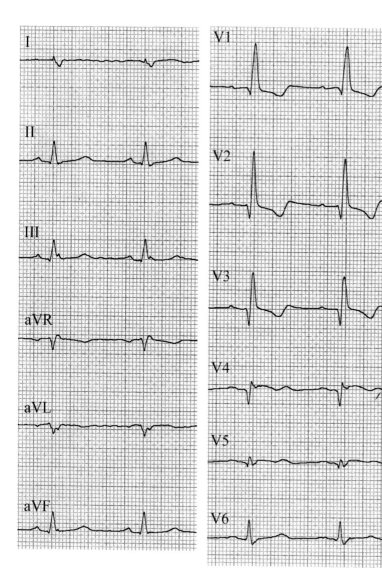

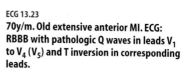

ECG 13.23

**70y/m. Old extensive anterior MI. ECG:
RBBB with pathologic Q waves in leads V$_1$
to V$_4$ (V$_5$) and T inversion in corresponding
leads.**

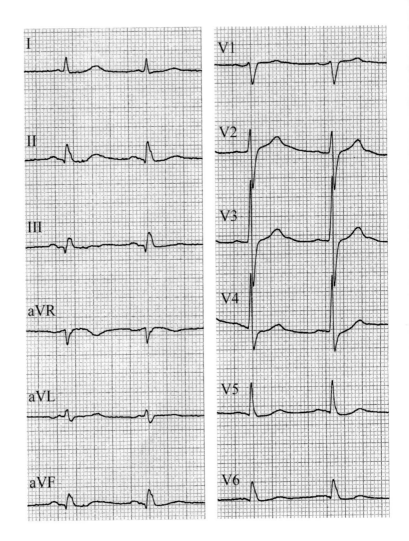

ECG 13.24
**81y/m. Old inferior MI, masked by LPFB. ECG:
ÂQRS$_F$ about + 60°. Non pathologic Q waves
in II, aVF and III. Slurred R downstroke in
V$_5$/V$_6$. Absent S wave in V$_5$/V$_6$. Coro: three-
vessel disease, occluded RCA, EF 50%, inferolateral hypokinesia.**

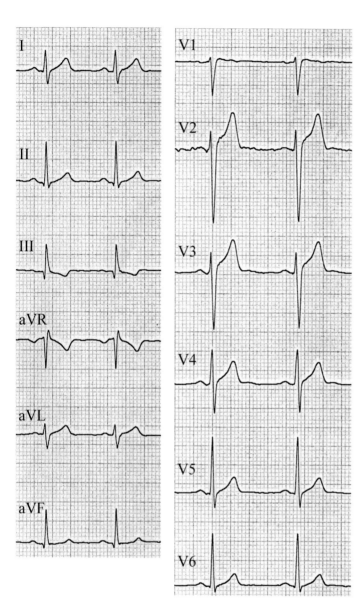

ECG 13.25

27y/m. Normal variant. No heart disease. ECG: ÂQRS_F + 80°. Small Q waves in inferior leads. No slurred R downstroke in V_6.

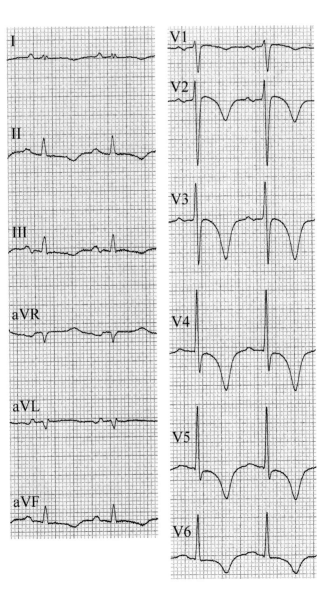

ECG 13.26

69y/m. Acute 16-hour-old non-Q wave MI. ECG: no pathologic Q waves but deep negative T waves in all precordial and limb leads except in aVL (aVR). Coro: 90% stenosis of a dominating LAD. Anterior hypokinesia to akinesia. EF 50%. PTCA.

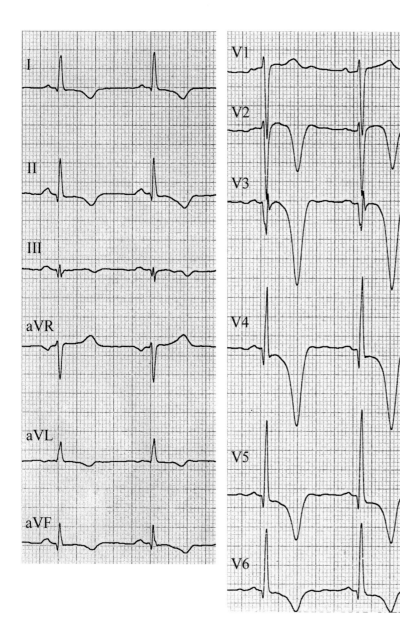

ECG 13.27

70y/m. Acute 1-day-old Q wave or non-Q wave MI? ECG: 1) Very deep symmetric T waves in leads V$_2$ to V$_6$ (and in aVL, I, II, aVF). 2) However pathologic Q wave in V$_3$ and suspect Q waves in V$_4$/V$_6$ and inferiorly. Coro: closed LAD, 50% stenosis of RCA. Extensive anterolateral akinesia. EF 30%.

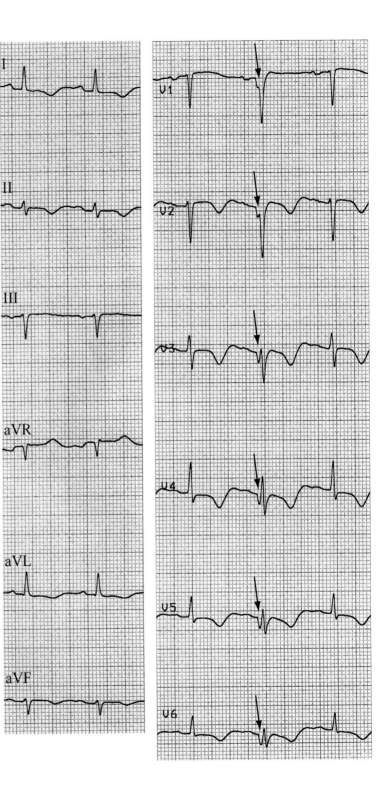

ECG 13.28
67y/f. Old non-Q wave MI. ECG: negative symmetric or symmetroid T waves in V_2 to V_6 and in aVL, I, II, aVF. No Q waves in SR. However, a late VPB (note the shorter PQ interval in the second beat) reveals QS in V_2 and pathologic Q waves in V_3 to V_6 ($\downarrow$). The patient refused Coro.

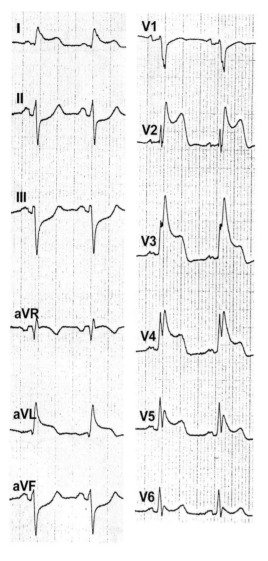

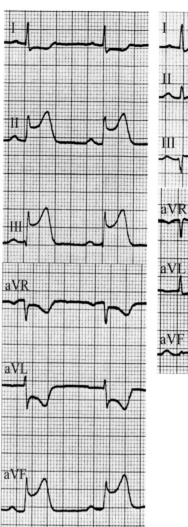

ECG 13.29

42y/m. Severe angina attacks at rest (Prinzmetal angina).
ECG: paroxysmal extensive ST elevation in leads I, aVL and
V$_2$ to V$_5$, reversible. Coro: subtotal proximal stenosis of
LAD, normal EF.

ECG 13.30a

48y/m. Severe angina attacks at rest (Prinzmetal angina). Limb leads: impressive ST elevation in the inferior leads (and V$_6$; not shown).

ECG 13.30b

Same patient. ST elevation almost reversible within 10 min. Coro: 90% RCA stenosis. PTCA.

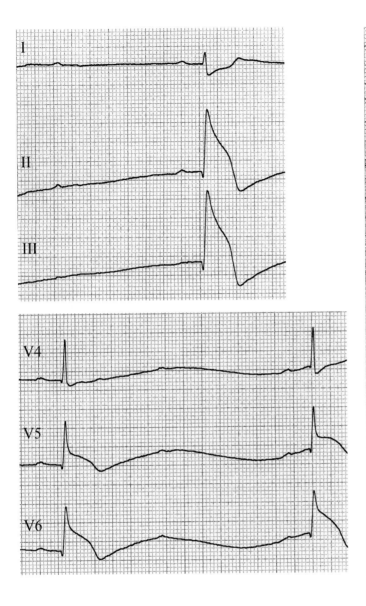

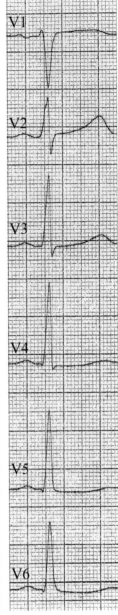

ECG 13.31

55y/m. Angina at rest during ECG registration (leads I, II, III and V$_4$ to V$_6$). Sinus bradycardia, striking ST elevation in the inferolateral leads and intermittent 2 : 1 AV block (ventricular rate 25/min). Coro: coronary two-vessel disease, two severe RCA stenoses with spasm and a similar ECG during PTCA.

ECG 13.32a

Short Story/Case Report 2. ECG before CABG: with exception of possible LVH and unspecific alteration of repolarization, within normal limits.

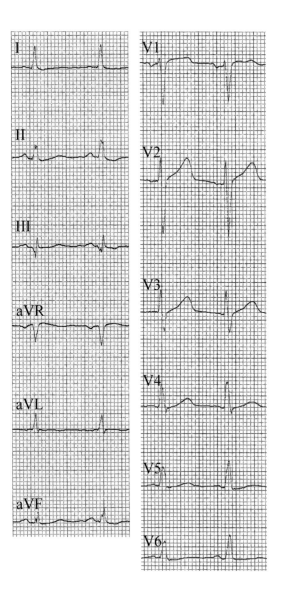

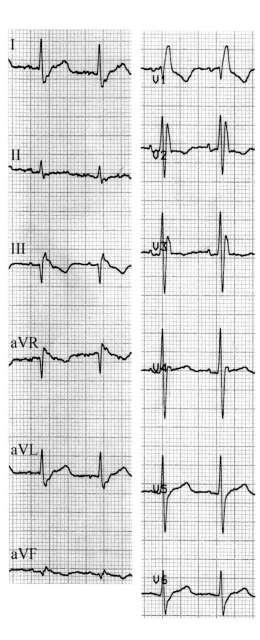

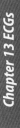

ECG 13.32b
Same patient. ECG after CABG: the extensive inferolateral MI is not visible in the ECG. Compared to ECG 13.32a, only a pathologic Q wave in lead III and a reduced R amplitude in V_5/V_6 can be observed.

ECG 13.32c
Same patient. ECG after heart transplantation: with exception of RBBB, ECG within normal limits. Echo: within normal limits.

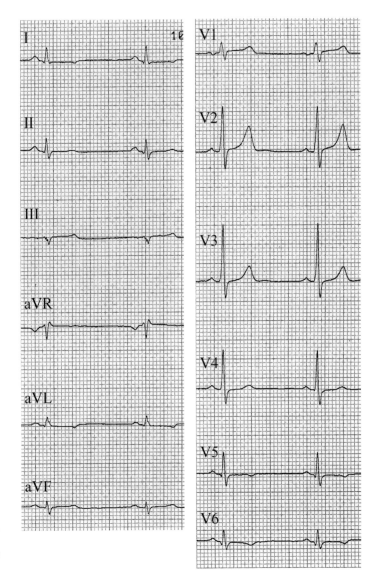

ECG 13.33
36y/m. 7-day-old posterior MI with lateral involvement. ECG: high R waves in V_1 to V_3 ($\geq$ 0.04 sec), symmetric T waves: mirror image of posterior MI. Decrease of R amplitude and increase of Q amplitude from V_5 to V_6, negative T waves in V_5/V_6. Coro: Closed CX, posterolateral hypokinesia, EF 50%.

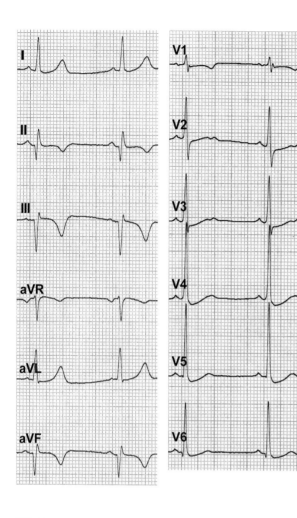

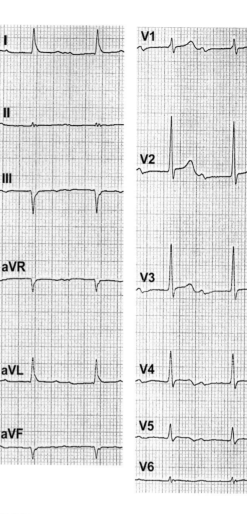

ECG 13.34

57y/m. 2-day-old inferoposterior MI. ECG: broad Q waves in inferior limb leads, broad R waves in V$_1$ to V$_3$ (R > S in V$_1$). Slight ST elevation in III, ST depression in V$_1$ to V$_6$. Symmetric negative T waves in III/aVF/II. Coro: three-vessel disease, closed RCA. Inferior akinesia, posterior hypokinesia. EF 55%.

ECG 13.35

70y/m. 6-year-old posterior MI, 2-year-old inferior MI. ECG: AV block 1° (PQ 0.38 sec). Broad R wave V$_1$ to V$_3$. QS in III/aVF. Small notched QRS in V$_6$: lateral involvement? Slight ST elevation in V$_1$ to V$_6$, together with decreased R amplitude due to pericardial effusion of unknown etiology. Coro: severe three-vessel disease with closed CX and RCA. Inferoposterior hypokinesia, EF 62%(!).

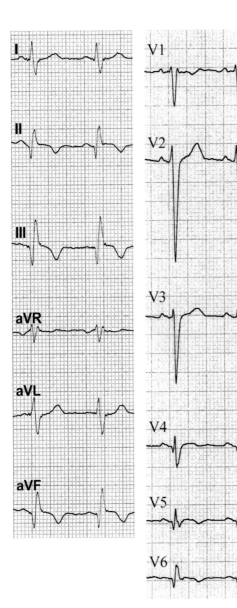

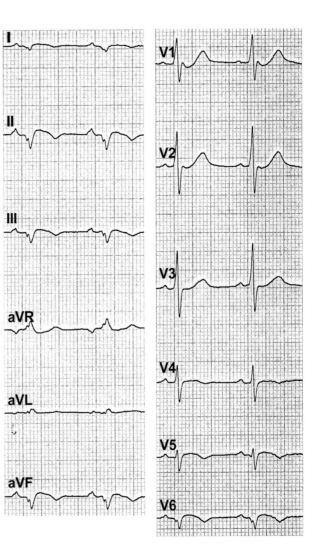

ECG 13.36

60y/m. 5-day-old inferolateral MI. ECG: Q waves in inferior and lateral leads, with symmetric negative T waves (rSr′ in V$_1$: incomplete RBBB). Coro: three-vessel disease, closed RCA. Inferolateral akinesia, EF 48%.

ECG 13.37

73y/m. 9-day-old inferoposterolateral MI. ECG: SR with a strange frontal QRS vector: QS in I, II, aVF and III. QS also in V$_6$. qrS in V$_5$. Tall R waves in V$_1$/V$_2$(V$_3$). Slight ST elevation and negative T waves in the leads with QS, and in V$_5$. In the ECG the infarct size is overestimated. Coro: closed CX, EF 55% (!).

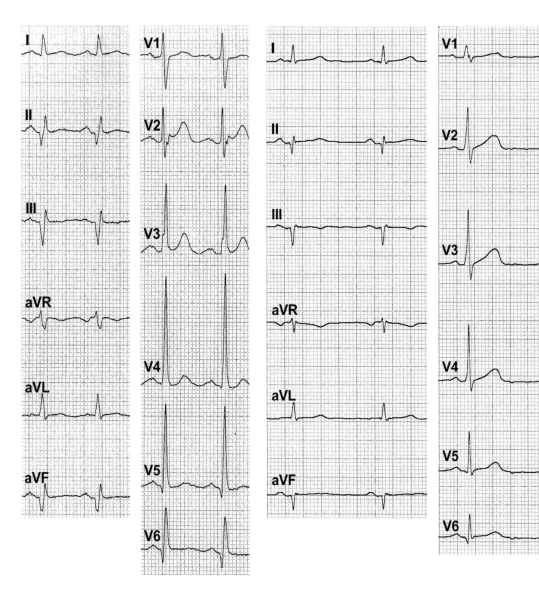

ECG 13.38

66y/m. Some years old inferoposterior MI with lateral involvement. LVH. ECG: Q in II, aVF, III, V$_6$. Tall R waves in V$_2$/V$_3$(V$_1$). LVH.

ECG 13.39

53y/m. One-month-old inferoposterior MI. ECG: Q in II, aVF. rS in III. Tall R waves in V$_1$ to V$_3$. Increasing Q and decreasing R from V$_5$ to V$_6$ may indicate lateral involvement. Coro: one-vessel disease, closed CX. EF 62%.

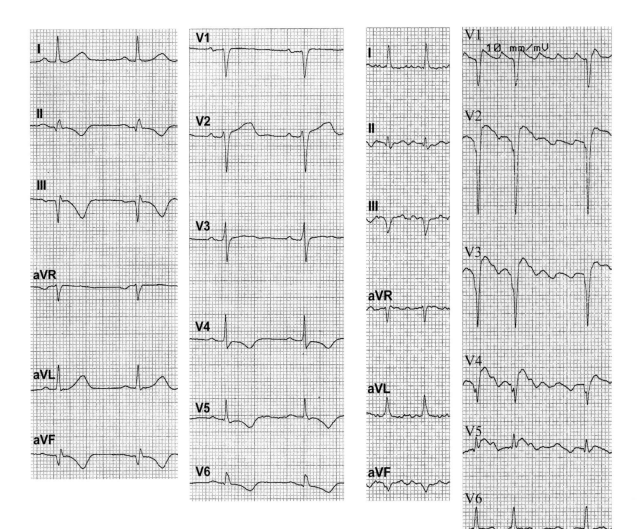

ECG 13.40

52y/m. 2-month-old inferior MI. ECG: Q in aVF, III (II), with negative T waves. Ischemic T waves also in lateral leads. Reduced R in V$_6$ may indicate lateral involvement. Coro: closed RCA, EF 39%(!).

ECG 13.41

63y/m. 6-year-old inferior and 3-day-old anterior MI. ECG: atrial flutter type 1 with irregular AV conduction. QS in III/aVF. QS in V$_1$ to V$_4$, ST elevation in V$_2$ to V$_5$. Coro: three-vessel disease, inferior hypokinesia to akinesia, anterior akinesia, EF 45%.

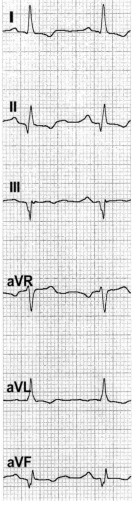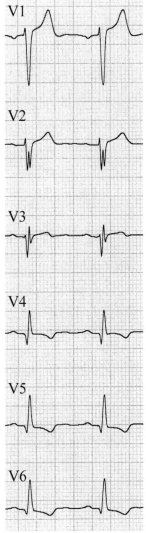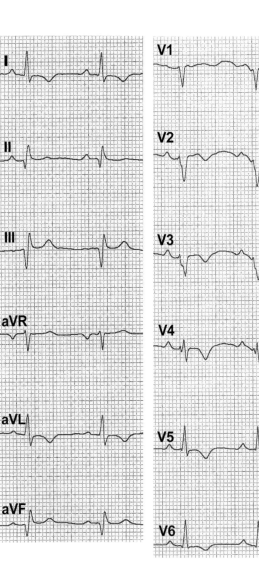

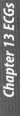

ECG 13.42

64y/m. 6-year-old inferior MI, 3-month-old anterior MI. ECG:
Q waves in III, aVF (II). Notched QRS in V_2/V_3, Q (0.04 sec) in V_4 (V_5).
Negative T in V_4 to V_6 (V_3) and some limb leads. Coro: two-vessel
disease, inferior and anterior akinesia, EF 35%.

ECG 13.43

59y/m. 3-year-old inferior MI, 17-day-old anterior MI. ECG: Q in III,
aVF, II with positive T. Poor R progression in V_2 to V_4, notched QRS in
V_2 to V_4. Negative T in V_2 to V_6, I and aVL. Coro: two-vessel disease,
inferior akinesia, anterior hypokinesia. EF 43%. By definition, the
anterior MI is a non-Q-wave infarction, but additionally diagnosable
by the rsR'(S) complex in V_4 (V_5); see section Special Infarction
Patterns.

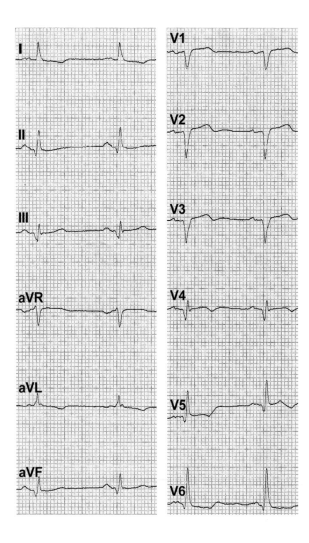

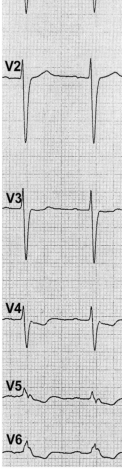

ECG 13.44

85y/m. Two MI occurred several years ago (anterior and inferior). No angina, heart failure. ECG: Q in III, aVF (II). QS in V_2/V_3 (V_1), Q in V_4(V_5). T negative in V_4 to V_6, terminally negative T in V_3. Echo: severely decreased EF.

ECG 13.45

73y/m. Several MI in the history. ECG: the infarctions are masking each other, but significant intraventricular conduction disturbance in all limb leads and V_5/V_6 is present (imitating LBBB in V_6). Decreasing R wave from V_2 to V_4/V_5. Note the negative (symmetrical) T waves inferiorly and in leads V_4 to V_6. Coro: severe three-vessel disease. EF 20%.

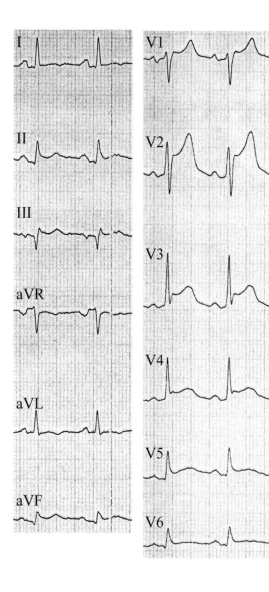

ECG 13.46

68y/m. 4-month-old inferior MI. Coro: three-vessel disease, inferior hypokinesia. EF 70%. Two days after aortocoronary bypass operation severe chest pain, pericardial friction. Re-coro: all four bypasses open. ECG: PQ depression in III/aVF, V$_5$/V$_6$. Slight ST elevation in I, II *and* aVF. Frontal mean ST vector + 75°. ST elevation in precordial leads (5 mm in V$_2$), in V$_5$/V$_6$ (V$_4$) arising directly from the R wave(!). Diagnosis: acute pericarditis (Dressler syndrome?).

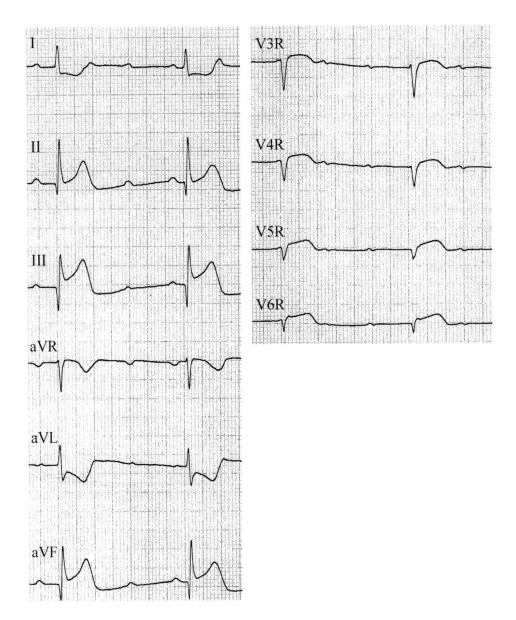

ECG 13.47

52y/f. 13-hour-old, acute inferior MI. EF 62%. ECG (limb leads only): complete AV block, AV junctional escape rhythm. 0.03 sec broad but deep Q waves in II, aVF, III, with slight ST elevation. Right precordial leads (V_3R to V_6R) show RV 'infarction'. Coro: one-vessel disease, closed RCA. PTCA.

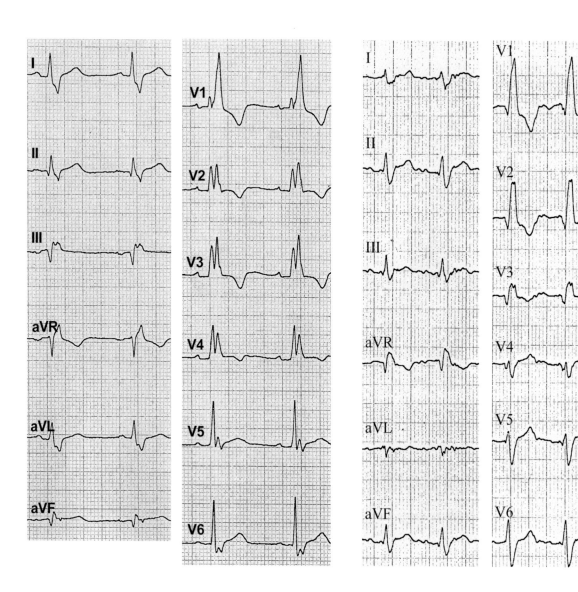

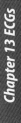

ECG 13.48
58y/m. Bronchial carcinoma, old inferoposterior MI. ECG: SR, RBBB.
Q waves inferiorly (only in III ≥ 40 msec), without T negativity. Tall
'primary' R waves in V₂/V₃ due to RBBB or posterior involvement.
Coro: severe three-vessel disease, closed RCA, inferoposterior
hypokinesia, EF 55%.

ECG 13.49
78y/m. 3-month-old anterior MI. ECG: SR, RBBB. Pathologic
Q waves in V₃/V₄ (rSR′ in V₁/V₂?). Vertical (LV) ÅQRS_F possibly due to loss of also lateral potentials.

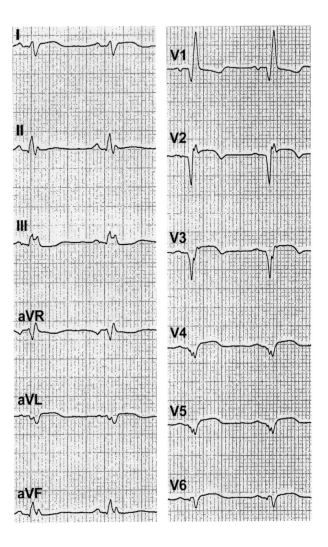

ECG 13.50
62y/m. 10-day-old extensive anterior MI. ECG: SR, RBBB. Pathologic Q waves V_1 to V_3, QS waves V_4 to V_5 (qrS in V_6) and aVL. ST elevation in V_2 to V_6 and I/aVL: aneurysm or 'acute' stage. Coro: severe three-vessel disease, anterolateral akinesia, EF 40%.

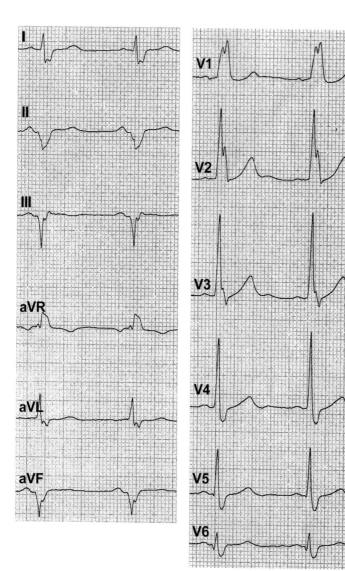

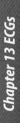

ECG 13.51

64y/m. One-year-old inferoposterior MI. ECG: SR, RBBB, broad Q/QS inferiorly, very tall first part of QRS in V$_1$ to V$_3$ due to additional posterior MI. Q and small R in V$_6$: possible lateral involvement. Coro: one-vessel-disease, closed great RCA, inferoposterior akinesia, EF 43%.

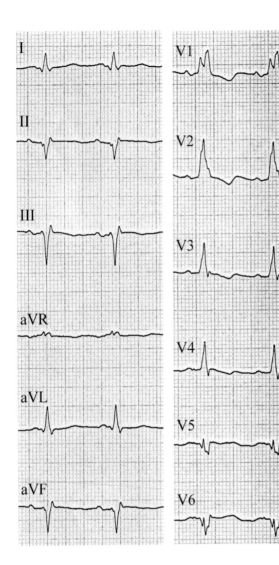
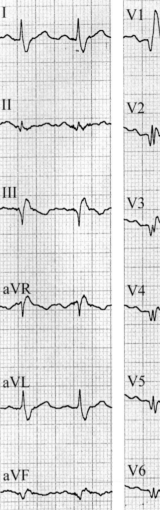
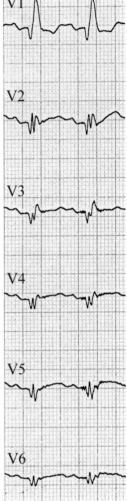

ECG 13.52

73y/m. CHD. ECG: old posterolateral MI. RBBB. SR, pathologic Q wave in II (rS in aVF/III), tall first part of R in V$_1$/V$_2$, notched broad Q wave in V$_6$ with small terminal R wave. Echo: severely depressed LV function.

ECG 13.53

74y/f. 1-year-old inferior and 6-year-old anterior MI. ECG: inferior and extensive anterolateral MI. RBBB. Q in inferior limb leads and V$_1$ to V$_6$, laterally with small R waves. QRS notching in V$_2$ to V$_5$. Persisting ST elevation in V$_2$ to V$_6$ indicates aneurysm. Coro: severe three-vessel disease, inferior akinesia, anterolateral diskinesia, EF 35%.

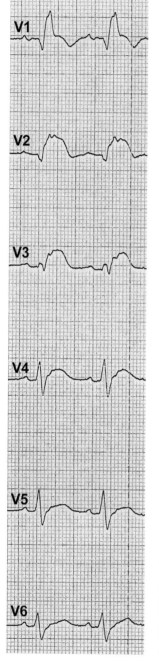

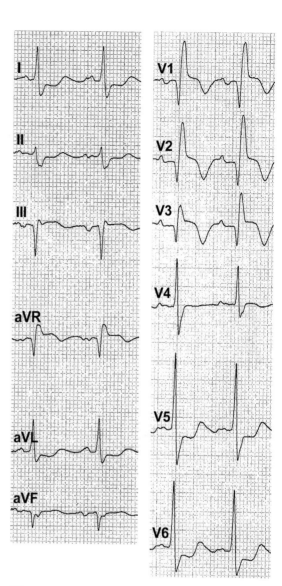

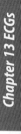

◄ ECG 13.54

84y/m. Several-hour-old acute anteroseptal MI. ECG (only precordial leads): SR, RBBB. Striking ST elevation in (V$_1$) V$_2$ to V$_4$ (V$_5$); pathologic Q waves in V$_1$/V$_2$. The ST elevation in V$_1$ is also pathologic, in presence of RBBB.

ECG 13.55 ▲

72y/m. CHD, 4-day-old anteroseptal MI, severe aortic stenosis. ECG: RBBB. Pathologic Q waves and ST elevation in V$_1$ to V$_3$. Minimal R waves in III, aVF. Tall R waves in V$_4$ to V$_5$ due to LVH. Coro: one-vessel disease, closed LAD, EF 20%(!).

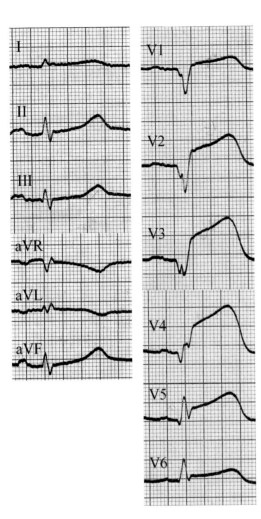

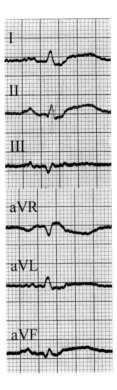

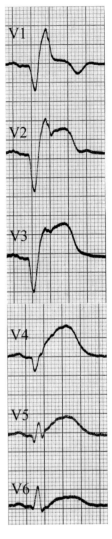

ECG 13.56a
59y/m. 1-day-old, acute extensive anterolateral MI. ECG (50 mm/sec!): MI, with QS in V$_1$ to V$_3$, pathalogic Q in V$_4$. Striking ST elevation V$_2$ to V$_5$ (V$_6$).

ECG 13.56b
Same patient. The ECG (50 mm/sec!) 4 days later shows reinfarction in the same region. Note also RBBB. No coro (ECGs from 1974).

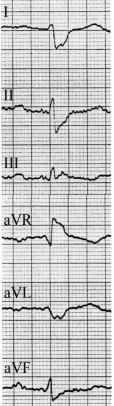

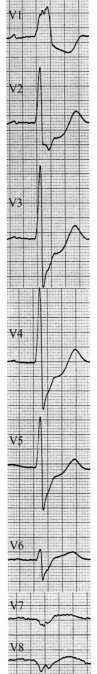

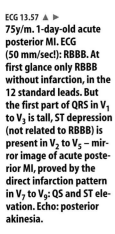

ECG 13.57 ▲ ▶

75y/m. 1-day-old acute posterior MI. ECG (50 mm/sec!): RBBB. At first glance only RBBB without infarction, in the 12 standard leads. But the first part of QRS in V_1 to V_3 is tall, ST depression (not related to RBBB) is present in V_2 to V_5 – mirror image of acute posterior MI, proved by the direct infarction pattern in V_7 to V_9: QS and ST elevation. Echo: posterior akinesia.

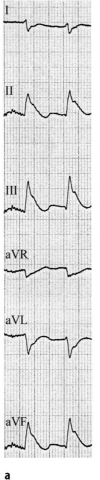

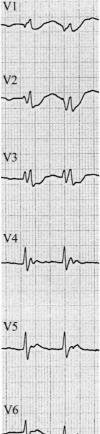

a

a

ECG 13.58a

88y/f. Several-hour-old, acute inferior MI + 'RV MI'. ECG: SR, AV block 2°, type Wenckebach (see leads V_4R to V_6R). RBBB. Striking ST elevation in II/ aVF/III.

b

ECG 13.58b

Same patient. Right precordial leads show RV 'infarction': ST elevation in V_4R to V_6R, Q wave in V_5R/V_6R.

ECG 13.59

63y/m. 2-day-old, acute inferoposterior infarction. Old anteroseptal MI. ECG: SR. AV block 1°. RBBB. Q waves in aVF/III, tall first part of QRS in V_2/V_3. Slight ST elevation in inferior limb leads (and V_5/V_6); ST depression in V_1 to V_3 (mirror image). In the presence of posterior MI: Q wave in V_1(!) as a possible sign of old anterior infarction. Coro: closed RCA, 70% CX stenosis, 50% LAD stenosis. EF 45%. Inferoposterior akinesia, septal hypokinesia.

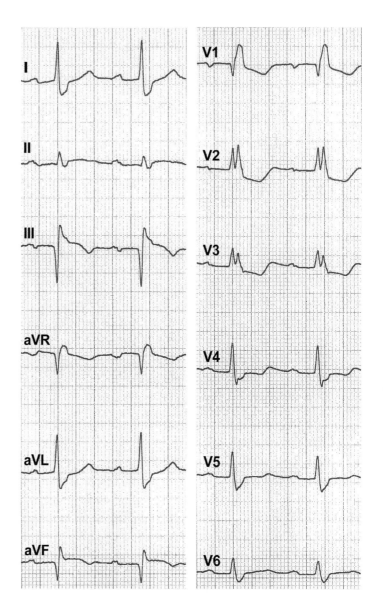

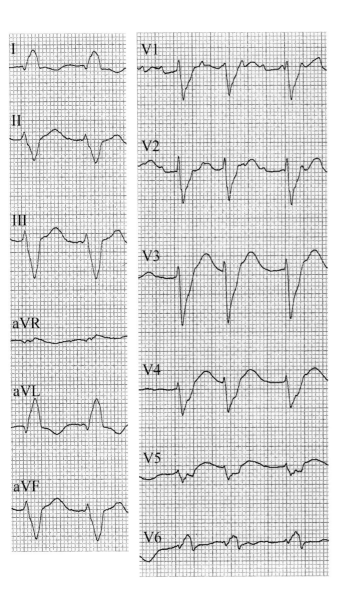

ECG 13.60

70y/f. 21(!)-year-old anterior MI. Coro 5 years before: closed LAD, LV EF 25%. ECG: atrial flutter with irregular conduction. LBBB. Pathologic Q waves (in LBBB) in I/aVL, reduced R in V$_5$, rsR's' in V$_6$. Decreasing R wave from V$_2$ to V$_5$. Actual echo: EF about 35%.

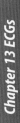

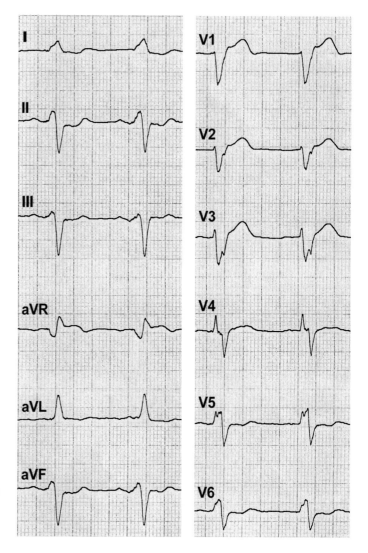

ECG 13.61

75y/m. 18-year-old extensive anterior MI. ECG: SR, LBBB. Pathologic notching in five precordial leads (V$_2$ to V$_6$), indicate anterior MI. Cabrera sign in V$_2$/V$_3$ (notched S upstroke). Inferior MI not diagnosable. Echo: apical dyskinesia, lateral and inferior akinesia, EF 25%.

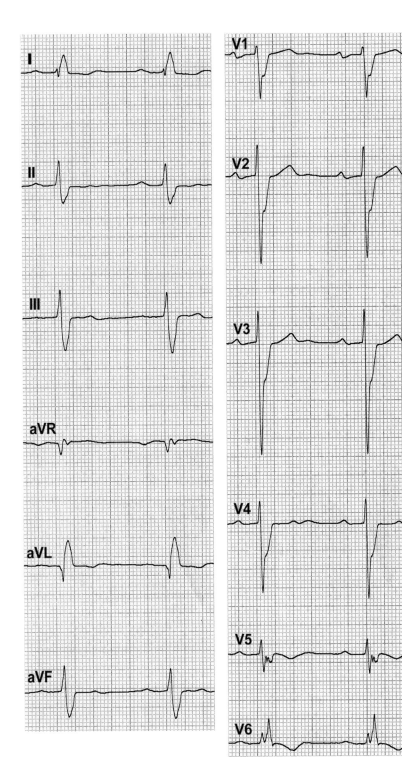

ECG 13.62

67y/m. Anterior, lateral, inferoposterior MI 20 years, 5 years, and 4 years ago. ECG: SR, AV block 1°. LBBB. Q in aVL, rsR' in I, notched QRS in V$_5$/V$_6$; Cabrera sign in V$_1$ to V$_4$. High R wave in V$_2$/V$_3$, decreasing to V$_5$. Coro: severe three-vessel disease, EF 25%.

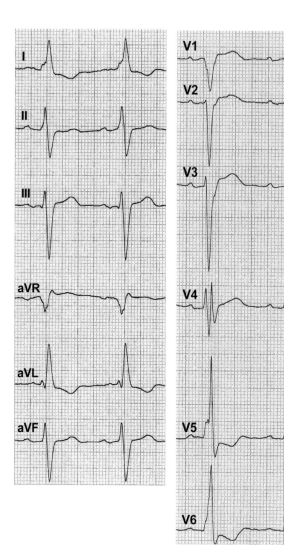

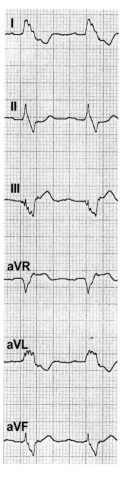

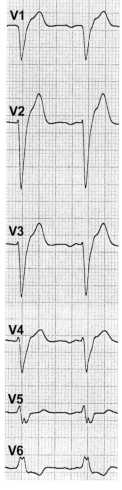

ECG 13.63

72y/f. 1-year-old anterior MI, 6-month-old inferior MI. ECG: SR, AV block 1°, LBBB. Slurred R upstroke in I, rsR' in aVL, Cabrera sign V_2/V_3, notched QRS in $V_4/V_5/(V_6)$. Inferior MI not diagnosable. Coro: two-vessel disease, 90% LAD stenosis, closed RCA. Inferior akinesia, anterior dyskinesia, EF 25%.

ECG 13.64

85y/m. At least two MI some years ago. CABG 13 years ago. ECG: SR (artifact: pseudo-p in V_3 to V_6), LBBB, in precordial leads similar/equal to 'uncomplicated' LBBB. Notched QRS in all limb leads, especially in I/III/aVL. Coro: severest three-vessel disease (all vessels closed, three of five bypasses open). Inferior akinesia, anterior hypokinesia. EF 40%.

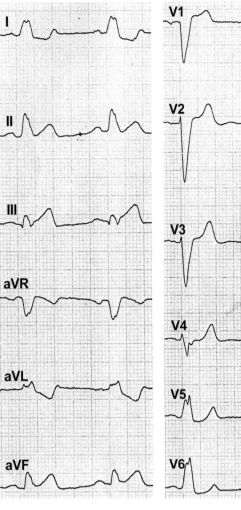

ECG 13.65
57y/m. Acute chest pain of 2 h duration. ECG: typical LBBB.
Slight but pathologic (concordant) ST elevation in leads aVF
and III, suggesting acute inferior infarction. Coro: two 90%
stenoses of RCA, inferior hypokinesia. The inferior lesion
was reversible after PTCA.

237

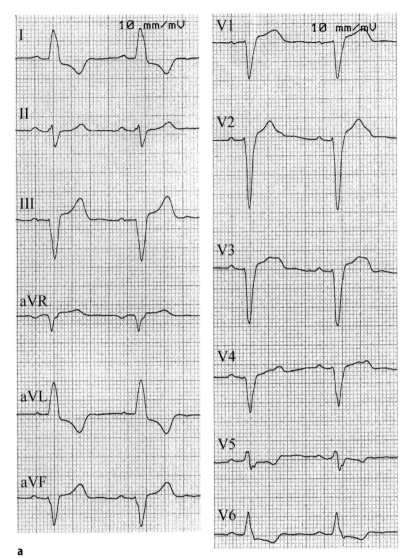

ECG 13.66a
68y/m. ECG: before AMI: SR, LBBB (incomplete?) without additional abnormalities.

a

a

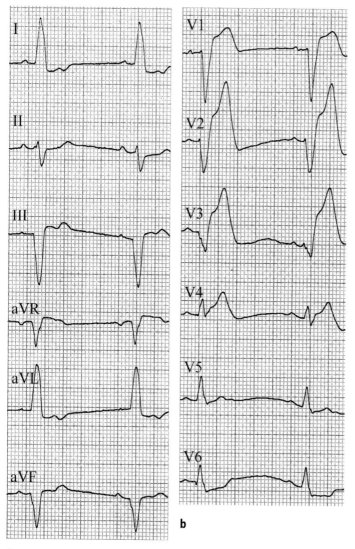

b

b

ECG 13.66b
Same patient. ECG (8 hours after MI): SR, LBBB.
ST elevation up to 8 mm in V_2/V_3 (V_1/V_4). Giant T in
V_2/V_3. No significant additional QRS abnormalities.
Coro: closed LAD and CX. Anterolateral akinesia,
posterior hypokinesia. EF 35%.

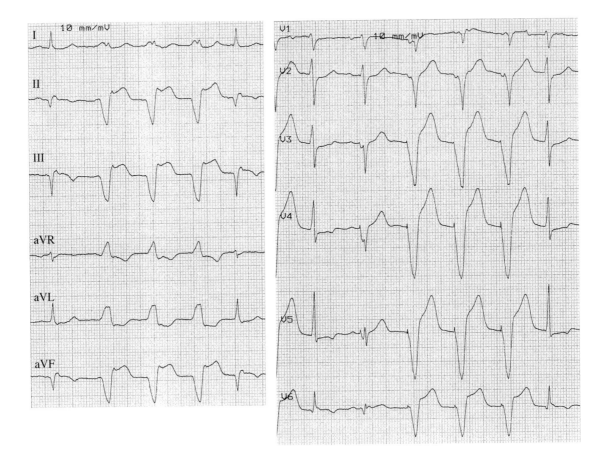

ECG 13.67

75y/m. Old inferior MI with aneurysm. In SR leads II, aVF and III reveal old inferior MI (ST elevation due to aneurysm), while during pacemaker rhythm there is the usual pattern of LBBB with QS complexes in these leads. The LBBB pattern in the precordial leads is common for paced beats, with a QS complex in all leads. The not-paced QRS are normal. The second precordial QRS complex imitates a loss of anterior potentials, however this is a fusion beat between spontaneous beat and paced beat.

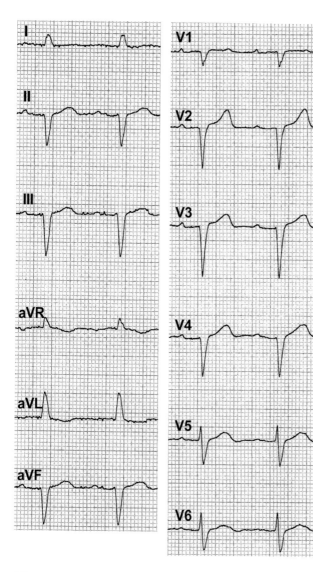

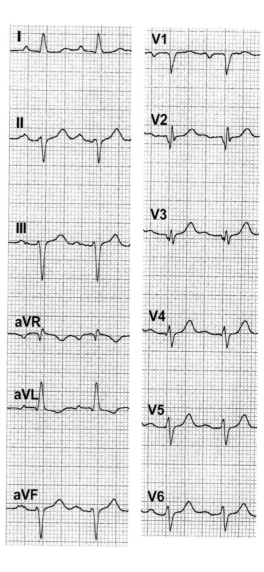

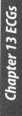

ECG 13.68

81y/f. Old anterior MI, partially masked by LAFB. ECG: LAFB, AV block 1°. Absence of 'smooth' transition zone generally present in LAFB, but abrupt change from a minimal R wave (up to V$_4$), to an R wave of 3–4 mm in V$_5$. Echo: anterior akinesia, EF 30%.

ECG 13.69

71y/m. Old anteroseptal MI. ECG: LAFB, AV block 1°. Pathologic Q waves in V$_2$/V$_3$ (V$_4$). No T wave abnormality. In a variant of LAFB, Q waves in anteroseptal leads are small.

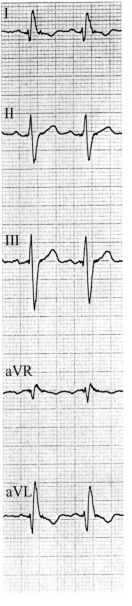

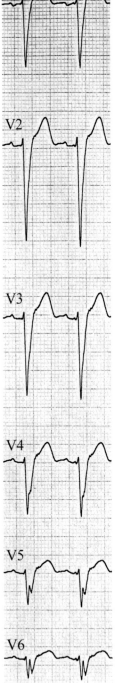

ECG 13.70 ▲ ▶

71y/f. Old anterior MI. ECG: LAFB. Notching of QRS in V₅/V₆ (V₄), rsR′ in I, aVL. Decrease of the (small) R amplitude from V₂ to V₆. Echo: extensive anterior hypokinesia, severely depressed LV function.

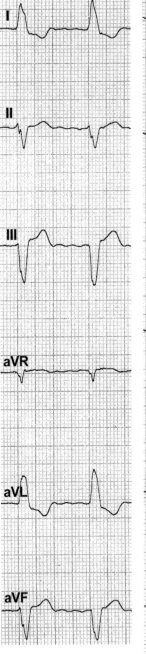

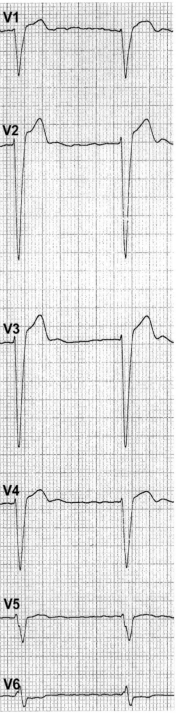

ECG 13.71 ▲ ▶

75y/f. 7-year-old anterior MI. ECG: atrial fibrillation, LAFB. Slight decrease of R wave from V₂ to V₅. Slight notching of QRS in V₅/V₆. Echo: anterolateral akinesia, EF 35%.

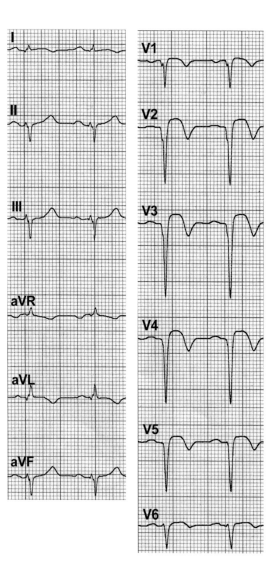

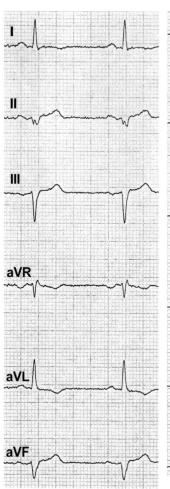

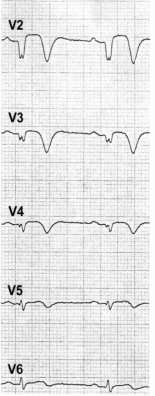

ECG 13.72

60y/m. 6-weeks-old, 'acute' anterior infarction. ECG: LAFB, QS in V$_1$/V$_2$ with initial notching, only minimal R waves in V$_3$ to V$_6$, ST elevation and T negativity in (V$_1$) V$_2$ to V$_6$ (and I, aVL). Coro: two-vessel disease, 90% stenosis LAD, anterior hypokinesia to akinesia, EF 55%.

ECG 13.73

43y/m. 3-week-old, 'acute' anterior infarction. ECG: LAFB, QS (with notching) in V$_1$ to V$_4$, slight ST elevation and T negativity in V$_1$ to V$_6$. Coro: two-vessel disease, closed LAD. Anterior akinesia, EF 49%.

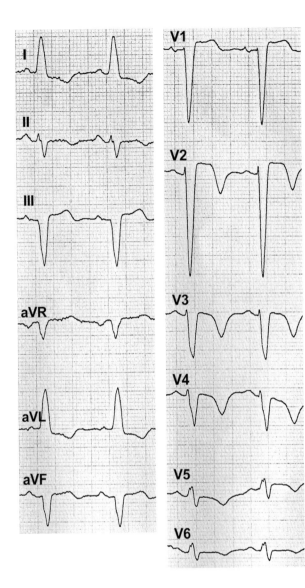

ECG 13.74

72y/f. 4-day-old, acute anterior infarction. ECG: LAFB, non-Q wave anterior infarction, however with probable reduction of R in V_3/V_4 and R notching in V_5/V_6. Slight ST elevation in V_1/V_2, deep negative T waves in V_2 to V_4 (V_5/V_6). Possibly, LAFB masks a Q-wave infarction. Echo: anterior hypokinesia, EF about 50%.

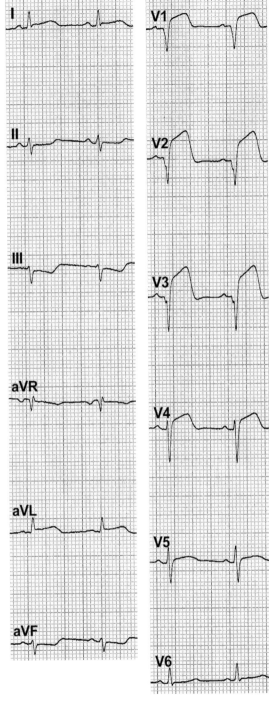

ECG 13.75a

72y/f. 3-day-old, acute anterior infarction. ECG: LAFB. QS in V_1 to V_3 (notching in V_2/V_3), ST elevation in V_1 to V_4 (V_5) and I/aVL. Echo: anterior akinesia, EF about 48%.

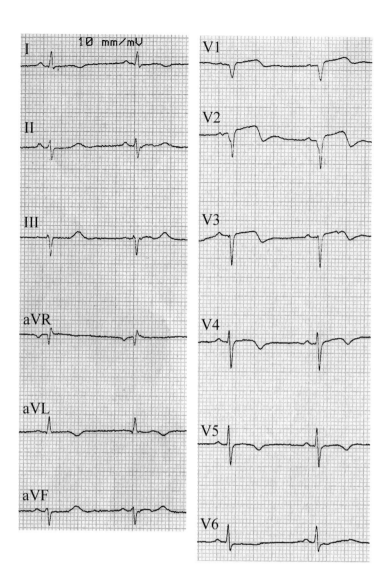

ECG 13.75b
Same patient, ECG 2 months later: QS in V₁/V₂,
minimal q in V₃/V₄. ST isoelectric, T negative in V₂
to V₅, I and aVL. Echo: Anterior hypokinesia, EF
58% (recovery of hibernating myocardium).

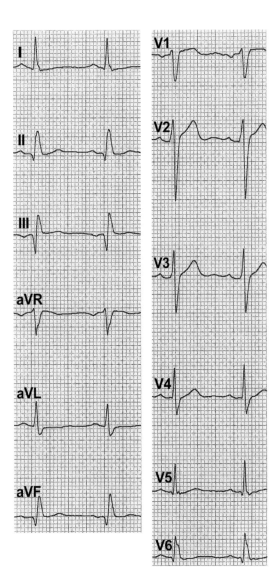

ECG 13.76
66y/m. 9-year-old inferior MI. ECG: LPFB with ÅQRS$_F$ + 40°, and Q waves in inferior leads; Q duration ≥ 0.04 sec only in lead III. Relative tall R waves in III/aVF. Preterminal slurred R downstroke in V$_6$. Coro: three-vessel disease, extensive inferior akinesia, EF 45%.

ECG 13.77 ▶
52y/f. Marfan syndrome. 8-year-old inferior infarction. ECG: atrial fibrillation. LPFB with ÅQRS$_F$ + 80°, masking inferior MI. Small Q waves and tall R waves in inferior leads. Terminal slurred R downstroke in V$_6$. Negative T waves inferiorly. Coro: closed RCA, normal LCA. Extensive inferior akinesia, EF 43%.

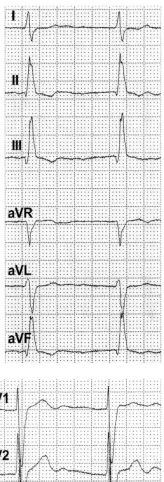

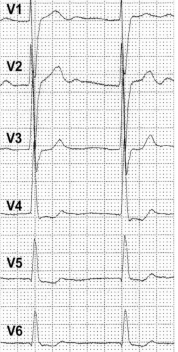

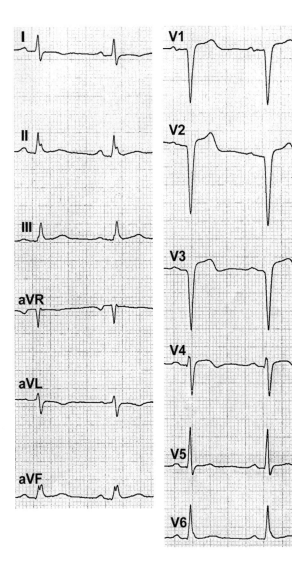

ECG 13.78

48y/m. Several-year-old inferior MI, acute 1-day-old anteroseptal MI. ECG: LPFB. ÅQRS$_F$ + 75°. Slurred R downstroke in II, aVF, V$_6$. No Q wave inferiorly! Additionally pattern of (acute) anteroseptal MI with QS in V$_1$ to V$_3$ and ST elevation in V$_1$ to V$_4$. The frontal QRS axis is due to LPFB, and not to an extensive anterolateral MI. Complete masking of inferior MI by LPFB. Coro: Closed RCA, stenosis 70% of LAD. Inferior akinesia, septoapical hypokinesia to akinesia, EF 45%.

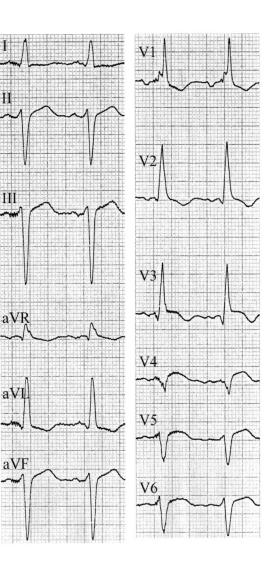

ECG 13.79

77y/f. 2-day-old, acute anterior infarction. ECG: LAFB and RBBB. Pathologic Q waves in V$_2$,V$_3$. QS with slurring in V$_4$. ST elevation in V$_2$ to V$_4$ (V$_5$/V$_6$). Echo: Extensive anterior akinesia, EF about 40%.

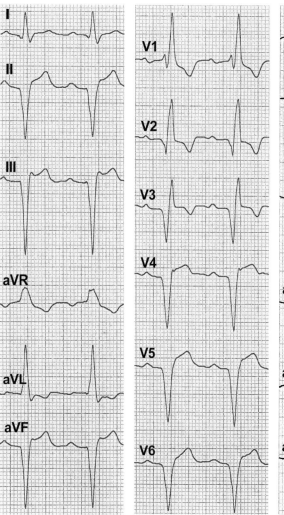

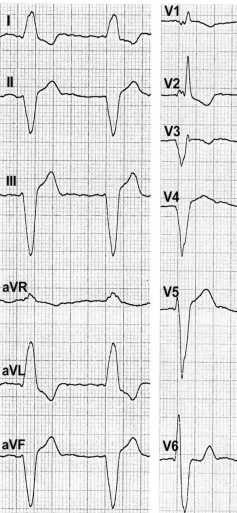

ECG 13.80

76y/m. Coronary and valvular HD (moderate aortic stenosis). Anterior and inferior MI 1 and 2 years ago. ECG: AV block 1°. RBBB + possible LAFB. Pathologic Q waves in V_2/V_3 and QS in V_4 to V_6 indicate extensive anterolateral MI. In this case ST elevation in V_3 to V_6 does not indicate a recent MI, but an old MI with anterolateral aneurysm. QS waves in the inferior leads are consistent with old inferior MI (not masked by LAFB). Coro: three-vessel disease. EF improved from 30% to 50% within one year, without surgical intervention or PTCA.

ECG 13.81

84y/m. Coronary and valvular heart disease (aortic valve replacement 16 years ago). 1-week-old anterior MI. ECG: atrial fibrillation. LAFB + RBBB. *Note:* leads V_1 and V_2 are mixed up! Pathologic Q waves in (real) V_2/V_3 and QS in V_4 (minimal Q waves in V_5/V_6 are not normal in LAFB) are typical for old anterior infarction. ST elevations in (V_3) V_4 to V_6 (and in the inferior leads) are probably due to LVH in LAFB (with a very wide QRS), and not to a more recent infarction stage. Echo: LV EF 45%, LV mass index 270 g/m².

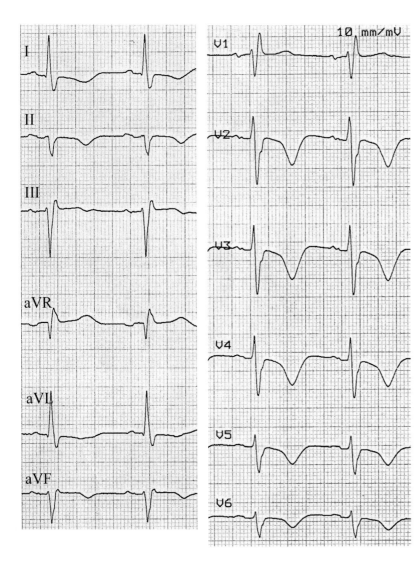

ECG 13.82
76/m. 3-day-old non-Q wave MI. ECG: RBBB (+ LAFB?). No pathologic Q waves. Negative, deep and symmetric T waves in V_2 to V_6 (and II) with long QT. Minimal ST depression in V_3 to V_6. Reduction of R waves in V_4 to V_6 probably due to RBBB (and possible LAFB). Echo: anterior hypokinesia, EF about 50%.

ECG 13.83

67y/m, Hypertensive and coronary HD, 3-year-old inferior MI. ECG: RBBB + LPFB. LPFB masks inferior MI. Only small Q waves in III, aVF. Note the slurred R downstroke and the small S wave in V$_6$ (in presence of RBBB), both typical for LPFB. Giant S waves in V$_2$ due to LVH. Autopsy: old inferior MI, LVH. RCA closed, stenoses in the other coronary arteries.

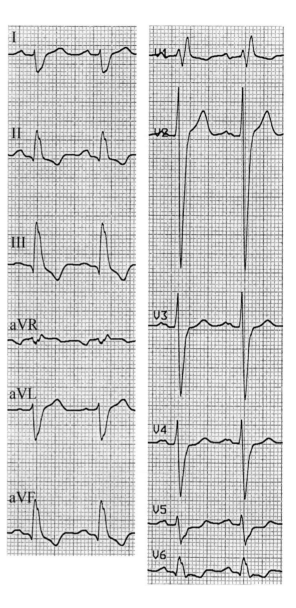

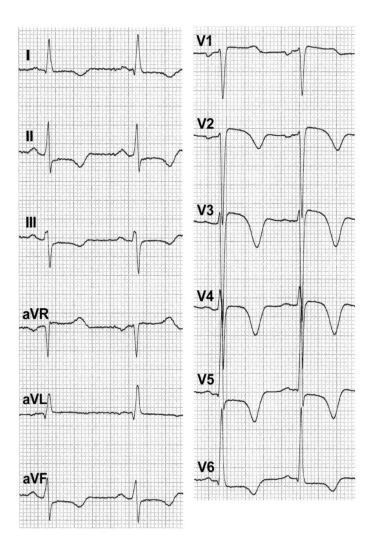

ECG 13.84

**47y/m. 6-hour-old, acute non-Q wave MI. ECG: normal
Q waves in I, aVL, V_5/V_6. Deep (symmetric) negative
T waves in leads V_2 to V_6 and in some limb leads.
ST elevation in V_1 to V_3, ST depression inferolaterally.
Coro: one-vessel disease, 90% stenosis of LAD.
Anterior hypokinesia, EF 55%.**

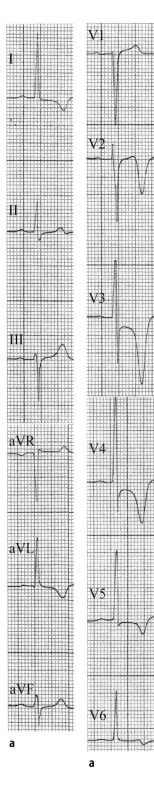

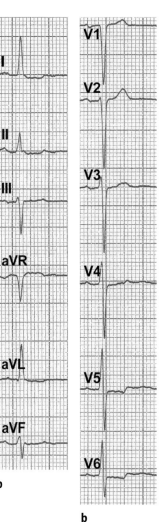

b

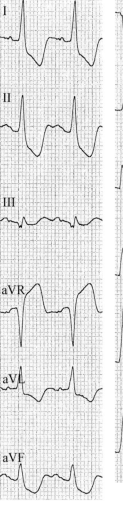

b

ECG 13.85b ▲
Same patient. 19 years after operation the patient is well, LVH has decreased.

◄ ECG 13.85a
46y/m. Short Story/Case Report 3. Asymptomatic moderate to severe aortic valve stenosis. Acute 1–2-day-old MI. ECG: apparent LVH. ST depression 2 mm in V$_3$ to V$_4$ (V$_5$) and deep symmetric T waves in V$_2$ to V$_4$ (V$_5$, I/aVL). The ECG is very similar to that in hypertrophic apical cardiomyopathy. Coro: subtotal stenosis of LAD, extensive anterolateral akinesia, described as aneurysm. LV EF 40%. After AC-bypassing of LAD and aortic valve replacement, LV function *normalized* (hibernating myocardium!) within 3 weeks.

ECG 13.86 ▲
82y/f. Angina for 2 weeks. 6-hour-old anterior MI. ECG: excessive ST depression in leads V$_3$ to V$_6$ (7 mm in V$_5$) and leads I, II, aVF (aVL), with negative (or biphasic) T waves. No Q wave, except in lead III. Strange purely positive QRS configuration in V$_2$. Coro: 80% stem stenosis, subtotal stenoses of middle LAD and CX, closed RCA. PTCA/stenting of stem. Anterolateral akinesia, EF 34%. Normalization of repolarization within 1 day (not shown). Echo 3 days later: EF 50%.

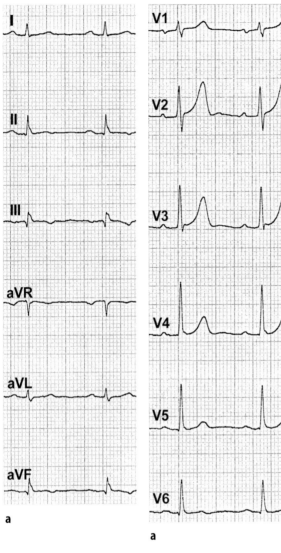

a

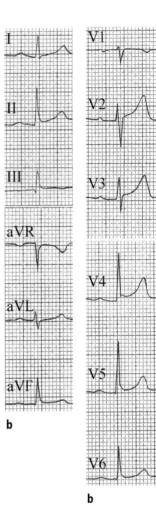

b

ECG 13.87a
57y/m. Short Story/Case Report 4. ECG: nonsignificant Q waves (< 0.04 sec) in II, aVF, III, with symmetric negative T waves. R waves in V_1 to $V_3 \geq 0.04$ sec, with high symmetric T waves. Overall the ECG suggests old posteroinferior infarction.

ECG 13.87b
Same patient. Normal ECG 3 years before.

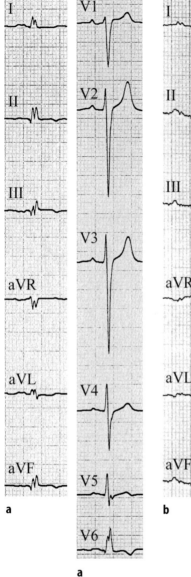

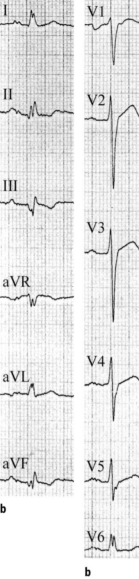

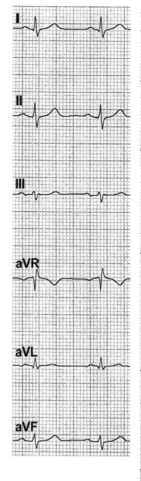

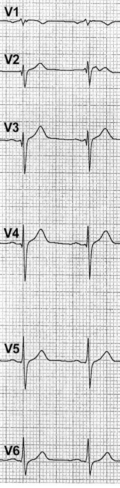

a

b

a

b

ECG 13.88a
85y/f. Old (inferior) infarction of unknown date. ECG: Peripheral low voltage. Notched QRS in all limb leads and V₆.
Nonsignificant Q waves, negative symmetric T waves in II, aVF, III. Slight ST elevation inferiorly. Echo: EF 40%.

ECG 13.88b
Same patient. The ECG 5 months later reveals a typical pattern of inferior infarction.

ECG 13.89
48y/m. 2-year-old (anterior) infarction. ECG: small pathologic Q waves (rsr'S' respectively) in V₂/V₃ (V₄). Normal T waves. Coro: subtotal proximal stenosis of LAD. Slight anterior hypokinesia, EF 60%.

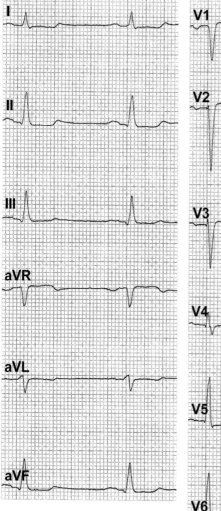

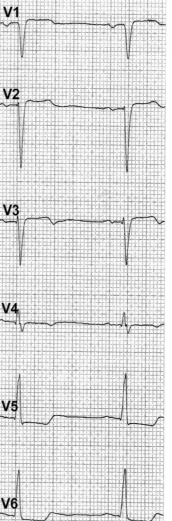

ECG 13.90

62y/m. 10-day-old (anterior) infarction. ECG: small pathologic Q waves in V$_2$/V$_3$, slightly notched QRS in V$_4$. Symmetric negative T waves in V$_3$/V$_4$ (deeper in V$_3$). Coro: two 90% stenoses of LAD, anterior akinesia. EF 40%.

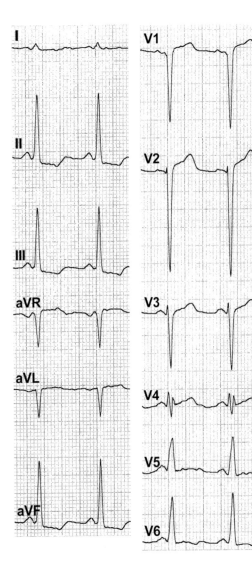

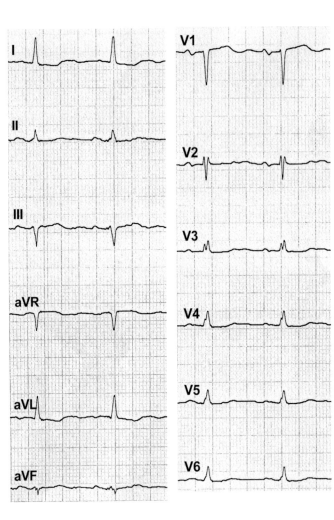

ECG 13.91

71y/f. 3-year-old (anterior) MI. ECG: small Q waves in V_2/V_3. (q)RSr' in V_4. Slurred R upstroke in V_5 (V_6). Coro: 90% stenosis of LAD, anteroapical akinesia, EF 52%.

ECG 13.92

71y/m. 8-year-old anterior MI during ACB operation. ECG: small physiologic Q wave in aVL. rSr' type in V_2, notched R waves in V_3 to V_6, decreased R waves in V_4 to V_6. Actual Coro: severe three-vessel disease. Apical dyskinesia, lateral hypokinesia. EF 45%.

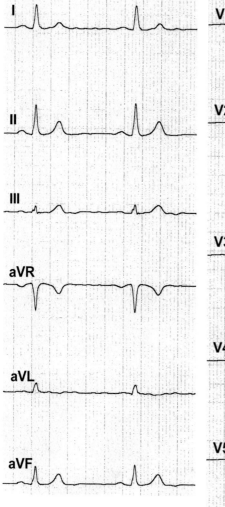

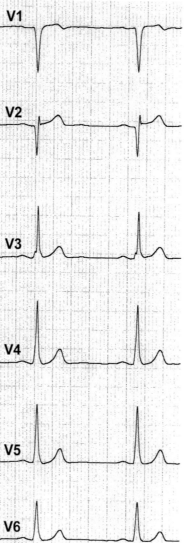

ECG 13.93

52y/m. 7-year-old anteroseptal MI. ECG: Qr in V_2, slurred R upstroke in V_3. Otherwise ECG within normal limits. Note: a QS complex in V_1/V_2 may be a rare normal variant, a Qr type in V_2 is pathologic. The diagnosis of 'atypical incomplete RBBB' would be false, because there is no r' in V_1 and no terminal R wave in aVR. Coro: proximal stenosis of LAD. Anteroseptal hypokinesia. EF 62%.

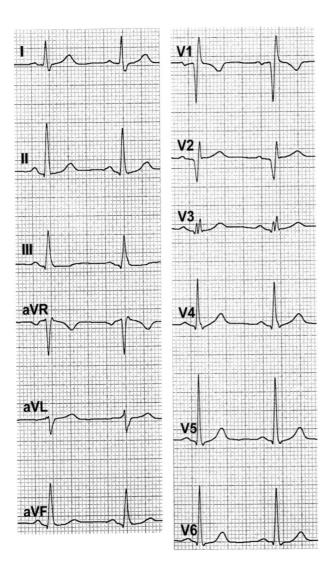

ECG 13.94

75y/f. 3-year-old anteroseptal MI during ACB operation. ECG: Qr (Q > 0.04 sec) in V_1/V_2 and qrsR'(s') in V_3 indicate old anteroseptal MI. The r' in V_2/V_3 is due to 'peri-infarction block' (see text), possibly also the r' in V_1 (see the only small terminal R wave in aVR). Echo: anteroseptal akinesia, EF 62%.

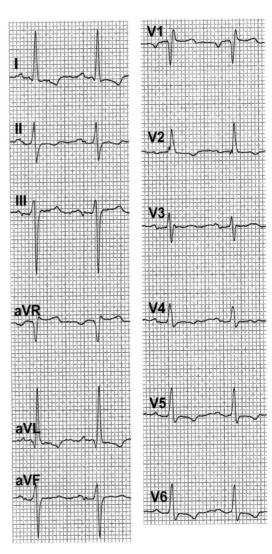

ECG 13.95

76y/m. Severe three-vessel disease, preoperative EF 68%. Perioperative anteroseptal infarction, intermittently with pathologic anteroseptal Q waves and ST elevation. ECG: Qr in V_1, (q)R in V_2, RSr' in V_3. Echo: anterior hypokinesia, EF about 55%.

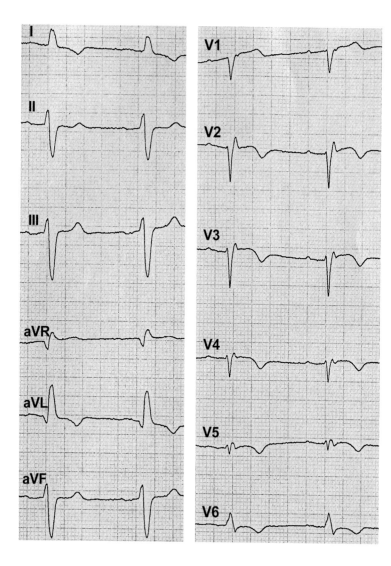

ECG 13.96

64y/m. 16-year-old anterior MI. Anterolateral aneurysm. ECG: no pathologic Q waves. LAFB, PQ 0.02 sec. rSr' in V_2 to V_5 (rsr's' in V_5), with reduced R amplitude in V_4 to V_5 (V_6). Symmetric negative T waves (slight ST elevation in V_2 to V_4 compatible with aneurysm?). Echo: extensive anterolateral akinesia, EF 30%.

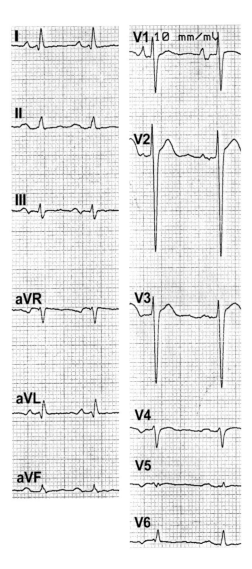

ECG 13.97

71y/f. 2-month-old apicolateral(-posterior) MI. ECG: SR, first beat in precordial leads: atrial premature beat. No pathologic Q waves. rSr' in I, aVL. Relative high R waves in V_1, V_2. R reduction from V_2 to V_5, notched QRS in V_5. Echo: apicolateral akinesia, EF 25%.

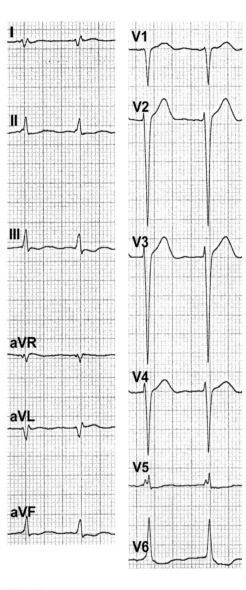

ECG 13.98

78y/f. 9-year-old anterior infarction. ECG: atrial fibrillation. ÂQRS$_F$ + 95°. No pathologic Q waves, rSr' in I, aVL. No R progression from V_2 to V_4. Notched R wave in V_5 (however in the 'displaced' transition zone). Vertical frontal QRS axis probably due to loss of anterolateral potentials. Echo: anterolateral hypokinesia to akinesia, EF 34%. Differential diagnosis, based only on the precordial leads: RV and/or LV dilatation, possible LVH (deep S waves in V_2/V_3 (V_4).

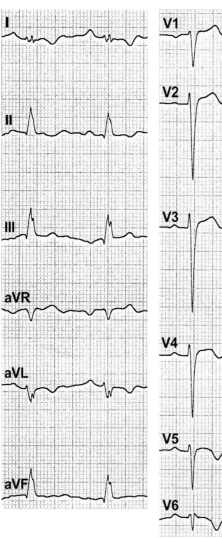
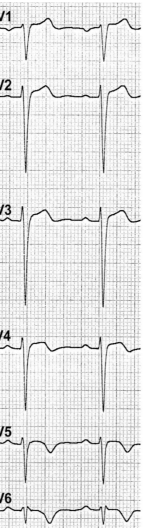
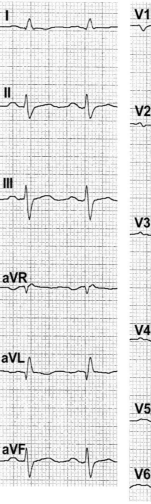
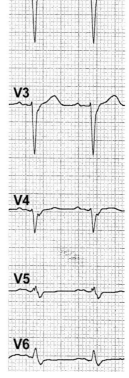

ECG 13.99

57y/m. 9-year-old anterolateral infarction. ECG: no pathologic Q waves, rsr's' in I. Notched QRS in most limb leads. R reduction from V_3 to V_6, rSr' in V_6. Symmetric negative T waves in V_5 and V_6 (I/aVL). Vertical QRS axis due to loss of lateral potentials. Coro: severe three-vessel disease. EF 24%. Anterolateral akinesia.

ECG 13.100

56y/m. 4-month-old anterolateral infarction. ECG: no pathologic Q waves (however relatively broad Q in aVL). Regression of small R wave from V_2 to V_4. Fine notching of S in V_4 (V_3), notched small R wave in V_5. No T negativity. Coro: 90% proximal LCA (stem) stenosis. Extensive anterolateral akinesia. EF 40%.

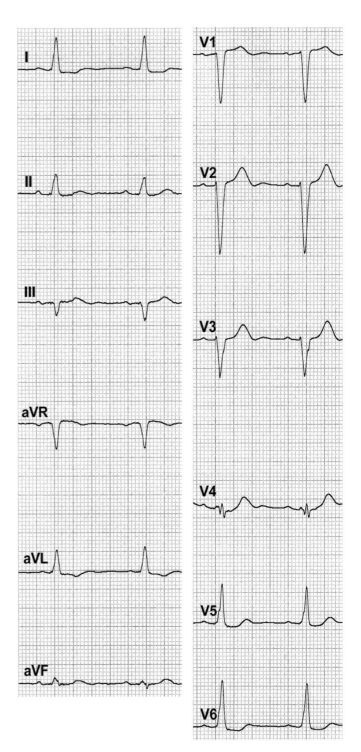

ECG 13.101

76y/f. Old anterior infarction. ECG: normal QRS in limb leads. Absent progression of R wave from V$_1$ to V$_3$, rsr's' in V$_4$. Minimal QRS notching in V$_3$ and V$_5$. Echo: apical hypokinesia to akinesia, EF 60%.

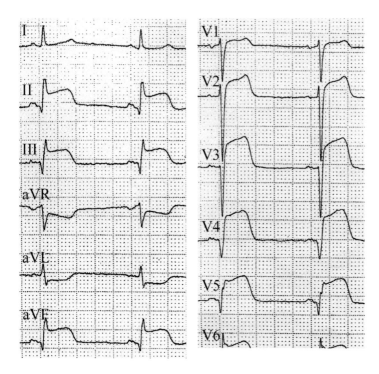

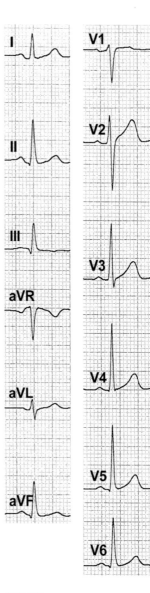

ECG 13.102

45y/f. Acute extensive MI. ECG written 20 min after onset of chest pain (lead V$_6$ partially lacking): striking ST elevations inferiorly and in V$_2$ to V$_6$, with pathologic Q waves in III, aVF and V$_4$/V$_5$. The patient died 30 min later, during transfer to the invasive center, due to cardiogenic shock.

ECG 13.103

39y/m. Mild angina. Coro: complete obstruction of middle part LAD. EF 80%. Good collateralization from first diagonal branch and RCA. ECG: Normal.

Chapter 14
Differential Diagnosis of Pathologic Q waves

At a Glance

The Q wave (Q > R), the QS wave (purely negative QRS complex) and the q wave (Q < R) have for decades preoccupied not only cardiologists but also physicians in many other disciplines of medicine. In 1987 Goldberger [1] published an interesting article about normal and noninfarct Q waves. A reappraisal of this important subject seems appropriate, with some new (and some old) supplementary information.

ECG

Definition of Normal Q Wave

The *normal Q wave* is always a *q wave* that it is smaller than the following R wave (ECG 14.1). The normal q wave is due to the depolarization of the interventricular septum. Its duration is usually a few to 15 msec and never exceeds 20–25 msec (excluding the 'normal variants' (see section 2 below and Chapter 3 The Normal ECG and its Normal Variants). Often there is no q wave in many leads because the projection of the septal vector on these leads is positive and is therefore manifested in the first 15 msec of the R wave. In the *normal* ECG, in lead aVR there is always a predominantly *negative QRS complex*. Lead aVR is situated at - 150° in the frontal plane and shows a *mirror image* of the usual QRS complex. We find a Qr or even a QS complex (ECGs 14.2 and 14.3), or an rS or rSr' configuration.

Definition of (Formally) Pathologic Q Wave

'Classically', the *pathologic* Q wave (that should indicate old myocardial infarction (MI)) is defined as a Q wave of duration ≥ 0.04 sec – *this does not make much sense*. Although in practice formally broad Q waves are important for the diagnosis of old MI, the MI may evolve with smaller Q waves, or without Q waves (non-Q wave infarction). Furthermore, there are many conditions other than MI with abnormal or striking Q waves.

Some infarct patterns are described in section 1. (For details about Q wave infarction, complex and 'unusual' patterns of MI, and non-Q wave infarction, see Chapter 13 Myocardial Infarction). Sections 8–17 (and in The Full Picture) present differential diagnoses of the abnormal Q wave more or less in order of prevalence, irrespective of the duration of the Q wave and the QRS complex.

Throughout this chapter please note that Q is stated in capitals if the Q wave is greater than the r wave, and in lower case if the q wave is smaller than the R wave. In undetermined cases or general descriptions, capital Q is used. Pure negative QRS complexes are described as QS (as usual).

1 Myocardial Infarction

Generally the Q waves in MI develop in combination with chest pain. In many patients the evolution of MI can be followed, based on significant ST elevations in the ECG and elevated serum levels of creatine phosphokinase (CPK), its myocardial-specific fractions and/or troponin, in the acute phase. However, in patients with silent infarction, Q waves – or their mirror image (in true posterior infarction) – may be the only indicators of myocardial necrosis.

There are some ECG criteria that *favor* infarction.

1.1 New Q Waves

The appearance of *new Q or q waves* within a short time is a very important (and often forgotten) sign of infarction. These q waves must not fulfill the usual criteria for infarction, i.e. a duration of at least 40 msec (see Short Story/Case Report 4 in Chapter 13 Myocardial Infarction). Alterations of the repolarization may sustain the diagnosis, in which case at least one previous ECG must be available. It is often laborious to search for an old ECG. Sometimes an ECG was written by a former family physician during a check-up for life assurance or military service. In some professions (e.g. pilot of an airplane) ECGs are mandatory in some countries.

1.2 ST Elevation

An ST elevation of $\geq$ 2 mm in some leads is typical for acute MI. In old larger anterolateral infarctions persisting ST elevations are typical of an aneurysm. Occasionally, modest ST elevation in V_3 to V_5, combined with a borderline q wave, may be the only sign of an anterior infarction. ST elevations in the inferior leads, associated with new Q waves, are typical for acute inferior MI. Minimal ST elevations have no special importance if the Q waves are not due to infarction, but are due to something like left ventricular hypertrophy. Remember that ST elevations in leads V_2/V_3 (up to 3 mm) without pathologic q waves represent a frequent normal variant, especially in sinus bradycardia.

1.3 Negative T Waves

Persisting symmetric negative (so-called 'coronary') T waves may be a hint of myocardial infarction, even associated with only borderline q waves. Of course chest pain and multiple risk factors for coronary heart disease (CHD) favor the diagnosis of infarction. For detection of hypokinetic or akinetic areas an echo is often useful. ECGs 14.4 and 14.5 show typical patterns of an old *inferior MI* and of an old *anterior MI,* respectively.

2 Normal Variants

These are fully discussed in Chapter 3 The Normal ECG and its Normal Variants.

2.1 Frontal Plane

A Q wave with a duration of more than 30 msec or a QS wave may be seen in lead III (ECG 14.6) and sometimes also in lead aVF, because of projections. The T wave may be positive or negative, but is always asymmetric. A broad Q wave in lead aVL based on projections is rare, a significant Q wave in lead II as a normal variant is extremely rare.

2.2 Horizontal Plane

A QS wave in lead V_1 and/or V_2 (never in V_3) may be due to erroneous placing of the leads one intercostal space too high,

but is also found with correct placing of the leads (ECG 14.7). With a change from supine to an upright body position, the R voltage in the precordial leads may decrease considerably (clockwise rotation). ECG 14.8b shows an extraordinary loss of positive QRS deflections (compared to ECG 14.8a), resulting in QS waves up to V_5. In both conditions (ECGs 14.8a–b) clinical and anamnestic findings, and especially an echo, help to assure a normal variant.

3 Left Ventricular Hypertrophy

i. Left ventricular hypertrophy may also be responsible for abnormal q or Q waves (or even QS waves) in lead III, more rarely in lead aVF, and very occasionally in lead II (ECGs 14.9 and 14.10). The T waves are generally positive and asymmetric. Other ECG signs or an echo confirm the diagnoses.

ii. In some cases of left ventricular hypertrophy, especially in patients with aortic valve incompetence, the q waves in V_4 to V_6 may measure up to 3 mm but the duration does not exceed 25 msec. In these cases left ventricular hypertrophy is obvious, based on very tall R waves in these leads.

4 False Lead Poling

False poling of the limb leads produces 'pseudo-abnormal' Q waves. It is striking that the upper limb leads in particular are often subject to exchange, especially in emergency situations. The inversion of lead I is not instantly recognized by some physicians. We find in *lead I* the *mirror image* of the *usual QRS complex,* often with 'pathologic' Q waves and negative T waves, mimicking infarction, but always combined with a negative p wave, in sinus rhythm (ECG 14.11). A glance at the precordial leads confirms that these leads do not reveal any signs of infarction and, in more than 99% of cases, do not show the typical pattern of *situs inversus.* For other false limb-lead poling see Chapter 32 Rare ECGs. In that chapter all possible lead misplacements are listed, for a left and for a vertical QRS axis.

5 Left Bundle-Branch Block

In LBBB a left-axis deviation is common and occasionally associated with a QS complex in III (and aVF), mostly with positive and asymmetric T waves. In V_1 to V_4 a QS complex may be present, although much more rarely than an rS complex (mostly with very small r waves). The diagnosis of LBBB is made on the basis of a QRS duration of 140 msec or more and other typical signs (ECG 14.12, with QS in V_1 to V_3). A q wave (qR complex) in leads I or aVL or V_5/V_6 is very rare. If there is a qR complex in at least three of these leads, old infarction is quite certain.

6 Pre-Excitation (Wolff-Parkinson-White Syndrome)

In patients with pre-excitation over a posteroseptal pathway, the delta wave and the following parts of the QRS complex are usually negative in leads III and aVF, resulting in a QS complex with a duration of 110 msec or more. The T waves are always positive and asymmetric in both leads. The shortened PQ interval and the altered QRS complexes (the delta wave included) in the other leads confirm the correct diagnoses (ECG 14.13).

7 Hypertrophic Obstructive Cardiomyopathy

In some patients with hypertrophic obstructive cardiomyopathy (HOCM), striking Q waves of different grades may be encountered.

i. The q waves are only minimally prolonged in leads I (aVL) and V_4 to V_6 (ECG 14.14).
ii. The q or Q waves have a duration of 40 msec or more, in the same leads (ECG 14.15).
iii. The main QRS vector is oriented to the right, backwards and upwards in a spectacular manner, resulting in negative QRS complexes in all leads except in aVR (and aVL), in combination with Q or even QS waves (ECG 14.16). In these extremely rare cases the diagnosis of infarction is occasionally made erroneously. However the T waves are positive and asymmetric, discordant to the negative QRS complexes. The patients are generally young and reveal typical clinical findings of HOCM.

The abnormal Q waves in HOCM can be explained by septal hypertrophy. In cases of extensive QS configuration there is an additional excessive conduction disturbance in the whole left ventricle, due to the chaotic orientation of the muscle fibers.

In many patients with HOCM abnormal q waves are missing. The ECG then shows 'simple left ventricular hypertrophy', an LBBB, or may be even normal.

The Full Picture

ECG Special

8 Congenital Corrected Transposition of the Great Arteries

In this very rare congenital anomaly not only is there inversion of the great arteries (aorta and pulmonary artery) but also of the ventricles. The ventricular excitation begins at the septal endocardium of the right-sided left ventricle. Thus the septal vector is not directed as it usually is from the left to the right, but more or less from the right to the left, and backwards. This leads to the so-called 'inversion' of q waves in the precordial leads. We find a q wave in lead V_1 but no q wave in lead V_6 (ECG 14.17). Due to variable rotation of the heart, this sign is found in only about 40% of cases. However, Preter et al [2] documented this ECG sign in five of seven patients with this anomaly.

9 Situs Inversus

This is another very rare congenital anomaly in which the heart is displaced to the left hemithorax like a mirror image. Often cardiac function is normal. In the ECG the inversion of the atria leads to the same alterations in the frontal plane as in the case of false poling of the upper limb leads – lead I is inverted. The inversion of the ventricles consequently produces a typical pattern in the precordial leads. In contrast to the typical increase of the R waves and the decrease of the S waves from V_3 to V_6, we observe decreasing and small r waves and tall S waves in V_3 to V_6 (ECG 14.18). The ECG can be 'normalized' if a) the upper limb leads are exchanged, and b) if the precordial electrodes are placed at the right side of the thorax in an otherwise usual manner. It is said that really good physicians make the diagnosis before studying the ECG, by heart palpitation, percussion and auscultation. The diagnosis is confirmed by thoracic x-ray (and echocardiogram).

10 Q Waves after Pneumectomy

In a minority of patients the dislocation and/or rotation of the heart due to pneumectomy leads to pathologic Q waves in the anterior or inferior leads (see also ECG 32.8 and 32.9 Chapter 32 Rare ECGs).

11 Q Waves in Pneumothorax

The same reason (dislocation and/or rotation of the heart) may provoke pathologic Q waves in the precordial leads in left pneumothorax [3].

12 Q Waves after Pericardectomy

Wood et al [4] published a case of 'reversible MI' in a patient after pericardectomy. The ECG showed striking Q and QS complexes in leads V_1 to V_3 and slight ST elevations in V_1 to V_6. The left ventricular ejection fraction (EF) was 20%–25%, serial evaluation of creatine kinase and troponin I remained normal. The cardiac damage was attributed to 'myocarditis induced by operative trauma'. ECG and EF normalized within 2 weeks.

13 Q Waves in Amyloidosis of the Heart

In heart amyloidosis the ECG pattern of old anterior and/or inferior infarction with significant Q waves or with a QS complex is encountered in about 30% of cases. ECG 14.19 demonstrates striking Q waves in leads V_2 to V_6. In a patient with thickened left ventricular wall (pseudohypertrophy) in the echo (without regional hypokinesia), and pathologic Q waves without signs of left ventricular hypertrophy in the ECG, amyloidosis of the heart should be considered. However, the combination of decreased QRS voltage and increased left ventricular mass is a much more frequent finding [5,6].

14 Pseudo-Q Wave due to Retrograde Atrial Activation

In AV junctional rhythm the atria are activated retrogradely and the direction of the p vector is inverse. In rare cases the p wave falls immediately before or into the beginning of the QRS complex and imitates Q waves in the inferior (and possibly in the lateral precordial) leads (ECG 14.20).

15 A Rarity: Q Waves in Muscular Dystrophy Steinert

Short Story/Case Report 1

In August 2001 the young resident Doctor Steiner showed a fairly common ECG to the author with a little smile (ECG 14.21); the author unfortunately overlooked that little smile and made the diagnosis of an old posterolateral infarction. Doctor Steiner's smile became broader: the patient was 20 years old and had never had a chest pain. He suffered from musculodystrophia *Steinert*.

Peripheral muscular dystrophy of the type *Duchenne* is often associated with hypertrophic (and dilating) cardiomyopathy. Generally concomitant cardiac dystrophy is most accentuated in the *posterior and basal* (lateral) region of the left ventricle, resulting in a hypokinetic zone, consequently leading to the pattern of an old posterior(-lateral) infarction (ECG 14.21). Also other heredofamilial neuromyopathic disorders as musculodystrophia Steinert (ECG 14.21), myotonic muscular dystrophy, and Friedreich ataxia, may be combined with cardiomyopathy and occasionally with patterns of old MI [7].

16 QR Complex in Lead V₁

In patients with massive pulmonary embolism a QR complex in lead V_1 (instead of the common RSR' (rSr') complex) can be observed in 10%–14% [8,9]; ECG 14.22 shows an example. Also a QS complex may be seen in V_1 (and V_2) that is explained by an extensive rotation of the heart [1]. A QR complex in lead V_1 is also found in right ventricular hypertrophy.

17 Q Wave in Lead V₁ in Right Atrial Dilatation

Last but not least a gem of an abnormal q wave due to right atrial dilatation, in the presence of atrial fibrillation; this is shown in ECG 14.23. Rarely, acute or chronic *extensive dilatation* of the right atrium may be the cause of the q in a *qR complex* in lead V_1. Why? In dogs and humans an electrode placed epicardially in the middle of the (normal) right atrium does not reflect the ventricular septal vector positively – as expected – but with a small negative deflection [10]. Thus in a dilated right atrium, lead V_1 may *act* as an 'epicardial right atrial electrode' and therefore shows the same alteration: the QRS complex is registered through a dilated right atrium. The R of the qR wave corresponds to hypertrophic right ventricular myocardium above the 'crista terminalis', activated with latency. Sodi Pallares et al [10] found a qR complex in lead V_1 (and V_2, very rarely up to V_4) in patients with severe mitral stenosis with tricuspid regurgitation, acute pulmonary embolism, atrial septal defects, and tetralogy of Fallot – all conditions with a markedly dilated right atrium.

ECG 14.23 shows a Q wave in lead V_1 due to severe right atrial dilatation in a person with severe mitral stenosis with tricuspid incompetence. The Q wave generally disappears after regression of right atrial dilatation, after surgical or drug treatment.

It is fascinating that in exceptional cases an *alteration of the QRS complex* may indicate an *alteration of an atrium*; and this in the presence of *atrial fibrillation* (ECG 14.23).

References

1. Goldberger AL. Normal and noninfarct Q wave. Cardiol Clin 1987;5:1357–66
2. Preter B, Gurtner HP, Fuchs WA, Weber JW. Zur korrigierten Transposition der grossen Gefässe. Cardiologia 1965;46:163–72
3. Raev D. A case of spontaneous left-sided pneumothorax with ECG changes resembling acute myocardial infarction. Internat J Cardiol 1996;56:197–9
4. Wood DE, Crumbley AJ, Pereira NL. Reversible left ventricular dysfunction simulating a myocardial infarction after pericardectomy. Heart 2002;88:183–4
5. Carroll JD, Gaasch WH, McAdam KPWJ. Amyloid cardiomyopathy: characterization by a distinctive voltage/mass relation, Amer J Cardiol 1982;49:9–13
6. Sivaram CA, Jugdutt BI, Amy RWM, Basualdo CA, et al. Amyloidosis of the heart. Combined use of two-dimensional echocardiography and electrocardiography in snoninvasive screening before biopsy. Clin Cardiol 1985;8:511–8
7. Neurologic disorders and heart disease. In: Braunwald E (ed). Heart Disease, fifth edn. Philadelphia: WB Saunders Company 1997;2:pp1865–1877
8. Weber DM, Phillips JH Jr. A re-evaluation of electrocardiographic changes accompanying acute pulmonary embolism. Am J Med Sci 1966;251:381–98
9. Kucher N, Walpoth N, Wustmann K, et al. QR in V1 – an ECG sign associated with right ventricular strain and adverse clinical outcome in acute pulmonary embolism. Europ Heart J 2003;24:1113–9
10. Sodi Pallares D, Bisteni A, Herrmann GR. Some views of the significance of qR and QR type complexes in right precordial leads in the absence of myocardial infarction. Am Heart J 1952;43:716–34

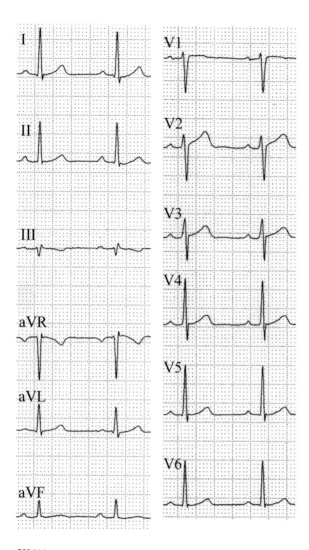

ECG 14.1

35 y/m. Lung carcinoma. ECG: normal, with small q waves in leads I/II/ aVL and V$_5$/V$_6$.

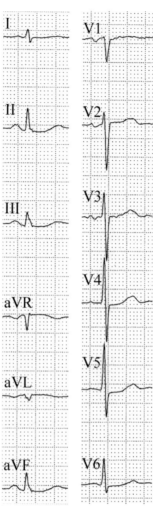

ECG 14.2

Qr configuration in lead aVR in a normal ECG.

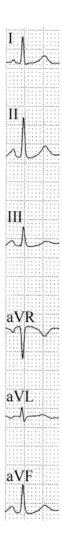

ECG 14.3

QS configuration in lead aVR in a normal ECG.

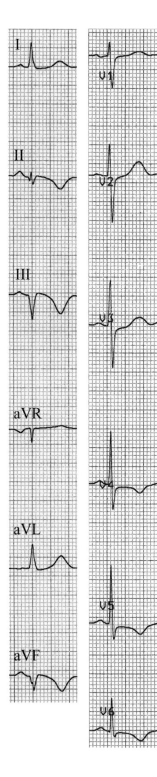

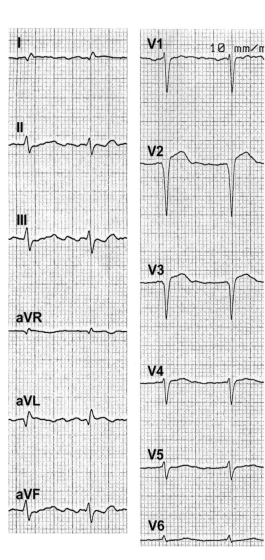

ECG 14.4
69 y/f. 4-day-old inferior infarction. ECG: QS in leads III/aVF, qrs in lead II, combined with deep symmetric negative T waves. Slight ST depression and negative T waves in V$_4$ to V$_6$. QT prolonged. Coro: great right coronary artery (RCA) closed. Percutaneous transluminal coronary angioplasty (PTCA).

ECG 14.5
66 y/m. 4-week-old anterolateral MI. ECG: atrial fibrillation. QS complex in leads V$_2$ to V$_3$ and pathologic Q waves in I and aVL. Reduction of R amplitude in V$_4$ to V$_6$. Slight ST elevation in leads V$_2$ to V$_3$ (V$_4$, I, aVL) due to extensive anterolateral dyskinesia.

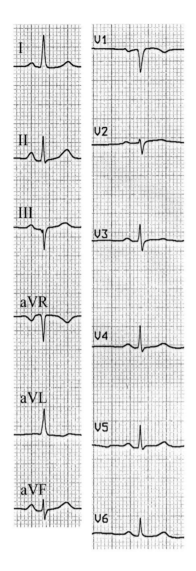

ECG 14.6
67 y/f. Obese patient (body mass index 32), no heart disease. ECG: QS (with initial 'notch') complex in lead III, with asymmetric to symmetric positive T wave. Relatively small amplitude of QRS in precordial leads (obesity). Echo: normal.

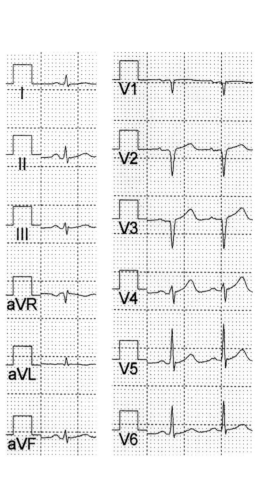

ECG 14.7
74 y/m. No heart disease, no risk factors for CHD. ECG (half calibration): QS in V_1/V_2, minimal r wave in V_3. Echo: normal.

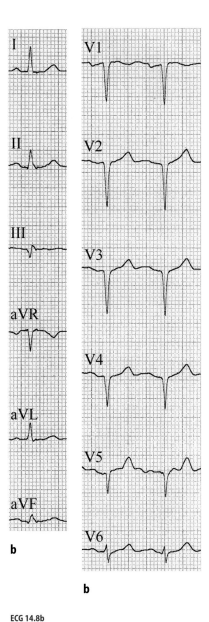

a

a

b

b

ECG 14.8a
68 y/f. Terminal renal failure. ECG (as usual in *supine* position): QRS clockwise rotation in precordial leads (artifact in V₄: 'p' wave). Additionally QS in III/aVF.

ECG 14.8b
Same patient. ECG (*upright* position for exercise test): complete loss of r waves (QS) from (V₁) V₂ to V₅. qR in the inferior leads.

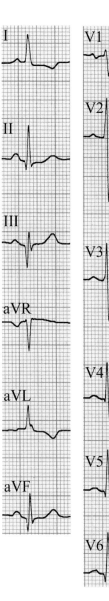

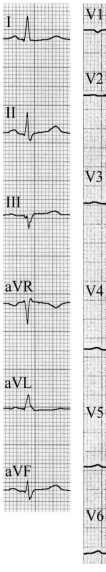

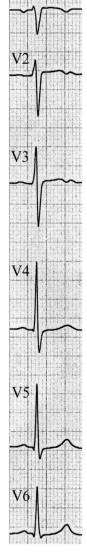

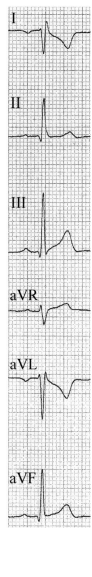

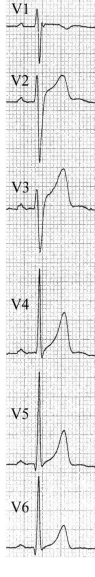

ECG 14.9

49y/f. Hypertension. ECG: left atrial enlargement. Deep and 40 msec broad Q waves in III/aVF. No classical signs for left ventricular hypertrophy. Alteration of repolarization ('systolic overload'). Echo: left ventricular hypertrophy (left ventricular mass 135 g/m^2), left ventricular function normal, no inferior hypokinesia.

ECG 14.10

52 y/m. 3 months after valve replacement (severe aortic regurgitation). ECG: QS with initial 'notching' in III. Small q in II/aVF. In contrast to the ECG 4 months before: no signs of left ventricular hypertrophy. Echo: regression of left ventricular hypertrophy (left ventricular mass 165 g/m^2 to 140 g/m^2). Coro (4 months before): normal coronary arteries, left ventricular ejection fraction 50%.

ECG 14.11

False poling (exchange of upper limb leads).

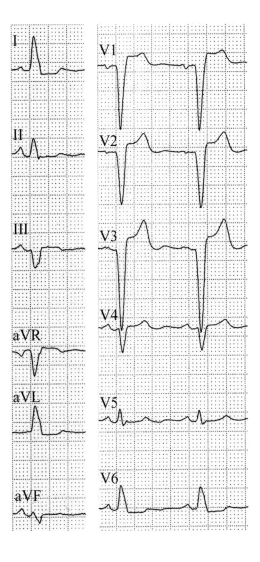

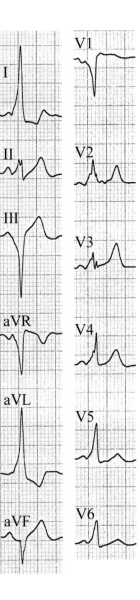

ECG 14.12
54 y/f. Surgical problem. Small heart. Echo normal. LBBB of unclear origin (QRS 130 msec) with QS in V$_1$ to V$_3$ and small r in V$_4$.

ECG 14.13
33 y/m. ECG: QS in leads III and aVF. Note that in aVF the PQ interval seems to be normal. Reason: the delta wave is iso-electric in this lead. Overall the ECG is very typical for *pre-excita-tion*.

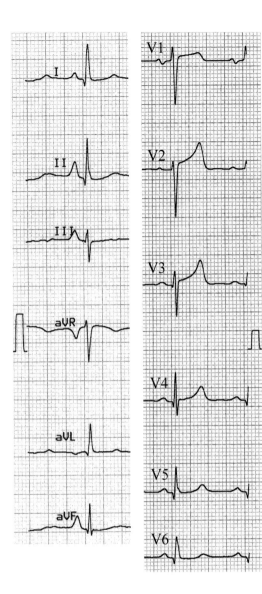

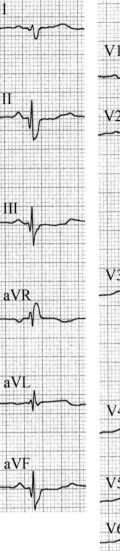

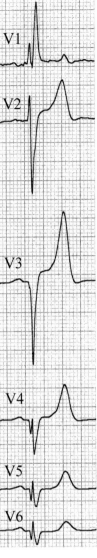

ECG 14.14

40 y/m. HOCM (systolic mean gradient 50 mmHg). ECG (*half calibration* in precordial leads!): atypical left atrial enlargement (p pseudo-pulmonale). Q waves pronounced in V$_4$ to V$_6$ (V$_3$). Sokolow index positive (44 mm), ST elevation in V$_1$ to V$_4$ (up to 4 mm).

ECG 14.15

30 y/m. Severe HOCM. ECG: deep Q waves in II, aVF, III and V$_4$ to V$_6$. QS complex in V$_3$. Positive T waves in these leads. RBBB.

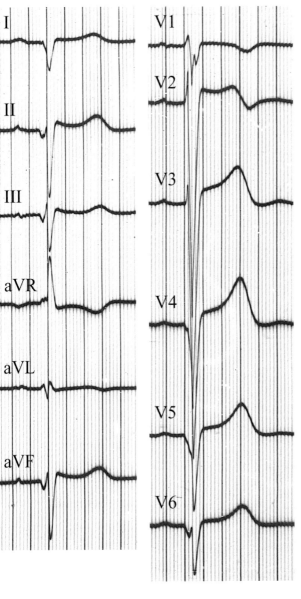

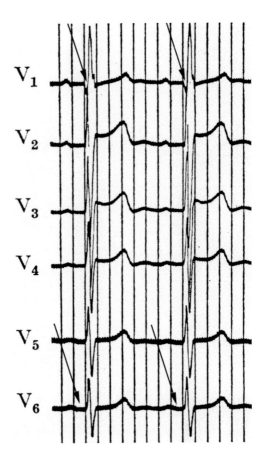

ECG 14.16

22 y/m. Severe HOCM. ECG (50 mm/sec): sinus rhythm. Striking QRS vector in the limb and precordial leads. ÅQRS$_F$ about - 130°, with a positive QRS complex only in lead aVR (and aVL). Giant S waves in V$_2$/V$_3$. QS complexes in leads I, II, V$_4$ to V$_6$, as in extensive lateral MI (however, positive discordant T waves).

ECG 14.17

22 y/f. Congenital corrected transposition of the great vessels, with ventricular septal defect grade IIIa (proven by heart catheterization and angiography). ECG (precordial leads, 50 mm/sec): so-called 'Q inversion': q wave in V$_1$ but no q wave in V$_6$ (arrows).

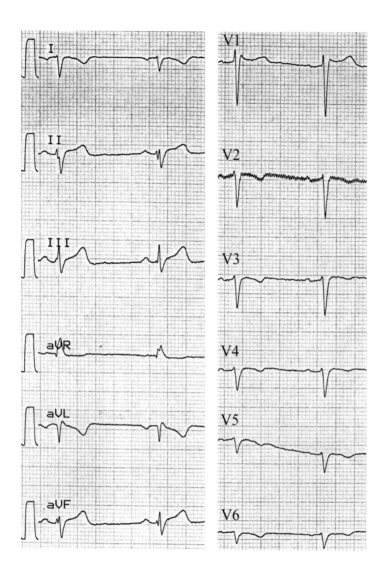

ECG 14.18

40 y/m. Situs inversus. The anomaly was detected at the age of 20 years, during a routine check. The patient had never had cardiac symptoms. ECG: typical inversion of p waves and QRS complexes in lead I (similar or identical as in false poling of the upper limb leads). rS complex in all precordial leads, with decreasing r amplitude from V_1 to V_6. ST/T alterations.

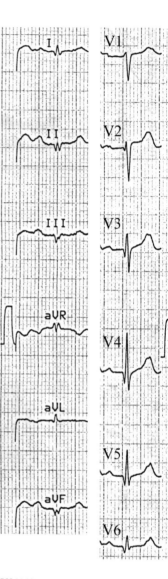

ECG 14.19

73 y/m. Amyloidosis of the heart. ECG: sinus rhythm, 103/min. AV block 1°. Peripheral low voltage. ÂQRS$_F$ - 90°. Prominent q waves in V_2 to V_6.

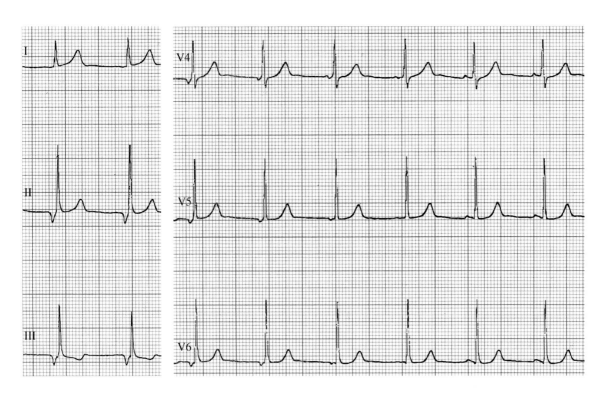

ECG 14.20

Pseudo-Q wave in AV junctional rhythm. The negative deflection immediately before the QRS complex corresponds to negative p waves but may be confounded with q waves. Note that the pseudo-Q waves disappear during change to sinus rhythm (leads V$_4$ to V$_6$).

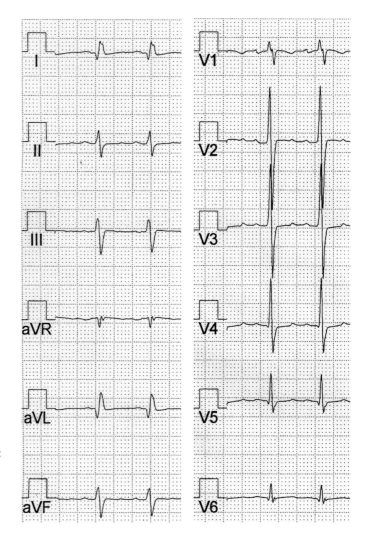

ECG 14.21

18 y/m. Steinert disease. ECG (half voltage(!)
1 mV=5 mm): sinus rhythm, 117/min. ÅQRS$_F$ - 15°. Deep
and broad Q waves in aVL and I (40 and 30 msec respectively). Prominent R wave in V$_1$ (50 msec), very tall R
(and S) waves in V$_2$/V$_3$. Relatively small R wave and
1.5 mm deep q wave in V$_6$. *Interpretation:* the giant R
and S amplitudes in V$_2$/V$_3$ (R + S=68 mm/62 mm) reflect
biventricular hypertrophy (positive Katz-Wachtel sign).
The pathologic Q waves (and high 'mirror-image'
R waves) are consistent with posterolateral dyskinesia
found in the echo. The left ventricle (mass 200 g/m^2)
and the right ventricle were hypertrophic.

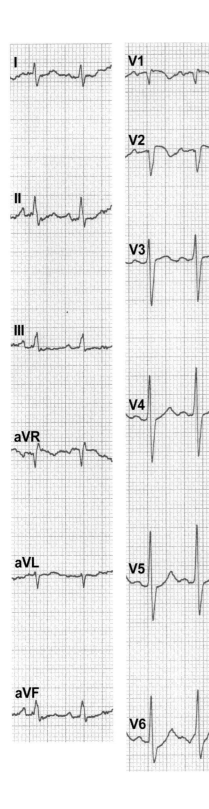

ECG 14.22

57 y/f. Acute massive pulmonary embolism (proven by spiral tomography). ECG: Qr complex in lead V$_1$, QS complex in V$_2$. Other 'typical' signs for acute PE: a) sinus rate 100/min; b) S$_I$/R$_{III}$; c) QRS clockwise rotation; d) negative T waves in V$_2$/V$_3$ (V$_1$/V$_4$). Also ST elevation in V$_1$ is frequently found associated with the QR type.

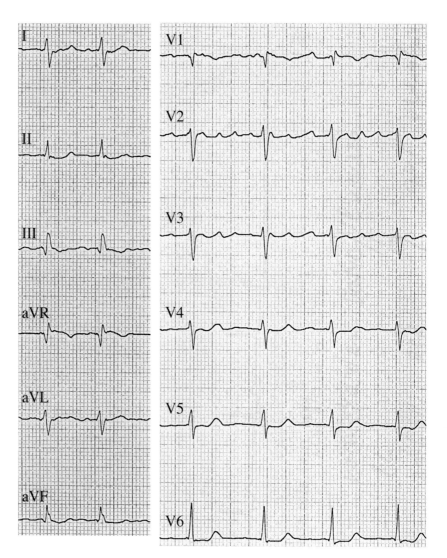

ECG 14.23

72 y/f. Severe mitral stenosis with pulmonary hypertension, right ventricular failure and tricuspid regurgitation. Mitral valvulotomy 24 years previously. ECG: atrial fibrillation. Q wave (Qr complex) in V$_1$, due to right atrial enlargement (for explanation see section 17). The q wave disappeared after diuretic therapy and regression of the heart size.

Chapter 15
Acute and Chronic Pericarditis

At a Glance

Compared with myocardial infarction (MI), pericarditis is quite a rare disease. Acute pericarditis is generally of viral or unknown etiology. The main symptom is a sharp (occasionally dull) pain of quite sudden onset, in the heart region, that varies with breathing and with different body positions. The pain may radiate to the neck and the scapular region. ECG alterations can be detected in about 90% of the cases if serial ECGs are available.

Etiology

Acute pericarditis is usually of unknown origin (in this case called 'idiopathic pericarditis') or has viral etiology. Chronic pericarditis is associated with many conditions. A summary of etiologies, specified for acute/subacute and subacute/chronic pericarditis, is presented in Table 15.1.

ECG

1 Acute Pericarditis

In acute pericarditis four (or five) stages can be distinguished (theoretically). Not all stages are always present in the same patient:

i.   acute, very early stage: PQ depression, positive T wave
ii. acute stage: ST elevation (*plus* PQ depression), positive T wave
iii. intermediate stage: ST and PQ isoelectric, flattened T waves
iv. subacute stage: negative T waves, ST and PQ isoelectrical
v.   (postpericarditis: normal ECG.)

PQ depression (a slightly descending segment between the end of the p wave and the beginning of the QRS complex) is seen as an isolated ECG sign in the very early stage (stage 1) of pericarditis in about 50% of cases, at best, in our experience (ECG 15.1). This alteration is extremely rare in acute MI (AMI). ECGs 15.2–15.3 show the more common combination of PQ depression with ST elevation in stage 2 pericarditis.

ST elevation generally does not exceed 2.0 mm and may be present in the majority of the 12 standard leads, with the exception of lead aVR, where ST is always depressed, and of lead V_1, where ST may be depressed. In the precordial leads the ST elevation may be accentuated more midprecordially (V_3 to V_5) or more laterally (V_5 and V_6). In contrast to the pattern in AMI (where the ST elevation generally arises from the R downstroke and is mostly of higher amplitude), the ST segment frequently arises from the S wave in the midprecordial leads. However, in the limb leads and in the lateral leads V_5/V_6 the ST elevation often arises from the R downstroke – as in acute infarction.

The frontal ST vector is between + 30° and + 70°. Thus the ST segment is elevated in leads aVF, II *and* I, a condition that is never seen in AMI.

In contrast to the ECG pattern of MI, the ECG during the evolution of acute pericarditis shows no reduction of the R wave, and no development of pathologic Q waves.

The negative T waves in subacute pericarditis (stage 4) are generally symmetric (as in ischemia) and are best detectable in the precordial leads (ECG 15.4). They may last for days or several weeks.

T negativity can only be interpreted correctly if a series of ECGs demonstrate at least one of the typical preceding ECG signs: ST elevation or PQ depression. ECG 15.5 shows a 'mixed' pattern of acute and subacute stage, with ST elevation and beginning T negativity.

Arrhythmias are very rarely provoked by pericarditis (except sinus tachycardia). If arrhythmias occur one has to look for coexisting organic heart disease. This may be concomitant myocarditis (very rare in viral or idiopathic pericarditis) or heart disease of any origin.

2 Chronic Pericarditis

In chronic pericardial diseases there are no specific ECG signs. T negativity is rather common. A massive pericardial effusion may lead to peripheral low voltage. In cardiac *tamponade* 'electric alternans' may be present. *Constrictive* pericarditis and cardiac tamponade result in diastolic dysfunction of the left ventricle (LV) and/or the right ventricle (RV).

The Full Picture

Idiopathic or viral acute pericarditis is an out-of-hospital disease. A young physician in general practice may therefore encounter more patients with pericarditis within just a few years than he saw during all of his postgraduate in-hospital training. Indeed, only those patients with complications (e.g. great pericardial effusion) or with pericarditis of other etiologies (e.g. bacterial, renal insufficiency, malignant tumor, tuberculosis, following heart operation) are treated in a hospital.

3 Etiology and Prevalence

The etiology of pericarditis is manifold (Table 15.1).

ECG Special ———————————————

4 PQ Depression

Acute pericarditis provokes transmural injury of the atria, leading to an STa vector. Because the atrial walls are thin, the vector points to the opposite direction of the p vector. This produces depression of the 'PQ' segment.

This slightly descending segment between the end of the p wave and the onset of the QRS complex is very typical for acute pericarditis and is found in about 50% of cases – more often in the earliest stage of pericarditis [1,2]. PQ depression is generally seen in leads V_3 to V_5 and sometimes in the frontal leads. In conditions other than pericarditis PQ depression is due to an enhanced 'STa' and follows high p waves in the frontal leads, for instance in individuals with enhanced sympathetic tone, where the negative 'STa' also influences the early ventricular repolarization, inducing ST depression and not ST elevation.

5 ST Elevation and ST Vector

ST elevation corresponds to injury of subepicardial myocardium and T negativity to a reaction of the same substrate leading to ECG signs equal or similar to those with ischemic origin. The *directions* of the ST and T vectors are different in pericarditis compared to AMI and subacute MI. The ST vector in AMI points to the injured area (inferiorly or anteriorly), whereas the (smaller) ST vector in acute pericarditis often has a more intermediate direction, due to the generalized inflammation of the pericardium. This leads to the characteristic behavior of ST elevation in the frontal leads, different in both diseases. Together with the different amplitude of ST elevation, the frontal ST vector represents the most important difference in the ECG in acute pericarditis and AMI (see section 6.1.3).

6 Differential Diagnosis of Acute Pericarditis versus Acute MI

Astonishingly, ECG signs are seen in about 90% of patients with idiopathic or viral pericarditis [1,3], based on *serial* ECG registrations, whereas AMI can only be diagnosed in 60%–70% in the ECG. Important differences in amplitude, configuration, and localization of the ST segment in the different ECG leads allow the correct diagnosis to be made in most cases. Moreover, the ECG evolution in pericarditis and MI is completely different.

Acute/subacute pericarditis
Common
– Idiopathic
– Viral: coxsackievirus A and B, echovirus, adenovirus
– Bacterial: staphylococcus, streptococcus, pneumococcus
– Myocardial infarction [12]
– Heart surgery
– Chest trauma
Rare
– Viral: mononucleosis, varicella, mumps virus, hepatitis B, Epstein-Barr virus
– Bacterial: Bacteroides fragilis, Bifidobacterium [13], Borrelia burgdorferi (Lyme disease), Brucella, Clostridium, Escherichia coli, Fusobacterium, Gram-negative sepsis, Klebsiella, meningococcus [14], Mycoplasma, Neisseria gonorrhoea, Neisseria meningitidis, Proteus, Pseudomonas, Salmonella
– Pulmonary embolism (in 4% of cases) [15]
– Fungal: Candida, Histoplasma
– Other infections: amoebiasis [16], echinococcosis, leishmaniasis (kala azar) [17], toxoplasmosis
– Acute rheumatic fever
– Other conditions: dissecting aortic aneurysm, radiation, pacemaker implantation [18]
– Drugs: procainamide, phenytoin, hydralazine, phenylbutazone, doxorubicin, clozapine [19], penicillin with eosinophilia.
– Eosinophilic [20,21]

Subacute/chronic pericarditis and chronic pericardial diseases
Common
– Uremia (treated and untreated)
– Neoplasias: lung, breast, melanoma, leukemia, Hodgkin disease, lymphoma
– Tuberculosis
– Myxedema
– Delayed injury: postpercardiotomy syndrome
Rare
– Infections: AIDS, amoebiasis, amyloidosis, inflammatory bowel disease, sarcoidosis
– Radiation
– Autoimmune disorders: dermatomyositis, periarteritis nodosa, rheumatoid arthritis, scleroderma, systemic lupus erythematosus
– Delayed injury: postmyocardial infarction syndrome (Dressler syndrome)
– Primary tumors: mesothelioma, sarcoma
– Chylopericardium [22]
– Pacemaker implantation [23]

6.1 ST Elevation

6.1.1 Amplitude of ST Elevation

In acute pericarditis the ST elevation is generally 1–2 mm and rarely exceeds 2.5 mm. In the typical pattern of AMI the ST elevation often exceeds 2.5 mm and may reach more than 10 mm.

6.1.2 Configuration of ST Elevation

We have learnt from many ECG books that in most cases of acute pericarditis the ST segment is concave-upward, arising from the S wave, whereas in AMI it is usually convex-upward, arising directly from the R downstroke (so-called monophasic deformation). This statement is *not* correct; in anterior AMI, ST elevation may also arise from an S wave in leads V_1 to V_3, and in acute pericarditis ST elevation often arises from the R wave, in limb leads, and in leads V_5/V_6. Moreover, the differentiation of ST configuration (convex/concave) is not reliable. The behavior of the frontal ST vector is much more important.

6.1.3 ST Elevation in Frontal ECG Leads and Frontal ST Vector

The frontal ST vector in acute pericarditis is the best criterion for differentiation from an infarction pattern. The ST vector in acute pericarditis is + 30° to + 70° (Figure 15.1a), in acute inferior infarction + 80° to + 120° (Figure 15.1b) and in extensive acute anterior infarction - 40° to + 10° (Figure 15.1c). Therefore, in acute pericarditis we find ST elevation in leads I, II *and* aVF, in lead aVR ST depression is present. The ST may be isoelectric or also slightly elevated in lead III or in lead aVL, depending on the ST vector, pointing more to the right (up to + 70°) or more to the left (up to + 30°). ECG 15.3 demonstrates a frontal ST vector of + 30° with ST elevation in leads aVL, I, II and aVF, combined with only slight ST elevation in the precordial leads (and ST depression in V_1).

This ST vector is extremely rare in AMI. In inferior AMI we find ST elevation in leads aVF, III and often II (in lead aVL ST is depressed). In anterior or anterolateral AMI there is ST elevation in leads aVL, I and sometimes II, but never in aVF or III, where ST is isoelectric or depressed.

6.1.4 ST Elevation in Horizontal Leads

In acute pericarditis ST elevation may be present in all precordial leads, with the exception of lead V_1 where ST may be depressed (ECG 15.6), or be accentuated in the midprecordial (V_3 to V_4) or lateral leads (V_5 to V_6). In AMI the localization of ST elevation depends on the extension of anterior infarction (anteroseptal: V_1 to V_3/V_4; anteroapical: V_1 to V_4; anterolateral:

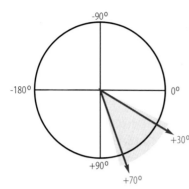

Figure 15.1a
Frontal ST vector in acute pericarditis

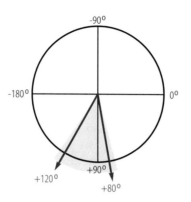

Figure 15.1b
Frontal ST vector in acute inferior myocardial infarction

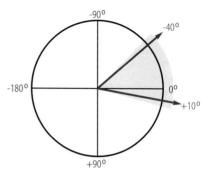

Figure 15.1c
Frontal ST vector in acute anterior myocardial infarction

V_1 to V_6; strictly lateral: V_5 and V_6). In none of the anterior AMI patterns do we ever find an ST depression in lead V_1. ST depression in V_1 and V_2/V_3 is common in acute strict posterior infarction, as a mirror image of ST elevation in the dorsal leads V_7 to V_9.

In a patient with subacute MI a sudden second elevation of the ST segment reflects local pericarditis (or new ischemia) or may be a precursor of imminent myocardial perforation [4]. ST elevation in the right precordial leads has been described due to acute pericarditis [5]. However, in this case transmural injury (acute right ventricular MI) should not be overlooked. RV infarction occurs almost only associated with inferior LV infarction.

6.2   Pathologic Q Wave

In contrast to the ECG evolution in MI, in acute pericarditis there is no or only minimal reduction of R waves and no development of pathologic Q waves. If pericarditis occurs as a complication of AMI or subacute MI, the ECG may be troublesome.

6.3   PQ Depression

PQ depression is extremely rare in AMI, where it is due to atrial ischemia or infarction.

6.4   T-Wave Negativity

Negative T waves develop in subacute pericarditis in the majority of cases and are generally symmetric. T wave negativity is best seen in the precordial leads V_3 to V_6, whereas in MI negative T waves appear in the leads with pathologic Q waves. Moreover, T-wave negativity in pericarditis develops *after* the ST segment has returned to the isoelectric line (exception see ECG 15.5), whereas in infarction the T waves still become negative in the presence of ST elevation.

7   General Differential Diagnosis of ST Elevation

ST elevation is seen in acute pericarditis, acute and subacute MI, old infarction with aneurysm, Prinzmetal angina, mirror image of LV systolic overload and normal variants (including early repolarization). ST elevation is rarely encountered in hyperkalemia, hypercalcemia, cerebrovascular accidents, hypothermia, pneumothorax and hypertrophic obstructive cardiomyopathy [6]. Ginzton and Laks [7] studied 19 patients with acute pericarditis and 20 healthy individuals with ST elevation of the normal variant type (early repolarization included). They observed that an ST/T ratio of more or equal to 0.25 in lead V_6 identified the patients with pericarditis and excluded normal variants.

A major ST elevation in leads V_1/V_2 is an inherent component of the Brugada syndrome (Chapter 31 Special Waves, Signs and Phenomena).

Short Story/Case Report 1

In April 2001 an 83-year-old woman experienced dyspnea and a dull persisting pain in the heart region. On hospitalization two days later she presented a good general (subfebrile) state, with blood pressure 140/80 mmHg and pulse rate 80/min. The ECG (ECG 15.7) showed striking ST elevation of 2–2.5 mm in leads III, aVF, II and V_4 to V_6, arising from the R wave in the inferolateral leads (but also slight ST elevation in lead I!). An echocardiogram was not performed. In spite of only borderline elevated creatine phosphokinase (CPK) and troponin, AMI was diagnosed and thrombolysis was applied. Dyspnea was aggravated and because of pre-shock the patient was transferred to another hospital. An echocardiogram revealed a great pericardial effusion and normal function of LV and RV. By pericardial drainage, 400 ml of fluid (hematocrit 4%) were removed instantly, 300 ml in the following 24 h. The patient recovered and the ECG normalized (no pathologic Q waves). Coronary angiography was not performed. One year later the patient was still well, but etiology of the pericardial effusion remains obscure. In conclusion, the ECG was strikingly similar to that of infarction. However, the frontal ST vector was + 65° (with slight ST elevation in lead I). There was slight PQ depression in leads V_4 to V_6 (artifact in V_3).

The differential diagnosis of acute pericarditis should have been considered, especially on the basis of only borderline troponin and CPK levels. Had the echocardiogram been performed in time, the potentially dangerous (at this age) thrombolysis, which led to increase of pericardial effusion by bleeding, could have been avoided.

A short, positive and small deflection (about 1 mm) in the region of the J point (the end of the QRS complex and the beginning of the ST segment, which is elevated) is called the *stork-leg* sign. Figure 15.2 shows the reason for this description. If we inverse the ECG by 180°, it is similar to a stork standing on one leg (the inverted R wave), with the other leg drawn back to the body (the small 'J point deflection'). This special sign is seen in leads V_4 to V_6 and occasionally inferiorly and is quite diagnostic for acute pericarditis (ECG 15.8). In this ECG we miss PQ depression, possibly due to the short PQ interval. A depressed PQ interval could be hidden within the QRS complex.

Short Story/Case Report 2

In February 2000 the author received a telephone call from a close friend, a professor in psychosomatic medicine, who was on a skiing holiday in a small village. For several days he had felt ill in some way, and had suffered a dull retrosternal pain radiating sometimes to the scapula, the neck and both ears. The pain increased by deep breathing and with the Valsalva manoeuvre. Despite feeling ill he did about 20 km cross-country skiing per day. On the author's suggestion he visited the physician in the village who performed an ECG. In the opinion of this physician a subacute inferolateral MI could not be excluded (CPK was significantly elevated: 648 u/l (normal value up to 195). The troponin level, received later from an external lab, was normal). On the basis of the ECG transmitted by fax, the author appeased both of his colleagues. The moderate ST elevation arose from the S wave, the frontal ST vector was + 50° and the stork-leg sign was present (ECG 15.8). The further evolution was uneventful. Two weeks later the echocardiogram revealed a small pericardial effusion over the RV and the ECG had normalized; the patient felt well again. Serum diagnostics were not made (as is usual with a physician who becomes a patient), the elevated CPK value was attributed to the cross-country skiing. Coronary angiography was not performed. Why should this be? The patient had no risk factors for coronary heart disease … except for stress.

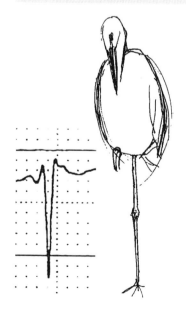

Figure 15.2
Stork-leg sign (design by Ursula Gertsch)

ECGs 15.9 and 15.10 show other examples of acute pericarditis with the stork-leg sign. The stork-leg sign is found in about 30% of cases. It may be present in some leads as a normal variant, without ST elevation in the lateral leads (ECG 15.11). Most probably the stork-leg sign is a variant of the 'Osborn wave' (see Chapter 31 Special Waves, Signs and Phenomena). In 'early repolarization' a concomitant similar phenomenon is localized also at the beginning of ST elevation, sometimes arising from the R wave (ECG 15.12).

8   Arrhythmias

Sinus tachycardia is the only arrhythmia related to acute pericarditis [8,9]. It may be present also without fever and can persist several weeks. All other arrhythmias, including atrial fibrillation, are connected with organic heart disease, e.g. with substantial myocardial involvement (perimyocarditis), which is rare in idiopathic or viral pericarditis, or with structural heart disease of any etiology. Spodick [10] makes the following statement: If your patient with arrhythmia has pericarditis, look carefully for heart disease.

9   Chronic Pericarditis

There are no typical ECG signs for chronic pericarditis, neither in its restrictive nor constrictive form. Slight ST elevation, similar to that in acute pericarditis may occur. In many cases negative T waves (symmetric or asymmetric) are present in the precordial and some frontal leads. Constrictive and restrictive pericarditis lead to diastolic heart failure [11]. In the advanced stage of constrictive pericarditis, atrial fibrillation is not uncommon and the frontal QRS axis may be vertical. A great pericardial effusion often produces peripheral low voltage. This alteration is never seen in cardiac tamponade, where the heart silhouette in x-rays may be unchanged.

10   Cardiac Tamponade

Electric alternans is sometimes seen in cardiac tamponade and in this case may represent an emergency situation (ECG 15.13). However, the diagnosis of this life-threatening complication is made on the basis of clinical findings and is confirmed by the echocardiogram. In the majority of cases with cardiac tamponade (especially after heart operations and in context with anticoagulation) the pericardial fluid or blood volume is relatively small (150–400 ml) and therefore very rarely leads to peripheral low voltage.

11   Clinical Findings in Acute Pericarditis

Classically, the symptoms of idiopathic and viral pericarditis are general malaise, thoracic pain and occasionally fever. Often the pain is of sudden onset, somewhat circumscript in the heart region, left from the sternal border or retrosternally, sharp or burning. It is accentuated by breathing, the recumbent position, or moving the thorax, and by the Valsalva maneuver, especially if there is concomitant pleuritis. Leaning forward often relieves pain. The pain may also be dull or oppressive, however, and may radiate to the throat, the neck or the trapezius ridge, thus imitating the pain of AMI. Pericardial friction can be heard in only about half of cases. It is advisable to auscultate the patient as often as possible, *not* over the apex but in the middle of the sternum at the second to fourth intercostal space, or at the left sternal border – and during inspiration and expiration.

(The references 12–23 are listed in Table 15.1, Etiology of pericarditis)

References

1. Spodick DH. Diagnostic electrocardiographic sequences in acute pericarditis: significance of PR segment and PR vector changes. Circulation 1973;48:575
2. Baljepally R, Spodick DH. PR-segment deviation as the initial electrocardiographic response in acute pericarditis. Am J Cardiol 1998;81:1505–6
3. Torija Martinez RN, Gonzalez Hermosilla JA. Acute nonspecific pericarditis. Arch Inst Cardiol Mex 1987;57:307–12
4. Hurst JW. Abnormalities of the S-T segment: Part II. Clin Cardiol 1997;20:595–600
5. Carson W. Maximal spatial ST vector of ST segment elevation in the right precordial leads on electrocardiogram due to acute pericarditis. Europ Heart J 1988;9:665–7
6. Khan IA, Ajatta FO, Ansari AW. Persistent ST segment elevation: a new ECG finding in hypertrophic cardiomyopathy. Am J Emerg Med 1999;17:296–9
7. Ginzton LE, Laks MM. The differential diagnosis of acute pericarditis from the normal variant: new electrocardiographic criteria. Circulation 1982;65:1004–9
8. Spodick DH. Arrhythmias during acute pericarditis: A prospective study of 100 consecutive cases. J Amer Med Assoc 1973;235:39–41
9. Spodick DH. Frequency of arrhythmias in patients with acute pericarditis determined by Holter monitoring. Amer J Cardiol 1984;53:842–5
10. Spodick DH. Significant arrhythmias during pericarditis are due to concomitant heart disease. JACC 1998;32:551 (reply by Danias on page 552)
11. Asher CR, Klein AA. Diastolic heart failure: restrictive cardiomyopathy, constrictive pericarditis and cardiac tamponade. Clinical and echocardiographic evaluation. Cardiol Rev 2002;10:218–29

12. Ajdinalp A, Wishniak A, van den Acker-Berman L. Pericarditis and pericardial effusion in acute ST-elevation myocardial infarction in the thrombolytic era. Isr Med Ass J 2002;4:181–3
13. Brook I. Pericarditis due to anaerobic bacteria. Cardiology 2002;97:55–8
14. Morgan DR, Spencer M, Crowe M, O'Keeffe DB. Primary (isolated) meningococcal pericarditis. Clin Cardiol 2002;25:305–7
15. Garty I, Mader R, Schonfeld S. Post pulmonary embolism pericarditis. A rare entity diagnosed by combined lung scanning and chest radiograph study. Clin Nucl Med 1994;19:519–21
16. Shamsuzzaman SM, Hashiguchi Y. Thoracic amebiasis. Clin Chest Med 2002;23:479–92
17. Mofredy A, Guerin JM, Leibinger F, Masmoudi R. Visceral leishmaniasis with pericarditis in a HIV-infected patient. Scand J Infect Dis 2002;34:151–3
18. Sivakumaran S, Irwin ME, Gulamhusein SS, Senaratne MP. Postpacemaker implant pericarditis: incidence and outcomes with active-fixation leads. Pacing Clin Electrophysiol 2002;25:833–7
19. Kay SE, Doery J, Sholl D. Clozapine associated pericarditis and elevated troponin I. Aust NZ J Psychiatr 2002;36:143–4
20. Li Q, Gupta D, Schroth G, et al. Images in cardiovascular medicine. Eosinophilic pericarditis and myocarditis. Circulation 2002;105:3066
21. Van den Bosch JM, Wagenaar SS, Westermann CJ. Asthma, eosinophilic pleuropneumonia, and pericarditis without vasculitis. Thorax 1986;41:571–2
22. England RW, Grathwohl KW, Powell GE. Constrictive pericarditis presenting as chylous ascites. J Clin Gastroenterol 2002;35:104–5
23. Elinav E, Leibowitz D. Constrictive pericarditis complicating endovascular pacemaker implantation. Pacing Clin Electrophysiol 2002;25:376–7

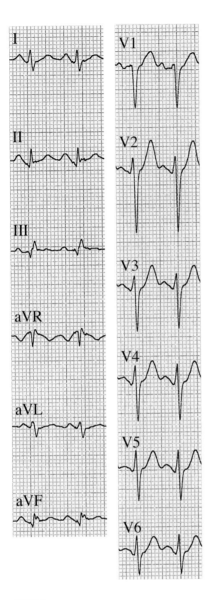

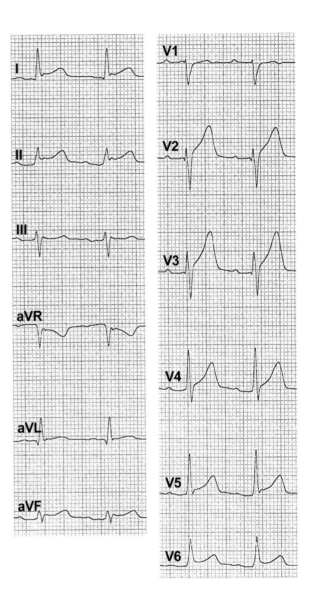

ECG 15.1

53y/m. ECG 6 h after onset of acute chest pain. Early acute stage of pericarditis with PQ depression in I, II, aVF and V₁ to V₆.

ECG 15.2

65y/m. Acute idiopathic pericarditis. ECG: ST elevation in leads I, II *and* aVF (frontal ST vector about + 50°) and in (V₂/V₃) V₄ to V₆. PQ depression in I, II, aVF, III and V₂ to V₆. Note the small Q waves in V₂/V₃, a normal variant on the basis of the normal coro.

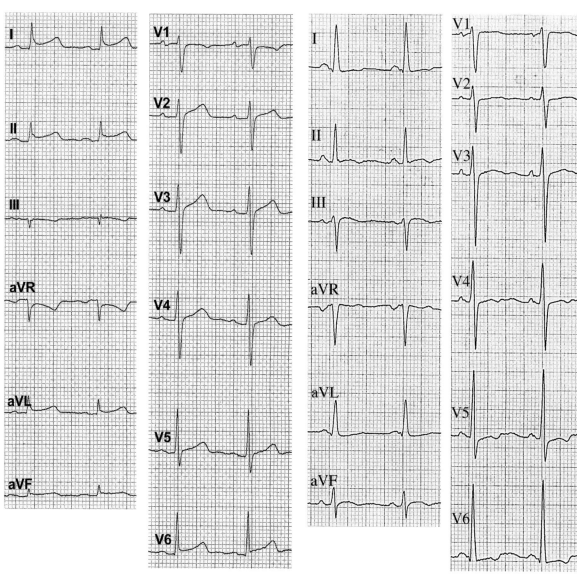

ECG 15.3

74y/m. Liver transplantation. Subacute pulmonary embolism with small pleural and pericardial effusion. ECG: frontal ST vector + 30°, ST elevation in aVL, I, II *and* aVF. Only slight ST elevation in (V$_2$/V$_3$/V$_4$) V$_5$/V$_6$. Note also PQ depression in I, II, aVF and V$_3$ to V$_6$.

ECG 15.4

60y/f. Subacute viral pericarditis. ECG: negative T waves in II and V$_3$ to V$_6$.

291

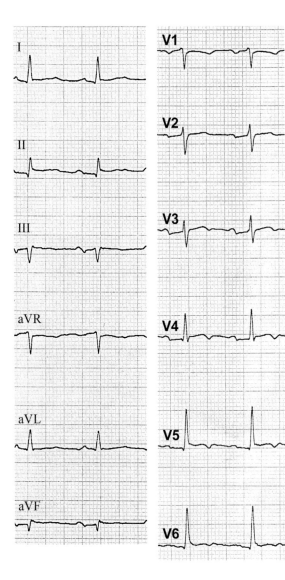
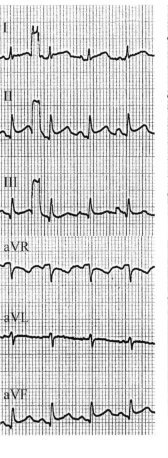
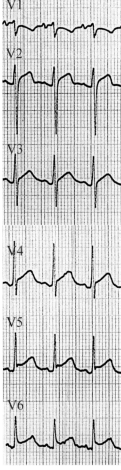

ECG 15.5

44y/m. Acute/subacute viral pericarditis. ECG: slight ST elevation in I, II *and* aVF, and in (V$_2$/V$_3$) V$_4$ to V$_6$, with beginning 'T negativity' in V$_3$ to V$_5$ (V$_6$). Note: 'negative T wave' *above* the isoelectric line. Slight ST depression in V$_1$.

ECG 15.6

28y/f. Acute viral pericarditis. ECG: frontal ST vector + 60°, with ST elevation in I, II, aVF and V$_2$ to V$_6$. *ST depression* in V$_1$(!) Typical PQ depression in II, aVF (I) and V$_2$ to V$_6$.

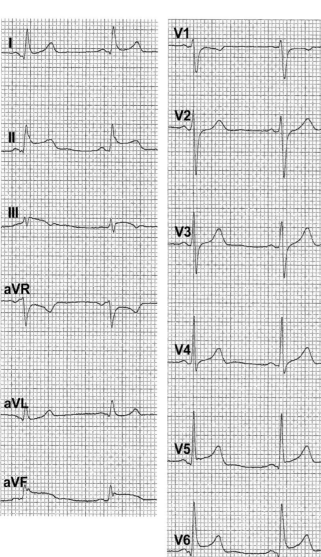

ECG 15.7

Short Story/Case Report 1. 83y/f. ECG: acute pericarditis mimicking inferior AMI. However, the frontal ST vector is + 60°, with ST elevation not only in II, aVF and III but additionally in I (and in V_5/V_6). Slight ST depression in V_1. No PQ depression, possibly due to the short PQ interval (130 msec).

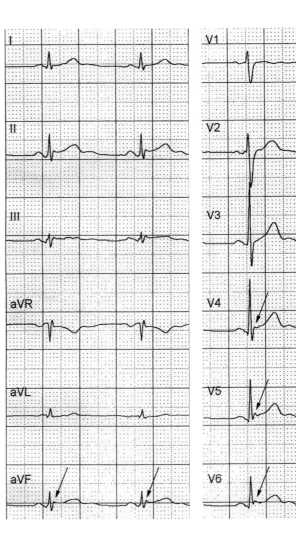

ECG 15.8
Short Story/Case Report 2. 62y/m.
Idiopathic acute pericarditis. ECG: frontal
ST vector + 50°. ST elevation in I, II, aVF, III
and V$_4$ to V$_6$ (V$_2$/V$_3$). _Stork-leg_ sign in aVF
and V$_4$ to V$_6$ (↓). Minimal PQ depression in
V$_4$/V$_5$ and in some limb leads (short PQ
interval).

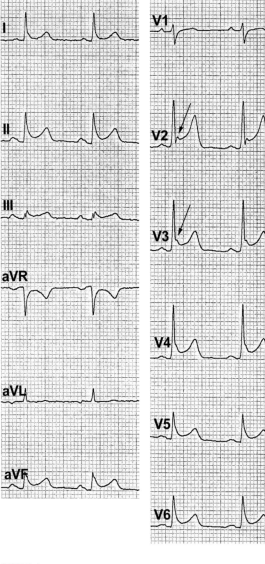

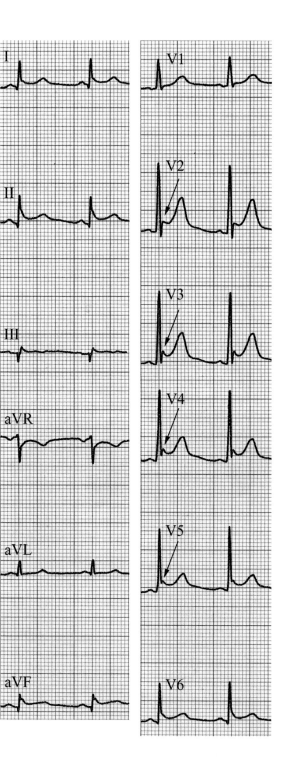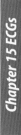

ECG 15.9 ▲

68y/f. Acute idiopathic pericarditis. ECG: frontal ST vector + 60°. ST elevation in I, II, aVF, III and V_2 to V_6. *Stork-leg* sign in V_2 (V_3), see arrows. Note that ST elevation arises exclusively from the R wave downstroke.

ECG 15.10 ▶

73y/m. Pericarditis 3 weeks after extensive *postero*inferior MI (Dressler syndrome). Tall R waves in V_1 to V_3 as mirror image of posterior MI, nonsignificant Q waves in II, aVF, III. Typical pattern of acute pericarditis. Frontal ST vector + 60°, with ST elevation in I, II, aVF, III, and (V_1) V_2 to V_6. *Stork-leg* sign in V_2 to V_5 (↓).

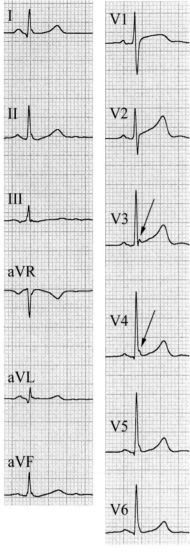

ECG 15.11
**57y/m. Normal heart. Stork-leg sign in V$_3$
(V$_4$) as a normal variant (arrows).**

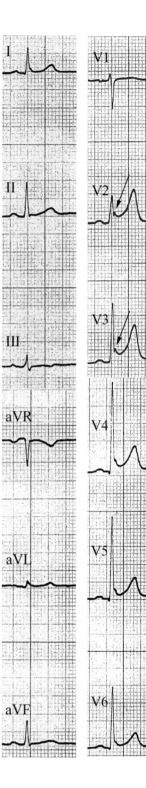

ECG 15.12
**57y/m. Normal heart. Variant of
Osborn wave in 'early repolarization'.
The Osborn waves arise from the
R wave downstroke, see leads V$_2$/V$_3$
(V$_4$ to V$_6$).**

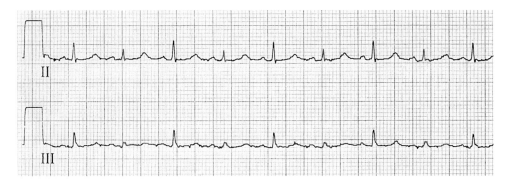

ECG 15.13
27y/m. Cardiac tamponade. Electric alternans of the QRS complex.

Chapter 16
Electrolyte Imbalances and Disturbances

At a Glance

Clinically important abnormalities of electrolytes concern potassium (K) more often than calcium (Ca). A pathologic cellular or serum level of sodium (Na) is not detectable in the ECG, and this is also the case for hypomagnesemia, which is often combined with hypokalemia. Generally there is a disappointingly low correlation (10%–30%) between the ECG and definitively pathologic serum levels of electrolytes. More importantly, severe or extreme electrolyte imbalance is detectable in the ECG in up to 90%. The recognition of typical ECG patterns or arrhythmias may even represent the first hint for a severe electrolyte disturbance. For instance, an extremely broad QRS may be due to hyperkalemia, and a ventricular tachycardia of the type torsade de pointes may indicate hypokalemia.

Note that in many cases of electrolyte imbalance the etiology is known in advance. In other instances, the reader may find a detailed checklist useful, such as the one provided in Appendix 1 at the end of this chapter.

ECG

1 Hyperkalemia (Hyperpotassemia)

Every physician is familiar with the typical tall and peaked, so-called 'tented' T waves of hyperkalemia, generally present in mild or moderate hyperkalemia. Surprisingly, the ECG pattern in *severe hyperkalemia* is not as well known, and sometimes it is not correctly interpreted. However, this ECG represents an urgent situation. It is characterized by *extremely broad QRS complexes* measuring up to 0.2 sec, or even 0.26 sec, with an atypical *bundle-branch block* pattern (ECGs 16.1 and 16.2). Additionally, a tall T wave is often seen. In rare cases a marked ST elevation is present, mimicking acute myocardial injury. Often the p wave is not visible, thus imitating a ventricular

rhythm (ECG 16.1). In reality sinus rhythm is present. The potassium induced 'intoxication' (also of the atria) inhibits a visible atrial depolarization. Life-threatening arrhythmias may develop, such as ventricular tachycardia and fibrillation, or ventricular asystole.

ECGs 16.3a–c illustrate the ECG patterns of a patient with terminal renal failure and severe hyperkalemia, that are regressing rapidly during hemodialysis.

The ECG in *moderate hyperkalemia* shows the well-known *tall, peaked* and *symmetric* ('tented') T waves, especially in the middle or lateral precordial leads (ECG 16.4), and less in the frontal leads.

2 Hypokalemia (Hypopotassemia)

The ECG in *severe hypokalemia* is characterized by a *fusion* of the T wave with a prominent U wave (ECGs 16.5 and 16.6). The QT interval cannot be measured, because the end of the T wave is not identifiable. The ST segment may be depressed or not (ECGs 16.5 and 16.6). ECG alterations similar to those due to hypokalemia are seen in patients under amiodarone (ECG 16.7). Similar to the true 'long QT syndromes' (Chapter 26 Ventricular tachycardias), other conditions with TU fusion favor episodes of polymorphous ventricular tachycardia of the type 'torsade de pointes' (see Short Story/Case Report 2). This type of ventricular tachycardia has a high rate (between 160 and 300/min) but generally converts into sinus rhythm spontaneously. However, longer episodes lead to syncope, and the tachycardia may degenerate into ventricular fibrillation.

3 Hypercalcemia

In *moderate-to-severe* hypercalcemia the ECG is characterized by a *shortened* QT interval, always at the expense of a *shortened* or *absent* ST segment (ECGs 16.8 and 16.9). Although the ECG pattern is striking and a glance at the ECG computer print (which indicates QTc time) often provides the diagnosis, this condition is often overlooked even by experienced ECG readers. There are several reasons for this:

i.   the pattern is rare
ii. the ECG looks *so* normal otherwise
iii. experienced ECG readers can be arrogant (!).

Hypercalcemia may be found in patients with primary or secondary hyperparathyroidism, tumors with or without metastases, acute and chronic renal failure, and other conditions.

4   Hypocalcemia

Hypocalcemia is a rare finding. In contrast to hypercalcemia, a *prolonged ST segment* is found in the ECG, with a consecutive *prolonged QT interval* (ECG 16.10). Isolated hypocalcemia is due to hypoalbuminemia, and disturbances in Parathormon and Vitamin D metabolism, generally in patients with chronic renal disease.

The *combination* of hypocalcemia and hyperkalemia is seen mostly in patients with chronic renal failure. The ECG shows a prolonged ST segment with *QT lengthening* and tall and somewhat *peaked* T waves (ECG 16.11).

5   Therapy of Potassium Imbalance

5.1   Severe Hyperkalemia

The fast recognition of the ECG pattern in severe hypokalemia allows a rapid and simple therapy: 10 ml of intravenous calcium gluconate (given slowly) normalizes within minutes both the cellular membrane potential and the ECG. Further therapy depends on the underlying disease, which is usually renal insufficiency or hyperglycemia.

5.2   Severe Hypokalemia

The therapy is potassium substitution that is generally complemented by magnesium substitution. Hypomagnesemia, not detectable in the ECG, often accompanies hypokalemia, especially if the potassium deficit is caused by diuretic drugs. A transient pacemaker may be useful.

The Full Picture

The action potential of the isolated heart muscle fiber is directly related to – or created by – shifts of the electrolytes sodium ions (Na^+), calcium ions (Ca^{2+}) and potassium ions (K^+). Only imbalance of potassium and/or calcium can be recognized in the ECG. Although the correlation between the serum level of these electrolytes in the serum and the alterations in the ECG is not at all strong, severe electrolyte disturbances can often be detected in the ECG. (A detailed list of the *etiologies* of electrolyte imbalance is given in Appendix 1 at the end of the text of this chapter.)

ECG Special

6   Hyperkalemia (Hyperpotassemia)

Tall, symmetric T waves in the ECG are generally recognized as a possible sign of hyperkalemia. Astonishingly, not all physicians – cardiologists included – consider the possibility of severe hyperkalemia on the basis of some typical and dangerous manifestations in the ECG.

ECGs 16.1, 16.2 and 16.3a show typical signs of *severe hyperkalemia* with an extremely broad QRS complex, measuring 180–260 msec and a bundle-branch-block-like pattern, that does not fulfill the criteria of either typical right bundle-branch block (RBBB) or left bundle-branch block (LBBB). Generally the R waves are decreased and the S waves are increased. Very rarely, there is a pronounced ST elevation (up to 8 mm!) which imitates acute myocardial infarction and which is called *dialyzable* current of injury. The T wave is deformed and broad and seems to arise from the QRS complex. The QT interval is generally prolonged.

Severe hyperkalemia greatly diminishes the atrial vectors. Thus the atrial depolarization can no longer be detected in the ECG. A ventricular rhythm (generally at a rate of 70–130/min) is simulated, in the presence of sinus rhythm (ECGs 16.1, 16.2, 16.3a).

Ventricular arrhythmias are not unusual, including ventricular premature beats (VPBs) and ventricular tachycardia that may degenerate into ventricular fibrillation.

Another less common sign of severe hyperkalemia is excessive bradycardia, due to atrioventricular (AV) block 2° and 3° [1], or sinoatrial (SA) block up to longer episodes of cardiac standstill (ECG 16.12b). Arrhythmic death from ventricular fibrillation occurs more often than from cardiac standstill. In some cases the ECG features are combined as in the case report that follows.

Short Story/Case Report 1 (or Tremendous 57 Minutes for a Young Patient and his Physicians)

In July 1997 heart transplantation was performed in a 19-year-old patient with Ivemark syndrome combined with situs inversus, single atrium and ventricle after total cavopulmonary connection. An erroneously transplanted heart with a distinct blood group (B–O mismatch) had severe consequences. Although the first 36 h postoperatively had been fairly uneventful, the still intubated patient showed a decrease in urine excretion as time progressed (that was only detected retrospectively); this was followed by a fall of blood pressure from 120/70 mmHg to 90/50 mmHg and increasing VPBs. The ECG done 40 min before the event showed sinus rhythm, a normal QRS, and runs of VPBs (ECG 16.12a). Just as the intensive care team arrived (a specialist in the field, a cardiologist and a surgeon) sudden ventricular asystole occurred, which was detectable on the ECG monitor. Cardiac massage was applied immediately (ECG 16.12b). After 13 min a slow 'VT' developed at a rate of 95/min, with strikingly broad QRS (ECG 16.12c). The cardiologist asked: What's the serum potassium level? Answer: Four hours ago it was normal (3.8 mmol/l). And now? Answer: Result on the way. (An urgent call to the lab.) Potassium 7.6 mmol/l 40 min before(!). Therapy: epinephrine and insulin and finally(!) calcium gluconate. Another 7 min later, the ECG showed sinus tachycardia with enormous ST elevation ('dialyzable injury') (ECG 16.12d). As there was no palpable pulse and the arterial catheter was obstructed, cardiac massage was continued. In the interval there was sinus rhythm with normal broad QRS and less elevated ST; in addition, there were episodes of ventricular

tachycardia with a maximal rate of 260/min (ECG 16.12e). The blood pressure had normalized 15 min later (measured over a new catheter), and the ECG showed sinus tachycardia without other ECG abnormalities (ECG 16.12f). Hemodialysis was begun. Thereafter the patient had many other severe complications, not related to electrolyte imbalance or arrhythmias [2]. Finally he recovered and was dismissed from the hospital 8 weeks after heart transplantation. Five years later he was in good health.

In conclusion: within a few hours progressive renal failure with severe hyperkalemia developed, with life-threatening consequences. The immediate recognition of strikingly broad QRS on the ECG monitor possibly saved the life of the patient on this occasion.

Moderate hyperkalemia is characterized by tall, peaked, so-called 'tented' T waves with a small basis of the T wave (ECG 16.3b, ECG 16.4). It must be mentioned that those T waves may also be present in severe hyperkalemia.

6.1 Differential Diagnosis of Tall and Peaked T waves

Prominent T waves exceeding a voltage of 0.8 mV are also seen in healthy individuals with dominating vagal tonus, most combined with sinus bradycardia. The T waves are high and peaked (but asymmetric and with a normal broad basis) in leads V_2/V_3 (and V_4), but generally of normal amplitude in leads V_5/V_6 (ECG 16.13).

Very tall and peaked, almost symmetric T waves, especially in leads V_2 to V_4, are typical for the earliest period of acute myocardial infarction. This alteration represents acute ischemia of the subendocardial layers of the left ventricle and is rarely captured by an ECG because it lasts only minutes. Generally heavy chest pain is present or develops within a short time, together with the appearance of ST elevation in the ECG.

6.2 Prevalence, Clinical Findings and Etiology of Hyperkalemia

Most cases of severe hyperkalemia are seen at the hospital emergency stations, sometimes transferred with a wrong diagnosis due to multiple symptoms such as nausea, vomiting, faintness, vertigo, para- or tetraparesis, syncope and rarely coma [3]. Out of the reported eight emergency patients (aged 44–75 years, mean 64 years) with a serum potassium level of

7.1–11.2 mmol/l, seven patients showed renal failure, and in all patients drugs were involved. Seven patients showed marked ECG signs including absent p wave; five patients had extremely broad QRS complexes. All but one patient (with severe heart failure due to valvular and coronary heart disease) were treated successfully.

Hyperkalemia is quite frequent in hospitalized patients, between 1% and 10%. However, the patient is under better control. Acker et al [4] described 242 episodes of hyperkalemia in patients, hospitalized in a division for renal diseases and consecutively with predominant renal failure. Drugs (in 63%) and hyperglycemia (in 49%) contributed to the development of hyperkalemia. Only a few patients showed rather severe hyperkalemia, and from the 161 episodes observed with ECG monitoring only six patients (8%) had a widened QRS complex and only 26 patients (36%) showed peaked T waves. There were no serious arrhythmias and no death occurred as a consequence of hyperkalemia. The correlation between the potassium level and the ECG was quite poor, very probably due to the low number of patients with excessive hyperkalemia.

Hyperkalemia is mainly due to renal insufficiency, in about 60% of cases. Other causes are hyperglycemia, metabolic acidosis (especially mineral acidosis), rapid tumor lysis, hypoaldosteronism, fasting, rhabdomyolysis and limb ischemia [5]. Many drugs aggravate or induce hyperkalemia [5]. These drugs include nonsteroidal anti-inflammatory agents (NSAIDs), spironolactone, amiloride and, in rare cases, angiotensin-converting enzyme (ACE) inhibitors, angiotensin II receptor blockers, heparin, beta-adrenergic blockers, alpha-adrenergic antagonists, cyclosporine and digoxin.

6.3 Therapy of Severe Hyperkalemia

After the emergency treatment of severe hyperkalemia by intravenous calcium gluconate 10 ml (0.22 mmol or 89 mg), with an effect lasting 30–60 min, further therapy depends on the underlying disease and should be managed by experienced physicians. They will decide if insulin, catecholamines, other drugs, or hemodialysis are indicated. Bicarbonate has little effect [5] but is still given in metabolic acidosis.

7 Hypokalemia (Hypopotassemia)

The correlation between the ECG and hypokalemia is somewhat stronger than for hyperkalemia [6–8] and leads to alterations of the repolarization. The typical fusion of the T wave with the U wave is generally seen in serum potassium levels below 2.6 mmol/l, and is often best detected in the mid-precordial leads (ECGs 16.5 and 16.6).

As mentioned, in TU fusion the end of the T wave cannot be identified. The QT interval has to be estimated. It has been argued that the correct QT time is often visible in lead aVL. We do not agree with this opinion, because the end of the T wave and the U wave may be isoelectric in this lead, by reason of projection.

Short Story/Case Report 2

In March 2000 a 19-year-old woman with bulimia and irregular intake of diuretic drugs suffered several episodes of syncope during the previous few weeks, with loss of consciousness lasting up to 10 min. On entry into hospital the patient had no complaints, her body weight was normal(!). The ECG showed sinus bradycardia alternating with AV dissociation, at a rate of 40–45/min (ECG 16.14a). The QTc (QTUc respectively) was 0.56 sec and there was a somewhat unusual fusion of the T wave with the U wave (ECG 16.14b). Potassium levels were 2.3 mmol/l (3.4–5.2), and magnesium levels 0.71 mmol/l (0.7–1.0). The patient was put on an ECG monitor and potassium (and magnesium) substitution was started. After a short time multiple (about 30) episodes of ventricular tachycardia occurred at a rate up to > 300/min lasting from 4 sec to a maximum of 22 sec. In some ECG stripes 'torsade de pointes' were identified (ECGs 16.14c–d), in other stripes a monomorphic ventricular tachycardia with the pattern of ventricular flutter (ECG 16.14e) was seen. The patient became dizzy on some occasions but lost consciousness only rarely for several seconds. Defibrillation was not necessary. After 4 h the episodes of ventricular tachycardia stopped. On the following day, the potassium level was within normal limits, the QTUc was still prolonged, and episodes of bradycardia AV dissociation persisted. Potassium was given orally and 3 days later the patient was dismissed with a normal ECG (sinus rhythm, rate 72/min, QTUc 0.46 sec) and a potassium serum level of 4.8 mmol/l. Psychiatric therapy was organized.

Conclusion: severe hypokalemia may represent a dangerous condition. Hypomagnesemia or a pre-existing prolonged QT (e.g. due to drugs) favor the development of torsade de pointes type of ventricular tachycardia. The treating physicians were very happy about the favorable outcome in this young woman, after episodes of ventricular tachycardia at rates up to 360/min (see ECG 16.14d).

In very rare cases of hypokalemia, a p wave of high amplitude in the inferior leads is seen, imitating right atrial enlargement ('p pseudo-pulmonale').

Moderate hypokalemia produces unspecific slight ST depression only, flattening of the T wave and some increasing of the U wave, without fusion of T and U.

7.1 Pathophysiology of Hyperkalemia and Hypokalemia

A detailed review article about the pathophysiologic mechanisms in hyperkalemia and hypokalemia was recently published by Halperin and Kamel [9].

8 Hypercalcemia

The most important shifts of calcium ions seem to occur during phase 2 of the action potential of a single heart muscle fiber. Phase 2 corresponds to the ST segment in the ECG. It seems logical that calcium imbalance influences the ST segment. A minimal decrease of the QRS duration, caused by hypercalcemia, is not measurable in the ECG.

The correlation between the calcium serum level and the ECG is poor [10]. However it is exciting to suspect, for instance, primary hyperparathyroidism on the basis of an ECG.

The only valuable ECG feature in hypercalcemia is the shortened QT interval, that is always decreased at the expense of the ST segment, which is shortened or absent [11]. This may be easily overlooked, more in ECG 16.9 than in ECG 16.8. In cases of doubt, the *QaT* interval (from the beginning of Q to the apex of T) is a more reliable measure than the QT time.

Short(est) Story/Case Report 3

Some years ago the author had the opportunity to diagnose hypercalcemia in a patient with left bundle-branch block (LBBB) – a rare combination, and not an easy diagnosis, as the ST segment in LBBB generally seems to be short because of the broad QRS. He missed it…

Arrhythmias in hypercalcemia are extremely rare. Ventricular arrhythmias, associated with sudden changes in blood pressure may occur during or after operation of parathyroid tumors, due to abrupt changes in serum and intracellular cal-

cium levels. Arrhythmias (e.g. SA block, sinus arrest, AV block 1°–3°, ventricular premature beats, ventricular tachycardia) may also arise by rapid injection of calcium, especially in fully digitalised patients. Lethal outcomes have been described in early publications.

9 Hypocalcemia (Isolated or Associated with Hyperkalemia)

Isolated hypocalcemia is rare [12]. Prolongation of the QaT interval is more specific than prolongation of the QT interval that may be influenced by other factors such as drugs. Moreover, the U wave may be 'absorbed' by the T wave. However, neither the prolonged QT interval nor this type of TU fusion in hypocalcemia predispose to ventricular tachycardia of the type torsade de pointes. The long QT is based on prolongation of 'phase 2', whereas in the 'long QT syndrome' and in TU fusion of hypokalemia 'phase 3' is affected.

The T wave is generally normal, in some cases it may be somewhat peaked (without concomitant hyperkalemia). But in most cases a prolonged QT in combination with tall and peaked T waves is due to hypocalcemia and hyperkalemia, especially in patients with renal failure.

10 Hypomagnesemia

It is generally acknowledged that hypomagnesemia is not detectable in the ECG. Due to its rather common association to hypokalemia, the serum level of magnesium should be determined in every case of hypokalemia, with or without ECG alterations.

11 Hypermagnesemia

In patients with intravenously administered magnesium sulfate, an increase of PQ interval and QRS duration has been described, as well as bradycardia due to AV block or SA block [13,14]. Too rapid injection of magnesium may induce cardiac asystole [15]. Opinions about the therapeutic effect of magnesium in arrhythmias are controversial [15,16].

Experimental hypermagnesemia in patients with normal QT interval induces – by blocking the slow sodium channel – slight prolongation of intra-atrial and AV-node conduction. During fast ventricular pacing a minor increase in QRS duration occurred, whereas a shortening of the QT interval was not observed [17,18].

12   Sodium Imbalance

Hypernatremia and hyponatremia do not induce detectable alterations in the ECG. This is astonishing, because the rapid transfer of sodium into the cell during phase 0 of the action potential (depolarization) of the single heart muscle fiber produces the most rapid and most evident change of the potential, corresponding to the initial part of the QRS complex. Theoretically one would expect that the amplitude and the slew rate of the QRS could be influenced.

13   New Classification of Antiarrhythmic Drugs

Over the last few decades there have been considerable increases in our knowledge about cellular electrolyte channels and the pathophysiologic mechanisms of antiarrhythmics and other drugs. Based on this progress, a new classification for antiarrhythmic drugs was proposed, called the 'Sicilian Gambit' [19]. This should replace the older one by Vaughan Williams [20,21]. Based on the statement of Garratt and Griffith [22] this new concept has had little influence on daily practice, hitherto. One may hope, however, that a more recent publication will help to propagate this fascinating approach [23].

References

1. Ohmae M, Rabkin SW. Hyperkalemia-induced bundle-branch block and complete heart block. Clin Cardiol 198;14:43–6
2. Mohacsi P, Rieben R, Sigurdsson G, et al. Successful treatment of a B-type allograft into an O-type man with 3 year clinical follow-up. Transplantation 2001;72:1328–30
3. Tamm M, Ritz R, Truniger B. Der hyperkaliämische Notfall: Ursache, Diagnose und Therapie. Schweiz med Wschr 1990;120:1031–6
4. Acker CG, Johnson JP, Palevsky PM, Greenberg A. Hyperkalemia in hospitalized patients. Arch Intern Med 1998;158:917–24
5. Greenberg A. Hyperkalemia: Treatment options. Sem in Nephrol 1998;18:46–57
6. Dreifus LS, Pick A. A clinical correlative study of the electrocardiogram in electrolyte imbalance. Circulation 1956;14:815
7. Surawicz B. Relationship of electrocardiogram and electrolytes. Am Heart J 1967;73:814
8. Fletcher GF, Hurst JW, Schlant RC. Electrocardiographic changes in severe hypokalemia. A reappraisal. Am J Cardiol 1967;20:628–31
9. Halperin ML, Kamel KS. Potassium. Lancet 1998;352:135–40
10. Bronsky D, Dubin A, Kushner DS, et al. Calcium and the electrocardiogram. III. The relationship of the intervals of the electrocardiogram to the level of serum calcium. Am J Cardiol 1961;7:840
11. Bronsky D, Dubin A, Waldstein SS, et al. Calcium and the electrocardiogram. I. The electrocardiographic manifestations of hyperparathyroidism and of marked hypercalcemia from various other etiologies. Amer J Cardiol 1961;7:833
12. Bronsky D, Dubin A, Waldstein SS et al. The electrocardiographic manifestations of hypoparathyroidism. Amer J Cardiol 1961;7:823
13. Miller JR, van Dellen TR. Electrocardiographic changes following the intravenous administration of magnesium sulfate. J Lab Clin Med 1941;26:1116
14. Smith PK. Pharmacologic actions of parenterally administered magnesium salts. Anesthesiology 1942;3:323
15. Brugada P. Magnesium: an antiarrhythmic drug, but only against very specific arrhythmias (Editorial). Eur Heart J 2000;21:1116
16. Stuehlinger HG. The wider use of magnesium (letter). Eur Heart J 2001;22:713–4
17. DiCarlo LA, Morady F, Buitleir M, et al. Effects of magnesium sulphate on cardiac conduction and refractoriness in humans. J Am Coll Cardiol 1986;7:1356–62
18. Kulick DL, Hong R, Ryzen E, et al. Electrophysiologic effects of intravenous magnesium in patients with normal conduction system and no clinical evidence of cardiac disease. Am Heart J 1988;115:367–73
19. The Task Force of the Working Group on Arrhythmias of the European Society of Cardiology. The 'Sicilian Gambit'. Review. Europ Heart J 1991;12:1112–31
20. Vaughan Williams EM. A classification of antiarrhythmic actions reassessed after a decade of new drugs. J Clin Pharmacol 1984;24:129–47
21. Vaughan Williams EM. Significance of classifying antiarrhythmic actions since the cardiac arrhythmia suppression trial. J Clin Pharmacol 1991;31:123–35
22. Garratt CJ, Griffith MJ. The Sicilian gambit: an opening move that loses the game? Eur Heart J 1996;17(3):341–3
23. Anon. The search for novel antiarrhythmic strategies. Sicilian Gambit. Eur Heart J 1998;19:1178–96

Appendix 1 Etiology

In many cases of electrolyte imbalance the etiology is known, often in advance. For other cases a checklist is useful:

Hyperkalemia

Increased intake/cut back

Cytolysis (hemolysis, rhabdomyolysis)

Tumor lysis

burns

Transfusion of blood

Distribution imbalance

Acidemia

Diabetic ketoacidosis

Hypertonicity (hyperosmolarity)

Decreased loss

1. Renal failure
2. Various

   Primary hypoaldosteronism
   - Addison disease
   - Adrenogenital syndrome

   Secondary hypoaldosteronism
   - Diabetic nephropathy
   - Systemic lupus erythematosus
   - Sickle cell anemia
   - Amyloidosis
   - Drugs (see list below)

Hypokalemia

Decreased intake

Anorexia

Distribution imbalance

Alkalosis (e.g. vomiting)

Catecholamines (stress-induced; drugs see below)

Anabolic state (myeloproliferative diseases)

Hypothermia

Increased loss

a) Extrarenal

Diarrhea

Vomiting

Villous adenoma

Lower GI fistulas

Vipoma (Verner-Morrison syndrome)

Sweating

Burns

b) Renal

1. Potassium-losing nephritis
2. Various

   Primary hyperaldosteronism
   - Conn syndrome (adrenal adenoma)
   - Adrenal carcinoma
   - Adrenocortical hyperplasia

   Secondary hyperaldosteronism
   - Renal artery stenosis
   - Hypovolemia
   - Renin-secreting tumor
   - Malignant hypertension

   Non-aldosterone mineralocorticoids
   - Liquorice
   - Chewing tobacco
   - Cushing syndrome
   - Liver cirrhosis

   Non-mineralocorticoid reasons
   - Acute renal failure
   - Hypomagnesemia

Hyperkalemia (continued)

Hereditary

Hyperkalemic periodic paralysis

Gordon syndrome

Pseudohypoaldosteronism (resistance to aldosterone)

Drugs

Spironolactone

Triamterene

Amiloride

ACE-inhibitors/angiotensin 1-antagonists

Nonsteroidal antiinflammatory drugs

Intravenous potassium

Heparin

Alpha-agonists

Beta-blockers

Succinylcholine

Arginine

Penicillin

Digitalis

Lithium

Cyclosporin

Trimethoprim

Somatostatin

Diazoxide

Cytostatic drugs (pentamidine and others)

Toxins

Palytoxin

Tetrodotoxin

Fluoride

Cocaine

Pseudohyperkalemia

High platelet count or white blood cell count

Tight tourniquet

Muscle-clenching

Hypokalemia (continued)

Hereditary

Hypokalemic periodic paralysis

Liddle syndrome (pseudohyperaldosteronism)

Renal tubular acidosis type 1 + 2

Bartter syndrome

Fanconi syndrome

Gitleman syndrome

Drugs

Loop diuretics

Thiazides

Carbonic anhydrase inhibitors

Insulin

Glucocorticoides

Aminoglycosides

Gentamicin

Amphotericin B

Laxatives

Cisplatin

Foscarnet sodium (virostatic drug)

Penicillin

$Beta_2$-adrenergic agonists

Alpha-adrenergic antagonists

Vitamin B12 in pernicious anemia

Cation exchangers

Barium

Toxins

Caffeine

Glue-sniffing

Carbenoxolone

Pseudohypokalemia

Acute myeloid leukemia (potassium uptake by abnormal cells)

Hypercalcemia

Increased intake

Milk-alkali syndrome

Hypervitaminosis D

Granulomatous diseases

- Sarcoidosis
- Tuberculosis
- Wegener granulomatosis
- Eosinophilic granuloma
- Histoplasmosis
- Berylliosis
- Silicon injection

Idiopathic hypercalcemia in infancy

Distribution imbalance

Malignancies

- Osteolytic metastases
- Paraneoplastic disorders

High bone turnover

- Immobilization
- Hyperthyroidism
- Acromegaly
- Pheochromocytoma
- Paget disease

Primary hyperparathyroidism

- Adenoma
- Carcinoma
- Hyperplasia
- Multiple endocrine neoplasia (see below)

Others

- Tertiary hyperparathyroidism
- Malabsorbtion
- Chronic renal failure
- after renal transplantation
- Addison disease

Hereditary

Familial hypocalciuric hypercalcemia

Multiple endocrine neoplasia (1 + 2)

Jansen disease

Drugs

Hypervitaminosis D

Hypervitaminosis A

Thiazides

Estrogens; Tamoxifen

Lithium

Aminophylline

Intoxication

Aluminium

Hypocalcemia

Decreased intake

Sprue

Cholestasis

Chronic pancreatitis

Vitamin D deficiency

- Malabsorption (see above)
- Sunlight deficiency
- Liver cirrhosis
- Nephrotic syndrome

Distribution imbalance and increased utilisation

Renal failure

Hypoalbuminemia

Hypoparathyroidism

- Hereditary forms (see below)
- Osteitis fibrosa after parathyroidectomy
- Hemochromatosis
- Hypomagnesemia

Increased utilisation

- Osteoplastic metastasis
- 'Hungry bones' syndrome
- Acute pancreatitis

Hyperphosphatemia

- Rhabdomyolysis
- Tumor lysis

Thyroidal cancer with calcitonin production

Hereditary

Idiopathic hypercalcuria

Vitamin D-dependent rickets (type I + II)

Hereditary hypoparathyroidism

Pseudohypoparathyroidism (PHP)

DiGeorge syndrome

Polyglandular autoimmune type 1 deficiency (in Finnish families)

Autosomal dominant hypocalcemia (ADH)

Drugs

Loop diuretics

Abuse of laxative drugs

Anticonvulsivant drugs (barbiturates, diphenylhydantoin, phenytoin)

Mithramycine

Calcitonin

Colchicine

Foscarnet-sodium

Transfusion of blood (citrate/EDTA)

Cytostatics

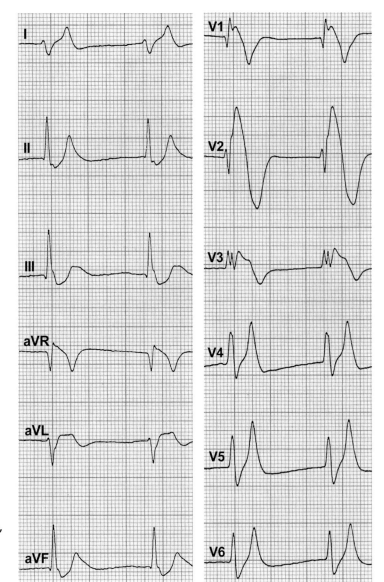

ECG 16.1

64y/f. Terminal renal failure. Hyperkalemia. ECG: very probably sinus rhythm, with invisible p waves, rate 54/min. Atypical RBBB pattern (QRS duration 0.16 sec). Striking ST elevation in leads V_1 to V_3 (I, aVR, aVL) as sign of 'dialyzable injury'. K^+ 8.7 mmol/l.

ECG 16.2

44y/f. Morbus Cushing after hypophysectomy, hypertension, diuretics containing amiloride. Hyperkalemia. ECG: monitor stripe. Very probable sinus rhythm with invisible p waves, rate 108/min. Atypical LBBB pattern, QRS duration about 0.18 sec. VT of moderate rate is imitated. K^+ 9.4 mmol/l.

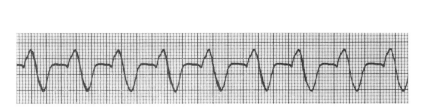

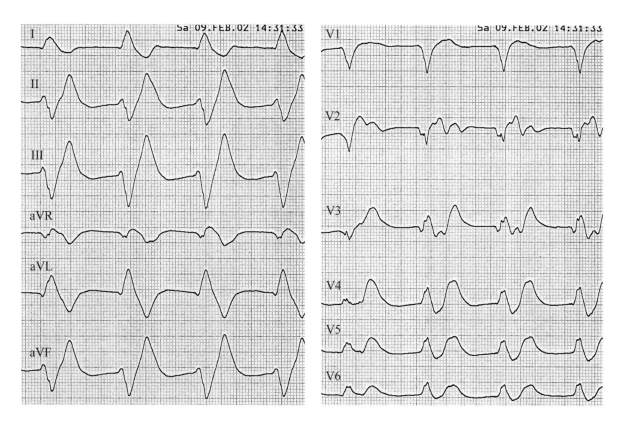

ECG 16.3a

60y/m. Terminal renal failure, hemodialysis (HD) three times weekly, for 2 years. Due to his birthday celebration, the patient came 2 days too late for HD. Hyperkalemia. ECG: probably sinus rhythm (without visible p waves), 58/min. Very broad LBBB-like QRS (240 msec), bizarre broad T waves, concordant to QRS in V_3 to V_6. K^+ 8.97 mmol/l (Ca^{2+} 0.96 mmol/l). Therapy: Immediate HD.

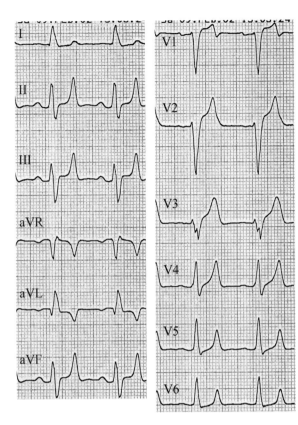

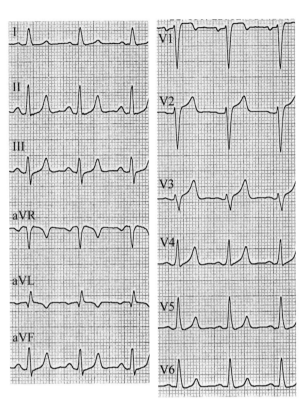

ECG 16.3b
Same patient. ECG after 30 min HD: sinus rhythm 78/min. Still slightly prolonged QRS duration, peaked and tall T waves, especially in the inferior leads. K+ 5.87 mmol/l (Ca²⁺ 1.13 mmol/l).

ECG 16.3c
Same patient. ECG after 60 min HD: normal broad QRS, peaky T waves in several leads. K+ 5.90 mmol/l (!) (Ca²⁺ 1.19 mmol/l).

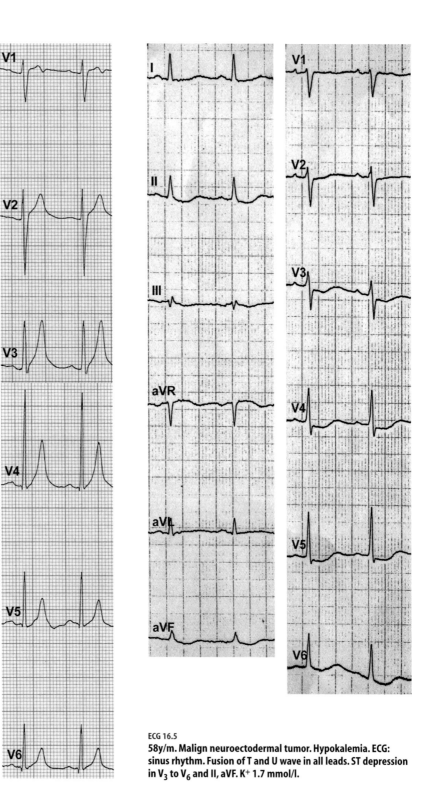

ECG 16.4
62y/m. 2 days after intestinal operation. Hyperkalemia. Sinus rhythm, rate 86/min. Normal QRS. Tall and peaky T waves in leads V$_3$ and V$_4$/V$_5$ (V$_6$). K$^+$ 5.8 mmol/l.

ECG 16.5
58y/m. Malign neuroectodermal tumor. Hypokalemia. ECG: sinus rhythm. Fusion of T and U wave in all leads. ST depression in V$_3$ to V$_6$ and II, aVF. K$^+$ 1.7 mmol/l.

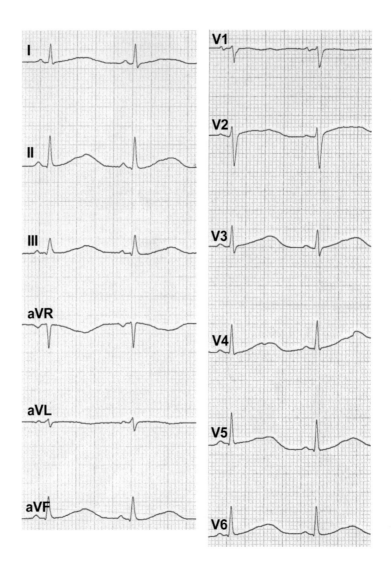

ECG 16.6
53y/f. Short syncope, antidepressants, and furosemide. Hypokalemia. ECG: almost complete TU fusion in all leads. No ST depression. K+ 2.8 mmol/l. Holter ECG: short episodes of VT type torsade de pointes.

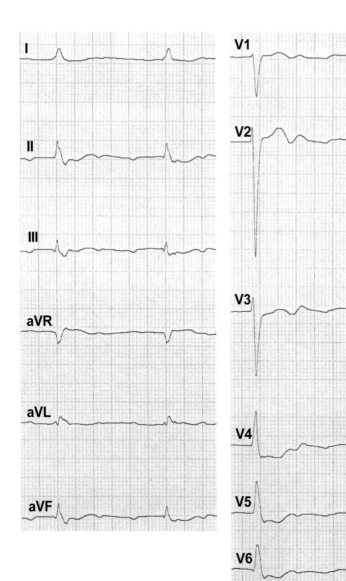

ECG 16.7

82y/m. Hypertension, diuretic drugs, amiodarone. ECG: atrial flutter with 3 : 1 AV block, ventricular rate 53/min. Fusion of T and U, with prominent U waves in V_3 to V_6 (I). Significant ST depression in V_4 to V_6 (also due to strain?). K+ normal. TU fusion due to amiodarone.

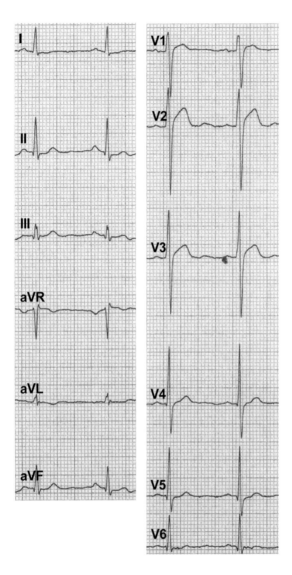

ECG 16.8

16y/m. Osteosarcoma. Hypercalcemia. ECG: sinus rhythm, rate 75/min. QT 308 msec, QTc 346 msec. The T wave immediately follows the QRS complex. Ca^{2+} (ionized) 1.32 mmol/l (normal 1.13–1.30).

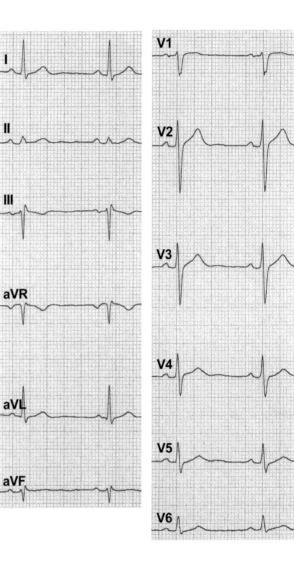

ECG 16.9

47y/m. Primary hyperparathyroidism. Hypercalcemia. ECG: sinus rhythm, rate 62/min. Only slightly reduced QT interval (368 msec, QTc 376 msec), but visually 'absent' ST segment. Ca^{2+} 2.88 mmol/l (normal up to 2.5).

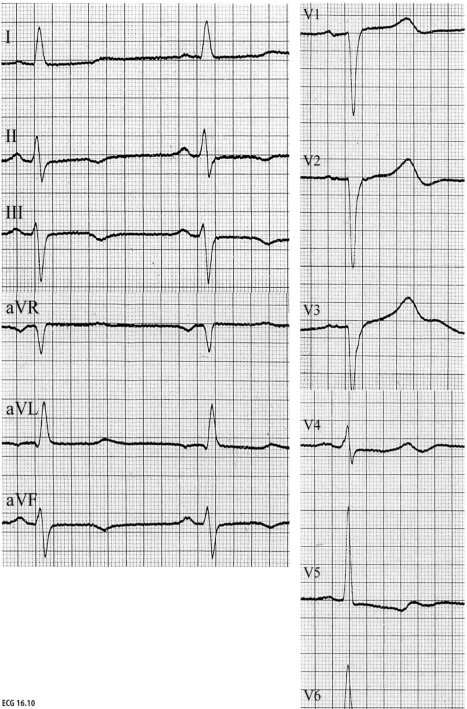

ECG 16.10
73y/f. Hypocalcemia. ECG (50 mm/sec): prolonged QT interval, with prolonged ST segment and 'late T wave'.

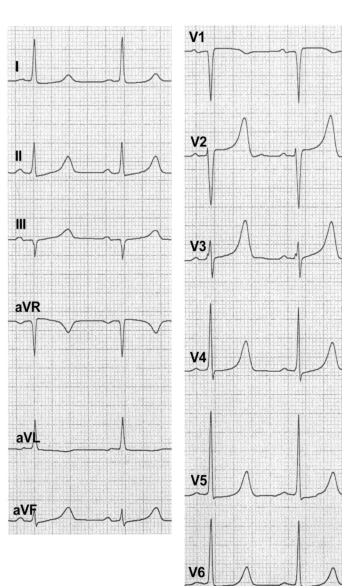

ECG 16.11
67y/f. Chronic renal failure. Hyperkalemia plus hypocalcemia. ECG: sinus rhythm, rate 63/min. QT interval 497 msec, QTc 510 msec. Tall and peaky T waves in V_2 to V_6 (II, aVF). No detectable U wave. K^+ 6.2 mmol/l. Ca^{2+} 1.4 mmol/l.

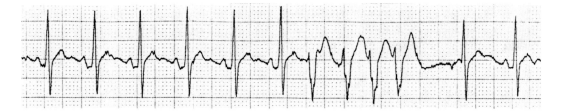

ECG 16.12a
Short Story/Case Report 1. Time 11:51. Monitor stripes. Hyperkalemia. Sinus tachycardia, normal broad QRS. Ventricular tachycardia of four beats.

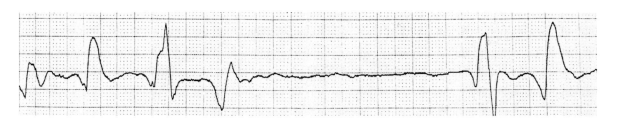

ECG 16.12b
Time 12:31. Ventricular asystole. The 'QRS complexes' are artifacts by heart massage, interference with QRS complexes is possible.

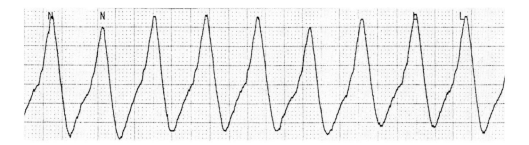

ECG 16.12c
Time 12:44. Regular rhythm (rate 107/min), with enormous broad QRS (> 180 msec), scarcely distinguishable from the T waves. It cannot be excluded that sinus rhythm is present with invisible p waves.

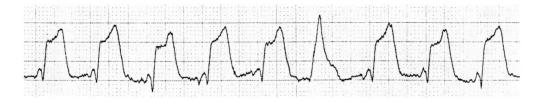

ECG 16.12d
Time 12:51. Supraventricular rhythm (sinus rhythm) with probably small QRS and tremendous ST elevation, mimicking acute infarction ('dialyzable injury').

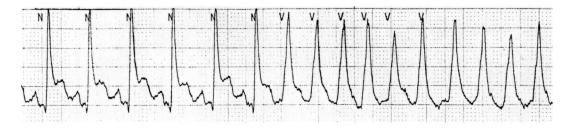

ECG 16.12e
Time 13:13. sinus rhythm with normal broad QRS, less elevated ST segment. Irregular ventricular tachycardia (mean rate about 210/min, maximal instantaneous rate about 260/min).

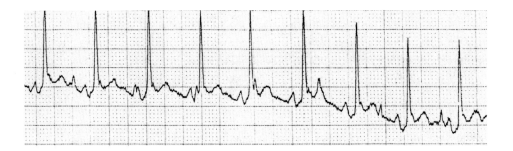

ECG 16.12f
Time 13:28. Sinus tachycardia 105/min, with normal QRS and repolarization.

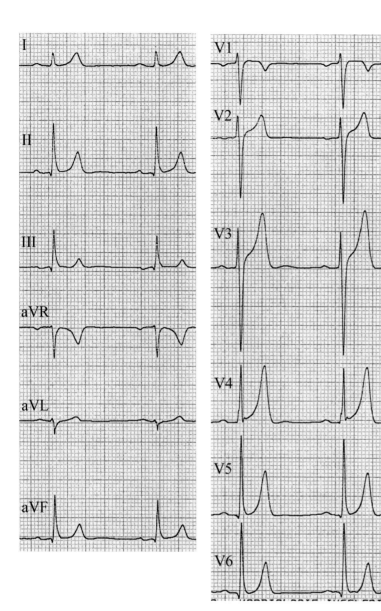

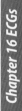

ECG 16.13

65y/m. Normal heart, normal renal function. Normal serum K+ and Ca2+. Sinus bradycardia 52/min. Tall T waves in leads V2 to V6, with a normal broad basis of the T waves. However the ECG is quite suggestive of moderate hyperkalemia!

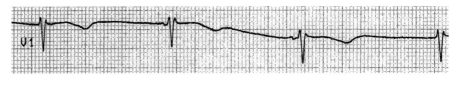

ECG 16.14a

Short Story/Case Report 2. Hypokalemia. (Rhythm strip V$_1$.) Bradycardic isorhythmic AV dissociation, rate 42/min.

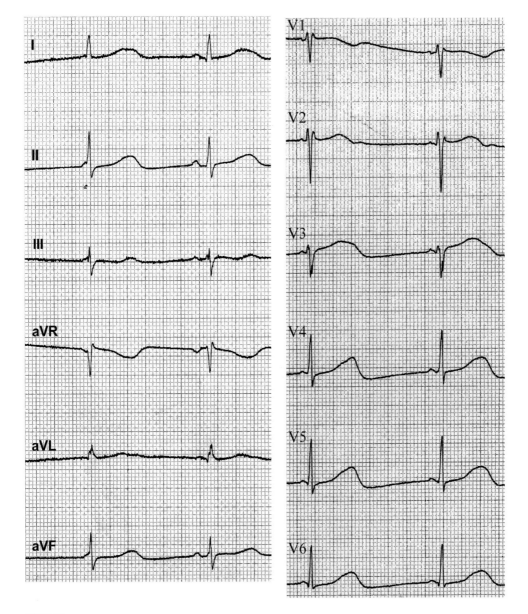

ECG 16.14b

Completely fused T and U waves. QT(U) 620 msec. QT(U)c 521 msec. Incomplete RBBB.

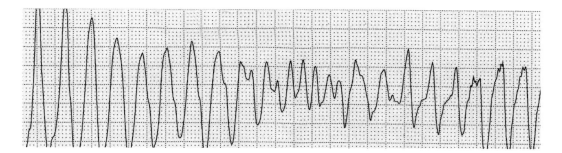

ECG 16.14c
(Rhythm strip.) VT of the type torsade de pointes, rate up to > 300/min.

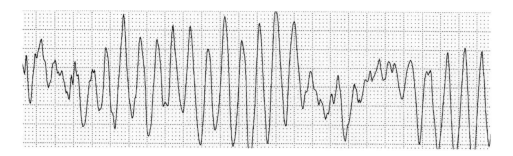

ECG 16.14d
(Rhythm strip.) VT of the type torsade de pointes, maximal instantaneous rate about 360/min.

ECG 16.14e
(Rhythm strip.) Almost regular VT with morphology of ventricular flutter, rate about 220/min.

Chapter 17
Alterations of Repolarization

At a Glance

This chapter is very short. Why? Pathologic negative T waves represent the most frequent isolated deformations of ventricular repolarization. However, T wave alterations not related to pathologic QRS complexes are very unspecific. The alterations of the ST segment are rarer and somewhat more specific.

ECG

1   ST Segment

1.1   ST Elevation

ST elevation in the *limb leads* produces ST depression in the opposite leads, as *mirror images*, so ST elevation in aVL >>> ST depression in aVF/III; and ST elevation in III/aVF >>> ST depression in aVL. In the *precordial leads* mirror images are less prominent and are restricted to the leads V_1/V_2 versus V_5/V_6 (in the case of left ventricular overload), and to the additional leads V_7 to V_9 *versus* (V_1) V_2/V_3 (in the case of acute posterior myocardial infarction (MI)).

Differential diagnosis of isolated *ST elevation* is relatively small (see Table 17.1).

1.2   ST Depression

The clinically most important ST depression occurs during *exercise testing* (in leads V_4 to V_6) as a marker of *ischemia*. ST depression at rest is relatively rare in pure ischemia. As mentioned above, significant ST depression in leads $V_2/V_3(V_1)$ corresponds to a mirror image of *acute posterior* MI but never to isolated 'anteroseptal ischemia', which cannot be identified in the ECG.

Table 17.1
Differential diagnosis of ST elevation

Condition	Typical signs
Acute myocardial infarction*	• ST arising from the R wave***
	• Amplitude 2–10 mm
	• Frontal ST vector inferior AMI 80° to 120°; anterior AMI about - 40° to + 10°
	• Evolution to Q-wave infarction
Prinzmetal angina	• Morphology and amplitude as in AMI
	• Reversible within 15–20 min
Early repolarization**	• ST arising from the R (or S) wave
	• Amplitude 1–5 mm
	• No evolution; healthy people, often young people
Vagotonia**	• Amplitude up to 4 mm in leads V_2/V_3
	• Mostly in sinus bradycardia
Pericarditis stage 2*	• ST mostly arising from S wave***
	• Amplitude < 2 mm
	• Frontal ST vector + 30° to + 70° (ST elevation in I *and* aVF!)
	• Evolution; no *pathologic Q wave!*
Mirror image of LV overload	• Amplitude up to 4 mm in leads V_2/V_3
	• High amplitude, mostly associated with LVH
Brugada syndrome	• Amplitude up to 3 mm in V_2, less in V_1/V_3
	• Combined with the pattern of incomplete RBBB
	• Suppressed by class I antiarrhythmic drugs
Other rare conditions	

AMI, acute myocardial infarction; LVH, left ventricular hypertrophy; RBBB, right bundle-branch block.
*See Chapter 13 Myocardial Infarction and Chapter 15 Pericarditis.
**See Chapter 3 The Normal ECG and its Normal Variants.
***A simplified 'rule' implies that in *acute MI* the elevated ST segment arises from the *R wave*, whereas in *acute pericarditis* (stage 2) the elevated ST segment arises from the *S wave*. This 'rule' leads to some confusion, because it is valid in about only 90% of cases of AMI, and in about 80% of cases of pericarditis.

In the ECG at rest ST depression in leads V_5/V_6 (and I/aVL), associated with asymmetric negative T waves in the same leads, is generally due to LV overload, with or without LV hypertrophy (LVH). In this case we often observe a mirror image in leads V_1/V_2.

Digitalis often leads to mild ST depression of about 1 mm, with a typical tub-like configuration. Slight ST depression (up to 1 mm) is found in many conditions and is therefore unspecific.

2   T Wave

2.1   T Negativity

Negative asymmetric T waves are a frequent *normal finding* in several limb leads. In these conditions, T negativity is related to the frontal QRS axis ($ÅQRS_F$). In vertical $ÅQRS_F$: T negativity in III, aVF(II). In left $ÅQRS_F$: T negativity in aVL. A negative T wave in *lead I* is *pathologic* in most cases. In the precordial leads, a negative T wave is only found in *lead V_1*, in *normal* hearts. There is an exception: occasionally a negative T wave may also be present in lead(s) V_2 (and V_3) in healthy men up to the age of 25 years and in healthy women up to the age of 35. However, in the presence of T-negativity in *leads V_2/V_3*, an abnormality of the *right ventricle* should be considered; such abnormalities include atrial septal defect, pulmonary embolism and arrhythmogenic right ventricle (see Table 17.2).

Table 17.2
Differential diagnosis of T negativity

- Classical non-Q infarction
- Ischemia without infarction
- Ventricular overload
- Normal variants
- Syndrome X
- Pericarditis (stages 3 and 4)
- Overload or diseases of the right ventricle
- Myocarditis
- Severe anemia
- Funnel chest
- Upright position
- Drugs
- Pancreatitis
- Hyperventilation
- Innumerable other diseases and conditions*

*It would not be useful to provide the full list of the hundreds of diseases and conditions concerned.

Negative T waves in some precordial leads are not only encountered in ischemia, but also in *countless* other conditions.

Negative T waves due to ischemia are called 'primary negative T waves' and T waves secondary due to ventricular hypertrophy are called 'secondary negative T waves'.

In *ischemia*, the negative T wave is generally *symmetric* (ECG 17.1), whereas in *LV overload* (often associated with LVH), the negative T wave is generally *asymmetric* (ECG 17.2). However, this rule is not reliable. For instance, negative symmetric T waves are also found in pericarditis (stages 3–4), in hypertrophic cardiomyopathy, and other diseases.

Differential diagnosis of asymmetric negative T waves is even much more extensive and includes normal hearts, inflammations, general diseases, drug effects, and so on.

Furthermore, asymmetric T waves may have a symmetric aspect at their apex (ECG 17.3). It would be absurd to diagnose LV overload, or LVH *and* ischemia, based on this pattern.

2.2   T Positivity

Positive T waves are rarely pathologic. Abnormally *tall symmetric* T waves are seen in moderate *hyperkalemia* (Chapter 16 Electrolyte Imbalances and Disturbances). In exceptional cases the same T morphology is observed in the earliest stage of MI and lasting only minutes.

Differential diagnosis: tall T waves in V_2/V_3 as normal variants, especially in sinus bradycardia.

Short Story/Case Report 1

In November 1998 a 65-year-old man with a history of stable angina felt a sudden, strong, typical chest pain during routine ECG registration. The excellent nurse was struck by the tall symmetric T waves in leads V_2/V_3 (ECG 17.4) and referred the patient immediately to the coronary care unit. There he developed an acute anterior infarction with a typical ECG within 20 min. Coronary angiography was performed 50 min after the onset of pain. The proximal left anterior descending artery (LAD) was closed. The result of percutaneous transluminal coronary angioplasty (PTCA) and stenting was excellent. The akinetic apical zone regressed to a slight hypokinesia.

ECG Special

In the section 'At a Glance' the most important alterations of repolarization were discussed. It does not make sense to discuss all patterns of so-called pathologic repolarization which lack all specificity in most instances. So for a change we can relax in an armchair (or in a rocking-chair, like a former President). It is sufficient for our purpose to touch on a few special items.

3 Special Remarks

3.1 Atypical Behavior of Repolarization in Acute Myocardial Infarction and Acute Pericarditis

As mentioned in the footnote to table 17.1 the repolarization in acute MI as well as in acute pericarditis may be atypical.

In *acute* MI, we may find an *elevated ST segment* arising from the *S wave* in the precordial *leads V_1 to V_3*, where the pre-existing S wave is generally of high amplitude

In *acute pericarditis*, the elevated ST segment arises from the R wave in the leads, where no S wave pre-exists. This may occur in leads V_5/V_6 and, depending on the frontal QRS axis, in leads aVL/I or in the inferior leads.

Consequently, in the same patient we may find patterns of ST elevation arising from the R wave and the S wave in different leads, in acute MI or in acute pericarditis (see ECGs in Chapter 13 Myocardial Infarction and Chapter 15 Pericarditis). As another consequence, recognition of the combination of acute MI and acute pericarditis is difficult or impossible, based on a single ECG.

Considering the anamnesis and clinical findings, the underlying condition of ST elevation can be determined in most cases. A striking ST elevation will correspond to acute MI in 99% of 60-year-old men with chest pain. In a patient of any age with a slight ST elevation in some precordial leads, and in lead I and aVF, acute pericarditis is present (see Chapter 15 Pericarditis). In a 20-year-old healthy and asymptomatic individual, the rare pattern of 'early repolarization' is very probable (see Chapter 3 The Normal ECG and its Normal Variants). ST elevation in leads V_1/V_2 (V_3) combined with the pattern of incomplete right bundle-branch block (iRBBB) is suggestive of the Brugada syndrome.

3.2 Patterns with Prolonged or Shortened QT Duration

Repolarization is altered *per se* in the presence of prolonged or shortened QT. In the congenital 'long QT syndrome' (Romano-Ward, Jervell and Lange-Nielsen) as well as in the acquired long QT (hypokalemia, antiarrhythmic drugs) the ST segment is often isoelectric but may show slight depression or even elevation. The T wave is generally fused with the U wave (see Chapter 16 Electrolyte Imbalance and 26 Ventricular Tachycardias). In the rare pattern of 'postsyncopal bradycardia syndrome' in association with bizarre QT(U) prolongation, we find abnormally broad and negative T waves in the precordial and in some limb leads (see ECG 32.17 Chapter 32 Rare ECGs). It is only in QT prolongation due to hypocalcemia that the T wave is often normal. Equally, in QT shortening due to hypercalcemia the T wave is normal, with the exception of a small T basis (see Chapter 16 Electrolyte Imbalance).

3.3 Giant Negative T Waves

Giant negative T waves (amplitude 5–15 mm) are relatively rare. In combination with LV hypertrophy they are found in some cases of left ventricular overload, in hypertrophic cardiomyopathy and in a large number of patients with apical hypertrophy (see ECG 5.14 in chapter 5 Left Ventricular Hypertrophy). In these cases the QT interval is often slightly prolonged.

Isolated giant negative T waves (without QRS alterations) are observed in the classical 'Non-Q wave infarction' pattern, in combination with cerebral diseases [1], in some cases of post-pacing T-negativity (Chatterjee phenomenon), after pulmonary edema [2] and in the so-called global T wave inversion, the latter predominantly in women and not associated with a bad prognosis, with the exception of a short QT interval in digitalised patients [3].

Giant negative T waves with an obvious or *excessive QT prolongation* represent a rare ECG pattern, formerly called 'postsyncopal bradycardia syndrome' (see above, and ECG 32.17 chapter 32 Rare ECGs). However, the pattern may arise without a previous syncope and may be combined with normocardia. In most cases a cerebral disease such as subarachnoidal hemorrhage, a cerebral insult or an epileptic attack precedes the appearance of the ECG alteration. The pathophysiologic mechanism is probably connected with hypothalamic dysfunction with consecutive hypertension, increased myocardial O_2 demand and coronary spasms. In an experimental set with cats it has been shown that a hypothalamic injury provokes subendocardial hemorrhage. In patients with an acute non-cardiac illness and deep T inversion in the precordial leads, a circumscript reversible left ventricular dysfunction was observed [4].

In some cases the etiology remains obscure and often the excessive QT (QTc) prolongation with very broad T waves is more striking than the amplitude of the negative T wave.

Finally it has to be mentioned that acute cerebral diseases may also lead to ST segment elevations in some rare cases [5].

References

1. Perron A, Bradey WJ. Electrocardiographic manifestations of CNS events. Am J Emerg Med 2001;19:332-3
2. Littman L. Large T wave inversion and QT prolongation associated with pulmonary edema: a report of nine cases. J Am Coll Cardiol 1999;34:1106-10
3. Walder LA, Spodick DH. Global T wave inversion: long term follow-up. J Am Coll Cardiol 1993;21:1652-6
4. Sharkey SW, Shear W, Hodges M, Herzog CA. Reversible myocardial contraction abnormalities in patients with acute non-cardiac illness. Chest 1998;114:98-105
5. Voegelin HP, Jutzi H, Gertsch M. EKG- und kardiale Veränderungen bei akutem Hirnschaden. Schweiz med Wschr 1989;119:461-6

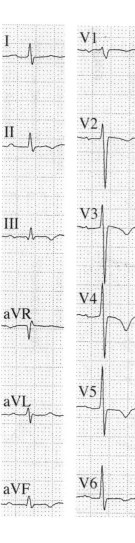

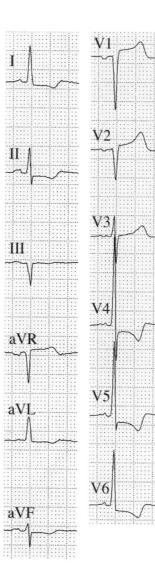

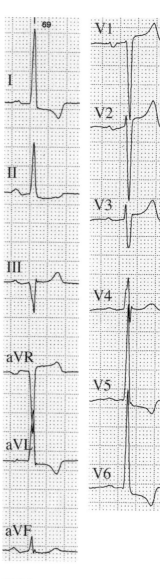

ECG 17.1
70y/m. Coronary heart disease, pulmonary emphysema. Typical chest pain 20 min before. ECG: symmetric negative T waves in leads V_1 to V_6. Note also peripheral near low voltage and AV block 1°. Coro: proximal 90% stenosis of LAD. Minimal apical hypokinesia.

ECG 17.2
52y/f. Hypertension and combined aortic valve disease. Normal coronary arteries. ECG: high R voltage in leads V_3/V_4. ST depression and negative asymmetric T waves in I, II, aVL, aVF and V_4 to V_6 (in V_4 the T wave is nearly symmetrical).

ECG 17.3
50y/m. Severe aortic valve disease with predominant regurgitation. Normal coronary arteries. ECG: LVH (positive Lyon index; positive Sokolow index; R amplitude in aVL 19 mm). ST depression in leads I, II, aVL, V_5, and V_6, with asymmetric T waves but symmetrical T waves.

327

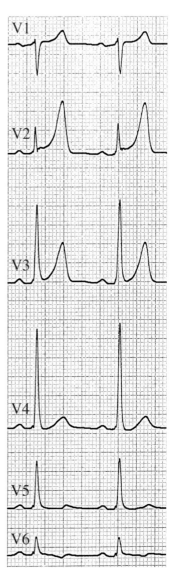

ECG 17.4
Short Story/Case Report 1. 65y/m. High symmetric T waves with slight ST elevation in leads V$_2$/V$_3$. Note: very similar T waves in these leads are seen as normal variants.

Chapter 18
Atrial Premature Beats

At a Glance

Atrial premature beats (APBs) are not much less frequent than ventricular premature beats (VPBs) but they are much more frequent than supraventricular PBs arising in the atrioventricular (AV) junction. Often APBs are not associated with heart disease. In up to 64% of healthy young individuals some APBs are found in an ambulatory ECG, in most cases without symptoms.

ECG

APBs are characterized by premature onset and a deformed p wave, indicating origin of a (mostly right) atrial 'focus', distant from the sinus node (ECG 18.1). A focus in the low right atrium, near the coronary sinus, leads to negative p waves in the inferior leads aVF, III (and II). The short PQ interval may be equal or slightly longer (> 0.12 sec) as in an atrioventricular junction (AVJ) beat. This p-wave morphology is more often seen in intermittent episodes of ectopic atrial rhythms (mostly in healthy hearts), or AV junction rhythms, than it is in isolated APBs. ECG 18.2 shows an example of ectopic atrial rhythm with negative p waves inferiorly and in leads V_2 to V_6 in an older patient with right ventricular hypertrophy (RVH). A negative p wave in I, aVL, and in V_6/V_5 may be due to either ectopic right or left atrial origin; only the latter is associated with a positive p wave in lead V_1.

As in VPBs, prematurity is not constant. In contrast to VPBs, the pause after the APB generally does not show full compensation (also in VPBs compensation is not always complete). If the p wave falls into the T wave of the preceding cardiac cycle, it may be difficult to identify. Whereas the first APB in ECG 18.3 (with a short PQ interval and negative p waves in V_3 to V_6) is clearly visible, the second, very early APB is only detectable by a peak on the T wave in V_1 (and V_2), due to superimposed p wave. There is aberration with a right bundle-branch block (RBBB) pattern. The last beat may be interpreted as postextrasystolic atrial escape, from the same focus as the first APB.

After early APBs, an aberration (ECGs 18.3 and 18.8) or AV block 1° can be observed. If the APB occurs very early it may be completely AV blocked (ECG 18.4). In these cases the false diagnosis of sinoatrial (SA) block is occasionally made.

The Full Picture

The clinical and prognostic impact of APBs is rather modest. APBs may provoke symptoms; APBs with aberrant conduction may be confounded with VPBs; and APBs may induce atrial tachycardia and atrial fibrillation. However, the correct *diagnosis* of APBs is not always easy.

ECG Special

ECG 18.5 does not reflect an atrial trigeminus – which might be diagnosed at a first glance – but a short polymorphous atrial tachycardia (see lead III) with AV block 2° type high degree.

The p waves 1, 4 and 6 are more or less hidden within the T wave; the p waves 3, 5 and 7 appear immediately after the QRS. After the eighth p wave (the seventh is not AV conducted) the tachycardia stops.

In contrast to some cases with ventricular bigeminy (or the extremely rare AV junctional bigeminy), the rare atrial bigeminy (ECG 18.6) is not registered by the 'patient', because there is neither AV dissociation nor retrograde atrial activation.

Atrial trigeminy (ECG 18.7) and quadrigeminy are very rare.

In APBs with *aberration*, an RBBB pattern is more frequent than an LBBB pattern. In ECG 18.8 the very early atrial depolarization is diagnosed by a minimal irregularity at the end of the T wave in V_1, and by a discrete increase of T wave amplitude in leads V_5 and V_6. The PQ interval is longer than in sinus beats and there is RBBB aberration. Moreover, there is no compensatory pause ('interponated' atrial APB). If, in a supraventricular PB, a p wave is not detectable, aberration may be difficult to distinguish from a VPB. The duration of the compensatory pause is not always a reliable factor for discrimination. The different QRS morphology in the precordial leads V_1 to V_6 allows a correct diagnosis in most cases (for details see Chapter 25 Ventricular Premature Beats).

1   Prevalence and Clinical Findings

Although APBs occur in about 65% of normal individuals, only 2% show more than 100 APBs in 24 h [1,2]. Folarin et al [3] observed 303 male military aviators. They found the following occurrences of APBs: rare ones in 73%, occasional in 2.6%, frequent in 2.3% and very frequent isolated (> 10% of normal beats) in 0.3%. In many instances APBs are combined with heart diseases and other diseases [4] but do not give any hint of the etiology, if they are not associated with alterations of QRS and/or repolarization. In contrast to VPBs, the prevalence of APBs is not related to coronary artery disease [5,6]. An increased risk for stroke in men with high frequency of atrial ectopic beats (≥ 219 in 24 h) has been described [7]. In pathologic conditions APBs occur more often in the presence of dilated atria. The incidence of the number of APBs increases as one gets older, but much less than the incidence of VPBs (that are often associated with hypertension and coronary heart disease).

In association with heart disease (perhaps in the first few days after a heart operation, or during viral infections), the arrhythmia often disappears spontaneously or after healing of the infection.

In patients with paroxysmal atrial fibrillation (AF) an elevated number of APBs (inducing AF) has been found [8], and can be treated by a sophisticated atrial pacemaker (Chapter 21 Atrial Fibrillation), often in combination with antiarrhythmic drugs, thus reducing AF episodes [9]. Principally, APBs not only initiate but also terminate atrial tachycardias [10].

Isolated or repetitive APBs impair cardiac output only in special conditions such as AV blocked APBs in bigeminy and longer runs at a high rate, corresponding to atrial tachycardia.

Short runs of APBs with a moderate rate (ECG 18.9) occasionally occur in healthy hearts. *Longer, rapid* salvos of APBs corresponding to more or less irregular *atrial tachycardia* (ECG 18.10) may cause discomfort, palpitations and anxiety.

2   Therapy

In asymptomatic patients short and also long runs of APBs should not be treated with antiarrhythmic drugs, generally, because of their potential proarrhythmic effects.

If antiarrhythmic drug therapy is necessary, many cardiologists prefer small doses of a beta-blocker or digitalis. For patients with preserved LV function, small doses of flecainide or propafenone can be used.

Short Story/Case Report 1

Some years ago a 62-year-old medical specialist, with a good reputation in internal medicine, told the author that in his opinion the ECG was a 'method for the foxes' and that it never helped him to arrive at a correct diagnosis. The author warmly congratulated him on this modern concept. In October 2000 the author received a long letter from this specialist. An ECG with a rhythm strip was enclosed (ECG 18.11). The 39-year-old patient, the physician's *daughter*, suffered from tachycardic palpitations, associated with vertigo and near-syncope. The physician made the diagnosis: basically normal ECG; sinus arrhythmia; atypical AV reentry tachycardia with AV dissociation and perhaps AV block. The author was very eager to analyze such an unusual arrhythmia, and made the diagnosis: basically normal ECG; APBs in salvos up to 12 beats, at a rate of about 150/min. The author proposed: therapy with atenolol (25 mg or 12.5 mg); investigation of infectious parameters; echo/Doppler; Holter ECG; exercise ECG. After this a decision about a definitive therapy.

Conclusion: the ECG may suddenly become important when a near relative shows symptoms ...

References

1. Brodsky M, Wu D, Denes P, Kanakis Ch, Rosen KM. Arrhythmias documented by 24-hour continuous electrocardiographic monitoring in 50 male medical students without apparent heart disease. Am J Cardiol 1977;39:390–5
2. Sobotka PA, Mayer JH, Bauernfeind RA, et al. Arrhythmias documented by 24-hour continuous ambulatory electrocardiographic monitoring in young women without apparent heart disease. Am Heart J 1981;101:753–9
3. Folarin VA, Fitzsimmons PJ, Kruyer WB. Holter monitor findings in asymptomatic male military aviators without structural heart disease. Aviat Space Environ Med 2001;72:836–8
4. Zipes DP. Specific arrhythmias: diagnosis and treatment. In: Braunwald E (ed) Heart disease: a textbook of cardiovascular medicine, Fifth edn. Philadelphia:WB Saunders 1997, pp 650–2
5. Chiang BN, Perlman LV, Ostrander LD, Epstein FH. Relationship of premature systoles to coronary heart disease and sudden death in the Tecumseh epidemiologic study. Ann Intern Med 1969;70:1159–66
6. Hinkle LE, Carver ST, Stevens M. The frequency of asymptomatic disturbances of cardiac rhythm and conduction in middle-aged men. Am J Cardiol 1969;24:629–50
7. Engstrom G, Hedblad B, Juul-Moller S, et al. Cardiac arrythmias and stroke: increased risk in men with high frequency of atrial ectopic beats. Stroke 2000;31:2925–9
8. Waktare JE, Hnatkova K, Sopher SM, et al. The role of atrial ectopics in initiating paroxysmal atrial fibrillation. Eur Heart J 2001;22:333–9
9. Wellens HJJ, Lau CP, Lüderitz B et al, for the Metrix investigators. Atrioverter: An implantable device for the treatment of atrial fibrillation. Circulation 1998;98:1651–6
10. Littmann L. The power of PACs. J Electrocardiol 2000;33:287–90

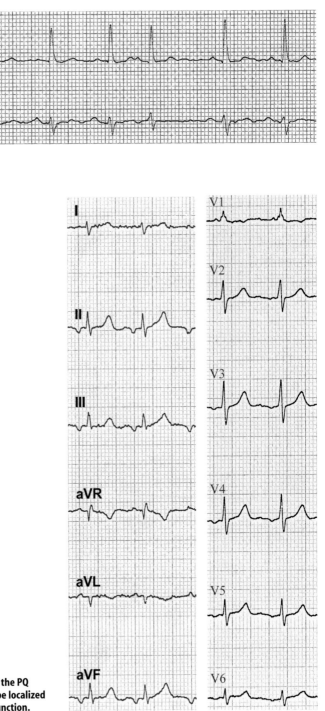

ECG 18.1
Atrial premature beat (leads aVL/aVF).

ECG 18.2
67y/m. RVH due to chronic obstructive pneumopathy. As the PQ interval is about 0.12 sec, the origin of the rhythm may be localized to the inferior portion of the right atrium, or to the AV junction.

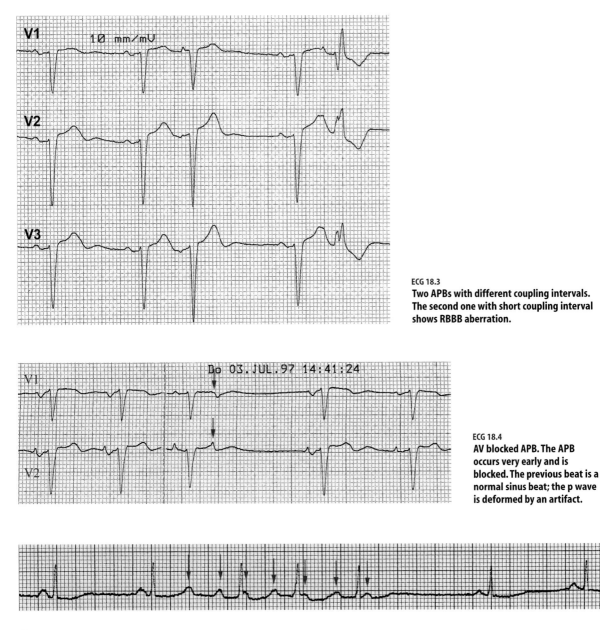

ECG 18.3
Two APBs with different coupling intervals.
The second one with short coupling interval
shows RBBB aberration.

ECG 18.4
AV blocked APB. The APB
occurs very early and is
blocked. The previous beat is a
normal sinus beat; the p wave
is deformed by an artifact.

ECG 18.5
Lead I. Short atrial tachycardia (seven p waves) with AV block 2°, mimicking an atrial triplet.

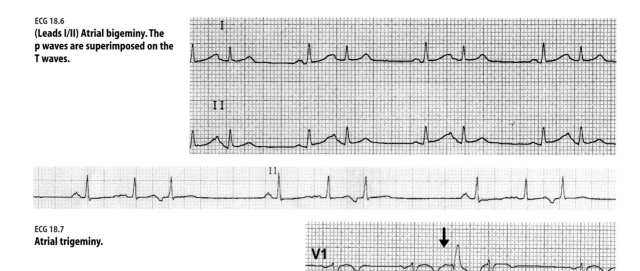

ECG 18.6
(Leads I/II) Atrial bigeminy. The p waves are superimposed on the T waves.

ECG 18.7
Atrial trigeminy.

ECG 18.8
Interponated APB with RBBB aberration (p wave: see [↓]).

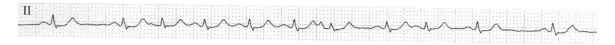

II

ECG 18.9
Run of APBs ('atrial tachycardia') with a moderate rate, irregular.

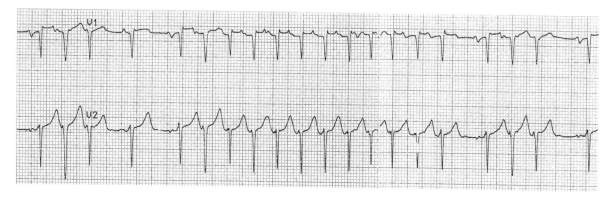

ECG 18.10
61y/m. Wegener disease. Leads V₁/V₂. Run of 11 APBs, slightly irregular atrial tachycardia at a rate of 185/min, preceded and followed by an atrial couplet.

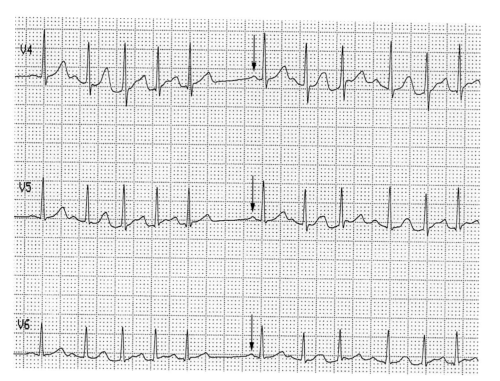

ECG 18.11
Short Story/Case Report 1. 39y/f. ECG (leads V₄ to V₆): only one sinusoidal beat (↓), runs of APBs, maximal instantaneous rate 165/min.

Chapter 19
Atrial Tachycardia

At a Glance

Atrial tachycardias are not frequent if atrial fibrillation (Chapter 21) and atrial flutter (Chapter 20) are excluded. The types of atrial tachycardia differ with respect to morphology of the p wave, atrial rate, atrioventricular conduction, duration of the arrhythmia, hemodynamic consequences, electrophysiologic mechanisms, and etiology.

ECG

In all atrial tachycardias the p waves precede the QRS complex, but p morphology is different from sinusal p waves. Most atrial tachycardias are regular. Based on clinical significance, atrial tachycardias may be classified in the following way.

1 'Salvos' of Atrial Premature Beats

The episodes of APBs (often 3–5 beats) are generally of moderate rate (110–150/min) and are often without symptoms. ECG 19.1 shows a longer episode of 8 beats.

2 'Benign' Atrial Tachycardia

This regular tachycardia is characterized by a relatively *short duration* (from several seconds to minutes), a *moderate rate* (< 150/min) and occurs in otherwise *healthy* hearts (ECG 19.2). Therapy is only needed if there are symptoms (mostly palpitations).

3 Atrial Tachycardia of Medium Duration and High Rate

The tachycardia lasts minutes to days, the rate is (individually) between 150 and 200/min (maximally 280/min) (ECG 19.3). The symptoms are malaise, palpitations, dizziness, presyncope or even syncope requiring drug therapy or catheter ablation. The tachycardia occurs in healthy individuals and in patients with heart disease. ECG 19.3 demonstrates that drug conversion with adenosine may also cause the treating physician's heart to tremble.

4 'Incessant' Atrial Tachycardia

The duration of this rare type of longstanding tachycardia is days to months. If the tachycardia lasts months and its rate is 150/min or more, it may induce a considerable reduction in the function of the left (and/or right) ventricle, and even chronic heart failure. The arrhythmia may have its origin in the right or left atrium and is often resistant to drugs. Restoration of sinus rhythm by catheter ablation may normalize heart function in otherwise healthy hearts, after weeks or months. However, this tachycardia also occurs in patients with heart diseases where ablation does not completely resolve the problem.

5 Atrial Tachycardia with Atrioventricular Block 2°

The tachycardia usually shows 2 : 1 atrioventricular (AV) block and is often associated with heart disease (ECG 19.4). It may also be due to *digitalis intoxication*. In the conventional ECG, differentiation from atrial flutter type 2 (with 2 : 1 AV block) is often impossible.

6 Multifocal Ectopic Atrial Tachycardia (Chaotic Atrial Mechanism)

This *completely irregular* tachycardia is very rare. The rate is 100–140/min (or less than 100/min). The morphology of the p waves changes from beat to beat, so do the PQ and the R–R intervals (ECG 19.5). The arrhythmia 'per se' has modest haemo-dynamic consequences. However, its usual association with *severe obstructive lung disease* is responsible for a bad progno-sis (details in the next section and in Chapter 32 Rare ECGs).

The Full Picture

The sequence of atrial tachycardias in the section At a Glance is based on clinical significance, but the series of atrial tachy-cardias in this section corresponds to the usual classification, with inclusion of some electrophysiologic mechanisms.

ECG Special

7   Ectopic (Focal) Atrial Tachycardia

Ectopic (focal) atrial tachycardia is due to enhanced auto-maticity of an ectopic atrial focus [1]. The morphology of the p waves depends on the localization of the ectopic centre. P is negative or positive in the inferior leads III and aVF. Often this *regular* tachycardia is of short duration (up to 30 sec), with a rate generally between 110 and 150/min. Therefore the tachy-cardia is called *benign slow atrial tachycardia*. It is especially seen in young people. Rates up to 180/min are rare. The *rare incessant form*, with a duration of weeks or months, is often associated with organic heart disease [2] but the tachycardia itself may lead to ventricular dilatation and heart failure [3,4], that is at least partially reversible after catheter ablation.

At the beginning of the tachycardia, aberrant conduction may be present (mostly right bundle-branch block, RBBB) that disappears after some beats, at the same rate. A longer tachy-cardia often shows some changes in the rate. Alterations of the repolarization are common and may persist for hours after conversion of the tachycardia. Short episodes are harmless and generally occur in healthy individuals. Long episodes (inces-sant form) are more often associated with organic heart dis-ease. Vagal maneuvers do not influence the atrial rate, but may induce AV block 2°. Adenosine is sometimes successful. In problematic cases catheter ablation is the best therapy.

8   Atrial Reentry Tachycardia

The reentry circuit consists of two distinct intra-atrial func-tional pathways [5]. Again the p wave is different from a sinusal p and may be positive or negative in III and aVF. The tachycar-dia is introduced by an atrial premature beat (APB). In contrast to the focal type, p wave morphology often changes, according to variations within the circuit. Moreover, at the beginning of the tachycardia an increase of the rate can be observed (so-called 'warming up effect'). Generally the rate is higher than in ectopic atrial tachycardia and may reach 240/min. Josephson [6] found an incidence of 6% in 260 patients with paroxysmal supraventricular tachycardia, studied invasively. Atrial reentry tachycardia is found in otherwise healthy hearts but also in patients with congenital and other heart diseases. Vagal maneuvers and adenosine are rarely successful. With a conven-tional ECG the differentiation between the two types of atrial tachycardia, mentioned above, is not possible in most cases.

9   Repetitive Paroxysmal Atrial Tachycardia

This arrhythmia is very rare. It is defined by excessively fre-quent paroxysms of a slightly irregular atrial tachycardia with a rate of 130–150/min. A more or less incessant tachycardia may be present, frequently interrupted by some sinus beats. The therapy depends on the symptoms and on the underlying heart disease.

10   Paroxysmal Atrial Tachycardia with AV Block

Atrial tachycardias rarely show an AV block 1°. The term 'atrial tachycardia with block' is reserved for the presence of AV block 2° and, extremely rarely, AV block 3°. The mechanism of tachy-cardia is probably an 'ectopic focus'. Triggered activity is dis-cussed in the case of digitalis intoxication [7], where the tachy-cardia is not paroxysmal. The rate is often between 150 and 200/min, with a range of 110–240/min. Usually AV block 2 : 1 is present (ECG 19.4), rarely with superimposed Wenckebach phenomenon (leading to irregularity of the ventricular action) or AV block 3 : 1. Often the atrial rhythm is slightly irregular. Occasionally an alternating slight 'regular irregularity' is found: the (AV blocked) p wave after the QRS shows a shorter distance to the previous (conducted) p than to the following (again conducted) p wave. The mechanism for this behavior is the same as in 'ventriculophasic sinus arrhythmia' (Chapter 12 AV Block and AV Dissociation The Full Picture). Differentiating between the arrhythmia and atrial flutter with 2 : 1 AV block, especially of type 2 (where 'saw-tooth' waves are lacking, with a preserved isoelectric line between the flutter waves) is often not possible. However, the differentiation is clinically important in *one* condition: in atrial flutter, digitalis is often helpful for slowing the ventricular rate. If atrial tachycardia with AV block is due to *digitalis intoxication*, digitalis is obsolete.

11 Left Atrial Tachycardia

This arrhythmia is very rare. Rates can be as high as 150–200/min and may cause severe symptoms. The ECG is characterized by negative p waves in lead I (and often in aVL) and by positive p waves in lead V_1 (ECG 19.6). Mirowski's ancient criteria [8,9] have been modified [10,11], because a similar p morphology may be observed also in cases with ectopic *right* atrial tachycardia, but with a biphasic p wave in lead V_1. The reason for the positive p wave in lead V_1 in left atrial rhythm is atypical activation of both atria. First the left atrium is activated eccentrically (vector directed anteriorly and to the right), followed by the activation of the right atrium, with a similar vector. A 100% differentiation between right and left atrial origin is necessary, of course, if ablation therapy is taken in consideration.

12 Multifocal Atrial Tachycardia (Chaotic Atrial Tachycardia)

This arrhythmia is also very rare and is also called *chaotic* atrial tachycardia or chaotic atrial mechanism. The rate is about 110–150/min (if less than 100/min, it is correctly called chaotic atrial mechanism; ECG 19.5). The definition depends on at least three (often more than 10) different p morphologies in one lead, and variable P–P, R–R and PQ intervals. As the absence of a dominant atrial centre is also mandatory, *sinus rhythm with salvos of atrial PBs* should *not* be misdiagnosed as multifocal/chaotic atrial tachycardia/mechanism. AV block 1° may occur in some beats, as well as singular AV junctional escape beats. The arrhythmia lasts for minutes or for days. It may change to atrial flutter or atrial fibrillation (which is exceptional in our experience). Multifocal atrial tachycardia has generally moderate hemodynamic consequences; its bad progno-

sis is based on frequent association with severe chronic obstructive pulmonary disease [12,13]. In this context up to 50% of patients die within 6 months of the underlying disease. Diabetes, hypertensive heart disease and hypokalemia may rarely be associated with the arrhythmia [13].

ECG 19.7 shows an example of a complex atrial tachycardia that fulfills the criteria of multifocal atrial tachycardia on one hand and shows features of paroxysmal atrial tachycardia with AV block on the other hand.

13 Accelerated Atrial Rhythm

As the rate of accelerated atrial rhythm generally does not exceed 100/min, the term tachycardia is not used. The abnormal rhythm is characterized by episodes of atrial rhythm with abnormal p waves at a rate slightly above that of sinus rhythm. The arrhythmia is occasionally seen in Holter ECGs, its clinical relevance is zero.

14 Closing Remarks

A new – but not yet definitive – nomenclature for atrial tachycardias, and especially atrial flutter, has been proposed [14] (see also Chapter 20 Atrial Flutter).

References

1. Gillette PC, Garson A Jr. Electrophysiologic and pharmacologic characteristics of automatic ectopical atrial tachycardia. Circulation 1977;56:571–5
2. Wu D, Denes P, Amat-y-Leon F, et al. Clinical, electrocardiographic and electrophysiologic observations in patients with paroxysmal supraventricular tachycardia. Am J Cardiol 1978;41:1045–51
3. Packer DL, Bardy GH, Worley SJ, et al. Tachycardia-induced cardiomyopathy: a reversible form of left ventricular dysfunction. Am J Cardiol 1986;57:563–70
4. Gillette PC, Smith RT, Garson A Jr, et al. Chronic supraventricular tachycardia. A curable cause of congestive cardiomyopathy. J Ammer Med Assoc 1985;253:391–2
5. Goldreyer BN, Bigger JT Jr. Site of reentry in paroxysmal supraventricular tachycardia in man. Circulation 1971;43:15–26
6. Josephson ME. Clinical cardiac electrophysiology, 2nd edition. Philadelphia: Lea & Febiger, 1993
7. Lown B, Wyatt NF, Levine HD. Paroxysmal atrial tachycardia with block. Circulation 1960;21:129
8. Mirowski M, Neill HB, Taussig HB. Left atrial ectopic rhythm in mirror-image dextrocardia and in normally placed malformed hearts. Report on twelve cases with 'dome and dart' P-waves. Circulation 1963;27:864–77
9. Mirowski M. Left atrial rhythm: diagnostic criteria and differentiation from nodal arrhythmias. Am J Cardiol 1966;17:203–10

10. Spodick D. Left atrial rhythm. Am Heart J 1971;81;146
11. Khalilulla M, Shrestha NK, Padmavati S. Left atrial rhythm in man. An experimental study. J Electrocardiol 1978,11:375–8
12. McCord J, Borzak S. Multifocal atrial tachycardia. Chest 1998;113:203–9
13. Kastor JA. Multifocal atrial tachycardia. N Engl J Med 1990;322:1713–7
14. Saouidi N, Cosio F, Waldo A, et al. A classification of atrial and regular atrial tachycardia according to electrophysiological mechanisms and anatomical bases. Europ Heart J 2001;22:1162–82

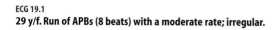

II

ECG 19.1
29 y/f. Run of APBs (8 beats) with a moderate rate; irregular.

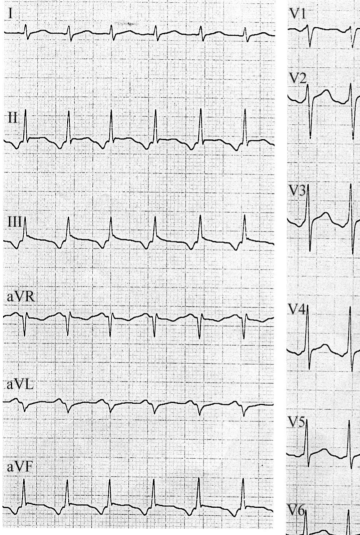

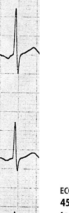

ECG 19.2
45 y/m. Healthy, no symptoms. ECG: atrial tachycardia, rate 127/min. Negative p waves in inferior limb leads and V_1 to V_5 (V_6). PQ 0.1 sec. Note ST elevation, due to also inverse atrial repolarization.

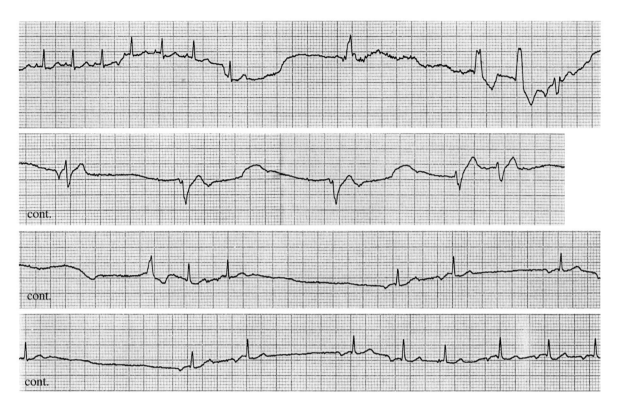

ECG 19.3

52 y/m. Several episodes with rapid palpitations, duration minutes to 2 h. Rarely vertigo. Otherwise healthy heart. *Continuous rhythm-stripe* (monitor lead): atrial tachycardia (EPI (electrophysiologic investigation): atrial reentry tachycardia), rate 160/min. Conversion with 6 mg adenosine i.v. Note several episodes of significant bradycardia (pauses up to 2.5 s), due to sinus standstill or sinoatrial block, with ventricular and atrial escape beats. Finally ectopic atrial rhythm.

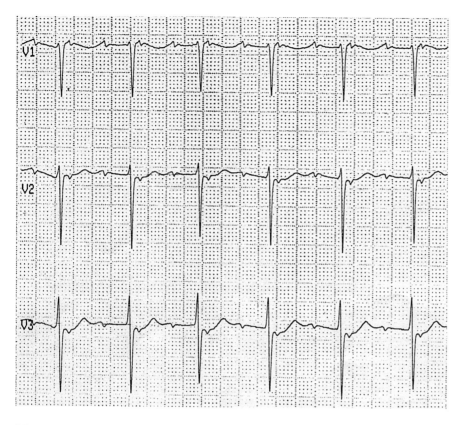

ECG 19.4

85 y/f. (leads V$_1$ to V$_3$) Coronary and hypertensive heart disease. Mild renal failure (creatinine 130 mmol/l, creatinine clearance not known). Serum digoxin level 5.7 mmol/l. ECG: atrial tachycardia, rate 156/min, with 2 : 1 AV block. The conducted beats show AV block 1°. Rare VPBs and relatively mild ST depression in V$_3$ to V$_6$ (not shown). Normalization of the rhythm within 7 days (over Wenckebach and AV block 1°).

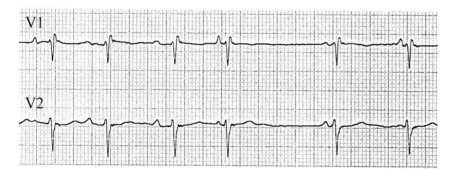

ECG 19.5

64 y/m. Coronary artery disease. ECG (leads V$_1$/V$_2$): chaotic atrial rhythm, instantaneous rate 50–107/min. Note the 'absolute ventricular arrhythmia', the six different p waves in six cycles and the varying PQ intervals.

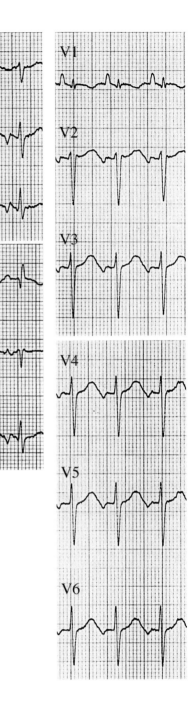

ECG 19.6
54 y/f. Left atrial tachycardia. Palpitations for years. ECG (courtesy of Reto Candinas). Atrial tachycardia, rate 125/min. Note the negative p waves in leads I, II and V$_2$ to V$_6$, and the high positive p wave in V$_1$. EPI: focus in the proximal right lower lung vein. Ablation.

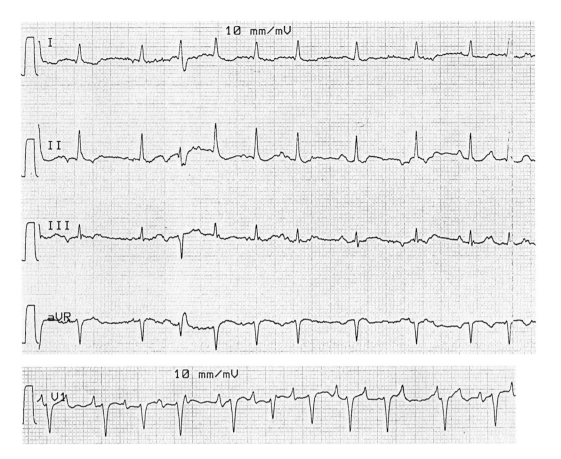

ECG 19.7

74 y/f. Complex atrial tachycardia. ECG: leads I to aVR and V₁. In the limb leads an absolute arrhythmia of ventricular action is observed, in the presence of at least five different p configurations. The third beat (after a relative long R–R interval) is an Ashman beat with RBBB configuration. Lead V₁ reveals an irregular atrial tachycardia (rate 150–180/min) with a morphologically predominant centre (peaky positive p waves), but also at least three other p configurations. The ventricular rate is slower due to AV block 2° of Wenckebach type, with different duration of the two Wenckebach periods and different behavior of the PQ interval.

Chapter 20
Atrial Flutter

At a Glance

Atrial flutter is eight times rarer than atrial fibrillation, and in old patients about 15 times rarer. The arrhythmia may last for some beats, some minutes, hours, months, or even years. Symptoms preferentially depend on the ventricular rate, which is determined by atrioventricular conduction. The etiology of atrial flutter is as manifold as that of atrial fibrillation.

ECG

The (atrial) rate of atrial flutter is between 230 and 330/min, often between 240 and 300/min, and stable in an individual patient. Atrial impulses are commonly blocked within the atrioventricular (AV) node in a 2 : 1 mode (2 : 1 AV block), resulting in a ventricular rate of about 140 to 150/min. Atrial rate is slowed by a dilated right atrium, by an excessive intra-atrial conduction disturbance, and by drugs such as amiodarone (in the last case to less than 200/min). Preexisting or rate-dependent right bundle-branch block (RBBB) (or rarely left bundle-branch block (LBBB)) may be present, masking the flutter waves and mimicking ventricular tachycardia at a first glance. A tachycardia with small or broad QRS, especially with RBBB configuration, with a rate of 130 to 160/min represents atrial flutter in 70% of the cases (ECG 20.1).

1   Morphologic Types of Atrial Flutter

There are two types of atrial flutter (for a new nomenclature see next section).

1.1   Common Type (Type 1) (in 85%)

Typical flutter waves show a 'saw-tooth' or 'picket fence' appearance in leads III and aVF (and II), where the isoelectric line cannot be identified anymore, and flutter waves or p-like waves

in some other leads, are well visible in V$_1$ (ECGs 20.2 and 20.3). On many occasions the ventricular response is irregular, due to varying AV block 2° (2 : 1 to 4 : 1 or higher), sometimes with a superimposed Wenckebach mechanism (ECG 20.4), occasionally mimicking absolute arrhythmia as in atrial fibrillation. However, in a longer rhythm strip a 'regular irregularity' can be recognized in all cases.

'Regular irregularity' may also indicate atrial flutter with changing AV-conduction if the flutter waves cannot be identified (ECG 20.5). *1 : 1 conduction is rare, but important.* It may occur in children, but also in adults during sympathetic stimulation, for example during exercise (ECG 20.6a), with 2 : 1 AV block after exercise (ECG 20.6b), in the early phase of quinidine therapy, and in patients with pre-excitation (Wolff-Parkinson-White syndrome). A ventricular response of about 300/min represents a dangerous condition. Moreover, ventricular fibrillation may develop.

1.2   Uncommon Type (Type 2) (in 15%)

The diagnosis of this rather rare type may be difficult because the 'saw-tooth' configuration is lacking. 'Type 2'-flutter waves are p-wave-like in all leads, and positive in leads III and aVF, with a more or less preserved isoelectric line (ECG 20.7). The atrial rate is also stable and may be faster, between 240/min and 380/min. The AV conduction shows the same variations as in the common type.

Due to the p-wave-like flutter waves, uncommon atrial flutter is easily confounded with atrial tachycardia. Because atrial tachycardia with incomplete AV block may be due to digitalis intoxication, it is dangerous to give digitalis in such a case. Although the rate of atrial tachycardia rarely exceeds 210/min, differentiation between a fast atrial tachycardia and atrial flutter, especially of the uncommon type, is sometimes very difficult. Clinical findings and the patient's history should be considered. Moreover, one has to check if the patient is already under digitalis.

In common and uncommon atrial flutter, the electrophysiologic mechanism is a macro-reentry within the right atrium.

The Full Picture

Recently the electrophysiologic mechanisms of atrial flutter have been re-evaluated. This means on the one hand that the ECG diagnosis has become more complex, and on the other that the clinical problems related to atrial flutter remain unchanged.

2   Nomenclature

During the last 10 years considerable progress has been made in the analysis of electrophysiologic mechanisms of atrial flutter and atrial tachycardias, based on special stimulation protocols and on non-contact mapping systems and electroanatomical contact systems [1–4].

The classification in atrial flutter type 1 and type 2 seems to be too simple. Based on electrophysiologic investigations, a new nomenclature was recently proposed by an expert group of the Working Group of Arrhythmias from the European and the North American Society of Pacing and Electrophysiology [4]. The following well-characterized modes of atrial flutter are distinguished (Table 20.1).

Table 20.2 demonstrates the atrial flutter patterns in the ECG (as far as they are known) of the different types.

Evidently, the same electrophysiologic mechanism may provide different flutter configurations in the ECG and, conversely, the same pattern in the ECG may be based on different mechanisms.

Interestingly, for people with *reverse* typical flutter, the typical flutter can be induced in the lab in about 50%. Lesion tachycardia is based on a scar due to atriotomy, to placement of a baffle (Mustard, Senning), to an excessively dilated right atrium, or to ablation of atrial fibrillation.

Some features of 'focal' atrial tachycardia (that may be due to enhanced automaticity, triggered activity and reentry!), fibrillatory conduction, reentrant sinus tachycardia, and inappropriate sinus tachycardia are also discussed in the publication of Saoudi et al [4].

Table 20.1
New nomenclature of atrial flutter (derived from [4])

- Typical flutter (formerly type 1 flutter) ECG: 'saw-tooth'/'picket fence'
- Reverse typical flutter (formerly type 2 flutter)
- Lesion makro-reentrant tachycardia ('incisional' flutter)
- Lower loop flutter
- Double-wave re-entry
- Right atrial free wall makro-reentry without atriotomy
- Left atrial macro-reentrant tachycardia (primary circuit in the left atrium)

Table 20.2
Corresponding ECG patterns (derived from [4])

Mode of atrial flutter	ECG
Typical flutter	- 'Saw-tooth' configuration, dominant negative in III, aVF
Reverse typical flutter	- Broad positive flutter waves in III, aVF - Negative flutter waves in V_1 - Similar pattern to typical flutter possible
Lesion tachycardia	- Often similar pattern to typical flutter in right atrial atriotomy tachycardia - Low voltage flutter waves - Any pattern
Lower loop flutter	?
Double-wave reentry	?
RA makro-reentry without atriotomy	?
Left atrial macro-reentrant tachycardia	- Similar or identical to typical flutter - Positive flutter waves in V_1 - P waves with isoelectrical line

The new classification, and especially the underlying mechanisms, are highly interesting. However, there has been only a modest impact on practical rhythmology, drug treatment included, hitherto.

The duties of the *practitioner* are:

i. to recognize atrial flutter (in aberration and in cases with hidden flutter waves) and to treat patients in context of the underlying disease and symptoms.
ii. to send selected patients to the electrophysiology lab
iii. to take note, if possible, of new developments (and nomenclatures) in this field. Electrophysiology becomes 'fractionated' more and more, like our daily lives.

The duties of the *electrophysiologist* are:

i. to determine the correct substrate and mechanism and to treat the patient with ablation
ii. to provide detailed information about the practical significance and importance of the findings.

3   Etiology

Overall, short-lasting atrial flutter is most frequently seen in patients after cardiac surgery [5,6], especially after valve replacement. Flutter of any duration occurs in many other heart diseases such as acute myocardial infarction, hypertension, hyperthyroidism, mitral valve lesions, cardiomyopathies of all etiologies, myopericarditis, and acute pulmonary embolism. The arrhythmia may also be associated with a special variant of the 'sick sinus syndrome', the 'bradycardia/tachycardia type' (Chapter 22 Sick Sinus Syndrome), but it is rare in chronic cor pulmonale [7] and in otherwise healthy hearts ('lone atrial flutter'). Granada et al [8] describe a prevalence of atrial flutter in 1.7% of 181 patients. In all the conditions mentioned here, atrial flutter is much more rare than atrial fibrillation.

ECG Special ─────────────────

In type 1 flutter with 2 : 1 AV block the 'saw-tooth'-like flutter waves are generally detectable in the inferior leads, if they are not masked by a bundle-branch block. In type 2 flutter with 2 : 1 AV block the p-like flutter waves are often placed *alternately in the middle between the QRS complexes, and completely hidden within the QRS complexes* (ECG 20.8a). In these cases the misdiagnosis of atrial tachycardia or even sinus tachycardia with

1 : 1 AV conduction is often made. Carotis sinus massage, enhancing AV block, may resolve the problem (ECG 20.8b). In sinus rhythm, vagal maneuvers slow the rate during a short time, whereas a ventricular tachycardia remains unchanged. Occasionally, type 2 flutter may only be diagnosed by careful analysis. ECG 20.9 shows an example with right bundle-branch block (RBBB). Even so, type 2 flutter cannot always be diagnosed at a first glance (ECG 20.10).

Thus, in a tachycardia with a rate of about 130–160/min and with detectable p wave-like deflections just in the middle between the QRS complexes, atrial flutter type 2 (or atrial tachycardia) with 2 : 1 AV block should always be excluded. In some cases every second flutter wave appears just at the end of the QRS complex, thus simulating incomplete right bundle-branch block in lead V_1 (ECG 20.11). In hospital conditions, an esophageal lead or right atrial catheter lead helps resolving diagnostic problems by demonstrating the presence or absence of flutter waves.

Extremely short flutter is only exceptionally detected, mostly in Holter ECGs (ECGs 20.12 and 20.13).

If a physician cannot distinguish between flutter with irregular ventricular response and atrial fibrillation, his diagnosis will be 'fibrillo–flutter'. Mixed *flutter–fibrillation* does indeed exist. Flutter-like episodes alternate with typical fibrillation, the atrial rate is high (about 400/min) and the ventricular response is almost completely irregular (ECG 20.14). On one hand, in the right atrium (and the left?) there are flutter circuits (with changing directions and velocity); on the other hand, a portion of the right atrium (and the left?) is fibrillating. According to a recent publication [4] the mechanisms are even more complex.

4   Clinical Significance

Every physician is aware of the symptoms and hemodynamic consequences of atrial flutter. Untreated flutter often shows a ventricular rate (about 130–160/min) that is too high, whereas drugs often provoke a ventricular response that is too slow by impairing AV conduction. Both conditions reduce cardiac output. Moreover, abrupt changes in heart rate may lead to palpitations and may even result in an inability to work. As is the case with every longstanding tachycardia, incessant flutter with 2 : 1 AV block may lead to a 'tachycardia-induced cardiomyopathy'.

In the experience of most physicians, atrial flutter sometimes, though rarely, provokes thromboembolic events. Thus, long-term anticoagulation does not seem to be indicated normally. However, flutter and fibrillation, or mixed flutter–fibrillation, are not that rare in the same individual. Periods of atrial fibrillation may remain undiscovered. Moreover, a recent publication reported an astonishingly high incidence of thrombotic material and/or spontaneous contrast in the left atrium and left appendage in 34% of cases, detected by transesophageal echocardiogram [9]. Wood et al [10] found, in 86 patients, an annual incidence of thromboembolic events of 3%. In a reader's comment, Densem [11] mentioned a 2.2% incidence of cardioversion-related thromboembolic events, and proposed that the 'anticoagulation guidelines of atrial fibrillation' issued by the American College of Chest physicians (international normalized ratio (INR) of 2–3, 3 weeks before and 4 weeks after cardioversion), should be applied to flutter also. In a recent review, based on eight studies, Lip and Kamath [12] reported a risk rate of 2.2% for embolism in non-anticoagulated or insufficiently anticoagulated patients after electroconversion (partially due to stunning atria after direct current (DC) shock). Therefore they recommend the same anticoagulation practice before and after DC shock, as for people with atrial fibrillation. Lip and Kamath surmise that the data for permanent anticoagulation in chronic atrial flutter are not yet completely convincing.

5 Pathophysiology and Therapeutic Consequences

The increasing age of the general population seems to influence the atrial rate in atrial flutter. The formerly 'classical' rate of about 300/min is seen mostly in younger patients. In older people, atrial rates of 220–270 are quite usual. This is probably due to age-related intra-atrial conduction disturbances, a dilated right atrium, and drugs, especially amiodarone, flecainide and procainamide.

In most patients with flutter an intra-atrial or inter-atrial conduction abnormality has been found, during intermittent sinus rhythm [13]. The rate of atrial flutter waves not only correlates with age and drugs, but also with atrial diameter. This can be explained by the underlying electrophysiologic mechanism, involving a makro-reentry circuit movement within the right atrium in both typical ('type 1') and inverse ('type 2') flutter. In a dilated right atrium the longer circuit results in a lower rate. Interestingly, rapid pacing (with a catheter placed in the right atrium) is more successful in type 1 flutter than in type 2 flutter, in 70% and 6% respectively [14]. Recent investigations [4] suggest that flutter type 2 is partially based on mechanism other than makro-reentry, which cannot be influenced by pacing.

Drugs like amiodarone, pronestyl, flecainide, and quinidine decrease the rate of atrial flutter to 200/min or even lower (ECG 20.15). Thus pronestyl and quinidine may induce a 1 : 1 AV conduction, whereas amiodarone impairs the conduction in the AV node enough for inhibiting 1 : 1 conduction.

Drug therapy and prophylaxis of atrial flutter is often unsatisfactory, and in cases of significant bradycardia or the 'bradycardia–tachycardia variant' of the 'sick sinus syndrome' a pacemaker is preferable. Today catheter-induced ablation is the best therapy for chronic atrial flutter and is successful in a high percentage of cases.

References

1. Rodriguez LM, Timmermans C, Nabar A, Hofstra L, Wellens HJ. Biatrial activation in isthmus dependent atrial flutter. Circulation 2001;104:2545–50
2. Marine JE, Korley VJ, Obioha Ngwu O, et al. Different patterns of interatrial conduction in clockwise and counterclockwise atrial flutter. Circulation 2001;104:1153–7
3. Ndrepepa G, Zrenner B, Weyerbrock S, et al. Activation patterns in the left atrium during counterclockwise and clockwise atrial flutter. J Cardiovasc Electrophysiol 2001;12:893–9
4. Saoudi N, Cosio F, Waldo A, et al. A classification of atrial flutter and regular atrial tachycardia according to electrophysiological mechanisms and anatomical bases. Eur Heart J 2001;22:1162–82
5. Angelini P, Feldman MI, Lufschanowski R, et al. Cardiac arrhythmias during and after heart surgery: Diagnosis and treatment. Prog Cardiovasc Dis 1974;16:469–95
6. Wells JL, MacLean WA, James TN, et al. Characterization of atrial flutter. Studies in man after open heart surgery using fixed atrial electrodes. Circulation 1979;60:665–73
7. Cosby RS, Herman LM. Atrial flutter and pulmonary disease. Geriatrics 1966;21:140–4
8. Granada J, Uribe W, Chyou PH, et al. Incidence and predictors of atrial flutter in the general population. JACC 2000;36:2242–6
9. Irani WN, Grayburn PA, Alfridi I. Prevalence of thrombus, spontaneous echocardiogram contrast, and atrial stunning in patients undergoing cardioversion of atrial flutter. A prospective study using transesophageal echocardiography. Circulation 1997;95:962–6
10. Wood KA, Eisenberg SJ, Kalman JM, et al. Risk of thromboembolism in chronic atrial flutter. Am J Cardiol 1997;79:1043–7
11. Densem CG. Patients undergoing cardioversion of atrial flutter should be routinely anticoagulated. Am J Cardiol 1998;82:580–3
12. Lip GJH, Kamath S. Thromboprophylaxis in atrial flutter. Europ Heart J 2001;22:984–7
13. Josephson ME. Clinical cardiac electrophysiology. Philadelphia: Lea & Febiger, 1993
14. Baeriswyl G, Zimmermann M, Adamec R. Efficacy of rapid atrial pacing for conversion of atrial flutter in medically treated patients. Clin Cardiol 1994;17:246–50

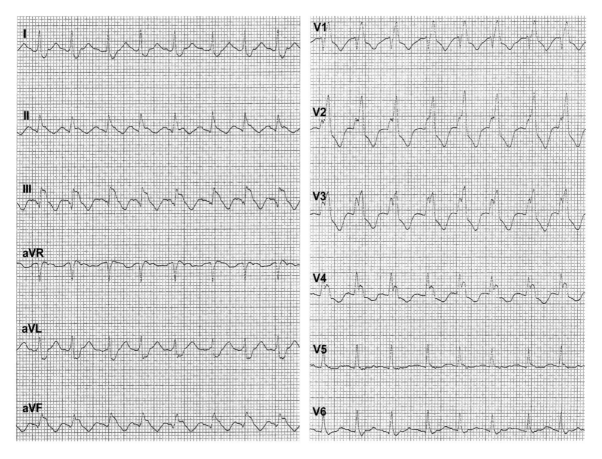

ECG 20.1

69y/m. Atrial flutter type 1 with 2 : 1 (or 3 : 1) AV block and RBBB. Atrial rate 270/min, ventricular rate 135/min (or slower). The 'saw-tooth' flutter waves (inferiorly) are partially hidden within the negative T waves and the QRS complex. (Note: the QRS complex in V$_5$ appears to be small, because the terminal part of QRS is almost isoelectric.)

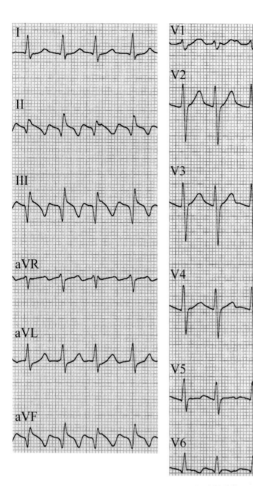

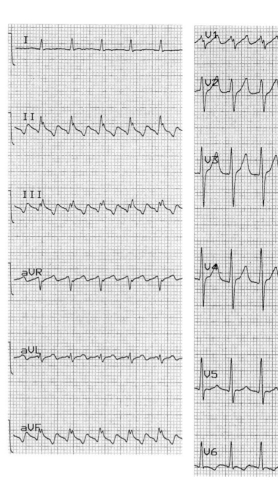

ECG 20.2

53y/m. Atrial flutter type 1 with 1 : 2 AV conduction (2 : 1 AV block). Atrial rate 270/min. Every second flutter wave is superimposed on the negative T waves in leads III/aVF/II, due to three old inferior myocardial infarctions (see Q waves in these leads).

ECG 20.3

73y/m. Atrial flutter type 1 with 2 : 1 AV block. Atrial rate 314/min, ventricular rate 157/min.

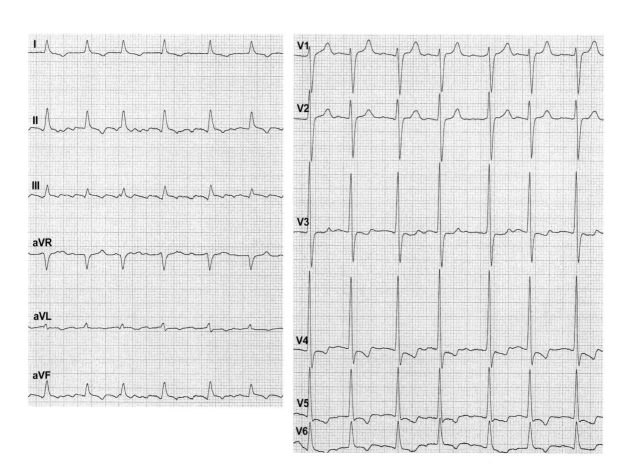

ECG 20.4

73y/m. Atrial flutter type 1 ('saw-tooth' pattern only minimal, see lead III) with AV-block 2 : 1 or 3 : 1, with superimposed Wenckebach phenomenon (interval between flutter waves and QRS changing). Atrial rate 276/min. LVH and LV overload.

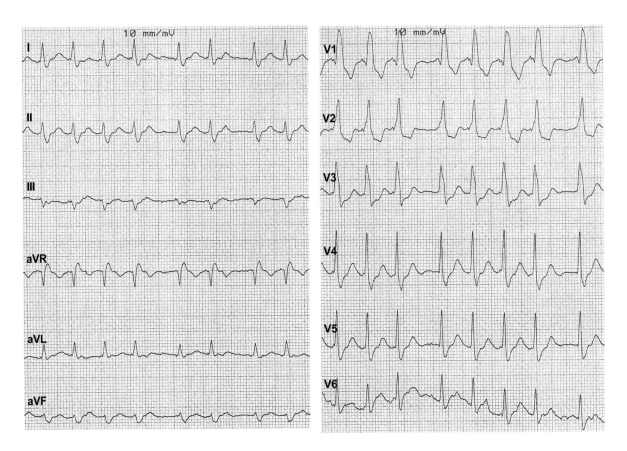

ECG 20.5

Atrial flutter without clearly detectable flutter waves, in a patient with RBBB. The diagnosis is made on the basis of 'regular irregularity', corresponding to 2 : 1 or 3 : 1 AV block. Flutter rate corresponds to the double of the instantaneous rate of the small R–R intervals=284/min.

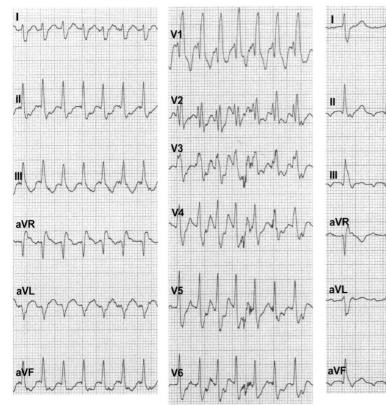

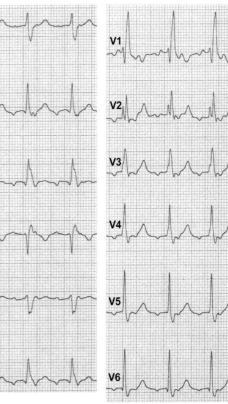

ECG 20.6a

47y/m. Tetralogy of Fallot, operated at the age of 26y. Atrial flutter with 1 : 1 conduction during exercise (9 MET (maximal exercise test)), ventricular rate 205/min. RBBB. The low atrial rate is caused by an excessively dilated right atrium.

ECG 20.6b

Same patient. At rest. Atrial flutter type 1 with AV block 2° 2 : 1. Atrial rate 204/min.

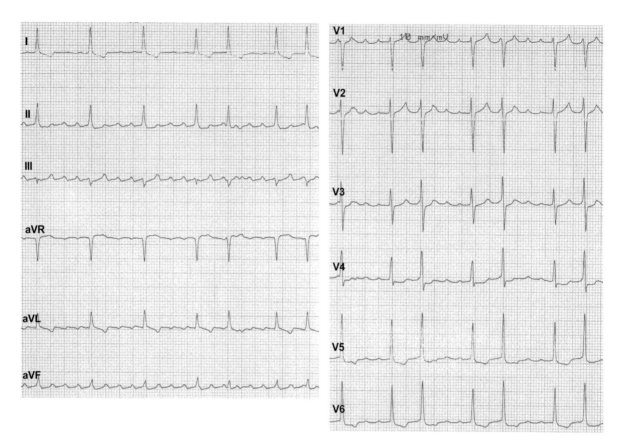

ECG 20.7

77y/f. Atrial flutter type 2 (positive flutter waves in III, aVF), with varying AV conduction (4 : 1 and 2 : 1 AV block, with superimposed Wenckebach phenomenon). Atrial rate 308/min, ventricular rate about 77/min and 144/min respectively.

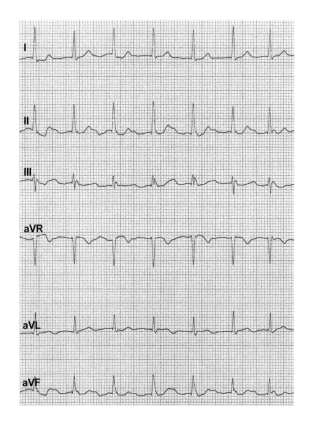

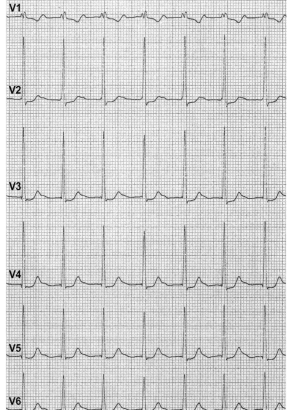

ECG 20.8a ▲ ▶

71y/m. Atrial flutter with 2 : 1 AV block. Alternating, one flutter wave is in the middle between the QRS complexes, the other hidden within QRS. Rather type 1 than type 2 flutter (no distinct isoelectric line in lead III).

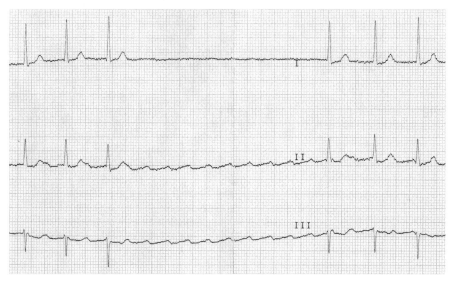

◀ ECG 20.8b

Same patient. Carotis sinus massage (leads I–III) enhances AV block to one episode of 11 : 1, unmasking the flutter waves (rate 197/min).

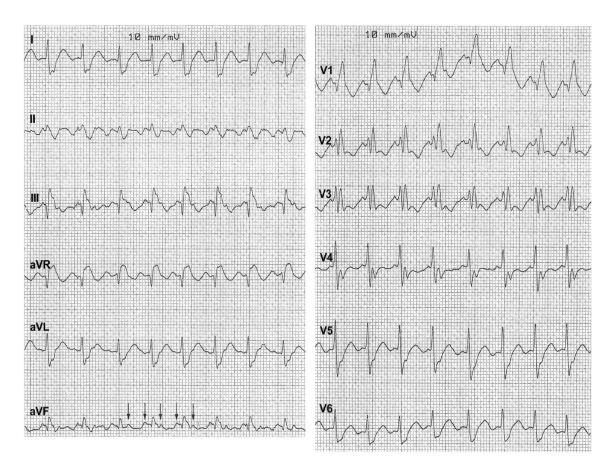

ECG 20.9

78y/m. Atrial flutter with 2 : 1 AV block, atrial rate 264/min. RBBB. Type 1 flutter seems to be present. However the 'pseudo-saw-tooth' pattern in II corresponds to the S wave of RBBB, and the negative deflection in III to the negative T wave. In lead aVF (and III) small positive flutter waves are detectable (↓), indicating type 2. Based on the 'p wave' in V_1 the arrhythmia was first interpreted as sinus tachycardia. However the 'p wave' is short and the 'p'–R interval only about 0.10 sec.

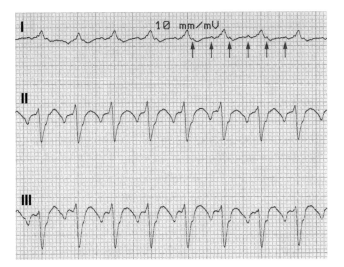

ECG 20.10

80y/m. (Leads I–III) Atrial flutter type 1 with 2 : 1 AV block, atrial rate 300/min. Negative flutter waves in the inferior leads _alternately_ hidden within the QRS. Positive flutter deflections clearly detectable in lead I (↑).

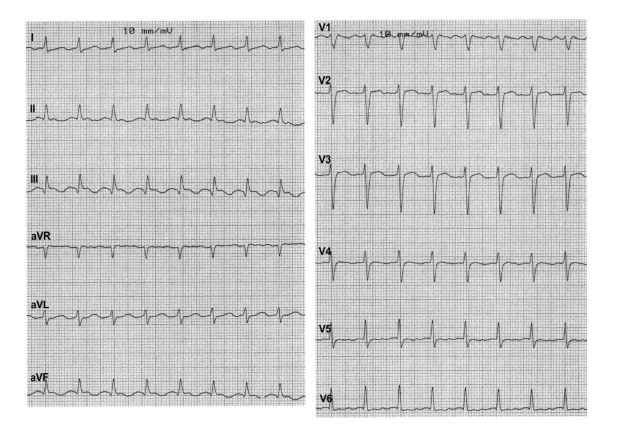

ECG 20.11

67y/m. Atrial flutter type 1 ('smooth saw-tooth'), with 2 : 1 AV block. Atrial rate 248/min. Flutter waves imitate iRBBB (pseudo-r') in lead V$_1$.

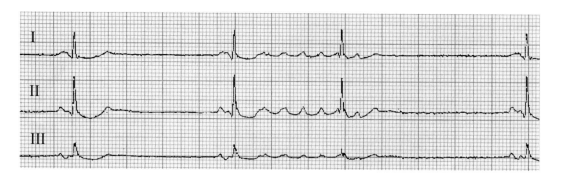

ECG 20.12
75y/m. Sinus bradycardia, interrupted by short paroxysmal flutter.

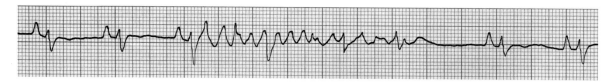

ECG 20.13
64y/m. Paroxysmal irregular flutter at a high rate (fibrillo–flutter?) in another patient. Ventricular irregularity excludes artifacts.

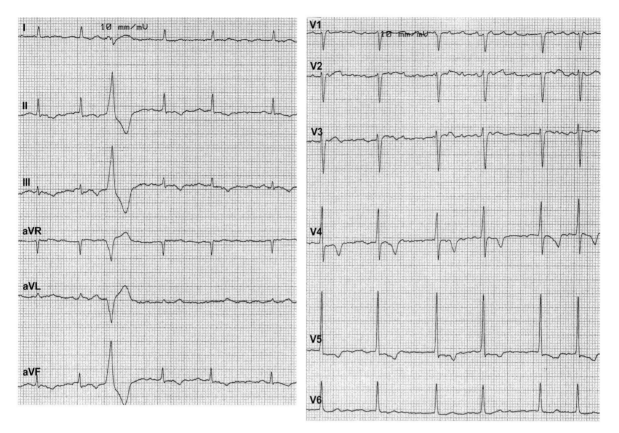

ECG 20.14

84y/m. Fibrillo–flutter. In lead V$_1$ flutter waves of variable configuration and at variable rates are seen. Absolute ventricular arrhythmia.

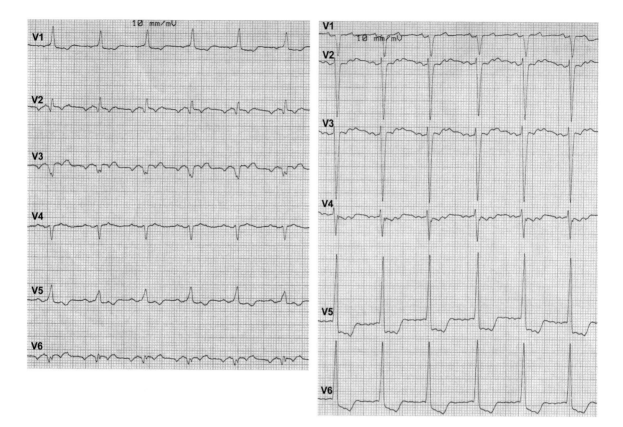

ECG 20.15

78y/m. Atrial flutter at a very slow rate, due to amiodarone, 164/min and 2 : 1 AV block. Deformation of the T wave and prolonged QT(U) interval (visible in V_2 to V_4) also induced by amiodarone. LVH and LV overload.

Chapter 21
Atrial Fibrillation

At a Glance

After ventricular premature beats (VPBs) and atrial premature beats (APBs), atrial fibrillation (AF) is the most frequent arrhythmia. Hemodynamics and symptoms are related to the ventricular rate and the loss of atrial contraction. The most important complication of AF is cerebral stroke. Moreover, AF is an independent risk factor for death. Therapy and prevention of AF are complex.

Etiology and Prevalence

The most common etiology in *chronic* AF is fibrosis of the atrial myocardium in older patients. Other etiologies include all diseases with chronic overload of the left atrium, such as hypertensive heart disease, cardiomyopathies of the left ventricle of any origin, left-sided valvular diseases (especially mitral stenosis), and many other conditions such as hyperthyroidism, infections, and alcohol abuse. The prevalence of AF is 0.5%–0.8% at age 51–60 years, and 9% at age 80–89 years.

Transient AF is often seen after open heart surgery (especially aortic and mitral valve surgery), in the acute stage of myocardial infarction, and also in hyperthyreosis and alcohol abuse. AF occasionally occurs in an otherwise normal heart, but in this case it is known as 'lone atrial fibrillation'.

ECG

The single reliable diagnostic ECG feature in AF is the *absolutely irregular ventricular response*, also called 'absolute arrhythmia' (ECG 21.1). This compulsory sign is always detectable in a rhythm strip. Note the pitfalls:

i.   In tachyventricular AF, the rhythm may be almost regular (pseudo-regularization; ECG 21.2).

ii. In the very rare combination of AF with complete atrioventricular (AV) block and escape rhythm, the ventricular rhythm is regular.

iii. Of course we also find a regular ventricular rhythm in AF associated with ventricular pacing.

In most cases of AF, the *f waves* (fibrillatory waves) are clearly visible. The f waves are completely irregular in respect to rhythm and configuration and have a rate of 350–500 (up to 650) per min. They are best detectable in leads V_1, III and aVF. We distinguish between coarse f waves (ECG 21.3) and fine f waves (ECG 21.4), both of which can sometimes be present in the same patient (ECG 21.5). However, there are some conditions where f waves cannot be detected:

i.   At very fast ventricular rates the f waves are hidden within the QRS complex and the repolarization waves (ECG 21.2).

ii. The f waves may also be masked by a bundle-branch block (BBB) that leads to prolongation of the ventricular cycle (ECG 21.6).

iii. In the presence of fibrotic atria with only a small rest of myocardial fibers the f waves are very small (ECG 21.7) or may even be lacking. In all these conditions, the correct diagnosis is made by the detection of absolute ventricular arrhythmia. In the presence of coarse f waves, the damage of the atrial muscle is generally less than in the presence of fine f waves, and is associated with better short- and long-term success of direct current (DC) conversion.

1   Hemodynamics

Fortunately, not all atrial impulses (rate 350–650/min) reach the ventricles. Many of them are blocked in the AV node. The other impulses are conducted at random intervals to the ventricles, thus leading to absolute arrhythmic ventricular activity. A very fast (and irregular) ventricular activity has great clinical importance. Similarly to very early VPBs, in every ventricular beat of AF with high instantaneous rate, the preceding diastole is shortened considerably, thus inhibiting normal ventricular filling and consequently reducing the stroke volume – in extreme conditions to just a few milliliters. This means that not every QRS complex induces a ventricular contraction that is sufficient for a palpable peripheral arterial pulse. The result is a 'peripheral pulse deficit' that may reach > 50% of the heart (i.e. ventricular) rate. The greater the peripheral pulse deficit, the smaller the cardiac output per minute.

2 Clinical Significance

AF is not necessarily a disease with symptoms and complications. About 50% of patients have no restrictions in their daily life and never suffer complications. The loss of the so-called atrial kick does not always cause symptoms. Yet 50% of patients have symptoms, including reduced work capacity, palpitations, even near-syncope, and perhaps more severe complications, the major one being cerebral stroke. The origin of embolism is thrombotic material within dilated atria, especially in the appendages. Whereas small pulmonary embolism is mostly asymptomatic, peripheral embolism often has serious consequences depending on the affected organs (cerebrum, intestine, limbs, and very rarely the coronary arteries). Moreover, AF may evoke or aggravate heart failure and it also reduces survival, especially in patients with heart decompensation.

Symptoms are generally due to an irregular ventricular response that is either too slow or, more often, too fast. Syncope is rare and may occur with ventricular rates above about 230/min or during (spontaneous) conversion in sinus rhythm (ECG 21.8) due to a longer atrial and ventricular standstill.

3 Therapy

The therapeutic approach includes drugs, direct current conversion and ablation or a combination of them. In most patients with AF, anticoagulation is necessary. For details see next section.

The Full Picture

Besides ventricular tachycardia (VT) and atrioventricular block (AV block) atrial fibrillation (AF) represents one of the most important and most fascinating arrhythmias. The diagnosis is not always easy and the prevention and therapy of AF is one of the perpetual evergreens of national postgraduate sessions, international meetings and 'consensus' conferences.

4 Etiology and Prevalence

Based on the Framingham study, the prevalence of AF has increased in men aged 65–84 from 3.2% in the period 1968–1970 to 9.1% in the period 1987–1998. The reason for this is unclear. It cannot be explained only by the fact that AF increases with age, with at least a doubled incidence for each decade of age [1]. It suggests also that the most common etiology of chronic AF is a degenerative process of the atrial muscle fibers that are replaced by fibrotic tissue.

While up to 200 ventricular or supraventricular PBs per 24 h are found in about 40% of healthy individuals, AF is hardly ever encountered in an otherwise normal heart [2]. In 'lone atrial fibrillation' the cause for the arrhythmia is unknown and the left atrium has normal dimensions. 'Lone AF' may occasionally lead to dilatation of the left atrium and in such cases it can no longer be regarded as lone. Hyperthyreosis, sometimes in its oligosymptomatic form, is found in about 5% of AF in middle-aged patients and needs to be excluded serologically [3]. In patients with apparent hyperthyreosis, AF occurs in 10%–20%, often transiently. Other causes of AF are hypertension, infectious or dilating heart disease, mitral valvular disease (formerly mitral stenosis in the main), aortic valvular disease, constrictive pericarditis, and atrial septal defect in older patients, and many other rare diseases. It is not well known that digitalis intoxication may provoke AF [4] in rare instances.

Obviously, AF in most cases develops after overload and organic injury of the left atrium and represents a consequence of left heart disease. In diseases of the right heart (the most frequent one is chronic cor pulmonale), the arrhythmia is rare and may occur transiently, usually as a sign of respiratory infection, or of respiratory or heart failure.

Transient AF occurs in acute myocardial infarction in 7%–16% [5,6] whereas chronic AF is not common in chronic coronary heart disease without congestive heart failure. In the CASS study only 126 of 18 630 patients (0.6%) with coronary heart disease had AF [7], that is a lower prevalence than in a general population of a comparable age. AF was negatively correlated with the number of diseased coronary arteries – an astonishing and unexplained phenomenon. AF in its transient form is commonly found in patients after open heart surgery, especially mitral and aortic valve replacement (in 20%–30%), and after lung and other operations [8].

In pulmonary embolism, transient AF is encountered more rarely than atrial flutter, although an early study reports an incidence of 10% [9]. AF by no means excludes a healthy sinus node. Indeed, all in all AF is only rarely connected with the 'sick sinus syndrome', usually with its bradycardia–tachycardia variant (see Chapter 22 Sick Sinus Syndrome).

ECG Special

5   Aberration in Atrial Fibrillation

As for any other supraventricular rhythm, AF may be conducted to the ventricles with every known aberration, such as bundle-branch block or fascicular block. However, two conditions are of particular interest.

5.1   Ashman Beats

If a relatively long R–R interval is followed by a near QRS complex showing a bundle-branch block configuration, ventricular aberration is much more probable than a VPB. This phenomenon is explained by the prolongation of the refractory period of the bundles by instantaneous bradycardia [10] and was first described by Gouaux and Ashman as long ago as 1947 [11]. Ashman beats are most probable if the phenomenon can be observed several times on a longer rhythm strip. Right bundle-branch block (RBBB) aberration (ECG 21.9) is much more frequent than left bundle-branch block (LBBB) aberration (ECG 21.10), because the refractory period is longer in the right bundle than in the left. After an Ashman beat a compensatory pause is lacking. This is in contrast to a VPB, which is usually followed by a compensatory pause. In an experimental setting, Pritched et al [12] have shown that a stimulated VPB is followed by a compensatory pause, thus confirming the findings of

Langendorf and Pick [13]. In practice, however (non-laboratory conditions), a full compensation after a real VPB is often missed. The correct diagnosis may be difficult.

5.2   Atrial Fibrillation in Pre-excitation (Wolff-Parkinson-White Syndrome)

In both common 'orthodromic' and rare 'antidromic' reentry tachycardia, the accessory pathway (AP) and the AV junction represent the circuit for conduction. In the first type the AP is used for retrograde conduction, and in the second type for antegrade conduction. The conduction of AF antegradely over an AP is rare but may represent the most tremendous arrhythmia in patients with pre-excitation. If the refractory time in antegrade conduction is very short, an abnormally high number of atrial impulses reach the ventricles, causing excessive fast ventricular activity and possible degeneration into ventricular fibrillation (VF).

Often a cautious analysis of the ECG allows differentiation between a fast regular VT or a supraventricular tachycardia with bundle-branch block, and tachyventricular AF with a pre-excitation pattern (eventually with pseudo-regularization of the rhythm at a high rate). In the first conditions delta waves are absent; in the last case delta waves are always present, generally best visible in the precordial leads (ECG 21.11). It is important to know that AF may occur in young patients and even in children with the Wolff-Parkinson-White (WPW) syndrome, thus including the possibility of VF [14]. It is absolutely contraindicated to give digitalis or verapamil intravenously in AF combined with pre-excitation. Both drugs slow conduction in the AV node and may enhance conduction antegradely in the accessory pathway. Death due to antegradely conducted AF (or rarely atrial flutter with 1:1 conduction) along an accessory pathway, with consecutive VF, is a rare but tragic event, particularly in young persons. This is one reason more why patients with WPW syndrome should be investigated by invasive electrophysiology and ablation should be performed (see Chapter 24 Wolff-Parkinson-White Syndrome).

6   Regular Ventricular Action in AF

Besides the presence of complete AV block with a 'physiological' escape rhythm or a paced ventricular rhythm, there is a rare but interesting rhythm disturbance that also appears with a regular rhythm. In some patients with sick sinus syndrome or bradycardia after (heart) operations, AF may be observed in combination with episodes of a regular AV junctional rhythm, in the *absence* of complete AV block. When this is the case, AV junction fibers take over the heart rhythm, thanks to their intrinsic rate (ECG 21.12). This happens only rarely because in AF with a very slow ventricular response the AV node is also diseased and its intrinsic rate is depressed. For this situation the terms 'accelerated AV junction rhythm' and 'functional AV block' may be used. On exercise, more atrial impulses are conducted to the ventricles and the usual arrhythmic response of the ventricles reappears.

7 Interatrial Dissociation in AF

Fibrillation of the left atrium and sinus rhythm of the right atrium (one possibility of interatrial dissociation [15]) represents an extremely rare condition; we have seen three cases in 30 years after DC conversion attempts to correct atrial fibrillation. The ECG was characterized by small p waves of short duration (0.05 sec), corresponding to the normal depolarization of the right atrium and fine fibrillation waves in lead V_1, corresponding to fibrillation of the left atrium. The rhythm was regular, the ventricles following the sinus node.

8 Differential Diagnosis

If AF *and* flutter-like waves are present in the same ECG, the term 'fibrillo-flutter' is used. This indicates an incomplete 'flutter circuit' in the right atrium that is partially fibrillating (for electrophysiologic details, see [16]). Functionally and clinically fibrillo-flutter has to be interpreted as a special form of AF. Absolute ventricular arrhythmia indicates AF (and rarely fibrillo-flutter) in 99%.

There is only *one* other and very rare arrhythmia where absolute ventricular arrhythmia is also present. It is called *multifocal atrial arrhythmia* or *chaotic atrial rhythm*. This arrhythmia shows p waves and is defined by four criteria:

i.   absolute atrial arrhythmia, and consequently
ii. absolute ventricular arrhythmia
iii. multiple configurations of the p wave
iv. changing PQ intervals, AV block 1° included (AV escape beats may occur).

The mean atrial and corresponding ventricular rate is generally < 100/min (ECG 21.13). The arrhythmia lasts several minutes or hours, occasionally for days. There is no effective drug or electric therapy. Degeneration to AF has been described but is extremely rare. Chaotic atrial rhythm is seen in many rare conditions, the most common being severe cor pulmonale, with or without digi-

talis medication. In these patients the in-hospital mortality rate is about 45% due to the underlying disease [17]. In practice, the diagnosis of multifocal atrial arrhythmia is made too often. This statement contrasts with the opinion of McCord and Borzak [18]. The diagnosis should only be made if the arrhythmia is continuous for at least several minutes. In some instances, in the presence of sinus beats and repetitive atrial premature beats with different p wave configurations, the diagnosis of multifocal atrial arrhythmia is not correct. In these cases the prognosis is much better. Multifocal atrial rhythm/tachycardia is also described in children, especially in those with congenital heart disease [19,20].

9 Electrophysiology

AF is introduced by an early atrial premature beat, occurring at the potentially vulnerable phase of atrial repolarization ('p on Ta'). ECG 21.14 shows spontaneous conversion of AF. After two sinusal beats AF is reintroduced by a premature atrial beat.

In AF the atria are not activated by a single electrical impulse but exposed to multiple chaotic wavelets that are unable to induce a regular and normal rhythm. Atrial depolarization in AF is based on the non-homogeneity of conduction and responsiveness of the atrial tissue. Recently, Haissaguerre et al [21] have found that electric impulses originating from a fast focal activity in the proximal parts of lung veins may be conducted to the left atrium and may induce AF.

The conduction of the irregular electric impulses from the fibrillating atria to the ventricles is of special interest. In sinus rhythm the stimulus is delayed in the AV node, enabling complete diastolic filling of the ventricles and thus assuring optimal sequential atrioventricular contractions. In AF the majority of the atrial impulses are blocked in the AV node, in order to prevent an excessively high ventricular rate. Only a restricted number of impulses – generally about 20%–30% – are conducted to the ventricles, at random intervals, thus inducing absolute ventricular arrhythmia. The ventricular rate depends on the degree of the slowing-down capacity of the AV node that acts within very large limits and is influenced by vagal and sympathetic tone, by drugs and by organic lesions. The conduction of the atrial impulses in AF, through the AV node to the ventricles, represents an example of concealed conduction.

The mechanism of spontaneous conversion of AF (ECGs 21.8, 21.14 and 21.15) is not clearly understood. However it exists, much in contrast to the non-existing spontaneous conversion in ventricular fibrillation, where conversion would be incomparably more wholesome.

10   Clinical Significance

AF is an independent risk factor for death, with a relative risk of 1.5 for men and 1.9 for women [22]. In the presence of ventricular dysfunction, the increased mortality seems to be primarily due to heart failure [23] and stroke [1]. Also drug therapy with anticoagulants [24] especially with an INR (international normalized ration) of > 3.5 [25] and antiarrhythmic substances may contribute to mortality in some cases.

Cerebral stroke is the most severe complication of AF, with a strikingly increasing incidence with aging (1.15% at age 50–59 years and 23.5% at age 80–89 [1]). Stroke represents the main factor for morbidity, with more or less severely impaired quality of life.

A recent study on all hospitalizations in Scotland (5.1 million inhabitants) revealed a tremendous increase in hospitalization of patients with the principal diagnosis of atrial fibrillation during the last few years, and a corresponding increase in costs. The cause is probably the higher age of the population and, more importantly, a change in medical practice [26].

11   Therapy and Prevention

Therapeutic and prophylactic approaches are multiple and complex [27] and have been extensively evaluated in the ACS/AHA/ESC guidelines for the management of patients with atrial fibrillation [28]. In principal, both electric or drug therapy/prophylaxis, or a combination of them, is possible.

11.1 Electric and Drug Conversion

Conversion to sinus rhythm is either attempted with electric DC conversion (with 50–200 Joules) or with drugs, especially amiodarone, beta-blockers or, more recently, ibutilide [29]. If AF lasts for more than 24 h, oral anticoagulation for 3 weeks within therapeutic levels is *mandatory* before conversion is attempted, either electrically or with drugs. Anticoagulation should be continued for at least 3 months because thromboembolic events most often occur in the first 3 months after DC conversion [30].

11.2 Implantable Defibrillator

Some selected patients with paroxysmal AF are treated by an implantable defibrillator device. For several reasons the method is not yet generally used [31].

11.3 Maze Procedure and Catheter Ablation

With the surgical open-heart method (so-called 'maze procedure') a complicated 'canalization' within the right atrium is realized, thus isolating and abolishing regions with chaotic activity and allowing only one major route for an electrical impulse (the sinusal one) to travel from the top to the bottom of the heart [32]. A new interventional technique with mapping-guided ablation of lung veins was recently introduced by Haissaguerre et al [33].

11.4 Pacemaker

With a sophisticated atrial (or dual chamber) pacemaker device, the induction of AF is partly inhibited by atrial rate stabilization and pacing intervention on APBs [31,34].

11.5 Prevention of Recurrent AF

Attempts have been made to prevent recurrent AF with drugs such as beta-blockers, propafenone and amiodarone, and atrial pacing devices as mentioned above [35]. Calcium antagonists like verapamil and diltiazem are less effective. Quinidine has been abandoned, especially in large doses, due to its proarrhythmic effect (possible induction of VT, type torsade de pointes, with a mortality rate of a few percent per year). Digitalis has been classified as ineffective in more recent literature, but it has been used successfully by many cardiologists, alone or in combination with the other drugs mentioned here.

11.6 New-Onset Atrial Fibrillation

New onset AF is often an innocent condition, reversible in about 50% of people within 24 h, without therapy. During the last 12 years, the author has been consulted by five in-hospital colleagues who have themselves suffered new-onset AF.

Short Story/Case Report 1

In 1990 a 32-year-old man with an otherwise normal heart, had palpitations during a viral infection. The ECG showed AF. There was conversion without therapy after 8 h, with no relapse.

Short Story/Case Report 2

In 1992 a 38-year-old woman had palpitations after a party, where she had consumed an unusual amount of alcohol. She had a normal heart, but the ECG showed AF. She received therapy with propanolol 20 mg twice a day and there was conversion after 16 hours (whether post or propter). She was relapse-free, without drugs.

Short Story/Case Report 3

In 1998 a 53-year-old man had palpitations after alcohol excess. His heart was normal but the ECG showed AF. Therapy was refused. Conversion occurred after 10 hours. After reduced alcohol intake there was no relapse.

Short Story/Case Report 4

In 1999 a 60-year-old man had palpitations and near-syncope while taking a shower after vigorous jogging on a hot summer's day. He had a known mild mitral incompetence and a normal left atrium. ECG showed AF. There was spontaneous conversion after 30 min during ECG registration. No relapse occurred; no prophylaxis was given.

Short Story/Case Report 5

In 2001 a 63-year-old man had palpitations with malaise. He sought consultation 3 days later. This revealed untreated moderate hypertension and a slightly enlarged left ventricle and left atrium. The ECG revealed AF. Therapy was started with an ACE inhibitor, atenolol 50 mg and anticoagulation. The AF persisted. After 3 weeks, the patient refused electroconversion and amiodarone but accepted the addition of digitalis. Conversion occurred 1 week later. There had been no relapse with this therapy 14 months later.

Conclusion: none of these patients had complications and none was hospitalized. In most situations, new-onset AF can be treated conservatively.

11.7 Rate Control

For control of a fast ventricular rate, digitalis is effective at rest, while beta-blockers have a better effect during exercise. In drug refractory tachycardia, *catheter ablation of the AV node* (generally its slow pathway) with consecutive implantation of a pacemaker, is an established therapy. Pure and symptomatic bradycardia needs a pacemaker. In the bradycardia/tachycardia variant (with or without the sick sinus syndrome) pacemaker and drug therapy are combined.

11.8 Prevention of Thromboembolism

Oral anticoagulation is much more effective than aspirin. Today there is no upper age limit for anticoagulation if contraindications such as hypertension, anamnestic major bleeding complications and so on are taken closely into account, and the therapeutic level is held at an INR between (2.0?) 2.5 and 3.0 (3.5).

Overall the 'handling' of AF has remained problematic, in spite of numerous symposia and consensus sessions [27].

11.9 Drug Rate Control versus Electroconversion

For decades it was not known if either attempts to restore SR or rate control and anticoagulation with warfarine is better for survival of patients with AF. Running multicenter studies and trials as AFFIRM, PIAF, PAFAC and STAF should give a definitive answer to this important question [36]. The results of some studies (STAF, AFFIRM, RACE) have recently been published revealing no significant difference between the two therapeutic methods in the endpoints of death, cerebral stroke, major bleeding or cardiac arrest [37].

Probably these results will reduce a worldwide obsession to re-establish sinus rhythm in almost every patient with atrial fibrillation with DC conversions which reached another summit, comparable with the enthusiasm just after the introduction of this therapeutic method 35 years ago. Yet many physicians have the impression that the long-term results of preserving sinus rhythm with *antiarrhythmic drugs* have not improved so much during the last few decades, especially in patients older than 65 years with a markedly dilated left atrium and with AF lasting more than 6 months. However, several publications suggest better long-term results, especially with the use of amiodarone and propafenone [38,39]. DC conversion in patients with post-thyrotoxic AF reveals by far the best long-term results. In the study of Nakazawa et al [40] 67% of 106 patients with AF (lasting < 12 months in 87% of cases) were in sinus rhythm after a follow-up of 80.6 ± 37 months.

11.10 Final Remarks

Catheter-induced ablation [33] represents a promising step forward in the treatment of AF. However, complications related to the procedure and insufficient late results have restricted the general use of the method so far [27].

The main purpose of re-establishing sinus rhythm (by any method) is to achieve sufficient atrial contraction to prevent thromboembolism and to improve hemodynamics. However, in a dilated and fibrotic left atrium, contraction remains poor even after conversion; in this case neither goal is reached. Hence, there remain some important problems in the treatment and prevention of AF to be resolved in the future.

References

1. Kannel WB, Wolf PA, Benjamin EJ, Levy D. Prevalence, incidence, prognosis, and predisposing conditions for atrial fibrillation: population-based estimates. Am J Cardiol 1998;82:2N–9N
2. Kopecky SL, Gersh BJ, McGoon MD, et al. The natural history of lone atrial fibrillation. A population-based study over three decades. N Engl J Med 1987;317:669–74
3. Forfar JC, Miller HC, Toft AD. Occult thyrotoxicosis: a correctable cause of idiopathic atrial fibrillation. Am J Cardiol 1979;44:9–12
4. Irons GV, Orgain ES. Digitalis-induced arrhythmias and their management. Prog Cardiovasc Dis 1966;8:539
5. Sugiura T, Iwasaka T, Ogawa A, et al. Atrial fibrillation in acute myocardial infarction. Am J Cardiol 1985;56:27–9
6. Goldberg RJ, Seeley D, Becker RC, et al. Impact of atrial fibrillation on the in-hospital and long-term survival of patients with acute myocardial infarction: a community-wide perspective. Am Heart J 1990;119:996–1001
7. Cameron A, Schwartz MJ, Kronmal RA, Kosinski AS. Prevalence and significance of atrial fibrillation in coronary artery disease (CASS registry). Am J Cardiol 1988;61:714–7
8. Ommen SR, Odell JA, Stanton MS. Atrial arrhythmias after cardiothoracic surgery. N Engl J Med 1997;336:1429–34
9. Weber DM, Phillips JH. A re-evaluation of electrocardiographic changes accompanying acute pulmonary embolism. Am J Med Sci 1966;251:381
10. Marriott HJL, Sandler IA. Criteria, old and new, for differentiating between ectopic ventricular beats and aberrant ventricular conduction in the presence of atrial fibrillation. Prog Cardiovasc Dis 1966;9:18
11. Gouaux JL, Ashman R. Auricular fibrillation with aberration simulating ventricular paroxysmal tachycardia. Am Heart J 1947;34:366
12. Pritched ELC, Smith WM, Klein GJ, et al. The compensatory pause of atrial fibrillation. Circulation 1980;62:1021–5
13. Langendorf R, Pick A. Artificial pacing of the human heart: its contribution to the understanding of arrhythmias. Am J Cardiol 1971;28:516–25
14. Wellens HJJ, Durrer D. Wolff-Parkinson-White syndrome and atrial fibrillation: relation between refractory period of the accessory pathway and ventricular rate during atrial fibrillation. Am J Cardiol 1974;34:777–82
15. Zipes DP, DeJoseph RL. Dissimilar atrial rhythms in man and dog. Am J Cardiol 1973;32:618–28
16. Saoudi N, Cosio F, Waldo A, et al. A classification of atrial and regular atrial tachycardia according to electrophysiological mechanisms and anatomical bases. Eur Heart J 2001;22:1162–82
17. Scher DL, Arsura EL. Multifocal atrial tachycardia: mechanisms, clinical correlates, and treatment. Am Heart J 1989;118:574–80
18. McCord J, Borzak S. Multifocal atrial tachycardia. Chest 1998; 113:203–9
19. Liberthson RR, Colan SD. Multifocal or chaotic atrial rhythm: report of nine infants, delineation of clinical course and management, and review of the literature. Pediatr Cardiol 1982;2:179–84
20. Yeager SB, Hougen TJ, Levy AM. Sudden death in infants with chaotic atrial rhythm. Am J Dis Child 1984;138:689–92
21. Haissaguerre M, Jais P, Shah DC, Takahashi A. Spontaneous initiation of atrial fibrillation by ectopic beats originating in the pulmonary veins. N Engl J Med 1998;339:659–66
22. Benjamin EJ, Wolf PA, D'Agostino RB, et al. Impact of atrial fibrillation on the risk of death: the Framingham Heart Study. Circulation 1998;98:946–52
23. Dries DL, Exner DV, Gersh BJ, et al. Atrial fibrillation is associated with an increased risk for mortality and heart failure progression in patients with asymptomatic and symptomatic left ventricular systolic dysfunction: a retrospective analysis of the SOLVD trials. J Am Coll Cardiol 1998;32:695–703
24. Hart RG, Boop BS, Anderson DC. Oral anticoagulants and intracranial hemorrhage. Facts and hypotheses. Stroke 1995;26:1471–7
25. Chesebro JH, Siebers DO, Holland AE, et al. Bleeding during antithrombotic therapy in patients with atrial fibrillation. Arch Intern Med 1996;156:409–16
26. Stewart S, Macintyre K, MacLeod MMC, et al. Trends in hospital activity, morbidity and case fatality related to atrial fibrillation in Scotland, 1986–1996. Eur Heart J 2001;22:693–701
27. Falk RH. Atrial fibrillation. N Engl J Med 2001;344:1067–78
28. Fuster V, Ryden LE, Asinger RW, et al. ACC/AHA/ESC Guidelines for the management of patients with atrial fibrillation. Circulation 2001;104:2118–50
29. Murray KT. Ibutilide. Circulation 1998;97:493–7
30. Van Gelder IC, Crijns HJ, Van Gilst WH, et al. Prediction of uneventful cardioversion and maintenance of sinus rhythm from direct-current electrical cardioversion of chronic atrial fibrillation and flutter. Am J Cardiol 1991;68:41–6
31. Cooper JM, Katcher MS, Orlov MV. Current concepts. Implantable devices for the treatment of atrial fibrillation. New Engl J Med 2002;348:2062–8
32. Cox JL, Schuessler RB, D'Agustino HJ, et al. The surgical treatment of atrial fibrillation. III. Development of a definitive surgical procedure. J Thorac Cardiovasc Surg 1991;101:569–83
33. Haissaguerre M, Shah DC, Jais P, et al. Mapping-guided ablation of pulmonary veins to cure atrial fibrillation. Am J Cardiol 2000;86(9 Suppl I):K9–K19

34. Wellens HJJ, Lau CP, Lüderitz B, et al (For the METRIX investigators). Atroverter: An implantable device for the treatment of atrial fibrillation. Circulation 1998;98:1651–6

35. Alessie MA, Boyden PA, Camm AJ, Kléber AG, et al. Pathophysiology and prevention of atrial fibrillation. Circulation 2001;103:769–77

36. Wyse DG, Anderson JL, Antman EM, et al. Atrial fibrillation follow-up investigation of rhythm management: The AFFIRM study design. Am J Cardiol 1997;79:1198–202

37. Saxonhouse SJ, Curtis AB. Risks and benefits of rate control versus maintenance of sinus rhythm. Am J Cardiol 2003;91(suppl.):27D–32D

38. Tieleman RG, Gosselink AT, Crjins HJGM, et al. Efficacy, safety and determinants of conversion of atrial fibrillation and flutter with oral amiodarone. Am J Cardiol 1997;79:53–7

39. Kochiadakis GE, Marketon ME, Igoumenidis ME, et al. Amiodarone, sotalol, or propafenone in atrial fibrillation; which is preferred to maintain normal sinus rhythm? Pacing Clin Electrophysiol 2000;23:1883–7

40. Nakazawa D, Lythall DA, Noh J, et al. Is there a place for the late conversion of atrial fibrillation? A long-term follow-up study of patients with post-thyrotoxic atrial fibrillation. Europ Heart J 2000;21:327–33

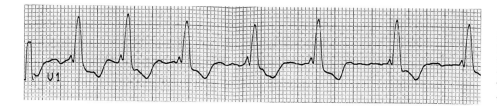

ECG 21.1
86y/f. Lead V_1. AF with the compulsory 'absolute ventricular arrhythmia'. The f waves are scarcely visible. RBBB.

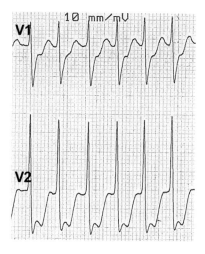

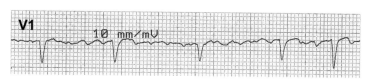

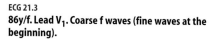

ECG 21.2
75y/m. Leads V_2 and V_3.
Pseudoregularization of ventricular rhythm in tachycardic AF, rate about 180/min. ST depression of 10 mm in V_2, probably due to true ischemia and tachycardia.

ECG 21.3
86y/f. Lead V_1. Coarse f waves (fine waves at the beginning).

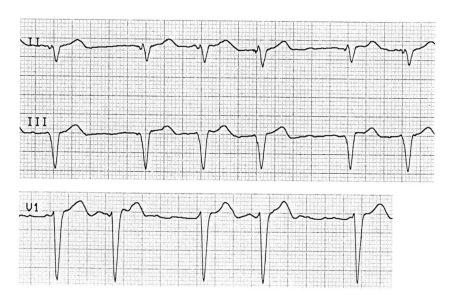

ECG 21.4
67y/m. Leads II, III, V_1. Fine f waves.

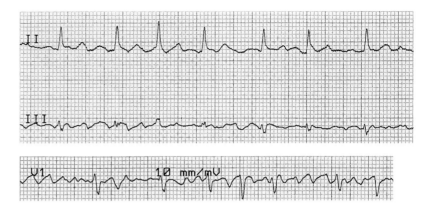

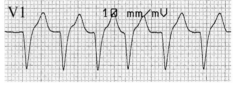

ECG 21.5
72y/f. Leads I, II, V$_1$. Coarse and fine f waves in the same patient.

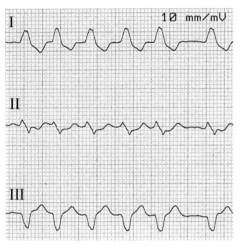

ECG 21.6
91y/f. Leads I, II, III, V$_1$. No visible f waves, in the presence of LBBB.

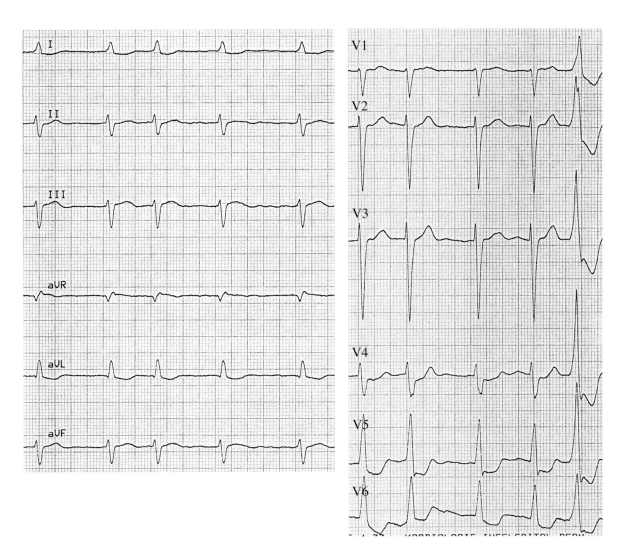

ECG 21.7

77y/m. Very small f waves in lead III (II, V₁). LVH and ST depression V₅/V₆ (V₄), The last beat is not an aberrant beat, but a VPB (positive QRS deflection in all precordial leads).

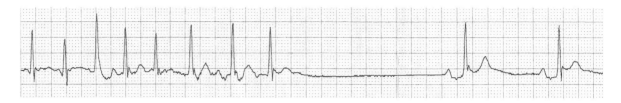

ECG 21.8
79y/m. Spontaneous conversion of AF. Ventricular pause before sinus rhythm 2.6 sec.

ECG 21.9
Lead II. RBBB aberration for two beats, where the rate is faster than in the other beats. Aberration occurs after a relatively long R–R interval.

ECG 21.10
Lead V$_2$. LBBB aberration for four beats, where the rhythm is slightly irregular and the rate relatively fast. Aberration occurs after a relatively long R–R interval. A VT could be excluded.

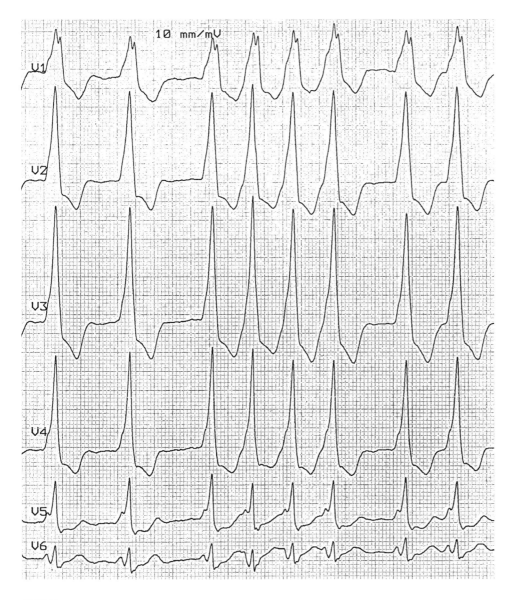

ECG 21.11

72y/m. ECG (V$_1$ to V$_6$): AF in pre-excitation (WPW syndrome). The delta wave in V$_6$ imitates a p wave.

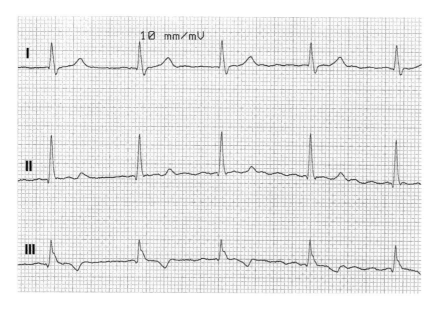

ECG 21.12

71y/f. AF *without ventricular arrhythmia*. The regular rhythm (rate 63/min) is due to an AV junctional escape (or 'accelerated') rhythm, *without* complete AV block. During mild exercise, the patient had AF at a ventricular irregular rate of about 80/min.

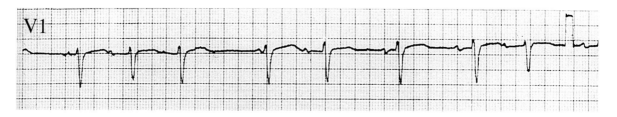

ECG 21.13

60y/m. Severe obstructive lung disease. Hypertension. Digoxin 0.125 mg/day, diuretics. ECG (lead V_1): chaotic/multifocal atrial rhythm with absolute ventricular arrhythmia. Instantaneous rate between 50/min and 85/min. P wave morphology is always different, so are the PQ intervals.

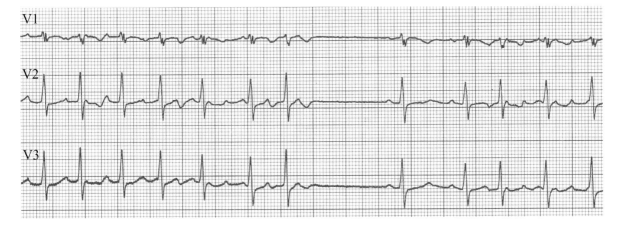

ECG 21.14
66y/f. AF (fibrillo-flutter) with spontaneous conversion. After two sinus beats an APB provokes AF again.

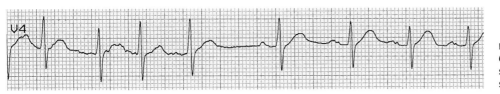

ECG 21.15
69y/m. ECG (lead V₄): spontaneous conversion of AF.

Chapter 22
Sick Sinus Syndrome (and Carotid Sinus Syndrome)

At a Glance

The sick sinus syndrome is a disease of the sinus node and occurs in middle-aged and older patients, with some exceptions. The most probable predominant etiology is a degenerative process of the sinus node with frequent involvement of the AV node. Other etiologies include coronary heart disease (CHD), infectious diseases, and other rare conditions. Clinically the etiology often remains unclear and is classified as 'unknown'. In the section 'The Full Picture' the carotid sinus syndrome, which is different from the sick sinus syndrome, is briefly discussed.

ECG

1 Characteristics

The sick sinus syndrome often represents a *collection* of ECG signs that include the features described below.

1.1 Sinus Bradycardia

At *rest,* a sinus rate of less than 50 per minute.

At *exercise,* or under drug-induced sympathetic stimulation (with adrenaline or isoprenalin), a sinus rate of less than 90 per minute.

1.2 Sinus Standstill/Arrest

See ECGs 22.1 and 22.2. In sinus arrest there is no impulse formation in the sinus node. In the ECG, sinus arrest can often not be distinguished from sinoatrial (SA) block 2° or complete SA block. Longer episodes with absent p waves favor sinus arrest. Periodic absence of p waves can be indicative of SA block 2°.

1.3 Exit Block or Sinoatrial Block

See ECG 22.3. SA block is a conduction block either within the sinus node, or between the sinus node and the surrounding fibers that normally conduct the sinus impulse to the atria and the atrioventricular (AV) node. Obviously in cases with episodes of ventricular asystole, the AV junction is also involved, because an AV junction escape rhythm does not arise. As in AV block, SA block is subdivided into SA block 1°, two or three forms of SA block 2°, and complete SA block. Commonly only the SA block type 2° with 2 : 1 or 3 : 1 block are diagnosed in the routine ECG or by Holter or monitor stripe. Longer episodes of complete SA block cannot be distinguished from sinus arrest.

1.4 Bradycardia–Tachycardia Variant

See ECGs 22.4 and 22.5. We find changes from *bradycardic* episodes (sinus arrest, SA block, sinus bradycardia) to episodes of *tachycardia,* including salvos of atrial premature beats, generally irregular atrial tachycardia, atrial flutter, atrial fibrillation and, rarely, AV nodal re-entry tachycardia. Episodes of tachycardia generally occur as a reaction to bradycardia or are induced by atrial premature beats. *Isolated atrial fibrillation* is in most cases a consequence of a hemodynamic overload or, in older people, of fibrosis of the *left* atrium. Let us remember that the sinus node is situated in the *right* atrium. Atrial fibrillation in chronic and acute cor pulmonale is rare indeed. There are cases, however, where atrial fibrillation represents a clinically important component of the sick sinus syndrome.

Often several signs of the sick sinus syndrome are detectable in the same patient (ECG 22.5).

1.5 AV Node and Bundle Branches

In many cases the AV node and in some cases the bundle branches are involved in the disease, with two consequences. Firstly, the AV node often fails to act as an escape pacemaker during episodes of SA block or sinus standstill. Secondly, an additional AV block of all degrees and a bundle-branch block are present in about 16% of cases of sick sinus syndrome. The progression to complete AV block is 2.6% per year.

2 Clinical Significance

The *diagnosis* of sick sinus syndrome is made on the basis of the ECG abnormalities mentioned above. The *clinical significance* of sick sinus syndrome depends on the severity of symptoms, such as palpitations, impaired work capacity, dizziness, presyncope, and syncope. Before therapy is performed, the correlation between the symptoms and the ECG abnormalities should be confirmed. Ambulatory ECG is the best diagnostic method; other parameters, such as electrophysiologic testing (determination of the sinus node recovery time (SNRT)) are not as reliable as previously thought.

The sick sinus syndrome may be a very *capricious* disease, with multiple attacks within a short time on one hand, and long normal intervals on the other. Thus the results of ambulatory ECGs may be falsely negative. In cases of doubt, long-term ambulatory monitoring for 1 week may be preferable.

3 Prognosis and Complications

The sick sinus syndrome is a chronic disease with a more or less rapid progression. The eventual episodes of syncope are generally shorter than those that occur in the presence of complete AV block with asystolic episodes. The most important *complication* of the disease is a *cerebral stroke*, especially in cases associated with atrial fibrillation. A stroke is best prevented by oral anticoagulation.

Compared to chronic (especially infra-His) complete AV block, the chance for survival is much better in the sick sinus syndrome. Survival in symptomatic sick sinus syndrome is impaired by stroke, heart failure, and complications of associated CHD.

4 Therapy

Drug therapy is a problem for patients with bradycardia and is impossible in cases of the bradycardia-tachycardia variant. A *pacemaker* is implanted in patients who have symptoms *plus* ECG abnormalities (dual chamber or atrial inhibited pacing in younger patients). Pacing generally eliminates many symptoms, thus improving quality of life, but does not significantly affect survival. In the bradycardia-tachycardia variant, antiarrhythmic drugs must be added to avoid tachycardic episodes. One or two episodes of cardiac asystole that occur in patients in the first days after a heart operation (or during or shortly after other operations) only rarely correspond to a diseased sinus node. They are mostly caused by enhanced vagal tone (ECG 22.6) and they disappear spontaneously. Temporary pacing is only needed in exceptional instances.

The Full Picture

5 Prevalence and Etiology

The first monograph about the syndrome was published in 1974 by Mary Irene Ferrer, the Queen of the sick sinus syndrome [1]. The sick sinus syndrome is a fascinating disease that is based on the abundance and capricious behavior of arrhythmic manifestations, on difficulties in finding the true diagnosis, and on the varied etiology.

Excluding the countless patients in the 'third world', the worldwide prevalence of symptomatic sick sinus syndrome can be estimated by the number of pacemakers implanted; this was 569 000 in 1997 and 601 000 in 1998. The sick sinus syndrome accounts for about 50% of pacemaker implantations. In about 300 000 patients a year, therefore, a symptomatic syndrome is diagnosed and treated with a pacemaker.

For unknown reasons, sick sinus syndrome occurs twice as often in women.

In practice, the definitive etiology often remains unknown. If there are no signs of CHD or cardiomyopathy of another etiology, the most frequent histopathologic finding is a degenerative fibrotic process that involves the fibers of the sinus node and its transitional cells, which can expand to the atrial fibers, the AV node, and even the bundle of His and its ramifications [2,3]. CHD is also a common cause for sick sinus syndrome that may be chronic or acute. The acute and generally reversible type is occasionally encountered in acute inferior myocardial infarction (MI). The sinus node has a potentially doubled coronary supply, with a dominant artery arising from the proximal right coronary artery and a 'reserve' artery arising from one of the great branches of the left coronary artery [4]. This guarantees the restoration of normal sinus node function within hours or a few days after inferior MI. Other etiologies include hypertensive and hypertrophic cardiomyopathy and, in rare cases, acute myocarditis, rheumatic heart disease, congenital heart disease (especially after Mustard operation for transposition of the great arteries), mitral valve prolapse, connective tissue diseases, myxedema, amyloidosis, hemochromatosis, scleroderma, and muscular dystrophy. Metastatic involvement of the sinus node in malignant tumors has been described, as well as the very rare familial version of the syndrome [1,5–7].

6   Pseudo versus True Sick Sinus Syndrome

Some ECG manifestations may be misinterpreted as true sick sinus syndrome.

6.1   Influence of Drugs

Drugs as beta-adrenergic blockers, digitalis, verapamil, diltiazem [8] and amiodarone [9] may lead to transient sinus node dysfunction or may unveil a hitherto silent sick sinus syndrome.

6.2   Abnormal Vagal Reaction After Invasive Procedures

Sinus bradycardia and even complete cardiac asystole lasting several seconds have occasionally been seen after heart opera-

tions and other operations or investigative procedures. These can occur with or without a longer decrease in blood pressure. In some cases neurovasal syncope occurs. The patient is usually observed on a monitor, and the problem normally resolves after atropine therapy, hydration, and/or 'antishock position'. The cause is an abnormal vagal reaction to pain, to aspiration of bronchial secretion, or to unknown agents. In these cases, true sick sinus syndrome can be detected only rarely.

Short Story/Case Report 1

A 68-year-old man had a sudden asystole while sitting on a chair, 36 h after an aortocoronary bypass operation. The nurse was alerted by the monitor and hurried to the patient who told her that he had probably slept for a moment. ECG stripe: sinus rhythm (mimicking atrial flutter) at a rate of 105/min. Sudden sinus arrest, first escape beat after ≥ 9.7 sec. After another short pause, sinus rhythm arose again (ECG 22.6). The patient was monitored for 48 h, then two Holter ECGs were performed. No other asystole occurred and the patient was dismissed without electrophysiologic investigation and without a pacemaker. He was well 4 years later but was lost to follow-up.

This case is extraordinary not only because of the long cardiac standstill. During vagal maneuvers (aspiration of tracheal secretion) the patient had no bradycardia. However, when sitting calmly on a chair sudden asystole occurred; the cause is not clear. An ECG artifact can be excluded by a discreet 'warming-up phenomenon' of the sinus node after the long pause and the occurrence of a second (short) pause. In view of the favorable outcome, the single episode of cardiac asystole corresponds to 'pseudo sick sinus syndrome', despite the prolonged cardiac standstill.

6.3   Excessive Sinus Bradycardia in Athletes

Athletes generally have sinus bradycardia at rest, occasionally at a rate of 25–30/min. In rare cases, an AV nodal or even ventricular escape rhythm is present. On exercise the sinus rate increases adequately. True sick sinus syndrome is extremely rare [10].

6.4   Atrial Premature Beats with AV Block

The pattern of AV blocked atrial premature beats (APBs) may imitate an SA block, especially if the premature p wave is hidden within the T wave. Precise analysis of the ECG, in most cases ambulatory ECG, allows the correct diagnosis to be made (ECG 22.7).

6.5 'Laboratory' Sick Sinus Syndrome

In a few patients without any symptoms related to sinus node dysfunction, electrophysiologic investigation reveals electric characteristics that are typical of sick sinus syndrome, such as prolonged sinus node recovery time (SNRT) and sinoatrial conduction time (SACT). These patients should not receive a pacemaker although clinical control is needed. The development of symptomatic sick sinus syndrome within months or years is possible.

6.6 Sinus Nodal Re-entry Tachycardia

Although the sinus node is involved in sinus nodal reentry tachycardia, this arrhythmia is not common in patients with sick sinus syndrome. It occurs in every age group, often in otherwise healthy individuals, and generally with a rate of about 130/min (80/min to 200/min!) [11]. This arrhythmia is often not diagnosed. Severe symptoms are rare however.

7 Hypersensitive Carotid Sinus Syndrome

With the postmicturition syndrome, 'swallow syncope', and other conditions, the hypersensitive carotid sinus syndrome belongs to the great family of neurally mediated syncopal syndromes [12]. The carotid sinus syndrome is found in older patients and is often associated with CHD [13]. Two types can be distinguished, cardioinhibitory and vasodepressor types, and they may be combined.

The mechanisms of carotid sinus syndrome include abnormal vagal function, baroreflex hypersensitivity, and hyper-responsiveness to acetylcholine. Rarely, the hypersensitive carotid sinus syndrome and the sick sinus syndrome are *combined*.

7.1 Cardioinhibitory Type

The cardioinhibitory type is defined as ventricular arrest of 3 sec or more that occurs spontaneously or after carotid sinus massage. The ventricular pause is more often due to sinus arrest or to SA block (absence of QRS *and* p; ECG 22.8) than to sinus or atrial rhythm with complete AV block without AV junctional or ventricular escape rhythm (absence of QRS com-

plexes and presence of p waves, ECG 22.9). Longer ventricular pauses lead to presyncope and syncope and are generally treated with a pacemaker, usually dual-chambered. Asymptomatic patients, especially older ones, with cardiac arrest of 3 sec or more, provoked by carotid sinus massage, should not be fitted with a pacemaker.

7.2 Vasodepressor Type

The vasodepressor type (vasodepressor carotid sinus hypersensitivity) is characterized by a decrease of systolic blood pressure of more than 30–50 mmHg, without rhythm disturbance, after carotid sinus massage. Symptomatic patients are treated with sodium retaining drugs and elastic support hose, and in some cases with radiation or surgical denervation of the carotid sinus.

8 Symptoms and Complications

Frequent *symptoms* include decreased exercise tolerance, dizziness, short blackouts, and palpitations. Occasionally, paroxysmal dyspnea, angina, or heart failure are encountered. It is interesting that the symptoms (even a stroke) may precede by years the moment of diagnosis or pacemaker implantation [14]. Because arrhythmias and symptoms often occur at wide intervals, diagnosis is often impossible on the basis of one Holter ECG. It is preferable to use an event Holter registration over 1–2 weeks, or an 'implantable' loop recorder (ILR) [15].

The most important complication is cerebral stroke, which affects 1%–3% per year [16] and is mostly associated with atrial fibrillation, and syncope that affects 40%–70% of patients.

9 Electrophysiologic Testing

The sinus node recovery time (SNRT) and the corrected SNRT (CSNRT; i.e. SNRT minus the basic cycle of sinus rhythm before atrial pacing) is prolonged to > 525 msec. Prolongation of the SA conduction time (SACT) may sustain the diagnosis [17]. Today the indication for a pacemaker implantation is seldom based on electrophysiologic data [18] but on ECG findings connected with relevant symptoms.

10 Therapy

Earlier publications [19,20] showed a striking reduction in complications (especially cerebral stroke) and mortality in patients treated with dual-chamber (DDD) pacemakers compared to ventricular inhibited (VVI) pacing. In later trials, such as the CTOPP [21], PASE [22], and MOST [23], these results were not confirmed. However, a substantial reduction in symptoms was found, together with a reduction of the pacemaker syndrome and improved quality of life, legitimating the use of DDD pacing [24]. Associated AV nodal disturbances and major intraventricular conduction disorders, such as bundle-branch blocks, are found in 16.6% of cases [25] and justify ventricular pacing substitution. In younger patients single atrial inhibited pacing (AAI) may be preferable. New onset conduction disturbances appear at a rate of 2.6% per year [25].

In practice, primary implanted VVI pacing devices have to be replaced by DDD devices in a substantial number of patients who have annoying symptoms.

All in all, conservative management is unrewarding. Only those patients with bradycardia who refuse a pacemaker should receive theophylline [26], with overall modest success. Alternatively, pindolol, a beta-blocker with intrinsic sympathicomimetic action, may influence bradycardia favorably [27].

References

1. Ferrer MI. The sick sinus syndrome. Mt Kisco, NY: Futura Publishing 1974
2. Kaplan BM, Langendorf R, Lev M, Pick A. Tachycardia–bradycardia syndrome (so-called "sick sinus syndrome"). Pathology, mechanisms and treatment. Am J Cardiol 1973;31:497–508
3. Rodriguez RD, Schocken DD. Update on sick sinus syndrome, a cardiac disorder of aging. Geriatrics 1990;45:26–30, 33–36
4. Kyriakidis MK, Kourouklis CB, Papaioannou JT, et al. Sinus node coronary arteries studied with angiography. Am J Cardiol 1983;51:749–50
5. Rubenstein JJ, Schulman CL, Yurchak PM, De Sanctis RW. Clinical spectrum of the sick sinus syndrome. Circulation 1972;46:5–13
6. Chou TC. Sinus Rhythm. In: Chou TC (ed). Electrocardiography in Clinical Practice, Adult and Pediatric, fourth edn. Philadelphia: WB Saunders 1991, pp 336–7
7. Mehta AV, Chidambaram B, Garrett A. Familial symptomatic sinus bradycardia: autosomal dominant inheritance. Pediatr Cardiol 1995;16:231–4
8. Crossen KJ, Cain ME. Assessment and management of sinus node dysfunction. Mod Concept Cardiovasc Dis 1986;55:43
9. Hoffmann A, Kappenberger L, Jost M, Burckhardt D. Effect of amiodarone on sinus node function in patients with sick sinus syndrome. Clin Cardiol 1987;10:451–2
10. Bertrand E, Le Gallais D, N'Dori R. The Flack test: a test exploring the sinus function in athletes. Apropos of 351 tests. Arch Mal Coeur Vaiss 1987;80:1533–9
11. Gomes JA, Mehta D, Langan MN. Sinus node reentrant tachycardia. Pacing Clin Electrophysiol 1995;18:1045–57
12. Benditt DG. Neurally mediated syncopal syndromes: pathophysiological concepts and clinical evaluation. Pacing Clin Electrophysiol 1997;20:572–84 (review)
13. Kenny RA, Richardson DA. Carotid sinus syndrome and falls in older adults. Am J Geriatr Cardiol 2001;10:97–9
14. Gurtner HP, Lenzinger HR, Dolder M. Clinical aspects of the sick sinus syndrome. In Luederitz B (ed). Cardiac pacing. Berlin: Springer 1976, pp 12–24
15. Mieszczanska H, Ibrahim B, Cohen TJ. Initial clinical experience with implantable loop recorders. J Invasive Cardiol 2001;13:802–4
16. Alt E, Lehmann G. Stroke and atrial fibrillation in sick sinus syndrome. Heart 1997;77:495–7
17. De Sisti A, Leclercq JF, Fiorello P, et al. Electrophysiologic characteristics of the atrium in sinus node dysfunction: atrial refractoriness and conduction. J Cardiovasc Electrophysiol 2000;11:30–3
18. Benditt DG, Gornick CC, Dunbar D, et al. Indications for electrophysiologic testing in the diagnosis and assessment of sinus node dysfunction. Circulation 1987;75:III93–102 (review)
19. Andersen HR, Thuesen L, Bagger JP, et al. Prospective randomized trial of atrial versus ventricular pacing in sick sinus syndrome. Lancet 1994;344:1523–8
20. Hesselson AB, Parsonnet V, Bernstein AD, Bonavita GJ. Deleterious effects of long-term single-chamber ventricular pacing in patients with sick sinus syndrome: the hidden benefits of dual-chamber pacing. J Am Coll Cardiol 1992;19:1542–9
21. Connolly II, Connolly SJ, Kerr CR, et al. Effects of physiologic pacing versus ventricular pacing on the risk of stroke and death due to cardiovascular causes. Canadian Trial of Physiologic Pacing (CTOPP) Trial Investigators. N Engl J Med 2000;342:1385–91
22. Lamas GA, Orav EJ, Stambler BS, et al. Quality of life and clinical outcome in elderly patients treated with ventricular pacing as compared with dual-chamber pacing. New Engl J Med 1998;338:1097–104
23. Lamas GA, Kerry L, Lee K, et al. The Mode Selection Trial in Sick-Sinus Dysfunction (MOST). New Engl J Med 2002;346:1854–62
24. Wong GC, Hadjis T. Single chamber ventricular compared with double chamber pacing: A review. Can J Cardiol 2002;18:301–7
25. Sutton R, Kenny RA. The natural history of sick sinus syndrome. Pacing Clin Electrophysiol 1986;9:1110–4
26. Saito D, Matsubara K, Yamanari H, et al. Effects of oral theophylline on sick sinus syndrome. J Am Coll Cardiol 1993;21:1199–204
27. Strickberger SA, Fish RD, Lamas GA, et al. Comparison of effects of propanolol versus pindolol on sinus rate and pacing frequency in sick sinus syndrome. Am J Cardiol 1993;71:53–6

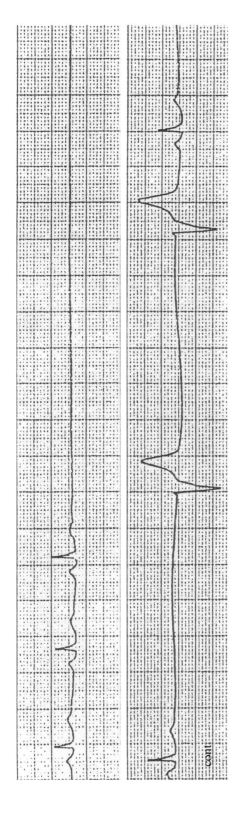

conti

ECG 22.1
Continuous stripe. Sinus standstill during about 7.5 sec. After another sinusal beat again sinus standstill. After two (probably) ventricular escape beats (instantaneous rate 21/min) one sinusal beat, then again sinus standstill.

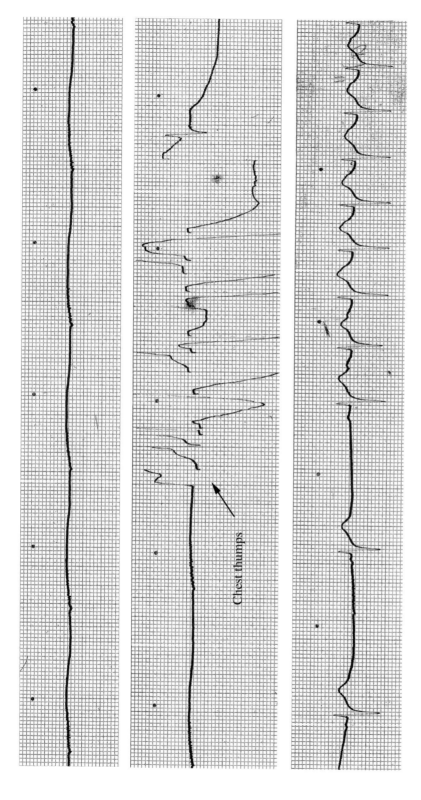

Chest thumps

ECG 22.2

Continuous stripe. Sinus standstill during > 17 sec, requiring short mechanical reanimation (chest thumps). After three ectopic atrial beats (rate 20–30/min), sinus rhythm arises (rate about 120/min). Another 3 possible QRS during chest thumping would reduce cardiac asystole by about 4 sec.

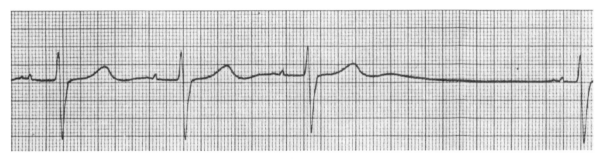

ECG 22.3
Paper speed 50 mm/sec. Sinus rhythm 92/min. 2 : 1 SA block. In this case the p3–p4 interval exceeds the double preceding p–p intervals by 55 msec.

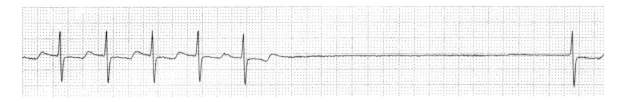

ECG 22.4
AV junctional rhythm (95/min) followed by an episode of sinus arrest (4.3 sec). After one AV junction escape beat another shorter sinus arrest occurs (not shown).

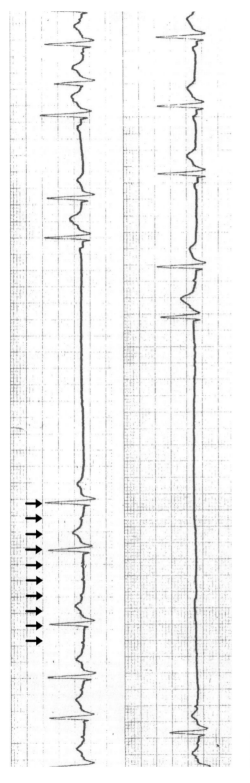

ECG 22.5

Bradycardia-tachycardia variant. Continuous stripe. Atrial flutter (irregular atrial action, rate about 300/min, see arrows) with changing AV conduction. Stop of atrial flutter, sinus arrest during 3.24 sec. Then sinusal beats and APBs. After a blocked APB a second episode of atrial standstill lasting 5.2 sec. Then one AV junction escape beat, one APB, sinus rhythm.

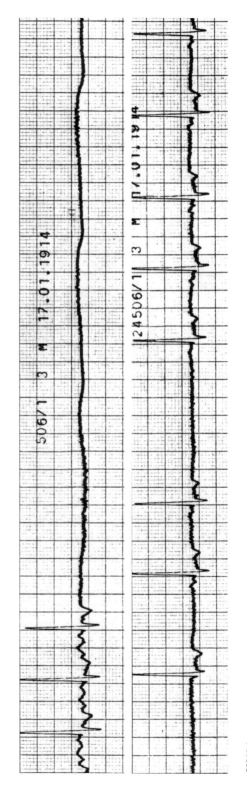
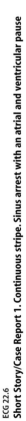

ECG 22.6

Short Story/Case Report 1. Continuous stripe. Sinus arrest with an atrial and ventricular pause

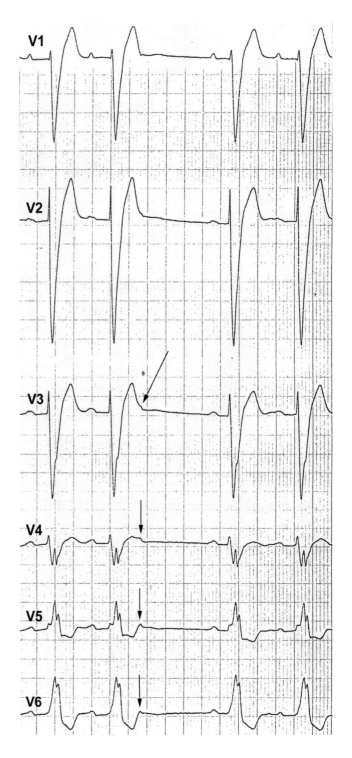

ECG 22.7
SR with AV block 1° and LBBB. AV blocked APB, with the
p wave detectable within/at the end of the T wave (arrow).
The p–p interval is almost doubled (minus 55 msec).

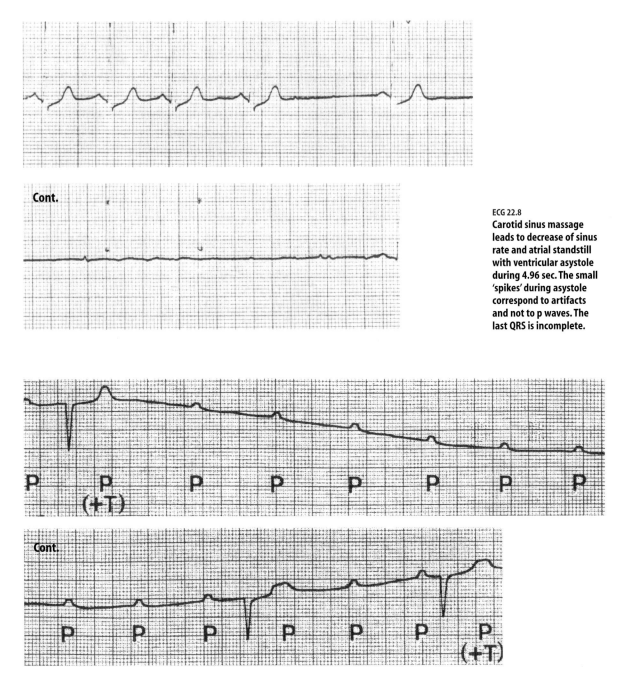

Cont.

ECG 22.8
Carotid sinus massage leads to decrease of sinus rate and atrial standstill with ventricular asystole during 4.96 sec. The small 'spikes' during asystole correspond to artifacts and not to p waves. The last QRS is incomplete.

Cont.

P   P   P   P   P   P   P   P
(+T)

P   P   P   P   P   P   P
(+T)

ECG 22.9
Carotid sinus massage induces complete AV block. After a ventricular asystole of 8.4 sec, two AV junction escape beats arise, and shortly later sinus rhythm (not shown).

Chapter 23
Atrioventricular Junctional Tachycardias

At a Glance

Some basic mechanisms of atrioventricular (AV) junctional tachycardias are presented in this section At a Glance. Why? For AV nodal reentrant tachycardia the enormous progress in electrophysiology and therapy of arrhythmias can be illustrated in an exemplary manner.

ECG

There are several types of AV junctional tachycardias. However every physician is particularly familiar with one type, the common *paroxysmal supraventricular tachycardia*, correctly called *AV nodal reentrant tachycardia* (AVNRT). (Note that the supraventricular (reentry) tachycardia in the WPW syndrome is called 'AV reentry tachycardia'.)

AVNRT is based on the *dual-pathway anatomy* of the AV node. In a minority of people, these two pathways are used functionally in sinus rhythm as well as in AVNRT.

1 Conduction in Sinus Rhythm

The sinus impulse is conducted over the *fast pathway beta*, antegradely. At the same time, the sinus impulse is conducted antegradely over the *slow pathway alpha*. However, it is blocked because the infra-AV nodal tissue is already activated by the sinus impulse over the fast pathway beta and is therefore refractory (Figure 23.1).

2 Conduction in AVNRT

In both pathways retrograde conduction is also possible. Under certain circumstances the two pathways are used as a *reentry circuit*, one pathway conducting *antegradely*, and the other *retrogradely*. The rate of this circuit movement is high, between 130 and 220/min, and the atria and the ventricles are activated almost simultaneously. AVNRT is usually introduced by an atrial premature beats (APB), often with AV block 1°.

There are *two* forms of AVNRT, one common and one rare. In both types the QRS complex is normal; right bundle-branch block (RBBB) aberration is rare. The tachycardia is mostly *absolutely regular*. The rate is between 130 and 240/min, often about 180/min.

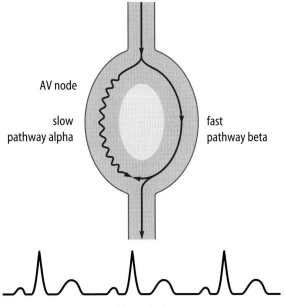

AV node

slow
pathway alpha

fast
pathway beta

Sinus rhythm

Figure 23.1
Dual AV pathway, in sinus rhythm.

3 Common Form of AVNRT

This tachycardia is *paroxysmal* and is responsible for > 90% of AVNRT, and for 50% of all regular supraventricular tachycardias. The slow pathway (alpha) is used for antegrade conduction, the fast pathway (beta) for retrograde conduction (Figure 23.2). Therefore, the atria (retrogradely) and the ventricles (antegradely) are activated practically at the same time. Indeed the p waves are *completely hidden* within the QRS complexes in about 70% of the cases (ECGs 23.1 and 23.2). There is always an opposite p vector, compared to the normal sinus p vector, in the frontal plane. The p waves are negative in leads III, aVF and often II, if they are not hidden within the QRS complex. In about 10% the p waves are superimposed at the end of the QRS complex and are detectable as *pseudo-s* waves in the inferior leads aVF and III and/or as *pseudo-r'* waves in lead V_1, imitating incomplete RBBB (ECGs 23.3a–b). In about 20% the p wave immediately follows the QRS complex and is visible within the ST segment or at the beginning of the T wave

(ECG 23.4) The RP interval is *always* shorter than the PR interval (RP < PR).

The beginning (commonly induced by an APB) and end of an episode of paroxysmal AVNRT are sudden ('light-switch effect') and are felt by most people who are otherwise generally healthy.

4 Rare Form of AVNRT

This tachycardia may be *paroxysmal* or *incessant* (lasting many hours or days) and is responsible for only 5% of AVNRT. The rare form of AVNRT occurs more likely in heart disease. As the fast pathway (beta) is used antegradely and the slow pathway (alpha) retrogradely, the retrograde activation of the atria occurs later (Figure 23.3). Consequently the negative p waves in the inferior leads aVF and III are often detectable, relatively late after the QRS complex. The RP interval is *longer* than the PR interval (RP > PR) (ECG 23.5). The incessant form is often resistant to drugs and may lead to heart failure after days or months.

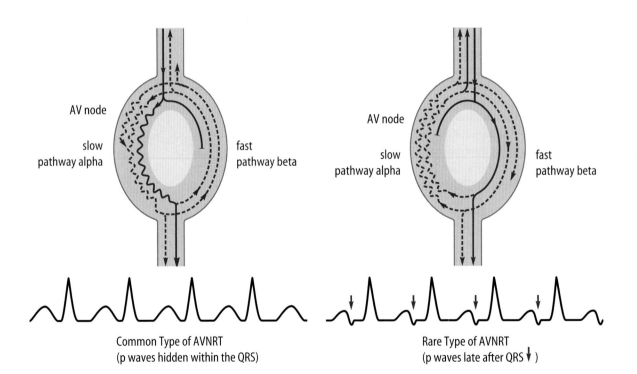

Common Type of AVNRT
(p waves hidden within the QRS)

Rare Type of AVNRT
(p waves late after QRS ↓)

Figure 23.2
In the common type of AVNRT the slow pathway alpha is used antegradely, and the fast pathway beta retrogradely.

Figure 23.3
In the rare type of AVNRT the fast pathway beta is used antegradely, and the slow pathway alpha retrogradely.

5   Differential Diagnosis

Theoretically, differential diagnosis includes all other forms of AV junction tachycardias and also atrial flutter and AV reentry tachycardia in the Wolff-Parkinson-White (WPW) syndrome. In practice the other types of AV junctional tachycardias (accelerated AV nodal rhythm, automatic junctional tachycardia, permanent junctional reciprocating tachycardia) are so rare, especially in adults, that only *atrial flutter* and *AV reentry tachycardia in WPW syndrome* are considered.

5.1   Atrial Flutter

Especially in flutter type 2 (with 1 : 1 or 1 : 2 AV conduction) the flutter waves are often not clearly detectable. Vagal maneuvers, especially carotid sinus massage, may enhance AV block and demask the flutter waves. In contrast, vagal maneuvers in AVNRT interrupt the tachycardia or have no effect. In sinus tachycardia with a high rate, carotid sinus massage slightly decreases the rate for a short time.

5.2   AV Reentry Tachycardia in the WPW Syndrome

As in the rare type of AVNRT, in the common WPW tachycardia the atria are activated with some latency, due to the longer conduction distance from ventricle to atrium. Thus the p waves appear *after* the QRS, usually with RP < PR. Furthermore, as in the rare form of AVNRT, RP > PR may be present. In AV reentry tachycardia in the WPW syndrome only one limb of the dual AV conduction is used (mostly the fast one, *antegradely*), the other part of the reentry circuit is the *accessory pathway*, distant from the AV node (mostly with *retrograde* conduction). The majority of people with WPW syndrome during sinus rhythm show a *shortened PQ interval* with the typical *delta wave* and more or less altered QRS and repolarization (Chapter 24 The WPW syndrome).

The previous remarks about differential diagnosis based on the ECG and especially on the behavior of the p wave, are theoretical to a certain degree. Every experienced cardiologist knows the obvious difficulties. In supraventricular tachycardias, especially at a *high rate* (and also without aberration), the p waves are often *not detectable*. In addition, an accessory pathway in the WPW syndrome may be occult during sinus rhythm. In fact, it is often impossible to differentiate between AVNRT, AV reentry tachycardia in the WPW syndrome, and even atrial flutter (with 1 : 1 or 1 : 2 AV conduction). In these cases an electrophysiologic investigation is mandatory for diagnosis (and of course for therapy).

5.3   Aberration

In the case of *aberration* (in general with RBBB pattern) a ventricular tachycardia may be assumed, especially on the basis of a monitor lead. However, aberration often occurs only during the first 3 to 10 beats (ECG 23.6a). ECG 23.6b shows *LBBB aberration* in the same patient. The different ECG signs in supraventricular tachycardias with RBBB or LBBB aberration (SVTab) and ventricular tachycardia (VT) are extensively discussed in Chapter 26 Ventricular Tachycardia.

6   Symptoms of AVNRT (Common Form)

Symptoms depend especially on the duration of the tachycardia. In general the episodes last minutes or up to an hour, and in exceptional cases they can last for many hours. Most patients suffer from tiresome palpitations and many patients feel the fast rate in the neck. This is due to the contraction of the right atrium against a closed tricuspid valve that provokes visible pulsation of the external jugular veins ('a waves').

7   Clinical Significance of AVNRT (Common Form)

A high rate and/or a long duration of AVNRT may lead to dizziness, presyncope, and occasionally syncope. Although the tachycardia is never directly life-threatening, it may be deleterious in situations like swimming or mountain climbing (if tachycardia is associated with enhanced sympathetic tone).

8 Etiology and Prevalence

Generally the common type of AVNRT is encountered in younger individuals with an otherwise *normal heart*, whereas the rare form is more often associated with *heart disease* [1–3]. It has been estimated that the common form of atrioventricular nodal reentrant tachycardia (AVNRT) is about eight times more frequent than all other AV tachycardias. The uncommon or atypical form of AVNRT (with RP > PR) is rare. Accelerated AV junctional rhythm, in its various forms, is not as rare. Automatic junctional tachycardia and the permanent form of junctional reciprocating tachycardia (also with RP > PR) are very rare, especially in adults.

ECG Special

9 Special Types of AV Junctional Tachycardias

9.1 Accelerated AV Junctional Rhythm

This rhythm was formerly called 'nonparoxysmal junctional tachycardia' [4]. Generally the rate is about 70–100/min (thus not fulfilling the definition of tachycardia) and rarely reaches 130/min. This may be the reason why the arrhythmia is sometimes not correctly diagnosed. The mechanism is enhancement of focal impulse discharge in the AV junction. In its *simple* presentation, the rhythm looks like an AV junctional escape rhythm, with a higher rate. It is seen more frequently in acute myocardial infarction (AMI) (especially of inferior localization) and after heart operations than it is in digitalis intoxication; it mostly indicates a heart disease. The arrhythmia may be *complex* due to different behavior of retrograde AV conduction and rarely due to antegrade incomplete or complete exit block. In retrograde exit block AV dissociation occurs, generally with a faster AV rate than the atrial (sinusal) rate. In the case of a wide QRS due to aberration, differentiation from accelerated *idioventricular* rhythm is difficult. Ventricular capture beats or fusion beats favor the latter diagnosis.

9.2 Automatic Junctional Tachycardia (AJT)

AJT is rare, based on enhanced automaticity in the AV junction, and is mostly associated with organic heart disease. The rate is between 120 and 220/min. In contrast to AVNRT, considerable changes in rate within a short time are common and occasionally there is an irregularity from beat to beat. Moreover, concomitant AV dissociation is more common than retrograde atrial activation (eventually with AV block 2°). Occasional ventricular capture may occur. AJT is resistant to vagal maneuvers [3].

9.3 Permanent Junctional Reciprocating Tachycardia (PJRT)

PJRT is often classified as a variant of the WPW syndrome, with an accessory pathway, but without delta wave. PJRT is also rare. The rhythm is regular, the rate is 130–220/min. The mechanism is 'between' that of AVNRT and that of AV reentry tachycardia in the WPW syndrome. In fact there is a circular movement with antegrade conduction over the AV node and retrograde conduction over a special perinodal pathway with decremental properties [5].

As in the uncommon type of AVNRT, and in AV reentry tachycardia in the WPW syndrome, the p waves can be detected clearly *after* the QRS. Thus the three arrhythmias cannot always be distinguished in the routine ECG. An irregular rhythm and AV dissociation strongly favors AJT. The absence of a delta wave in sinus rhythm favors AJT or PJRT, the presence of a delta wave allows the diagnosis of AV reentry tachycardia in WPW. In the (rare) cases with aberrant conduction (mostly RBBB) even the differentiation between supraventricular and ventricular origin of the tachycardia may be very difficult or impossible.

The following case report shows that also in a tachycardia at a moderate rate the ECG may be misleading.

Short Story/Case Report 1

In March 2001 an anxious 25-year-old woman was seen at the emergency unit for palpitations. Her general state was normal with the exception of a slight fever. The ECG showed a supraventricular tachycardia at a rate of 126/min (ECG 23.7a). The diagnosis of AVNRT was made, because negative p waves were supposed in lead II and aVF in the ST/T segment (arrows). Therapy was postponed in view of the relatively low rate of tachycardia. One hour later the patient had calmed down, the pulse rate was now 102/min, and the ECG revealed a *sinus rhythm*, with AV block 1° (ECG 23.7b). Retrospectively, the correct diagnosis should have been made already in lead V_1 of the ECG 23.7a where the negative deflection cannot be a T wave but represents a p wave. Mononucleosis was diagnosed later.

10 Prognosis

Sudden death in AVNRT is very rare. Wang et al [6] studied 290 patients with aborted sudden death. Thirteen of these patients (4.5%) had documented or strong presumptive evidence of supraventricular tachycardia that deteriorated into ventricular fibrillation; six had an accessory pathway, four had atrial fibrillation with enhanced AV conduction, and three had AVNRT (and nothing else? Remark of the author of this book). General opinion is that prognosis is good.

11 Therapy of AVNRT (Common Form)

Acute intravenous drug therapy is not without danger. The drug most often used is adenosine. However some precautions should be taken, as for instance a reduction of the dose using a central venous catheter [7,8]. Verapamil, formerly widely used, is potentially dangerous. Too rapid injection (within seconds) may induce a long-standing asystole, in this case requiring immediate heart massage and calcium intravenously, the latter effectual only with latency. In patients with supraventricular tachycardias and the Wolff-Parkinson-White syndrome the drug may induce ventricular fibrillation (see chapter 24 The WPW syndrome). Verapamil should only be used with great caution. It may be effectual a thousand times, in case 1001 it may be deleterious.

The author's experience with other drugs such as flecainide (contraindicated in patients with reduced ventricular function and renal failure), beta-blockers, amiodarone and other antiarrhythmic drugs is very restricted, in the therapy of AVNRT. In a patient with AVNRT resistant to the first drug, electroconversion is the preferred therapy [3]. Vagal maneuvers such as the Valsalva, and carotid massage, end the tachycardia in less than 40% of attempts.

Oral drug prophylaxis remains problematic. *Catheter-induced radiofrequency ablation* is used for AVNRT and troublesome or severe symptoms, and a first attempt is successful in nearly 95%. Generally the distal part of the *slow pathway* is interrupted. This *curative* therapy has caused a considerable reduction in urgent home visits by physicians, especially during the night.

12 Therapy of the Other Types of AV Junctional Tachycardias

The therapy of the other types of AV junctional tachycardias depends on the mechanism of the arrhythmia.

References

1. Akhtar M, Jazayeri MR, Sra J, et al. Atrioventricular nodal reentry. Clinical, electrophysiological, and therapeutic considerations. Circulation 1993;88:282–95
2. Pieper SJ, Stanton MS. Narrow QRS complex tachycardias. Mayo Clin Proc 1995;70:371–5
3. Kadish A, Passman R. Mechanisms and management of paroxysmal supraventricular tachycardia. Cardiol Rev 1999;7:254–64
4. Pick A, Dominguez P. Nonparoxysmal AV nodal tachycardia. Circulation 1957;16:1022
5. Coumel P. Junctional reciprocating tachycardias: The permanent and paroxysmal forms of AV nodal reciprocating tachycardias. J Electrocardiol 1975;8:79–90
6. Wang YS, Scheinman MM, Chien WW, et al. Patients with supraventricular tachycardia presenting with aborted sudden death: incidence, mechanism and long-term follow-up. J Am Coll Cardiol 1991;18:1711–9
7. Smally AJ. Preventing complications of adenosine administration. Ann Emerg Med 2002;39:347–8
8. Chang M, Wrenn K. Adenosine dose should be less when administered through a central line. J Emerg Med 2002;22:195–8

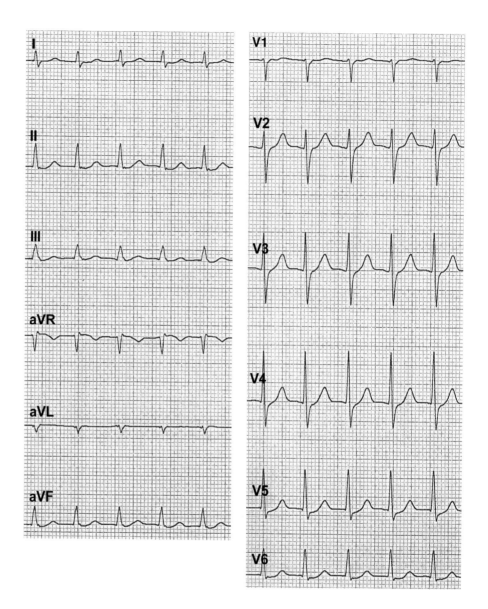

ECG 23.1
53 y/f. Otherwise healthy heart. AVNRT, rate 131/min, without visible retrograde atrial activation (no detectable p waves).

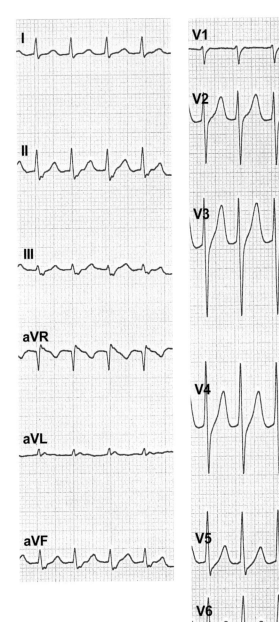

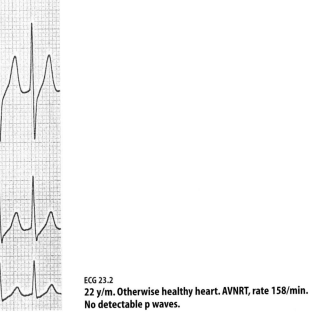

ECG 23.2
22 y/m. Otherwise healthy heart. AVNRT, rate 158/min.
No detectable p waves.

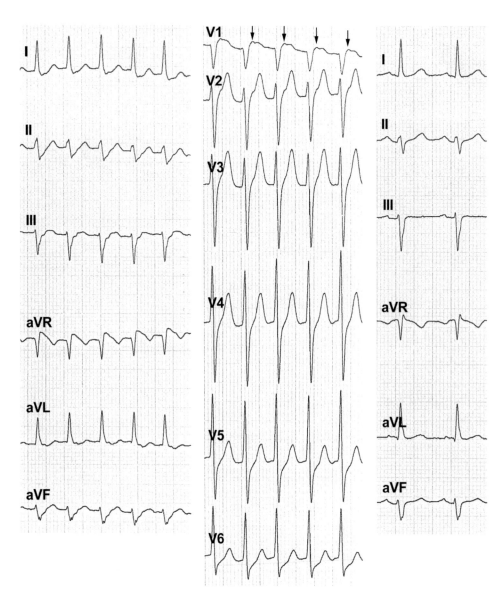
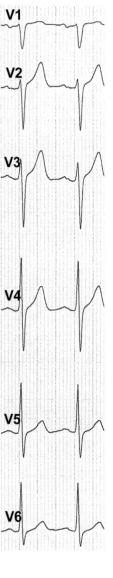

ECG 23.3a

28 y/f. Otherwise healthy heart. ECG: AVNRT, rate 173/min. The negative p waves are seen at the end of the QRS complex in II, aVF and III, formally broadening the S waves. Positive p wave after R in aVL. Moreover p is seen as a positive deflection in V₁, mimicking an r′ wave (see arrows), as in the pattern of incomplete RBBB. Compare with ECG 23.3b of the same patient in sinus rhythm.

ECG 23.3b

Same patient. Sinus rhythm. The S waves in the inferior leads are small, the pseudo-r′ in lead V₁ has disappeared.

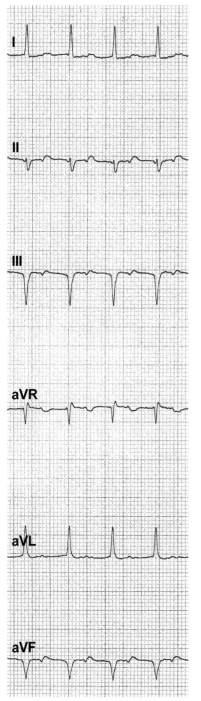

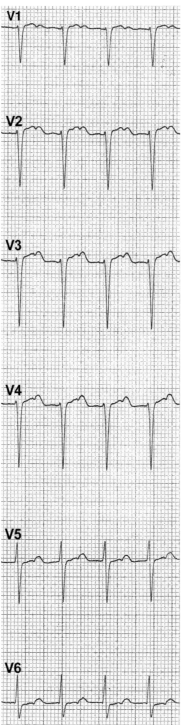

ECG 23.4
44 y/f. Hypertension. Moderate dilating cardiomyopathy. ECG: AVNRT, rate 126/min. The negative p waves are seen in the inferior leads and in all precordial leads, at the beginning of the T wave (the negative p waves in V_1/V_2 are unusual). Pathologic QRS configuration.

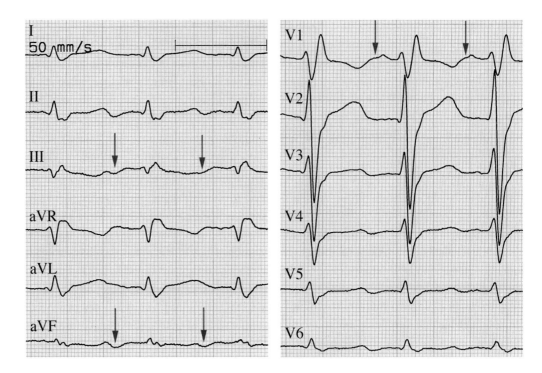

ECG 23.5

32 y/m. Otherwise normal heart. ECG: AVNRT, rare type, rate 118/min. The p waves (negative in III/aVF and positive in V_1) are seen *after* the T wave (RP > PR), see arrows.

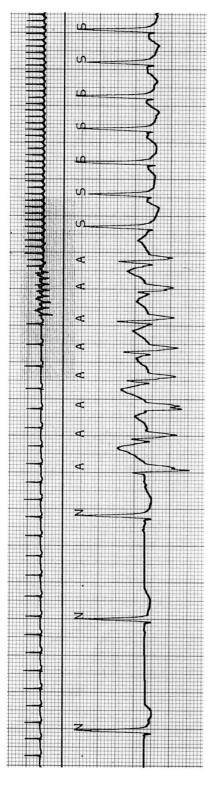

ECG 23.6a

52 y/m. Coronary heart disease. Supraventricular tachycardia with aberration. The first eight beats (rate 180/min) show RBBB aberration. After the rate decreases to 166/min, the QRS complexes normalize (N = normal beats, A = beats with aberration, S = supraventricular beats).

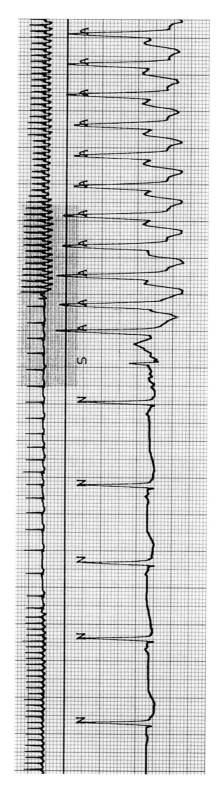

ECG 23.6b

Same patient. The first beat shows RBBB aberration, the following beats an LBBB aberration that remains in spite of the decrease of the rate from 194 to 185/min (N = normal beats, A = beats with aberration, S = supraventricular beat with RBBB aberration).

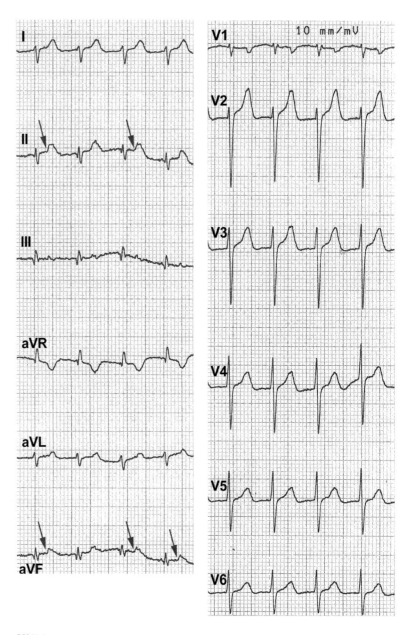

ECG 23.7a
Short Story/Case Report 1. Pseudo AVNRT. Arrows: mimicking of retrograde p waves.

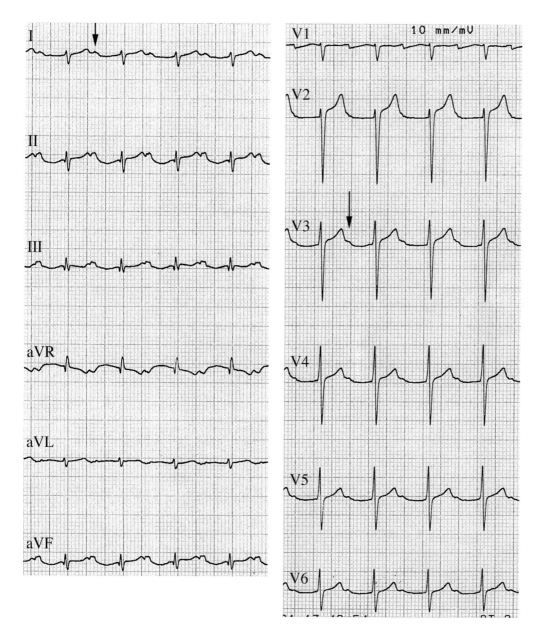

ECG 23.7b

Short Story/Case Report 1. With decrease of sinus rate, the p waves appear after the T wave (arrow), confirming sinus tachycardia. AV block 1°. The pattern of incomplete RBBB in lead V₁ has disappeared probably because of different lead placement.

Chapter 24
The Wolff-Parkinson-White Syndrome

At a Glance

Pre-excitation is based on an accessory conduction pathway between atrium and ventricle. In the human embryo there are three to four atrioventricular (AV) connections. Normally all the pathways (except the AV node and His system) undergo hypoplasia or fibrosis and lose conduction function. However, in about three people out of every 1000 in the population one so-called *accessory pathway* (AP) persists and may support antegrade and retrograde conduction. These individuals show, constantly or intermittently, an ECG pattern typical of pre-excitation, with a shortened PQ interval and a delta wave. About 40% of those with an AP suffer from tachycardia, in which this pathway is used. The term Wolff-Parkinson-White syndrome is used for patients with the pre-excitation/WPW pattern associated with *AP-related tachycardias*.

ECG

1   Pre-Excitation Pattern (WPW Pattern)

The pre-excitation pattern or 'WPW pattern' is characterized by:

i.   a shortened PQ interval (PQ ≤ 0.12 sec)
ii. typical delta waves
iii. deformation and prolongation of the whole QRS complex
iv. alterations of the repolarization.

The pre-excitation pattern corresponds to ventricular activation by atrial impulses, conducted along the 'AP' (fusion beats; see section 1.2 below), formerly called the bundle of Kent. Thus, the impulse *'bypasses'* the AV node and is conducted *faster* than normally to the ventricle (Figure 24.1). As a consequence of pre-excitation of the ventricles, the PQ interval is *shortened* and lasts 0.12 sec or less. Moreover, the abnormal 'eccentric' excitation of

the ventricles leads to a deformation of the whole QRS complex and also to alteration of the repolarization. The initial part of the deformed QRS is called *delta* wave, according to its similarity to the Greek letter 'delta' (ECG 24.1). The delta wave corresponds to the pre-excited portion of one or both ventricles.

1.1   Nomenclature

The traditional and simple old nomenclature differentiates between type A and type B. Type A shows an initially positive deflection in leads V_1/V_2 (corresponding to early activation of the posterior left ventricle), type B shows an initially negative deflection in V_1/V_2 (corresponding to early activation of the anterior/superior right ventricle). Patterns with a negative delta wave in the left lateral leads V_5/V_6 have been called type C.

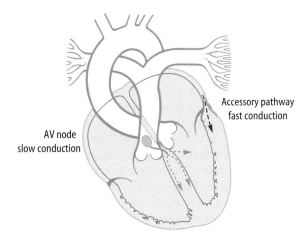

AV node
slow conduction

Accessory pathway
fast conduction

Figure 24.1
Pre-excitation over the eccentric accessory pathway.

The modern classification (see 'The Full Picture') considers more than a dozen different localizations of the APs.

The polarity of the delta wave and the configuration of the whole QRS complex depends on the localization (site of origin and insertion) of the accessory pathway, that may be left-sided or right-sided, in the septal region, posterior or anterior/lateral. Consequently, both delta wave and the following part of the QRS may be positive, negative, or biphasic in some leads. To a certain degree, the localization of an AP can be predicted by the vectors of the delta waves and the QRS.

1.2   ECG Patterns in Pre-Excitation

In WPW patients, three different QRS patterns can be seen in sinus rhythm:

i.   Most pre-excitation patterns represent *fusion beats*. The ventricles are activated at the same time along the AP and the AV node. The QRS configuration depends on the grade of activation along the AP and the AV node, respectively. The more ventricular tissue is activated along the AP, the more similar to the classical pre-excitation pattern the QRS complex is (ECG 24.1). The more ventricular tissue activated along the AV node, the more normal the configuration of the QRS complex (ECG 24.2). Thus, in the case of 90% ventricular activation along the AV node, the pre-excitation pattern may be difficult to detect. We may find an only modestly reduced PQ interval, only an 'abortive' delta wave, and a minor alteration of the whole QRS complex and the repolarization (ECG 24.2). Also, the same patient may show different grades of pre-excitation in his ECGs, with more or less typical pre-excitation.

ii.   In rare cases we find *full* pre-excitation in sinus rhythm. The ventricles are activated exclusively along the AP. The ECG pattern is very typical (ECG 24.3). However, full pre-excitation is present in antidromic AV reentry tachycardia and in some cases with atrial fibrillation.

iii. In about 30% of WPW patients, the *AP conducts only retrogradely*. The term 'concealed AP' is used. In theses cases the PQ interval and the QRS complex are normal and the diagnosis cannot be made on the basis of an ECG, but by electrophysiologic studies (in patients with paroxysmal supraventricular tachycardias). In contrast to the patients with manifest WPW pattern *and* syndrome, these patients have concomitant atrial fibrillation in only about 3% (*see* section 2.2 Atrial Fibrillation and ... below).

1.3   Differential Diagnosis of the WPW Pattern

1.3.1   Myocardial Infarction

In more than 50% the WPW pattern leads to pathologic Q waves that may be confounded with an old myocardial infarction (MI). However, the shortened PQ interval and the delta wave suggest the true diagnosis. Moreover, the T waves are discordant positive in the leads with pathologic Q waves and not concordant negative as usual in old myocardial infarction.

A complete negative QRS complex (QS) with a negative delta wave in leads III and aVF may imitate the pattern of an old inferior MI (ECG 24.4). Tall R waves in V_1 to V_3 suggest posterior MI (ECG 24.5), whereas the combination of such patterns imitates inferoposterior MI (ECG 24.6). Also lateral MI may be mimicked (ECG 24.7). In patients with pre-excitation the presence of an old infarction is not recognizable in general. The pattern of acute MI can occasionally be detected on the basis of striking ST elevations.

1.3.2   Left Ventricular Hypertrophy

Not uncommonly pre-excitation enhances the R wave voltage (especially in the precordial leads), thus suggesting left ventricular hypertrophy (LVH) (ECG 24.8). In these cases also the strain pattern with asymmetric negative T waves may be observed.

1.3.3   Pseudo-Delta Wave

Occasionally a 'pseudo-delta wave' is present in leads V_2 and V_3, and/or in the inferior leads, due to projection. In these cases the PQ interval and the QRS complex are normal (Chapter 3 The Normal ECG and its (Normal) Variants).

2   Tachycardias in the WPW Syndrome

2.1   Reentry Tachycardias

The typical tachycardias in the WPW syndrome are based on a *macro*-reentry using the AP and the AV node. Two types are distinguished:

i.   In > 90% the impulse is conducted *retrogradely* along the AP and *antegradely* along the AV node (Figure 24.2a). This type is called AV *orthodromic* reentrant tachycardia. Consequently, the QRS is *normal* (in the absence of an additional bundle-branch block) and a delta wave is always

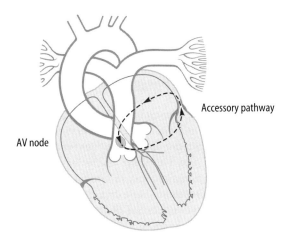

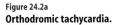

Figure 24.2a
Orthodromic tachycardia.

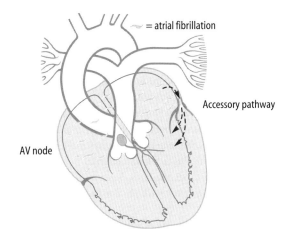

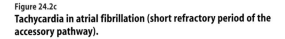

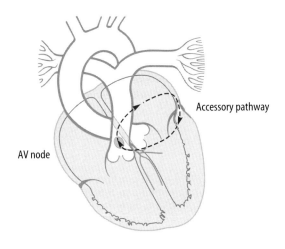

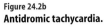

Figure 24.2b
Antidromic tachycardia.

responds to the typical WPW pattern, a delta wave included (ECG 24.10).

In both antidromic and orthodromic tachycardia the rhythm is *regular* and the rate is between 140 and 240/min (ECG 24.9) and occasionally reaches 250/min (ECG 24.11) or even 300/min. At rates up to 220/min *negative* p waves may be detected in the inferior leads III and aVF, due to retrograde atrial activation, with RP > PR.

2.2 Atrial Fibrillation and Atrial Flutter in the WPW Syndrome

In patients with manifest pre-excitation in the ECG, atrial fibrillation is not rare, and has even been described in children.

Tachycardias due to atrial fibrillation and atrial flutter do *not* represent a reentry tachycardia (see below). However, these arrhythmias are clinically very important, due to possible degeneration into *ventricular fibrillation,* in the case of a very short (antegrade) refractory period of the AP.

Only the AP is used for conduction, antegradely, and there is *no* retrograde conduction over the AV junction (Figure 24.2c). Therefore delta waves and wide, deformed QRS are present during tachycardia. In atrial fibrillation the ventricular rhythm is *absolutely irregular* (ECG 24.12a). ECG 24.12b was registered while the patient was being infused with procainamide. In ECG 24.12c (after conversion to sinus

missed (ECG 24.9). The distinction from AV nodal reentrant tachycardia is often not possible without electrophysiologic investigation. A negative p wave in lead V$_1$, shortening of the R–R interval in the case of disappearing ipsilateral bundle-branch block (BBB) and an RP > PR interval, favour WPW syndrome.

ii. In < 10% the AP is used *antegradely* and the AV node *retrogradely.* This type is called AV *antidromic* reentry tachycardia (Figure 24.2b). In these rare cases the QRS complex cor-

At a Glance

rhythm) the pre-excitation pattern is scarcely detectable, at first glance.

Atrial fibrillation with pre-excitation must be distinguished from monomorphic ventricular tachycardia, where the rhythm is regular. Rarely in ventricular tachycardia a slow upstroke of wide QRS may imitate a delta wave.

Ventricular rate in atrial fibrillation or atrial flutter depends on *antegrade conduction properties* of the AP. If the refractory period is very short, the ventricular rate may reach a rate of up to 300/min in atrial fibrillation and in atrial flutter with 1 : 1 conduction. At these extreme rates, degeneration into ventricular fibrillation may occur partially due to severely impaired coronary perfusion.

Although only a minority of patients with WPW tachycardia present a very fast antegrade conduction over the AP, allowing an extremely rapid ventricular response, the typical ECG pattern must be recognized (also for therapeutic reasons).

2.3 Therapy

The majority of patients with the WPW syndrome show symptoms that depend on the *duration* and the *rate* (especially) of tachycardia. The symptoms include palpitations, dizziness, presyncope and syncope. Symptomatic patients should undergo electrophysiologic evaluation and catheter ablation (success about 95%). In those patients who refuse ablation one has to resort to prophylactically active drugs such as flecainide, propafenone, and beta-blockers. For interrupting a WPW tachycardia we prefer electroconversion or procainamide.

2.4 Therapeutic Pitfalls

Drugs like *digitalis* or *verapamil* not only slow antegrade conduction along the AV node but may accelerate conduction along the AP, thus inducing an extremely high ventricular rate and degeneration into ventricular fibrillation. Many case reports have been published about adverse outcomes of trials of tachycardia conversion with these drugs. Digitalis and verapamil (especially intravenously) are *absolutely contraindicated* in patients with WPW syndrome.

This is also true for patients in whom a typical AV reentry tachycardia in known WPW syndrome (or in WPW tachycardia misdiagnosed as atrioventricular nodal reentrant tachycardia, AVNRT) has been interrupted successfully in the past, e.g. with verapamil. Such patients may suddenly present atrial flutter or fibrillation that may be difficult to diagnose in the ECG. Let us remember that atrial fibrillation is more frequent in patients with WPW than in a population without WPW (lifetime prevalence up to 32%). Atrial fibrillation may occur during a common regular WPW tachycardia, by enhanced sympathetic tone, left atrial stretch and impaired coronary flow.

The Full Picture

In 1913 Cohn and Fraser published the first ECG with ventricular pre-excitation in a patient with intermittent tachycardias [1]. In 1930, Louis Wolff, John Parkinson and Paul Dudley White described 11 patients who suffered from attacks of tachycardia associated with a short PR interval and a broad QRS during sinus rhythm [2]. This has subsequently been termed the Wolff-Parkinson-White (WPW) syndrome. In 1932 Holzmann proposed ventricular pre-excitation as the mechanism [3]. The WPW syndrome includes a WPW pattern in the ECG associated with paroxysmal tachycardia. The WPW pattern refers to the presence of pre-excitation without tachyarrhythmias.

3 Etiology

Most patients with the WPW syndrome have otherwise normal hearts, but some suffer from concomitant congenital heart diseases. Approximately 10% of patients with Ebstein's anomaly show the WPW syndrome (the majority of these accessory pathways are located in the right free wall and right posteroseptally) [4]. Other congenital heart diseases associated with the syndrome include atrial and ventricular septal defects, and coronary-sinus diverticula. In the WPW syndrome there is incomplete embryonic development of the process that leads to electric isolation of the ventricles from the atria. The precise pathogenesis of this defect is not known. Among the patients with the WPW syndrome, 3.4% show a familial form that is usually inherited as an autosomal dominant trait [5]. MacRae et al found a genetic defect on chromosome 7 in a large family with hypertrophic cardiomyopathy and the WPW syndrome [6]. In two additional families with the WPW syndrome and familial hypertrophic cardiomyopathy, a probable causative mutation was identified in a protein kinase gene on chromosome 7 [7]. Defective genes may result in the persistence of accessory conduction pathways that normally regress during cardiogenesis.

4 Anatomy and Localization of Accessory Pathways

Based on electrophysiologic studies the accessory pathway (AP) may be located anywhere along the AV groove or in the septum (Figure 24.3). The most frequent localizations are left lateral (50%), posteroseptal (30%), right anteroseptal (10%) and right lateral (10%). The analysis of the pre-excited QRS allows localization of the AP. The localization of an AP helps the planning of radiofrequency ablation. Transseptal puncture

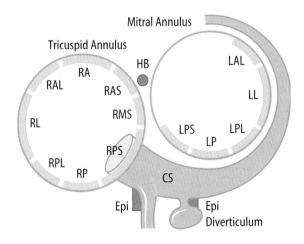

Figure 24.3
Diagram of accessory pathway location. Schematic cross-section of the ventricles at the level of the atrio-ventricular valve rings in left anterior oblique projection. CS, coronary sinus; Epi, epicardial; HB, His bundle; LAL, left anterolateral; LL, left lateral; LP, left posterior; LPL, left posterolateral; LPS, left postero-septal; RA, right anterior; RAL, right anterolateral; RAS, right anteroseptal; RL, right lateral; RMS, right midseptal; RP, right posterior; RPL, right posterolateral; RPS, right posteroseptal.

may be needed, the eventual proximity of the AP to the His bundle must be respected, and the suitable mapping catheter can be chosen.

The localization is based on analysis of the delta wave and QRS deflections in a 12-lead ECG that shows maximal pre-excitation. The reliability of the localization algorithm is decreased if pre-excitation is only partial or in the case of concomitant structural cardiac abnormalities (e.g. congenital heart disease, hypertrophic cardiomyopathy, myocardial infarction, bundle-branch block). Furthermore, the coexistence of multiple APs may render the localization difficult.

ECG Special

4.1 Algorithms

Several algorithms allow accurate localization of APs [8–10]. As mentioned above, it is important to assess the degree of pre-excitation first. The next important step is to assess the onset of the delta wave. A frequent mistake is failure to recognize the very onset of a delta wave when it is isoelectric, and to assess it erroneously as negative or positive. In ECG 24.13 the delta wave is isoelectric in aVF and the negative deflection in aVF occurs 60 msec after the onset of the delta wave in the other leads. Thus it is important to determine the real onset of the delta wave in observing all 12 ECG leads.

Two elements can be used for classifying AP localization:

i. the electrical vector of the delta wave itself (the vector of the initial 40 msec of the pre-excited QRS)
ii. the axis of the QRS complexes, mainly the precordial R/S transition.

Left- and right-sided pathways can be differentiated as shown in Table 24.1. R larger than S in V_1 (V_1 R/S > 1) indicates a left-sided AP (ECG 24.14). If R/S transition (in a pre-excited ECG!) occurs between V_2 and V_3 or later (transition > V_2), the AP is located on the right side. If the R/S transition occurs after V_1 and before V_2 or at V_2 (transition > V_1 and ≤ V_2), the AP can be either left- or right-sided, and further analysis is needed. The amplitude of the R and S waves in limb lead I can be assessed: R > S by 0.1 mV or more indicates a right-sided AP; R=S or R < S in lead I indicates a left-sided AP. A more precise location of AP can be derived from further analysis of the delta wave, as illustrated in Table 24.2. For example, the polarity of the delta wave in the inferior leads can help localizing the AP. Negative delta waves in leads II, III and aVF indicate a posterior (inferior) location; conversely positive delta waves in the inferior leads indicate an anterior (superior) location of the AP (ECG 24.14).

5 Degree of Pre-Excitation, Latent Pre-Excitation and Concealed Accessory Pathway

The degree of pre-excitation and consequently the degree of fusion depends on several factors:

i. Autonomic tone: sympathetic activation may shorten the conduction over the AV node thus decreasing pre-excitation.

Table 24.1
Algorithm to localize left-sided versus right-sided accessory pathway.

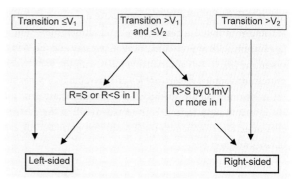

Table 24.2
Stepwise ECG algorithm for determination of accessory pathway (AP) location. AS, (right) anteroseptal; LAL, left anterolateral; LL, left lateral; LP, left posterior; LPL, left posterolateral; PSMA, posteroseptal mitral annulus; PSTA, posteroseptal tricuspid annulus; RA, right anterior; RAL, right anterolateral; RL, right lateral; RP, right posterior; RPL, right posterolateral. Modified from [8] with permission.

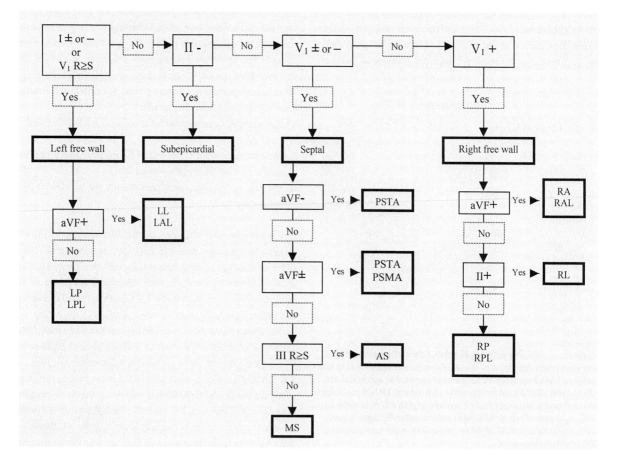

410

ii. Refractory period of the AP: if the AP has a long refractory period, a conduction block may occur during sinus tachycardia (ECGs 24.15, 24.16, 24.17a–b).

iii. Distance from the sinoatrial node to the atrial insertion of the AP: pre-excitation is sometimes absent or discrete when the bypass tract is remote from the sinus node (e.g. left lateral AP) (ECG 24.18), because the normal conduction over the AV node reaches the ventricle before a relevant part of the left ventricle is pre-excited. Right ventricular free wall and septal AP are closer to the sinus node, and their activation occurs quickly resulting in marked pre-excitation and in a shorter PR interval (ECGs 24.13 and 24.17b).

iv. Intra-atrial conduction delay: a normal PR interval does not necessarily mean pre-excitation through a Mahaim fibre (see below). It can occur in the setting of intra-atrial conduction delay, particularly if the AP is remote from the sinus node.

v. Rhythm mechanism and heart rate: an ectopic rhythm or an ectopic beat may modify the pre-excitation for two reasons: (a) the portion of pre-excited myocardium is increased if the ectopic focus is closer to the bypass tract than the sinus node; and (b) because of its decremental properties the conduction over the AV node will be slower following a premature beat or during an atrial tachycardia thus leading to an increase in the degree of pre-excitation.

Some of these factors can fluctuate in a given patient, accounting for labile pre-excitation or varying degree of pre-excitation. If the conduction time of the sinus impulse over the AP and over the AV node/His-Purkinje system is about the same, pre-excitation can be absent or only mild (latent pre-excitation) and difficult to diagnose (ECG 24.19). In ECGs 24.18 and 24.19 the absence of small (septal) Q waves in lead V_6 is a sign for a pre-excitation of the ventricle (absence of initial septal depolarization directed rightward).

Sometimes, conduction over the AP can be demasked; for example by increased vagal tone or antiarrhythmic drugs slowing the AV node conduction (e.g. verapamil, digoxin, beta-blockers), or by atrial premature beats.

APs do not always conduct in both directions, but may conduct in one direction only, either antegradely or retrogradely. *Concealed* AP refers to a bypass tract with conduction only in the retrograde direction, thus not leading to ventricular pre-excitation.

6 Repolarization Abnormalities

ST segment depression and T wave inversion are usually present in patients with pre-excitation (ECG 24.13). The vectors of the secondary ST–T wave changes are usually directed opposite to the vectors of the delta wave and the QRS complex. ST–T changes may mimic changes associated with left ventricular strain. ST depressions often increase during stress test and may be confused with ischemic related ST depressions (ECG 24.20a).

Following radiofrequency ablation of the AP, T wave inversion can be seen in the ECG leads exploring the area where the AP was localized. ECG 24.20b shows inverse T waves in leads II, III and aVF after radiofrequency ablation of a right posteroseptal AP. This manifestation of cardiac memory (Chatterjee effect) can persist several days after RF ablation.

7 Differential Diagnosis

The ECG pattern displayed by some patients with the WPW syndrome may mimic or mask the changes found in other cardiac conditions (see also above). A negative delta wave (presenting as a Q wave) may mimic an MI pattern (ECG 24.4). Pre-excitation by a left-sided AP leads to an early precordial transition with tall R waves in V_1/V_2, mimicking an old posterior MI (ECG 24.6). Conversely, in rare cases a delta wave may mask the presence of a previous MI.

The WPW pattern is occasionally seen in alternating beats and may suggest ventricular bigeminy (ECG 24.15). Conversely, ventricular bigeminy may be misdiagnosed as intermittent pre-excitation (ECG 24.21). If the WPW pattern persists for several beats only, the rhythm may be misdiagnosed as an accelerated idioventricular rhythm.

A bundle-branch or fascicular block pattern may sometimes mimic pre-excitation or make the localization of an AP more difficult (ECGs 24.22 and 24.23).

WPW associated with hypertrophic cardiomyopathy has been observed. Pre-excitation may be difficult to diagnose or may be ruled out on the basis of a 12-lead ECG (ECGs 23.17a–b).

8 Tachyarrhythmias Associated with the Wolff-Parkinson-White Syndrome

The prevalence of the WPW syndrome, defined as a WPW pattern in the ECG associated with AP-related arrhythmias, is substantially lower than that of the WPW pattern alone. Approximately 80% of patients with arrhythmias suffer from atrioventricular reentry tachycardias, 15% show atrial fibrillation and less than 5% suffer from atrial flutter, atrial tachycardia or atrioventricular nodal reentrant tachycardia (AVNRT).

8.1 Atrioventricular Reentry Tachycardias

In these arrhythmias the AP is a substrate for a macro-reentrant circuit, involving the normal AV node, His-Purkinje system, the atrial and the ventricular myocardium. Two forms of this type of arrhythmia in the WPW syndrome are orthodromic and antidromic atrioventricular reentry tachycardia (AVRT). These arrhythmias can usually be distinguished by the duration of the QRS complex and the presence or absence of a pre-excitation.

8.1.a Orthodromic Atrioventricular Reentry Tachycardia

In orthodromic AVRT the QRS complexes are usually narrow because antegrade conduction from the atria to the ventricles is via the normal conduction system. The tachycardia is initiated by either an atrial or ventricular premature beat. For example, an atrial premature beat can be blocked in the AP, whereas the impulse is conducted to the ventricle via the AV node/His-Purkinje system, with subsequently conduction of the impulse back to the atrium over the AP (ECG 24.24). Thus the polarity of the p wave is determined by the location of the atrial insertion of the AP (ECG 24.25). P waves arise always distinctly after the QRS, usually allowing differentiation between AVRT and AVNRT (during AVNRT the P wave is hidden within, partly merging with or close to the QRS). Because conduction to the atria occurs rapidly, the retrograde P wave is closer to the preceding QRS than to the following QRS (RP < PR), except in the case of slowly conducting AP (see below). The RP interval remains constant, regardless of the tachycardia cycle length. QRS alternans (beat-to-beat oscillation in QRS amplitude) may be present when the rate is very rapid.

Ventricular aberration is relatively common in AVRT. If there is an aberrant ventricular conduction, a typical bundle-branch block pattern (right or left BBB) is present (ECGs 24.24 and 24.26a). Sudden shortening of the cycle length at the onset of the tachycardia may lead to phase 3 aberration (the tachycardia cycle length is shorter than the refractory period of the AP). While the refractory period of the bundle branches rapidly shortens after onset of the AVRT, aberrations are usually short-lived (Ashman phenomenon, ECG 24.24). If an aberration persists longer, this is usually due to concealed retrograde conduction through one of the bundle branches (ECG 24.26a).

When episodes of both aberrant and nonaberrant conduction are present during tachycardia, it is interesting to compare the tachycardia cycle length under both circumstances. If a bundle branch block is on the same side as an AP, the rate is slower during aberrant ventricular conduction than during nonaberrant conduction, because the depolarization has to travel via the controlateral bundle branch and across the septum, making the circuit longer. Such a finding is specific for the diagnosis of orthodromic AVRT and allows localization of the AP. In ECG 24.24, as well as in ECGs 24.26a–b, the rate of tachycardia is slower during LBBB than with nonaberrant conduction. Thus, the diagnosis of an orthodromic AVRT with a retrograde limb using a left-sided AP can be established.

Orthodromic AVRT may often be distinguished from AVNRT on the basis of the timing of the retrograde p waves. However, it may be impossible to differentiate between AVRT and atrial tachycardia.

8.1.b Antidromic Atrioventricular Reentry Tachycardia

During antidromic AVRT, the antegrade conduction from the atria to the ventricles is via the AP, and the retrograde conduction from the ventricles to the atria is via the normal nodal His-Purkinje conduction system. Thus, the QRS complexes are fully pre-excited and the polarity of the QRS onset is the same as the delta wave polarity during sinus rhythm. QRS complexes are usually broader than during sinus rhythm and may resemble ventricular tachycardia. The width of the QRS and the repolarization often obscure retrograde P waves (ECG 24.10).

The initiation of antidromic AVRT by atrial premature beats requires that the atrial coupling interval is longer than the antegrade refractory period of the AP but shorter than the refractory period of the AV node/His-Purkinje system. The atrial premature beat is therefore blocked antegradely in the AV node but is conducted antegradely via the AP. Antidromic AVRT is far less common than orthodromic AVRT and usually occurs if AP has a short refractory period or/and if the AP is remote from the AV node (left free wall AP).

8.1.c Permanent Junctional Reentrant Tachycardia

Permanent (incessant) junctional reentrant tachycardia (PJRT) most often occurs in early childhood and is sometimes seen in young adults. PJRT is an orthodromic AVRT mediated by a concealed AP that has slow and decremental conduction properties. The AP is usually localized in the posteroseptal region. Slow retrograde conduction over the pathway causes the RP interval during PJRT to be longer than the PR interval. P waves resulting from retrograde conduction are inverted in leads II, III and aVF (ECG 24.27). Due to long retrograde conduction over the AP, the arrhythmia tends to be incessant, with a heart rate usually between 120 and 200/min. As a result of the rapid rates, some patients with PJRT may present with impaired left ventricular function (tachycardia-mediated cardiomyopathy). PJRT is often difficult to distinguish from ectopic atrial tachycardia.

8.2 Other Tachycardias Associated with an Accessory Pathway

Atrial tachycardia, AVNRT, atrial fibrillation, and atrial flutter, as well as ventricular tachycardia, can all coexist with an AP. Both AVNRT and atrial tachycardia can use the bystander AP to transmit impulses to the ventricle and may result in a pre-excited regular tachycardia. In these cases, the arrhythmia can not be distinguished from antidromic AVRT without electrophysiologic testing.

Because the AV node has decremental conduction properties, antegrade conduction time through the AV node is longer during atrial tachycardia or during typical AVNRT than during sinus rhythm, whereas the conduction time over the AP will remain the same. Consequently, the degree of ventricular pre-excitation will increase and the QRS will broaden.

8.2.1 Special Condition: Atrial Fibrillation

Atrial fibrillation occurs in 10%–30% of patients with WPW (see above). Most of the patients with pre-excitation do not present structural heart disease. Radiofrequency ablation of AP may often cure atrial fibrillation. Thus, the AP itself is related to the genesis of atrial fibrillation.

There are several characteristic ECG findings in patients, with a 'pre-excited atrial fibrillation' (ECG 24.12a):

i. there is a completely irregular rhythm
ii. the QRS complexes are wide, resembling those seen during sinus rhythm, with many beat-to-beat variations in the degree of fusion in some cases (ECG 24.12b)
iii. moreover, some QRS complexes may even be normal.

The degree of fusion or pre-excitation is not just related to the R–R interval, which means it is not only a rate-related phenomenon. This may result from concealed retrograde conduction into the AP or the AV node.

The shorter the refractory period of the AP, the more rapid is AV conduction. If the AP has a very short refractory period there is a risk that the ventricular rate will be very rapid and will degenerate into ventricular fibrillation.

Atrial flutter does not have the same causal association with accessory AV connections as AF and is rarely seen in patients with a WPW pattern. The ventricular rate is related to the AP refractory period. If the AP refractory period is short, 1 : 1 AV conduction over the AP can occur during atrial flutter. Atrial flutter with 1 : 1 AV conduction may be difficult to distinguish from ventricular tachycardia.

8.3 Ventricular Fibrillation and Sudden Death

If the AP has a very short antegrade refractory period (< 250 msec), a rapid ventricular response can occur during AF. Ventricular rates over 300/min may degenerate into ventricular fibrillation.

Drug therapy with agents slowing the AV node (especially digitalis and verapamil) may increase the risk of ventricular fibrillation in patients with pre-excitation.

9 Other Accessory Connections

The anatomic substrate for the classic pre-excitation is a bundle of myocytes that bridges the AV junction (bundle of Kent). Several other conducting pathways have been described (Figure 24.4), including:

i. Mahaim fibres of several types (fasciculoventricular, nodoventricular, atriofascicular, or atrioventricular) (see section 9.1)
ii. James fibres connecting the atria with the low AV node or with the bundle of His.

9.1 Mahaim Fibre and Mahaim Tachycardias

In 1937, during pathologic examinations of a heart, Mahaim and Benatt identified islands of conducting tissue extending from the His bundle tissue into the ventricular myocardium (fasciculoventricular connections) [11]. The expression 'Mahaim fibre' was subsequently expanded to include connections between the AV node and the ventricular myocardium (*nodoventricular* fibres), and later the *atriofascicular* and *atrioventricular* connections with decremental conduction (Figure 24.4), [12,13]. The true Mahaim (fasciculoventricular) fibres are encountered exceptionally and are not associated with reentry arrhythmias. The *nodoventricular* connections were initially presumed to be responsible for an antidromic AVRT with LBBB morphology, called Mahaim tachycardia. However, as the fasciculoventricular fibres, these nodofascicular fibres turned out to be extremely rare. The anatomic substrate for this LBBB morphology tachycardia (Mahaim tachycardia) was later found to be a slowly conducting atriofascicular or atrioventricular AP with decremental conduction properties (conduction slowing at faster heart rates).

Histologic examination of tissue from patients treated surgically demonstrated an AP with features similar to normal AV nodal tissue. The presence of nodal tissue in the AP may account for the decremental properties seen in this type of Mahaim fibre. Therefore, this type of AV connection with decremental properties has been referred to an *accessory* AV node. In fact, 'accessory AV nodes' with a right lateral or anterolateral localization have been described more recently.

Thus, the modern definition of Mahaim fibres includes two types of decremental right-sided APs (both arising from the atrial side of the tricuspid annulus but with different ventricular insertions), that may be responsible for Mahaim tachycardias [12,13]. In contrast to the WPW syndrome there is no delta wave with Mahaim fibre conduction.

The ECG at rest in patients with Mahaim fibres is usually normal, without pre-excitation. This is due to preferential ventricular activation via the AV node at normal heart rates at rest. Furthermore, some Mahaim fibres have decremental conduction similar to the AV node and conduction over the fibre will be slower with enhanced vagal tone or after an atrial ectopic beat. The antegrade conduction over the Mahaim fibre may become apparent only during incremental atrial pacing.

The usual arrhythmia in patients with a Mahaim tachycardia is a reentrant tachycardia using the Mahaim connection as the antegrade limb, and the AV node as the retrograde limb of the circuit [14]. Mahaim fibres can also function as a bystander pathway, conducting an impulse antegradely during an AV nodal reentrant tachycardia, atrial flutter, or atrial tachycardia.

Several conditions have been associated with Mahaim fibres, particularly other APs. Approximately 40% of the patients with Mahaim fibres have other accessory AV connections or dual AV nodal pathways. Mahaim fibres are also associated with Ebstein's anomaly. The typical ECG during Mahaim tachycardia shows a wide QRS tachycardia with fairly typical LBBB morphology, because the antegrade limb inserts into or near the right bundle branch (ECG 24.28).

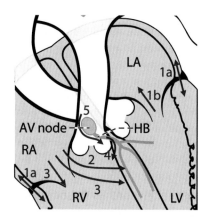

Figure 24.4
Different varieties of conducting bypass tracts. Arrows indicate the direction of propagation. (4) and (5) are extraordinarily rare. 1a) bundle of Kent; 1b) concealed accessory pathway (Kent); 2) atriofascicular fibre (Mahaim); 3) atrioventricular fibre (Mahaim accessory AV node; see text); 4) true Mahaim fibre; 5) James fibre. RA, right atrium; LA, left atrium; RV, right ventricle; LV, left ventricle; HB, His-bundle.

9.2 Lown-Ganong-Levine Syndrome

A short PR interval (< 0.12 sec) without ventricular pre-excitation and associated with paroxysmal tachycardias has been termed as the Lown-Ganong-Levine (LGL) syndrome. LGL was thought to be due to an AP called James bundle, which would link the atrium to the His bundle and bypass the normal AV node. Due to the fast conduction velocity over the AP, the impulse would reach the His-Purkinje system and ventricles before the activation via the AV node and without affecting the QRS complex morphology. However, the existence of an atriohissian AP was not clearly demonstrated. Today it is thought that the majority of patients with short PR interval, paroxysmal tachycardia and no pre-excitation show AVNRT in the setting of an enhanced conduction velocity over the AV node.

10 Therapy of the WPW Syndrome

Patients with the WPW syndrome are treated because of symptomatic arrhythmia on one hand, or because of the risk of a life-threatening arrhythmia on the other.

10.1 Acute Termination of Tachycardia

Manoeuvres that increase vagal tone and depress AV nodal function, such as carotid sinus massage and the Valsalva manoeuvre, may be sufficient to cause AV nodal block and thus terminate the tachycardia. If these procedures fail, intravenous adenosine is the drug of choice to terminate *orthodromic* AVRT. The drug of choice for *antidromic* AVRT is intravenous procainamide. In countries where procainamide is not available, adenosine or ibutilide may be alternative drugs. Antidromic AVRT can also degenerate into atrial fibrillation following drug administration, especially adenosine. Because APs supporting antidromic AVRT usually have short antegrade refractory periods, the ventricular response during pre-excited atrial fibrillation may be more dangerous than the primary arrhythmia.

Pre-excited atrial fibrillation may be complicated by ventricular fibrillation and requires rapid treatment. If the patient is haemodynamically unstable, DC cardioversion should immediately be performed. If the patient is stable, procainamide is the first choice therapy in the USA [15]. Although the class Ic antiarrhythmic drug, flecainide, is efficacious and is used in several countries [16], the parenteral formulation is not approved for use in the USA. Flecainide may organize atrial fibrillation into a slow atrial flutter with 1 : 1 AV conduction resulting in a very rapid ventricular rate. Furthermore, it may cause marked QRS widening at fast heart rates. The most interesting drug for termination of pre-excited AF is ibutilide, a class III antiarrhythmic drug that is only available for intravenous administration. It prolongs the refractoriness of the atrioventricular node, of the His-Purkinje system *and* of the AP. In one series of 22 patients with atrial fibrillation during an electrophysiologic study, ibutilide prolonged the shortest pre-excited R–R interval and terminated the arrhythmia in 95% [17].

During atrial fibrillation, beats conducted via the AV node may be conducted retrogradely to the AP, thereby blocking antegrade AP conduction and slowing the ventricular rate. Thus, all agents slowing AV node conduction without affecting the refractory period of the AP may increase the ventricular rate during atrial fibrillation, thus increasing the risk of ventricular fibrillation. They are contraindicated in pre-excited atrial fibrillation therefore. Verapamil is the most dangerous agent for precipitating ventricular fibrillation [18–20].

With intravenous verapamil a second mechanism is probably involved: hypotension produced by verapamil-induced vasodilatation is followed by a sympathetic discharge that may enhance AP conduction. Intravenous digoxin and beta-blockers have been described as being responsible for degeneration into ventricular fibrillation, but this is rare.

10.2 Chronic Therapy for Prevention

Radiofrequency ablation can cure more than 95% of patients; it has a low risk of complications, and is the first choice therapy in symptomatic patients (ECG 24.29), [21,22]. Pharmacological therapy may be preferred occasionally. Class Ic antiarrhythmic drugs are the drugs of choice for preventing orthodromic tachycardias [16]. Although sotalol can abolish tachycardias, the risk of torsade de pointes (4%) appears unacceptable for long-term therapy in this context. Amiodarone can abolish arrhythmias. However, it has a number of common adverse effects – a concern for patients with WPW who are often young and may require many years of therapy. Finally, beta-blockers can be used in patients with concealed AP or with an AP known to have a long refractory period. If the refractory period of the AP is not known, beta-blockers should be used with caution because of the risk of precipitating ventricular fibrillation in case of pre-excited atrial fibrillation. For the same reason, beta-blockers are contraindicated in patients with antidromic AVRT.

10.3 Treatment of Patients with an Asymptomatic WPW Pattern

Optimal management of patients with a WPW pattern without tachycardia is still a matter of debate [23,24]. On one hand, sudden cardiac death because of ventricular fibrillation is a rare, yet possible, outcome in these individuals. The underlying mechanism is atrial fibrillation with a very high ventricular rate, because of a short antegrade refractory period of the AP, deteriorating into ventricular fibrillation. On the other hand, there is a very low risk of serious complications from electrophysiologic studies and from ablation. Information on the antegrade refractory period of the AP is therefore important in order to recognize asymptomatic people at risk for dying suddenly.

Several noninvasive tests are available for identifying low and high risk patients. Our approach is first to perform an exercise test and look for conduction block over the AP. Sudden conduction block over the AP (from one beat to the next) with increasing heart rate during sinus rhythm (ECGs 24.15 and 24.16) indicates that the refractory period of the AP has been reached (long refractory period). We consider that the prognosis of these patients is excellent without any therapy. However, progressive decrease of pre-excitation over several beats may be due to acceleration of conduction in the AV node and decreased degree of pre-excitation. In these patients, as well as in the patients where pre-excitation persists during stress testing (ECG 24.19a), we perform an invasive study to determine the electrophysiologic properties and location of the AP. We recommend an ablation to all patients with a rapidly conducting AP (refractory period 250 msec or shorter). In the other patients, the decision depends on the localization of the AP and the feasibility of the ablation. In practice, ablation is performed in about 90% in these patients.

References

1. Cohn AE, Fraser FR. Paroxysmal tachycardia and the effect of stimulation of the vagus nerves by pressure. Heart 1913;5:93
2. Wolff L, Parkinson J, White PD. Bundle branch block with short P–R interval in healthy young people prone to paroxysmal tachycardia. Am Heart J 1930;5:685–704
3. Holzmann N, Scherf D. Über Elektrokardiogramme mit verkürzter Vorhof-Kammer-Distanz and positiven P-Zacken. Z Klin Med 1932;121:404
4. Deal BJ, Keane JF, Gillette PC, Garson A Jr. Wolff-Parkinson-White syndrome and supraventricular tachycardia during infancy: management and follow-up. J Am Coll Cardiol 1985;5:130–5
5. Massumi RA. Familial Wolff-Parkinson-White syndrome with cardiomyopathy. Am J Med 1967;43:951–5
6. MacRae CA, Ghaisas N, Kass S, et al. Familial Hypertrophic cardiomyopathy with Wolff-Parkinson-White syndrome maps to a locus on chromosome 7q3. J Clin Invest 1995;96:1216–20
7. Gollob MH, Green MS, Tang AS, et al. Identification of a gene responsible for familial Wolff-Parkinson-White syndrome. N Engl J Med 2001;344:1823–31
8. Arruda MS, McClelland JH, Wang X, et al. Development and validation of an ECG algorithm for identifying accessory pathway ablation site in Wolff-Parkinson-White syndrome. J Cardiovasc Electrophysiol 1998;9:2–12
9. d'Avila A, Brugada J, Skeberis V, et al. A fast and reliable algorithm to localize accessory pathways based on the polarity of the QRS complex on the surface ECG during sinus rhythm. Pacing Clin Electrophysiol 1995;18:1615–27
10. Chiang CE, Chen SA, Teo WS, et al. An accurate stepwise electrocardiographic algorithm for localization of accessory pathways in patients with Wolff-Parkinson-White syndrome from a comprehensive analysis of delta waves and R/S ratio during sinus rhythm. Am J Cardiol 1995;76:40–6
11. Mahaim I, Benatt A. Nouvelles recherches sur les connections supérieures de la branche du faisceau de His-Tawara avec cloison interventriculaire. Cardiologia 1937;1:61
12. Haissaguerre M, Cauchemez B, Marcus F, et al. Characteristics of the ventricular insertion sites of accessory pathways with anterograde decremental conduction properties. Circulation 1995;91:1077–85
13. Klein LS, Hackett FK, Zipes DP, Miles WM. Radiofrequency catheter ablation of Mahaim fibers at the tricuspid annulus. Circulation 1993;87:738–47
14. Aliot E, de Chillou C, Revault d'Allones G, et al. Mahaim tachycardias. Eur Heart J 1998;19 (Suppl E):E25–E31,E52–E53
15. Fuster V, Ryden LE, Asinger RW, et al. ACC/AHA/ESC guidelines for the management of patients with atrial fibrillation: executive summary. A Report of the American College of Cardiology/American Heart Association Task Force on Practice Guidelines and the European Society of Cardiology Committee for Practice Guidelines and Policy Conferences (Committee to Develop Guidelines for the Management of Patients With Atrial Fibrillation): developed in Collaboration With the North American Society of Pacing and Electrophysiology. J Am Coll Cardiol 2001;38:1231–66
16. Crozier I. Flecainide in the Wolff-Parkinson-White syndrome. Am J Cardiol 1992;70:26A–32A
17. Glatter KA, Dorostkar PC, Yang Y, et al. Electrophysiological effects of ibutilide in patients with accessory pathways. Circulation 2001;104:1933–9
18. Gulamhusein S, Ko P, Klein GJ. Ventricular fibrillation following verapamil in the Wolff-Parkinson-White syndrome. Am Heart J 1983;106(part 1):145–7
19. Gulamhusein S, Ko P, Carruthers SG, Klein GJ. Acceleration of the ventricular response during atrial fibrillation in the Wolff-Parkinson-White syndrome after verapamil. Circulation 1982;65:348–54
20. Michel B, Goy JJ, Kappenberger L. Syndrome de Wolff-Parkinson-White et verapamil: à propos d'un cas de fibrillation ventriculaire. Schweiz med Wschr 1989;119:630–4
21. Morady F. Radio-frequency ablation as treatment for cardiac arrhythmias. N Engl J Med 1999;340:534–44
22. Calkins H. Radiofrequency catheter ablation of supraventricular arrhythmias. Heart 2001;85:594–600
23. Schilling RJ. Which patient should be referred to an electrophysiologist: supraventricular tachycardia. Heart 2002;87:299–304
24. Wellens HJ, Rodriguez LM, Timmermans C, Smeets JP. The asymptomatic patient with the Wolff-Parkinson-White electrocardiogram. Pacing Clin Electrophysiol 1997;20:2082–6

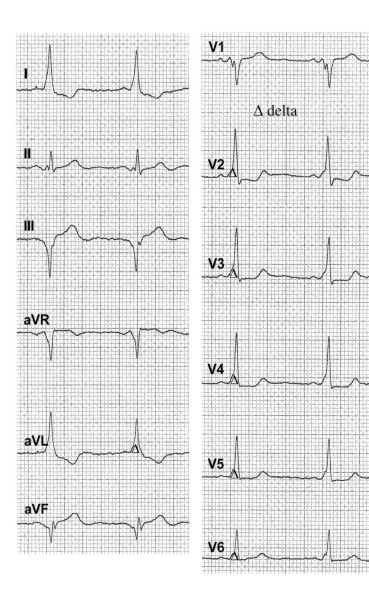

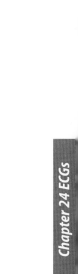

Δ delta

ECG 24.1
60 y/f. Sinus rhythm, typical pre-excitation with shortened PQ interval (0.11 sec) and (positive) delta wave, best seen in V$_2$ to V$_6$ (note: in aVF and III the delta waves are negative because of projections). QRS duration 160 msec. Alteration of repolarization.

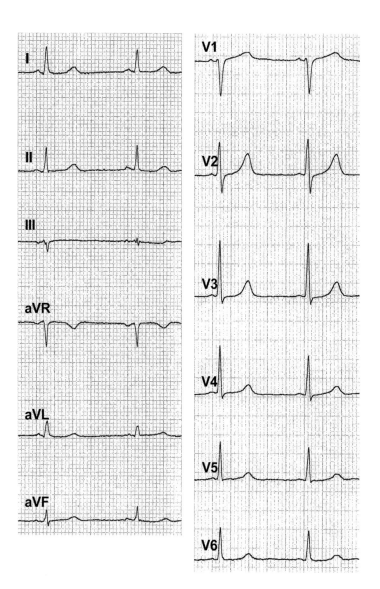

ECG 24.2

56 y/f. Sinus rhythm, PQ interval about 0.11 sec. Questionable 'abortive' delta waves in V$_2$/V$_3$. Similar patterns are seen as normal variants (pseudo-delta waves, due to projection of a normal QRS; Chapter 3), albeit with a normal PQ in this case.

ECG 24.3 ▶

6 y/f. 'Full' pre-excitation, with enormous deformation of QRS and of repolarization.

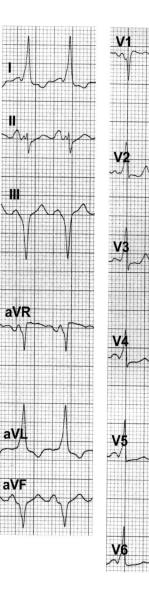

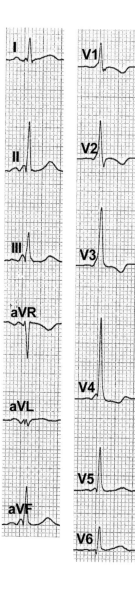

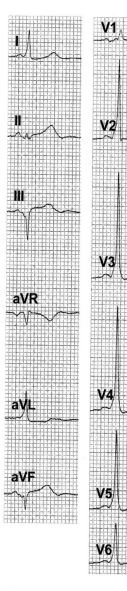

ECG 24.4
29 y/f. Sinus tachycardia, PQ 0.10 sec, delta waves. QS in III/aVF formally imitates inferior MI. Note: the T wave is positive.

ECG 24.5
24 y/m. Sinus rhythm, typical pre-excitation. Tall R waves in V_1 to V_3 imitate posterior MI. Note *biphasic* delta waves in several leads.

ECG 24.6
63 y/m. Sinus rhythm, typical pre-excitation. QS in III/aVF and tall R waves in V_1 to V_3 might be falsely interpreted as inferoposterior MI, and the giant R waves in V_2 to V_5 as concentric LVH.

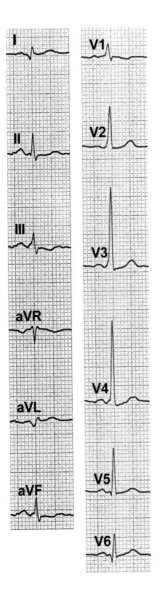

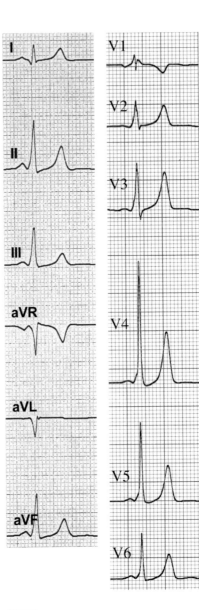

ECG 24.7
56 y/m. Sinus rhythm, typical pre-excitation. Significant Q waves in I/aVL (and V₆) and tall R waves in V₁ to V₃ imitate posterolateral MI.

ECG 24.8
57 y/m. Typical pre-excitation. Tall R wave in V₄ might suggest LVH.

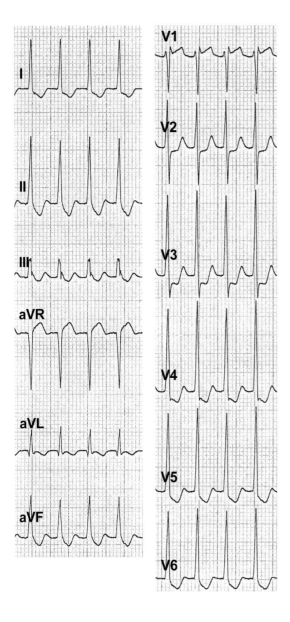

ECG 24.9

48 y/m. WPW syndrome. Orthodromic tachycardia, rate 185/min. The QRS are normal (no delta wave, because the AP is used retro-gradely). No visible p waves. Incomplete RBBB.

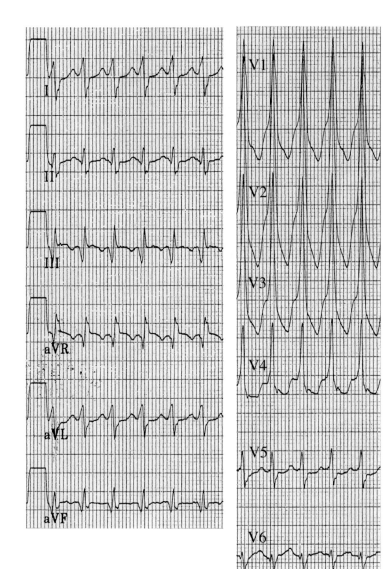

ECG 24.10
75 y/f. Antidromic AV reentry tachycardia, rate 185/min. The QRS complexes are fully pre-excitated and indicate the location of the accessory pathway (left lateral).

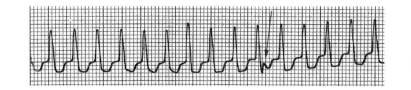

ECG 24.11
40 y/m. WPW syndrome. Rhythm strip. Orthodromic tachycardia, rate 238/min. Arrow: artifact.

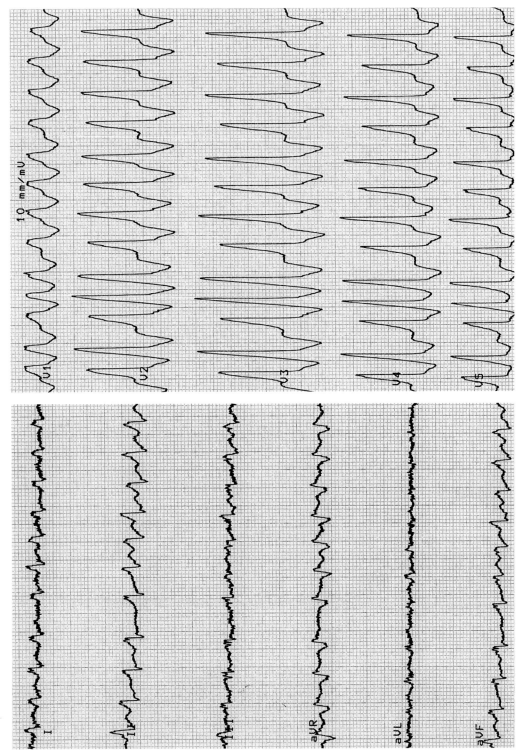

ECG 24.12a

45 y/f. Patient at the emergency unit because of a presyncope during palpitations. ECG: atrial fibrillation with absolute ventricular arrhythmia and wide QRS; maximal instantaneous rate 268/min. No clear delta waves, however relative slow R upstroke in many complexes (see leads V_2 to V_6). WPW syndrome was not known but diagnosed on the basis of this ECG.

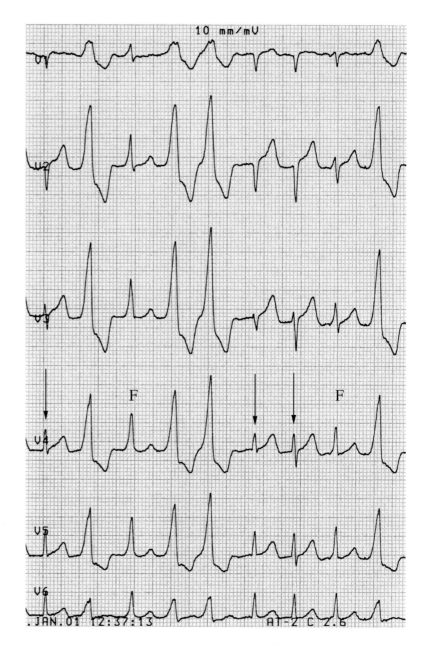

ECG 24.12b
Same patient. ECG (V$_1$ to V$_6$) during infusion of procainamide. Slower rate, persisting arrhythmia. Four QRS complexes show the pattern of 'full pre-excitation', three beats are conducted over the AV node (arrow), two beats are fusion beats (F).

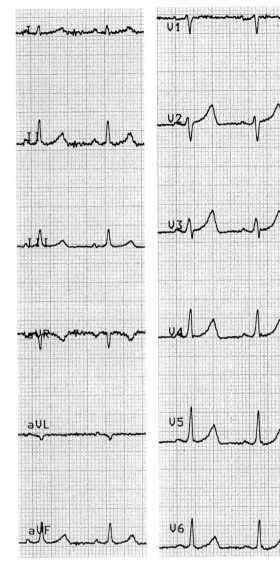

ECG 24.12c

Same patient. ECG after conversion to sinus rhythm with procainamide. Although the patient had a potentially life threatening arrhythmia, her ECG in sinus rhythm shows only a 'minor' pattern of pre-excitation, not recognizable at a first glance.

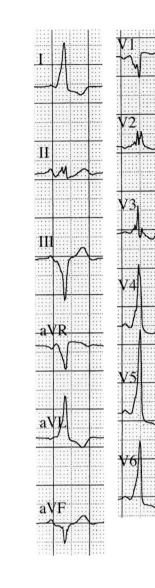

ECG 24.13

Pre-excitation in a patient with an accessory pathway, later ablated in the right posteroseptal location.

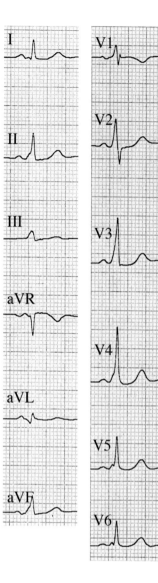

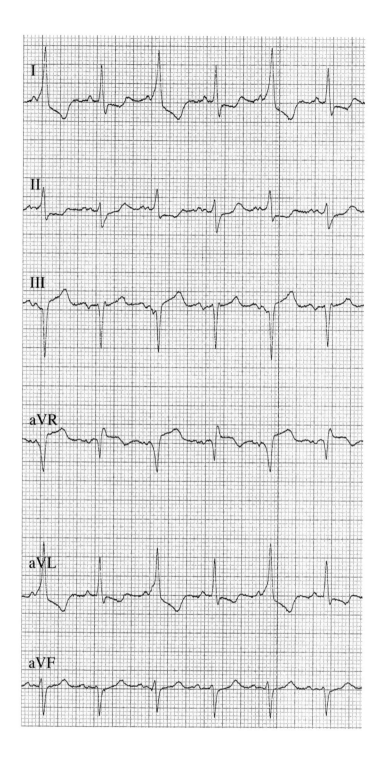

ECG 24.14 ▲

ECG showing borderline PQ interval (120 msec) and pre-excitation. In V_1, R is larger than S, allowing to classify this AP as left-sided. Since the delta wave is positive in II, III and aVF, the pre-excitation pattern is consistent with an anterolateral location. The PR is only slightly shortened because the atrial insertion of the pathway is anatomically far away from the sinus node.

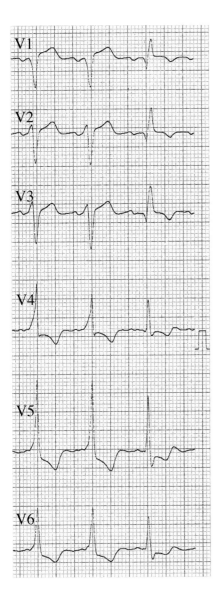

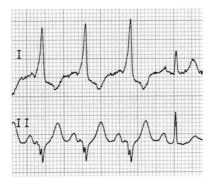

ECG 24.16
ECG during stress test showing marked pre-excitation during sinus tachycardia at 125/min. The location of the AP is right posteroseptal. Abrupt conduction block in the AP leads to disappearance of the delta wave, probably because the refractory period of the AP is just about the same as the sinus rhythm cycle length.

ECG 24.15 ◄ ▲
Intermittent pre-excitation, with presence of normal and short PQ interval, as well as non-pre-excited and pre-excited QRS. RBBB and left anterior fascicular block (LAFB) are seen in the nonpre-excited QRS complexes. The R' wave in V$_1$ due to the delayed depolarization of the right ventricle is not seen when a delta wave is present because of the pre-excitation of the right ventricle by a right-sided AP (note half calibration in the precordial leads).

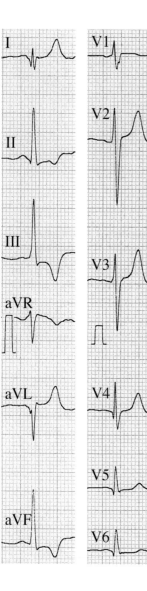

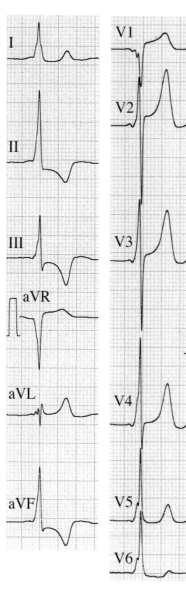

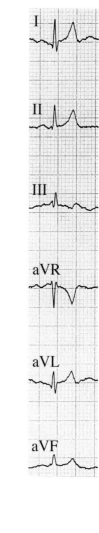

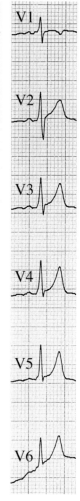

ECG 24.17a
ECG registered in a patient with hyper-trophic obstructive cardiomyopathy, showing a normal PR interval with no clear pre-excitation (note half calibration in the precordial leads). Q waves in V$_4$ to V$_6$ and aVL are probably due to the initial depolarization of the severely hypertrophied ventricular septum. The ST–T changes in II, III, and aVF are probably related to the cardiomyopathy.

ECG 24.17b
Same patient, pre-excitation over a right anteroseptal AP appears at a slower sinus rate (55/min). Intermittent pre-excitation in this case is due to the long refractory period of the AP, that cannot conduct antegradely at a faster sinus rate.

ECG 24.18
Mild pre-excitation with normal PR interval, due to atrial insertion of the AP far away from the sinus node. R > S in V$_1$ is consistent with left-sided AP.

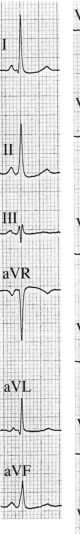
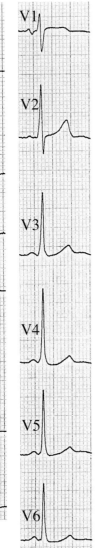

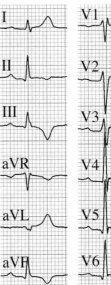

ECG 24.20b
ECG after radiofrequency ablation of the posteroseptal AP in the same patient, demonstrating T wave inversion in leads II, III, and aVF.

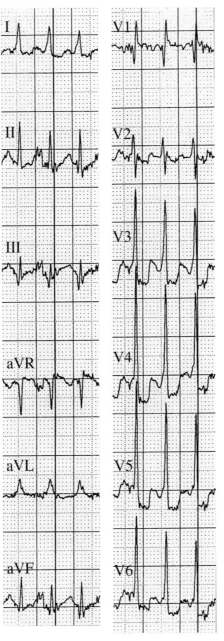

ECG 24.19
ECG registered in a 40-year-old man with an antegrade conducting AP left anterolateral. Recognition of pre-excitation and localization of the AP is more difficult because there is only mild pre-excitation. There are a shortened PQ interval (110 msec), 'abortive' delta waves and an absent Q wave in V_6, consistent with pre-excitation. The large R in V_2 is consistent with a pre-excitation of the left ventricular free wall. The delta wave is positive in aVF, consistent with the left anterolateral position of the AP. If the pre-excitation is not recognized, this ECG may be misdiagnosed as old posterior MI.

ECG 24.20a
ECG from the same patient as ECG 24.14 obtained during a stress test, showing persistence of delta waves during sinus tachycardia at 182/min and marked horizontal ST segment depressions in V_3 to V_6, due to WPW and not to ischemia. Coro: normal.

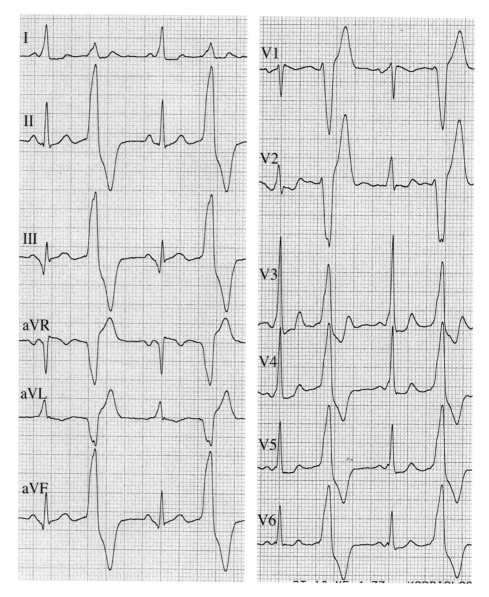

ECG 24.21

Ventricular bigeminy from the right ventricular outflow tract alternating with sinus beats with relatively short PR (0.14 sec) and pre-excited QRS. If pre-excitation is not recognized, the negative delta waves in aVF and III might be misdiagnosed as consistent with an old inferior scar.

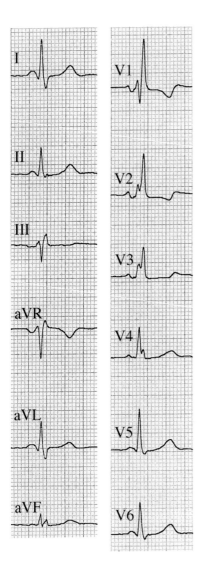

ECG 24.22
ECG showing sinus rhythm with short PR interval, probably due to enhanced atrioventricular conduction. RBBB is present, but there is no pre-excitation of the ventricle.

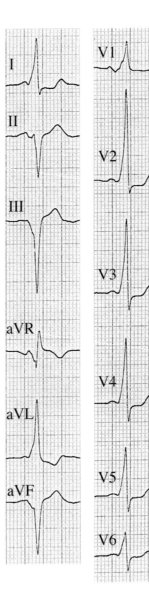

ECG 24.23
Pre-excitation over a left posterior or left posterolateral AP associated with LAFB. The clockwise rotation, usually present in left anterior fascicular block, is masked because of pre-excitation of the left ventricle.

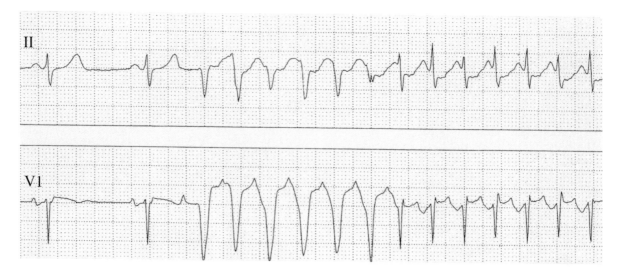

ECG 24.24

Initiation of orthodromic AVRT by an APB. Transient LBBB aberration is present (Ashman phenomenon). Since the tachycardia cycle length is longer (370 msec) during LBBB than with nonaberrant conduction (330 msec), this is an orthodromic AVRT with a retrograde limb using a left-sided accessory pathway. The cycle length is longer during aberrant ventricular conduction than during non-aberrant conduction, because the depolarization has to travel down via the controlateral bundle branch and across the septum, making the circuit longer.

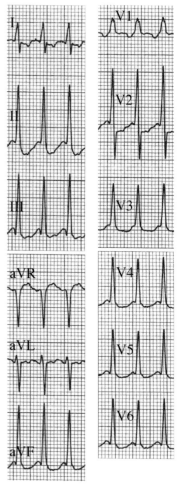

ECG 24.25

Narrow QRS tachycardia at a rate of 174/min during orthodromic AVRT. Retrograde P waves are negative in I and aVL, consistent with a retrograde limb of the circuit activating the left atrium first (left sided AP).

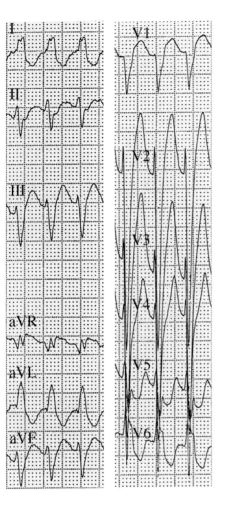

ECG 24.26a
Wide QRS tachycardia at a rate of 178/min, with typical LBBB morphology consistent with orthodromic AVRT with LBBB. Persisting aberration is probably due to concealed retrograde conduction up the left bundle branch, since phase 3 aberration usually disappears promptly because of shortening of the bundle branch refractory period.

ECG 24.26b
Same patient, 1 min later; narrow QRS tachycardia with a rate of 197/min.

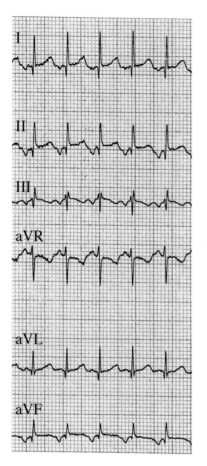

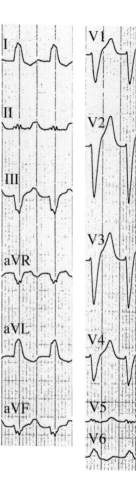

ECG 24.27 ◄

2y/m. Permanent junctional reentrant tachycardia (PJRT). Slow retrograde conduction over the pathway causes the RP interval to be longer than the PR interval. P waves resulting from retrograde conduction are inverted in leads II, III and aVF.

ECG 24.28 ►

Mahaim tachycardia with a wide QRS tachycardia with LBBB morphology. The substrate for this tachycardia was a decremental, slowly conducting AV fibre with a right anterolateral localization.

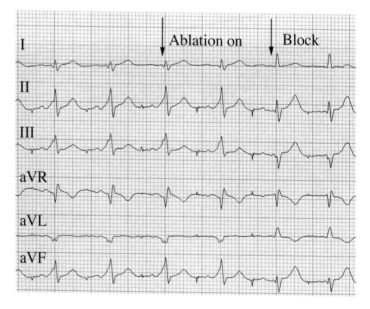

ECG 24.29 ►

Radiofrequency ablation: disappearance of the pre-excitation due to block of AP conduction shortly after onset of current application.

Chapter 25
Ventricular Premature Beats

At a Glance and The Full Picture

Both sections are combined because this chapter can be presented in a relatively concise manner. Ventricular premature beats (VPBs) represent by far the *most frequent* arrhythmia. They are found in about 60% of healthy people, in ambulatory ECGs, and in these cases the VPBs are generally single and monomorphic, not exceeding 100 (or 200?) per hour. In people with heart disease, VPBs occur in 80%–90%, either isolated or in salvos; they may be monomorphic or polymorphic.

ECG

1 Definition and Nomenclature

VPBs are characterized by a *premature broad QRS complex* (generally QRS duration ≥ 120 msec), without a preceding p wave occurring in a normal or prolonged PR interval. A p wave occurring immediately before a broad QRS is not conducted unless pre-excitation is present. Small QRS with only slightly altered configurations are encountered in VPBs arising in the interventricular septum.

In *bigeminy* (ECG 25.1) every normal beat is followed by one premature beat (1 : 1 extrasystole).

In *trigeminy* (ECG 25.2) every normal beat is followed by two premature beats.

In *quadrigeminy* every normal beat is followed by three premature beats.

In 2 : 1 extrasystole a premature beat occurs after two normal beats (ECG 25.3), and in 3 : 1 extrasystole a premature beat occurs after three normal ones (ECG 25.4).

Several textbooks fail to take into account the different sequences of normal and premature beats. However, the hemodynamics are more compromised (ECG 25.5) and the heart is generally sicker in trigeminy/quadrigeminy than in 2 : 1 or 3 : 1

extrasystole. ECG 25.6 shows another possibility – an example of the rare 2 : 2 extrasystole.

Two consecutive VPBs are called a couplet; three consecutive VPBs are called a triplet. Three or more consecutive VPBs are called ventricular tachycardia (see Chapter 26 Ventricular Tachycardias). With up to about four consecutive VPBs the expression salvos is also used. VPBs arise in one of the ventricles and occasionally in the interventricular septum and in the latter case may show a normal QRS duration.

1.1 Coupling Interval

In general the coupling intervals of VPBs show no differences, or only modest ones (up to about 60 msec). Changing coupling intervals are observed in polytopic VPBs. If frequent single (and generally monomorphic) VPBs show considerably different coupling intervals, ventricular parasystole is probable and can be confirmed by detecting an independent regular slower ventricular rhythm, with the help of a pair of dividers.

1.2 Compensatory Pause

In VPBs the ventricular impulses are conducted retrogradely to the atria, at least partially. About 50% are discharging the sinus node. If the impulse does not interfere with the SR, the next sinusal impulse is delivered after a normal interval. This cycle is called fully compensatory. However, a slightly earlier onset of the sinusal beat is common (not fully compensatory cycle).

1.3 Morphology and Origin

Monomorphic VPBs originate from the same focus and are called unifocal (ECG 25.7). Polymorphic VPBs may be unifocal with varying ventricular activation (the coupling interval is equal), or they may be multifocal (with varying coupling intervals) (ECGs 25.8a–b).

It is often stated that VPBs with a right bundle-branch block (RBBB)-like pattern originate in the left ventricle (LV) and that VPBs with a left bundle-branch block (LBBB)-like pattern originate in the right ventricle (RV). This concept contradicts the following reflection: as the diseases of the LV are far more frequent (overall) than those of the RV, the prevalence of VPBs with RBBB-like patterns should greatly exceed that of VPBs with LBBB-like patterns. Because this is not true, more complex mechanisms (such as the site of the breakthrough phenomenon of the electric impulse) are responsible for the QRS configuration. However, the concept of origination site is quite reliable in some conditions. In arrhythmogenic RV dysplasia we generally find VPBs or ventricular tachycardia (VT) with LBBB-like patterns, and when there are VPBs or VT originating in the outflow tract of the RV, LBBB-like patterns with vertical ÅQRS$_F$ are typical.

A superior QRS axis generally reflects an origin near the left posterior fascicle or at the base of one ventricle, and a vertical QRS axis generally reflects an origin near the left anterior fascicle or at the outflow tract.

In the relatively rare VPBs originating in the interventricular septum and conducted nearly normally over the right bundle branch and the left fascicles, the QRS complex is narrow. The QRS configuration may be altered, however.

1.4 Special Types

1.4.1 R-on-T Phenomenon

A VPB that falls on the T wave early (earlier than about 90% of the preceding QT interval), is called 'R on T'-VPB. Such a VPB may induce VT (ECG 25.9) or even ventricular fibrillation, especially in the ischemic myocardium (Chapter 31 Special Waves, Signs and Phenomena).

1.4.2 Interponated VPBs

Very occasionally, a VPB does not interfere with the following normal beat. We miss a postextrasystolic pause (ECG 25.10). Interponated (interpolated) VPBs do not have any special significance.

1.4.3 Fusion Beat

Simultaneous activation of the ventricles by a supraventricular and a ventricular center leads to a *fusion beat*. The QRS duration is between that of the supraventricular beat and that of the VPB. The morphology generally shows signs of the supraventricular and ventricular QRS complex, like a child that shows characteristics of both the mother *and* the father. Fusion is an important phenomenon which is seen in late (phase 4) VPBs, in pre-excitation, and as an additional diagnostic sign in VT (so-called 'Dressler beats'), accelerated idioventricular rhythm, and parasystole.

1.4.4 Concealed Bigeminy

In long rhythm strips with bigeminy, periods without bigeminy may be observed. If the number of supraventricular (mostly sinusal) beats between the VPBs is odd, concealed bigeminy can be assumed (ECG 25.11). After every second sinusal beat a premature beat is generated, but it is not conducted and is therefore invisible in the ECG. Concealed bigeminy does not impair the hemodynamics – as bigeminy often does – but it represents an additional disturbance of conduction. It may result from drug treatment of bigeminy. In this context let us remember the famous remark by Douglas Zipes: "Antiarrhythmic drugs make sick cells sicker."

2 Differential Diagnosis

VPBs need to be distinguished from supraventricular premature beats with a broad QRS. In supraventricular premature beats, broad QRS are caused by aberrant ventricular conduction, generally RBBB or LBBB aberrations. In many cases, a preceding p wave can be identified, with a normal or prolonged (sometimes minimally reduced) PR interval. Often the p waves are hidden within the T wave and can be detected by deformation of the T wave, which becomes either pointed or 'camelhump-like'. AV nodal premature beats with broad QRS (aberration) are very rare. In this case, p waves are hidden within the QRS complex due to retrograde activation of the atria, and differentiation from VPBs may be possible by respecting QRS morphology in the precordial leads.

3 Mechanism

VPBs are due to re-entry, enhanced automaticity, or triggered activity (see Chapter 26 Ventricular Tachycardias).

4 Prognosis

The prognosis of VPBs depends more on the underlying heart disease and its severity than on the frequency and morphology of VPBs. However, the prevalence of VPBs has been recognized as an independent risk factor for premature cardiac death.

Based on the Framingham study, men without clinically apparent coronary artery disease (CAD) and frequent VPBs (> 30 per hour) or complex ventricular arrhythmias, have a twofold increase of the risk for all-cause mortality and MI or death, due to CAD. However, in men with CAD and in women with and without CAD, complex and frequent ventricular arrhythmias are not associated with increased risk [1].

Bjerregaard et al [2] found in a small cohort of 237 apparently healthy people an increase in subsequent CAD in those individuals who had > 900 VPBs per day or VT in the 24-hour ECG. A total of 378 placebo patients enrolled on the European Infarction Study [3], who had pairs or runs of VPBs, showed a low 2-year mortality rate of 4%, but a high rate of 16.7% when ventricular arrhythmias were combined with impaired LV function. In the study by Vaage-Nilsen et al [4] the number of VPBs (> 10 per hour) registered 1 week and 1 month after acute MI had a predictive value for mortality. In the study by Statters et al [5] the frequency of VPBs (registered 6–10 days after acute MI) was significantly predictive for adverse cardiac events in 379 MI patients with early thrombolysis and 301 without, at a follow-up of 1–8 years. Schmidt et al [6] described the absence of heart rate turbulence after VPBs as an independent and potent postinfarction risk stratifier. In patients after coronary artery bypass grafting, the ventricular arrhythmias do not seem to predict premature sudden cardiac death [7]. In patients with idiopathic dilated cardiomyopathy, ventricular arrhythmias are significantly worse at predicting mortality than other factors, such as LV ejection fraction and stroke work index [8]. In a study of 617 patients (393 women, 224 men) with left ventricular hypertrophy (LVH), the 6-year cumulative incidence of all-cause mortality in men without ventricular arrhythmias was 12%, compared to 28% in men with frequent or complex ventricular arrhythmias. In women the corresponding values were 11% and 22% [9].

In a review, Podrid et al [10] reported for patients with cardiomyopathy of any etiology and heart failure a high prevalence of frequent VPBs (70%–95%) and of unsustained VT (40%–80%).

5   Therapy

For many years VPBs have been treated on the basis of their frequency, regardless of the myocardial function. The goal of therapy was to reduce the number of VPBs by 85% in 24 h. Two studies changed this appalling approach completely. Velebit et al [11] proved that various antiarrhythmic drugs have proarrhyhmic effects; effects that are most accentuated in Vaughan Williams Class I drugs. The results of the CAST study [12] hit the medical world like a bomb: patients treated with flecainide, encainide or moricizine showed a threefold mortality compared with the placebo group. Risk factors (besides the antiarrhythmic drug itself) were reduced LV function and probably reduced renal function (the latter is significant because flecainide is partly eliminated by the kidneys). From that point on, the 'cosmetic' therapy of VPBs was abandoned and the antiarrhythmic drugs of Vaughan Williams Class I [13,14] are now avoided whenever possible. If some therapy or prophylaxis is necessary, beta-blockers are preferable. In symptomatic patients, flecainide continues to be used by many cardiologists because of its potent antiarrhythmic action, albeit only in patients with preserved ventricular and normal renal function. This with a *maximum* dose of 100-50-100 mg a day; generally 50-50-50 mg are sufficient.

References

1. Bikkina M, Larson MG, Levy D. Prognostic implications of asymptomatic ventricular arrhythmias: the Framingham Heart Study. Ann Intern Med 1992;117:990–6
2. Bjerregaard P, Sorensen KE, Molgaard H. Predictive value of ventricular premature beats for subsequent ischemic heart disease in apparently healthy subjects. Eur Heart J 1991;12:597–601
3. Andresen D, Bethge KP, Boissel JP, et al. Importance of quantitative analysis of ventricular arrhythmias for predicting the prognosis in low-risk postmyocardial infarction patients. European Infarction Study (EIS) Group. Eur Heart J 1990;11:529–36
4. Vaage-Nilsen M, Rasmussen V, Hansen JF, et al. Prognostic implications of ventricular ectopy one week, one month, and sixteen months after an acute myocardial infarction. Danish Study Group on Verapamil in Myocardial Infarction. Clin Cardiol 1998;21:905–11
5. Statters DJ, Malik M, Redwood S, et al. Use of ventricular premature complexes for risk stratification after acute myocardial infarction in the thrombolytic era. Am J Cardiol 1996;77:133–8
6. Schmidt G, Malik M, Barthel P, et al. Heart-rate turbulence after ventricular premature beats as a predictor of mortality after acute myocardial infarction. Lancet 1999;353:1390–6
7. Pinto RP, Romerill DB, Nasser WK, et al. Prognosis of patients with frequent premature ventricular complexes and nonsustained ventricular tachycardia after coronary artery bypass graft surgery. Clin Cardiol 1996;19:321–4
8. De Maria R, Gavazzi A, Caroli A, et al. Ventricular arrhythmias in dilated cardiomyopathy as an independent prognostic hallmark. Italian Multicenter Cardiomyopathy Study (SPIC) Group. Am J Cardiol 1992;69:1451–7
9. Bikkina M, Larson MG, Levy D. Asymptomatic ventricular arrhythmias and mortality risk in subjects with left ventricular hypertrophy. J Am Coll Cardiol 1993;22:1111–6

10. Podrid PJ, Fogel RI, Fuchs TT. Ventricular arrhythmia in congestive heart failure. Am J Cardiol 1992;69:82G–95G (discussion of review 95G–96G)
11. Velebit V, Podrid P, Lown B, et al. Aggravation and provocation of ventricular arrhythmias by antiarrhythmic drugs. Circulation 1982;65:886–94
12. CAST (Cardiac Arrhythmia Suppression Trial). Preliminary report: effect of encainide and flecainide on mortality in a randomized trial arrhythmia suppression after myocardial infarction. N Engl J Med 1989;321:406–12
13. Vaughan Williams EM. A classification of antiarrhythmic actions reassessed after a decade of new drugs. J Clin Pharmacol 1984;24:129–47
14. Vaughan Williams EM. Significance of classifying antiarrhythmic actions since the cardiac arrhythmia suppression trial. J Clin Pharmacol 1991;31:123–35

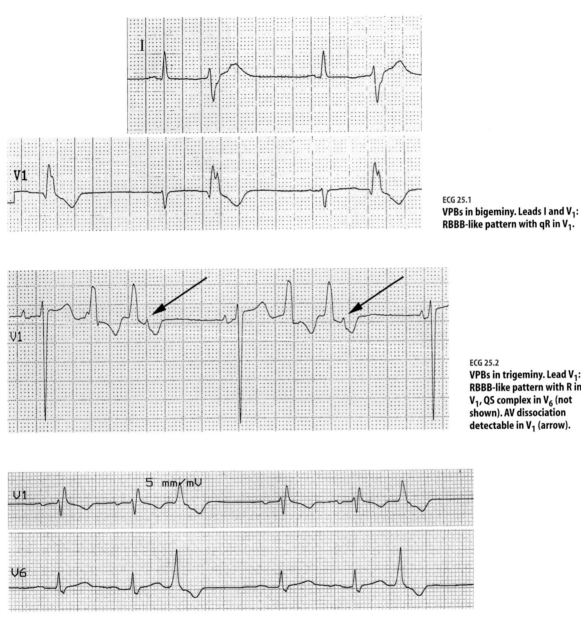

ECG 25.1
VPBs in bigeminy. Leads I and V$_1$: RBBB-like pattern with qR in V$_1$.

ECG 25.2
VPBs in trigeminy. Lead V$_1$: RBBB-like pattern with R in V$_1$, QS complex in V$_6$ (not shown). AV dissociation detectable in V$_1$ (arrow).

ECG 25.3
Leads V$_1$/ V$_6$. Ventricular 2 : 1 extrasystole. Purely positive QRS in the precordial leads. In sinus rhythm there is AV block 1° and incomplete RBBB.

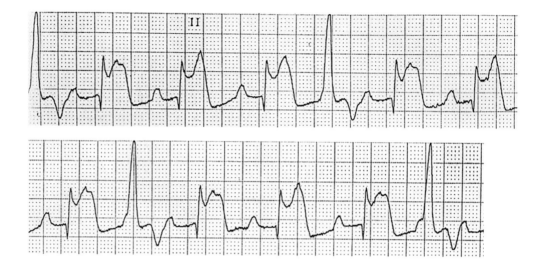

ECG 25.4

44y/m. Lead II, continuous stripe: ventricular 3 : 1 extrasystole in a patient with acute inferior MI. Note alternating repolarization (as a sign of ischemia), interrupted by VPB. Other stripes showed bigeminy. Thus concealed bigeminy is probably present.

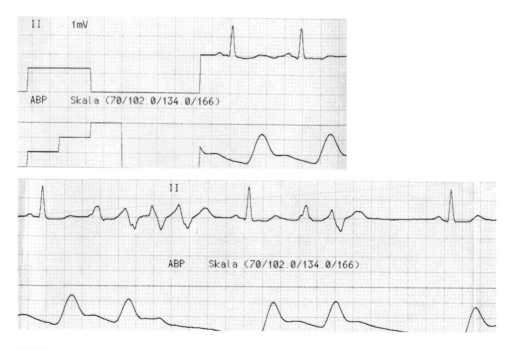

ECG 25.5

Continuous stripe. Upper stripe: rhythm. Lower stripe: blood pressure. In this case only the first VPB leads to normal LV contraction. The subsequent VPB(s) remain without hemodynamic response.

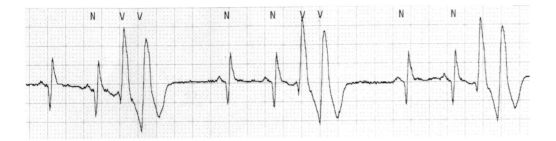

ECG 25.6 ▲
Monitor lead. Ventricular 2:2 extrasystole.

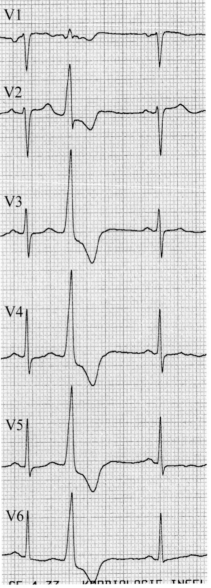

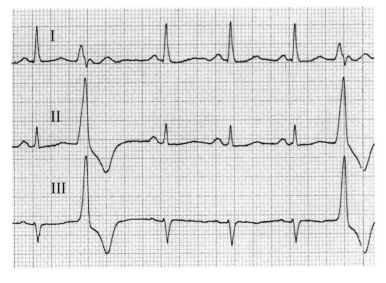

ECG 25.7 ▲ ▶
Monomorphic VPBs. Note almost exclusively positive QRS in precordial leads.

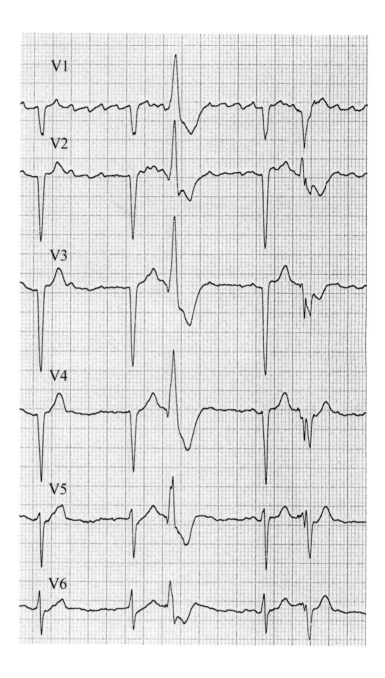

ECG 25.8a
76 y/m. ECG: polymorphic VPBs. Atrial fibrillation.

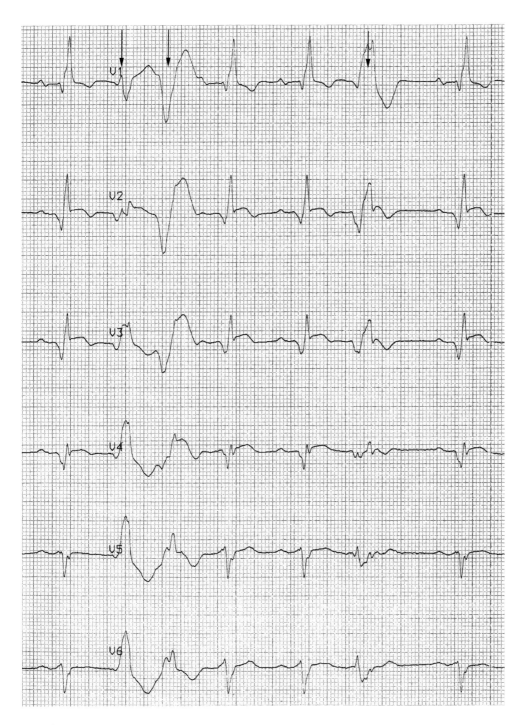

ECG 25.8b
70 y/m. ECG: polymorphic VPBs (arrows). Subacute anterior MI. RBBB.

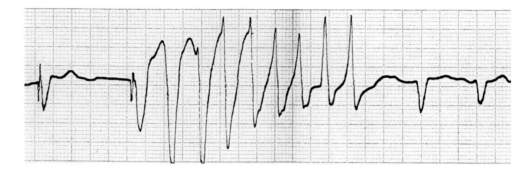

ECG 25.9
86 y/m. R on T. Rhythm strip. In this patient with a pacemaker, a VPB falling on the T wave immediately after the apex induces a short VT of the type torsade de pointes.

ECG 25.10
45 y/m. Uncomplicated AV channel. ECG, lead V$_4$ (4 days after surgical correction): interponated VPB in 2 : 1 sequence. Purely positive QRS in all precordial leads (not shown). No postextrasystolic pause. AV block 1° and RBBB. The PQ time (0.32 sec) is equal before and after VPB. Note that in interponated VPBs the PQ interval is generally prolonged in the postextrasystolic beat.

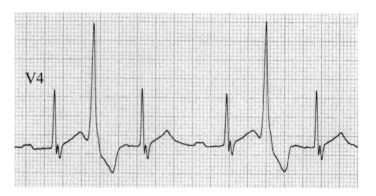

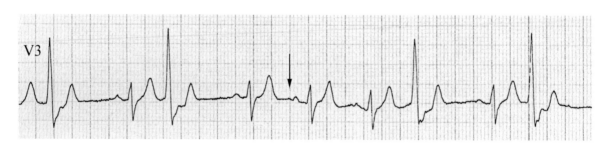

ECG 25.11
Concealed bigeminy (lead V$_3$). Ventricular VPBs in bigeminy, except during three consecutive sinusal beats. A blocked VPB (arrow) is very probable. In this case the coupling interval of the VPBs is not constant.

Chapter 26
Ventricular Tachycardia

At a Glance

Ventricular tachycardia (VT) is generally a severe arrhythmia that often impairs heart function considerably and may be a precursor of ventricular fibrillation. We distinguish the impact of VT on haemodynamics and on prognosis.

The haemodynamic response to VT depends on the pre-existing left (or right) ventricular ejection fraction and the rate and duration of tachycardia. The worse the ventricular function and the faster the rate, the worse the ventricular filling and output are. A VT of long duration (minutes to hours or even days) generally leads to a further haemodynamic deterioration.

The prognosis of VT is determined by the type and severity of the underlying cardiac disease.

ECG

1 Definition and Characteristics of Ventricular Tachycardia

Ventricular tachycardia is defined as ≥ three consecutive premature ventricular complexes with a QRS duration of > 0.12 sec (often ≥ 0.14 sec) and a rate between 100 to 240/min (exceptionally up to 300/min), generally 140 to 220/min. The QRS complexes are not preceded by atrial deflections. The tachycardia may be *sustained* (duration > 30 sec; often lasting minutes to hours) or *nonsustained* (duration < 30 sec; often shorter (ECG 26.1)). The repolarization is always altered, with ST elevation or depression and T inversion in some leads.

2 Types of Ventricular Tachycardia

There are three types of VT that *differ* in morphology, clinical significance and often in etiology.

2.1 Monomorphic VT

Monomorphic VT is the most frequent type. It may be sustained or nonsustained.

Sustained monomorphic VT has a rate of 130–240/min and is initiated by a ventricular premature beat (VPB). The tachycardia is regular or minimally irregular. If VT terminates spontaneously, it is followed by a 'post-tachycardia' pause (ECGs 26.2a–b), except in atrial fibrillation.

Monomorphic VT generally shows a left bundle-branch- or right bundle-branch block-like *QRS pattern* (atypical LBBB and RBBB respectively). ECGs 26.3a–b show two episodes of VT in the same patient with LBBB pattern, ECG 26.3c shows the ECG in this patient in sinus rhythm, with a pattern of RBBB + LAFB (left anterior fascicular block) and an extensive anterior myocardial infarction (MI). ECG 26.4a is an example of VT with RBBB-like pattern (and retrograde AV block 2°), ECG 26.4b shows the QRS configuration in sinus rhythm.

A VT with a rate above 200/min is called 'ventricular flutter' by some authors. Others only use the term 'ventricular flutter' if the morphology of VT has a sinus-like form, so that depolarization and repolarization can no longer be distinguished.

Atrioventricular dissociation, one or more fusion beats, capture beats or a retrograde AV block 2° (rare) indicate a *ventricular origin* of the tachycardia in a very high percentage of cases. ECGs 26.4a, 26.5 and 26.6 demonstrate retrograde AV block 2°.

Ventricular capture beats are intermittent supraventricular beats (mostly of sinusal origin) with a narrow (normal broad) QRS complex. Unfortunately, a retrograde AV block and fusion beats, as well as capture beats, are relatively rare phenomena during VT. *Atrial capture* means retrograde activation of the atria. It is always present in supraventricular tachycardia (SVT) and in > 60% of VT. However, in VT the p waves are mostly not detectable.

In *nonsustained* VT the QRS complexes may be monomorphic or more or less polymorphic.

2.1.1 Etiology of Monomorphic VT

The most current *etiology* of monomorphic VT is a coronary heart disease (CHD). However all diseases of the left ventricle, and also (but more rarely) diseases of the right ventricle as congenital heart diseases and arrhythmogenic RV dysplasia, can provoke this type of VT. It may even be seen in people without an apparent structural heart disease. This special type of tachycardia was formerly called *idiopathic* VT. In a substantial number of 'idiopathic VT' invasive electrophysiologic studies have revealed a 'focus' in the right ventricular outflow tract (RVOT), responsible for a typical ECG with LBBB-like pattern and frontal QRS right-axis deviation (ECG 26.7).

The *prognosis* of VT generally depends on the type and severity of the heart disease.

2.2 Polymorphic VT of Type 'Torsade de Pointes'

Torsade de pointes VT is characterized by a special ECG morphology. According to the term, the points of the QRS complexes gradually and repetitively change their polarity, 'twisting' around the isoelectric line, thus appearing as peaky R and S waves. This peculiarity is often not seen in a single lead. The rate can be *excessively* high at 200–300/min (ECGs 26.8 and 26.9), exceptionally as high as 400/min (ECG 26.10). A torsade de pointes type of tachycardia will usually terminate *spontaneously* after several seconds, even after minutes, despite a high rate; attacks lasting longer than 5–10 seconds lead to loss of consciousness, and a long-lasting attack may provoke organic (especially cerebral) damage. But in relatively rare cases, torsade de pointes type of tachycardia degenerates into *ventricular fibrillation*. This deleterious complication cannot be predicted. So anyone with this tachycardia should immediately be monitored and treated (generally with magnesium and potassium, and/or a pacemaker), with a defibrillator on standby.

2.2.1 Etiology of Torsade de Pointes VT

VT of the type torsade de pointes was first associated with the *congenital long QT* syndromes, the *Romano-Ward* syndrome (without deafness), and the *Jervell and Lange-Nielsen* syndrome (with deafness). The *acquired long QT* is far more frequent, arising from many conditions, and leading to a prolongation of the QT or QTU interval. The most common associated conditions arise from therapy with *diuretics* (that provoke

hypokalemia often combined with hypomagnesemia) and *antiarrhythmics* (especially of Vaughan Williams class Ia).

However, torsade de pointes have been observed in many other conditions, such as CHD with and without bradycardia, and with many other drugs (see The Full Picture).

2.3 Polymorphic VT (without 'Torsade de Pointes')

In many publications the term 'polymorphic' refers only to polymorphic VT of the type 'torsade de pointes'. However there are polymorphic VTs *without* torsade de pointes:

i. Polymorphous QRS complexes are not uncommon in nonsustained VT, especially if the tachycardia only lasts for some beats.
ii. Polymorphism of the QRS complexes without torsade de pointes is occasionally seen in patients with severe myocardial damage, and is associated with a bad prognosis. The rate is often not excessive (ECG 26.11). Degeneration into ventricular fibrillation is quite common. This VT type can also be observed in patients with cardiogenic shock shortly before death.

3 A Special Condition: Accelerated Idioventricular Rhythm

Accelerated idioventricular rhythm is *not* a VT, by definition, because its rate rarely exceeds 100/min. However, it does not represent an escape rhythm (as in the case of a low rate ventricular rhythm in the presence of complete AV block) and is therefore often not clearly identified. In most cases a ventricular rhythm (with broad QRS) arises during some beats (generally 2 to 10), suppressing the sinus rhythm by a slightly higher rate. At the beginning and the end of the ventricular rhythm, fusion beats may be observed (ECGs 26.12 and 26.13).

Accelerated idioventricular rhythm is seen especially in acute MI (in a high percentage of patients during the first hours after successful thrombolysis) and after coronary bypass operations; it is therefore accepted as a fairly reliable marker of myocardial ischemia.

4 Differential Diagnosis of 'Wide QRS' Tachycardias: VT *versus* SVT with Aberration

Not only VT but also supraventricular tachycardias (SVT) with *aberration* (SVTab) lead to broad QRS complexes (≥ 0.12 sec).

4.1 Types of SVT with Aberration (SVT with Wide QRS)

Three types of SVTab are distinguished.

4.1.1 SVTab with Bundle-Branch Block

SV tachycardias like atrial flutter, atrial fibrillation, AV tachycardia, and sinus tachycardia without detectable p waves with bundle-branch block (rarely bilateral bundle-branch block), represent the most common form of SVTab with wide QRS.

In all cases of wide QRS tachycardias at a moderate rate (110–150/min) a sinus tachycardia with bundle-branch block aberration should be excluded. The p wave may be hidden within the T wave of the preceding beat, especially in the presence of a long PQ interval.

4.1.2 SVTab in Wolff-Parkinson-White Syndrome

This rare condition only occurs by conduction antegradely through the accessory pathway, or in cases of additional bundle-branch block. *More than 90%* of the 'WPW tachycardias' show a narrow (normal) QRS.

4.1.3 SVT with other Aberrations

In some textbooks a third type of SVTab is mentioned – as an excuse for unidentifiable aberration – that is not connected with bundle-branch block or with the WPW syndrome. It also has to be mentioned that in rare cases a wide QRS may be present without aberration, for instance in severe ventricular hypertrophy and myocardial infarction.

4.2 Criteria for Differentiation Between VT and SVTab

Many morphologic ECG criteria have been published, concerning alterations of the QRS complex, that should allow the differentiation between VT and SVTab. In Table 26.2 the common characteristics are summarized. However, even experienced rhythmologists only achieve 85% accuracy, even if all 12 standard leads are available.

Those readers who have neither time nor leisure to learn all these rather complicated morphologic ECG signs may resort to a more simple approach.

Tchou et al [1] demonstrated in an intelligent publication that a positive answer to two *questions* may be more reliable than diagnosis based on other clinical and morphological criteria:

1. Did you recently suffer from a *myocardial infarction*?

2. Did you have those symptoms (due to tachycardia) only *after* myocardial infarction?

A positive answer to both questions predicted VT with great accuracy. The initial 'clinical' diagnosis in 31 patients (10 women, aged 27–79 years) with broad QRS tachycardias was VT in 17 and SVT in 14 patients. Electrophysiologic studies revealed 29 VTs and only two SVTs. Two of the 17 VTs proved to be SVT and, more important, all 14 SVTs proved to be VT. Based on the answers to the two questions above, 28 of 29 VTs and 2 of 2 SVTs were correctly diagnosed. Only one VT was taken for a SVT. Thus the 'two-question' method resulted in 95% diagnostic accuracy, whereas the 'clinical–morphologic' method had accuracy of about 50%. The study was slightly limited by the profile of the patient cohort: almost all had CAD (and MI) and were referred to hospital for electrophysiologic evaluation of broad QRS tachycardia. Furthermore, it should be mentioned that the primary ECG was not interpreted by an experienced rhythmologist.

4.3 Criteria for Differentiation Between VT and Artifacts

Artifacts may be misdiagnosed as wide complex tachycardias, especially in rhythm strips. Generally these are due to mechanical manoeuvres, such as teeth-brushing, knocking on the back during physiotherapy, or perhaps from insufficient skin/electrode contact. Careful analysis of the ECG allows identification of remnant QRS complexes (so-called 'notches') within the artifacts (see The Full Picture).

5 Therapy

As mentioned earlier, differentiation between VT and SVTab may be difficult or even impossible on the basis of the ECG. However, it would be extremely important to make the true diagnosis *before* drug treatment. Misdiagnosis of wide QRS tachycardia, like SVTab, in the presence of VT, may result in life-threatening complications. Take for example a VT that is misdiagnosed as SVT with bundle-branch block aberration and is treated intravenously with verapamil or another cardiodepressant drug. The tachycardia does not respond, but blood pressure falls dramatically, perhaps leading to death.

In all unclear cases, DC conversion is the *only* correct therapy! Of course, oxygen should be applied and cardiodepressant narcotics must be avoided. Some antiarrhythmic drugs can impair the effect of external direct current (DC) conversion. In the presence of VT, lidocaine is only successful in 20%–30%. Procainamide (success rate of about 80%) produces a fall in systolic blood pressure of 10–20 mmHg, or even more.

In summary, a wide QRS complex tachycardia at a high rate often needs *immediate* DC conversion. Unprofessional 'pretreatment' with antiarrhythmic drugs may not only be deleterious, but also may impair or inhibit the success of DC conversion.

The Full Picture

It is quite ambitious to discuss ventricular tachycardia, the differential diagnosis included, in just a few pages. The subject is covered by over 14 000 publications (PubMed in spring 2003), special meetings are dedicated to it and many chapters of books and even whole books discuss it at length.

6 Pathophysiology

Many mechanisms are responsible for the onset and maintenance of VT, the most important being reentry, enhanced automaticity, and triggered activity.

6.1 Reentry

Reentry is by far the most important mechanism for induction and maintenance of VT. Three conditions must be fulfilled to allow a 'circus movement' of conduction and consecutive excitation:

i. a circuit around an anatomic or functional obstacle
ii. unidirectional block within this circuit
iii. impaired conduction.

The *length* of the circuit is defined as the product of the conduction velocity and refractory period. In the heart, such a circuit is only possible if the conduction velocity is considerably slowed and the refractory period is shortened.

Table 26.1 demonstrates the formula in:

i. normal conditions
ii. in 'macro' reentry
iii. in 'micro' reentry.

Macro reentry occurs around a scar due to myocardial infarction (structural obstacle) or around an ischemic zone (functional obstacle).

Micro reentry occurs at a cellular basis, e.g. within the Purkinje conduction network. Multiple small and chaotic reentry circuits with so-called valvelets represent the electrophysiologic mechanism for ventricular fibrillation.

6.2 Enhanced Automaticity

The underlying mechanism for automaticity is *slow diastolic depolarization* that is inherent to all myocardial conduction fibres. In normal conditions the cells of the sinus node have the fastest diastolic depolarization, thus conducting the heart. Under pathologic circumstances, such as ischemia, fibres of the conduction system may accelerate diastolic depolarization. If a ventricular conduction fibre reaches the threshold for systolic depolarization earlier during diastole (compared with the sinus node), the ventricle overpaces the sinus node. If this occurs once, a ventricular premature beat is produced. If the process is repetitive, VT occurs. In this case, monomorphic VT is mainly maintained by reentry mechanisms. Enhanced automaticity is commonly found in sinus tachycardia, AV junctional rhythms, parasystole, and accelerated idioventricular rhythm.

Table 26.1
Length of the reentry circuit (conduction velocity × refractory period)

Normal*	Circuit length 4.0 m/sec × 0.3 sec = 1.2 m
Macro reentry	Circuit length 0.02 m/sec × 0.24 sec = 0.0048 m (i.e. 4.8 mm)
Micro reentry	Circuit length 0.001 m/sec × 0.2 sec = 0.0002 m (i.e. 0.2 mm)

* In normal conduction velocity, a reentry circuit is not possible.

6.3 Triggered Activity

Triggered activity is directly connected to the previous electrical cycle and may be manifest as *early* afterdepolarization (during the T wave of the previous repolarization) or as *late* afterdepolarization (after the T wave of the previous repolarization). The phenomenon may be single or repetitive. Triggered activity occurs in the presence of QT prolongation, e.g. in conditions of acute ischemia, hypokalemia, in congestive heart failure, and digitalis excess. The mechanism in polymorphous VT of the type 'torsade de pointes' is probably a combination of triggered activity, enhanced automaticity and reentry. For details about pathophysiology see the wonderful ECG Tutor produced by Gettes and co-workers [2].

6.4 Electrotonus

Electrotonus seems to be a basic mechanism for different forms of AV dissociation (e.g. isorhythmic, and with interference), *not* connected with complete AV block. Electrotonus probably plays a rule in many arrhythmias like VT and ventricular fibrillation. However, this mechanism is poorly understood overall – a promising subject for further research.

ECG Special ——————————————————

6.5 Onset of VT

The initiation of VT may be related to the previous rate, especially in patients without structural heart disease. The autonomic nervous system may play an important role [3]. In adrenergic-dependent VTs, the previous sinusal rate increases. Decreased heart-rate variability enhances the arrhythmia. It has also been observed that VT may be immediately preceded by a long R–R interval (by decreased sinusal rate or a postextrasystolic pause), thus leading to the *short-long-short* coupling intervals (ECGs 26.14 and 26.15) that may be based on the 'bigeminy rule'. The *second* 'short' coupling corresponds to the first VT beat.

Occasionally the VT begins with a fusion beat (ECG 26.16).

7 Types of Ventricular Tachycardia

Several morphologically different types of VT are distinguishable, often differing in etiology and clinical significance. These are monomorphic VT; polymorphic VT *with* torsade de pointes and *without* torsade de pointes; and special types of VT.

7.1 Monomorphic VT

Besides the common form of VT with an atypical LBBB or RBBB pattern, mainly due to coronary artery disease (CAD) and other cardiomyopathies, two special 'subtypes' with characteristic morphology and etiology have gained attention in recent decades.

i. The ECG in *monomorphic* VT in patients with *arrhythmogenic right ventricular dysplasia* [4,5,6] often show VPBs and episodes of VT with an LBBB-like pattern (ECG 26.17). The so-called *epsilon wave* is a typical sign for this condition and may occasionally be seen in routine ECGs with sinus rhythm in lead V_1. ECG 26.18 shows an epsilon wave in a patient with sarcoidosis, involving the right ventricle (confirmed by biopsy).

ii. *Monomorphic* (idiopathic) VT in young patients *without* structural heart disease [7,8,9] is the other type. Often the arrhythmogenic substrate is situated in the right ventricular *outflow tract* (RVOT). In these cases the ECG is characterized by an LBBB-like pattern with a vertical QRS axis (ECG 26.7). Idiopathic VT arising in the left ventricle, identical to *fascicular* tachycardia, is much rarer. It is found predominantly in young men and was first described by Zipes et al [10]. Its origin is generally found in the region of the left *posterior* fascicle and consequently there is a pattern of RBBB and left-axis deviation (ECG 26.19). In some rare cases the origin is localized in the left *anterior* fascicle. The ECG is then characterized by a pattern of RBBB and right-axis deviation. The QRS in the left *posterior* fascicular type is relatively small (≤ 140 msec). All types of idiopathic tachycardia respond to calcium antagonists (e.g. verapamil) but also to flecainide, sotalol, and amiodarone.

7.2 VT of the Type Torsade de Pointes

This type was first described by Dessertenne in 1966 [11] and has been discussed in At a Glance section 2.2. The acquired form, due to various conditions, occurs more frequently than the congenital forms, the *Romano-Ward* syndrome (without deafness) [12,13] and the *Jervell and Lange-Nielsen* syndrome (with deafness) [14]. Viskin published an excellent review about this subject [15].

7.3 Polymorphic VT Without Torsade de Pointes

In its nonsustained form, this arrhythmia occurs during rest or at exercise, often indicating heart disease, generally as polymorphic triplets.

Its sustained form is connected with a severely depressed ventricular function and is associated with a very bad prognosis.

7.4 Special Types of VT

Other types of tachycardia (parasystolic VT, bidirectional VT, double tachycardia) are extremely rare.

7.4.1 Parasystolic VT

Parasystolic VT is characterized by a regular interectopic interval, a variable interval of the parasystolic beats to the beats of basic rhythm and fusion beats. Intermittent failure of parasystolic beats to manifest is due to exit block (type 1 or 2) and may make the diagnosis difficult.

7.4.2 Bidirectional VT

Bidirectional VT may be seen in patients with severe heart disease or digitalis intoxication [16,17]. The ECG is characterized by alternations of ventricular complexes with opposite axis deviation. The origin of the VT is found in the first part of the left bundle branch or in the His bundle, the left ventricle is alternately activated over the left anterior and left posterior fascicle. ECG 26.20 shows a typical example. In this young patient, the tachycardic episodes could be provoked by exercise as well as by infusion with isoprenalin.

7.4.3 Double Tachycardia

Double tachycardia is the combination of VT and SVT (atrial or AV tachycardia). The ventricles are activated by the ventricular 'focus' and the atria follow the supraventricular tachycardia. Ventricular capture beats with the supraventricular rhythm may occur. In general double tachycardia is only detected with the help of oesophageal or intra-atrial leads. Double tachycardia during exercise was described by Eldar et al [18] in one patient with CAD and in two young individuals with no apparent heart disease.

7.4.4 Accelerated Idioventricular Rhythm

Accelerated idioventricular rhythm is generally not a tachycardic arrhythmia and occurs mainly in acute MI, especially during thrombolysis [19] and in the first 24 hours after coronary bypass operations. As the following case report demonstrates it may be difficult to classify a VT, and a VT may even need an unconventional therapy.

Short Story/Case Report 1

One Saturday morning in 1989 a 54-year-old man with a history of two MI was hospitalized because of left heart failure that was confirmed by clinical findings and x-rays. Blood pressure was 90/70 mmHg. The ECG showed a monomorphic ventricular tachycardia with a relatively slow rate of 120/min (ECG 26.21a). In a *retrospective* analysis, AV dissociation could be detected, with an atrial rate only a few beats below the VT rate. Left ventricular function seemed to be severely impaired (M-mode echo). The VT neither responded to lidocaine nor amiodarone, intravenously. In another attempt to restore sinus rhythm, five DC shocks were applied without success. On the Monday morning, the patient's general state was dramatically impaired, he was in shock with anuria and blood pressure of 70/50 mmHg. His arrhythmia, about 120 beats/min, had persisted for 48 h.

This case of relatively slow VT, unresponsive to antiarrhythmic drugs and DC shock, was discussed again, and it was decided to evaluate the effect of atrial overpacing as 'ultima ratio'. The cardiac index (determined by thermodilution) was 3.1 l/m². Right atrial pacing was successful at a rate some beats above the VT rate, with a PQ interval of 0.2 sec and a bundle-branch block pattern (ECG 26.21b). In the following 20 min, blood pressure slowly rose to 100/70 mmHg, the cardiac index increased to 4.2 l/m², and the patient was more alert. His cardiac state stabilized under constant atrial pacing, and 4 h later diuresis recovered. During repetitive short interruption of pacing, VT at a rate of 120/min reappeared immediately, with a rapid fall of blood pressure. Two short episodes of sinus tachycardia at a rate of 120–122/min were also observed. After 16 h the arrhythmia stopped, without using an antiarrhythmic drug. Coronary angiography revealed severe three-vessel disease and a left ventricular ejection fraction of 30%. The patient was operated on the next day (four bypasses), recovered, and was still alive 8 years later [20].

To conclude, in this patient with severe CHD, cardiogenic (arrhythmogenic) shock was reversible by atrial overpacing of a low rate VT – an apparently life-saving procedure. The VT may be classified as a relatively slow 'common' monomorphic VT or as an accelerated idioventricular rhythm, extremely atypical in duration and (high) rate. The VT, unresponsive to drugs and electroconversion, supports the latter diagnosis. (The method of atrial overpacing in VT was already described by Easly and Goldstein in 1968 [21].)

8 Differential Diagnosis of Regular Monomorphic 'Wide QRS Complex' Tachycardias: VT *versus* SVT with Aberration

8.1 General Remarks

Before leaping to the details of the ECG, it is convenient (also for experienced arrhythmia readers) to consider some general conditions of patients with a 'wide QRS complex' tachycardia.

8.1.1 Age and Prevalence

The *older* the patient, the more probable VT is. Occasionally atrial flutter with aberration (especially with a previously abnormal ECG) may cause diagnostic difficulties. The WPW syndrome is rare in the elderly.

In *young* patients, supraventricular tachycardias with *aberration* (SVTab) are more frequent than in older patients and may be connected with the WPW syndrome. However, many conditions are responsible for the preponderance of VT over SVTab, also in young patients. These include:

i.   myocardial infarction
ii. other LV cardiomyopathies
iii. RV outflow tract VT
iv. VT in right ventricular arrhythmogenic dysplasia
v.   malignant VT in Brugada syndrome
vi. fascicular tachycardia, especially in men.

Overall, VT is far more frequent than SVTab, occurring at a ratio of about 10 : 1.

8.1.2 Underlying Cardiac Disease

A patient with a significant heart disease, especially with involvement of the left ventricle, is much more prone to VT than to SVTab. The most frequent etiology of VT is CAD with myocardial infarction. Long-term survival is considerably impaired [22,23]. A patient with myocardial infarction and broad QRS tachycardia, who never suffered from a tachycardia before the infarction, has a 95% probability of developing VT.

However, Tchou's [1] results are based on a highly selected population.

9 Electrocardiographic Findings in Monomorphic VT

9.1 General Findings

9.1.1 AV Dissociation

AV dissociation strongly favors the presence of VT. Only in *automatic junctional tachycardia* (which is rare, especially in adults) is AV dissociation often present, due to retrograde AV block. In cases with aberrant ventricular conduction, a clear diagnosis can only be made with the help of His bundle and intra-atrial electrograms. The *absence* of AV dissociation does not exclude VT. In about 55% of occurrences of VT, AV dissociation is present. In about 25% there is retrograde 1 : 1 atrial activation and in 20% VA block 2°, 2 : 1 or Wenckebach, according to a study by Akhtar et al [24]. Wellens and Lie [25] published differing results on 45 patients, where 11 patients showed AV dissociation, 29 had retrograde 1 : 1 conduction and 5 had VA block 2°. Second degree VA block may be intermittent and its detection requires careful examination. Again, second degree VA block is also seen in automatic junctional tachycardia.

9.1.2 Fusion Beats and (Ventricular) Capture Beats

These phenomena are generally linked to the presence of AV dissociation. Both fusion beats (ECG 26.3b) and ventricular capture beats are rare, even in VT with a relatively slow rate. A long rhythm strip enhances the chance of detecting such a beat, confirming the diagnosis. Occasionally the VT begins with a fusion beat. The first beat of the VT in ECG 26.16 represents a fusion. The VT is stopped by the increase of the rate because the impulse in the reentry circuit meets with refractory tissue.

9.1.3 VA Block 2°

Based on the literature, retrograde AV block 2° occurs in 10%–20%. In practice, we have observed VA block 2° in only a few percent, although considering long rhythm strips, in many cases. Retrograde 2 : 1 AV block is more frequent (ECGs 26.4a and 26.5) than retrograde Wenckebach block (ECG 26.6).

9.1.4 Rate

The rate in VT is overall extremely variable and is useless for distinguishing SVTab. However, a rate of 130–160/min is always suspicious for atrial flutter with 2 : 1 AV block, where the flutter waves are hidden within a typical bundle-branch block pattern. Flutter may be unmasked by carotid artery massage in some cases.

9.1.5 Regularity

Monomorphic VT is said to be regular or slightly irregular. However, any irregularity is often minimal and detectable in only a few cases (by comparing several cycles – with the help of a pair of dividers – with the same number of other cycles). Moreover, also SVTab may be slightly irregular, in some cases. Note that a patient with SVTab may show a rate of 178/min and 1 h later a rate of 170/min. The same behaviour of the rate may be found in patients with VT too (also in untreated patients).

9.1.6 Comparison of 'Wide QRS' Tachycardia ECG with a *Previous* ECG Without Tachycardia

Whenever possible the wide QRS tachycardia ECG should be compared with a *previous* ECG without tachycardia. Often this is decisive for correct diagnosis. Consider the following examples:

i. The *previous* ECG shows *ventricular* premature beats with the same QRS configuration that is present during tachycardia. The diagnosis of VT is sure – if the PBs are really of ventricular origin (!).

ii. The *previous* ECG (without tachycardia, mostly sinus rhythm) shows the *same* wide QRS configuration (that means a bundle-branch block) as the wide QRS complex tachycardia; the diagnosis of SVTab is sure.

iii. The *previous* ECG shows an LBBB and the wide QRS complex tachycardia ECG shows an RBBB-like pattern (or vice versa); the diagnosis of VT is sure. Explanation: a bundle branch, blocked at a low rate, will not conduct at a high rate. Caution: very rarely, in the previous ECG (without tachycardia) we find an RBBB and during tachycardia a pattern of RBBB + LAFB, simulating an LBBB pattern in the limb leads. However, VT patterns are seen that simulate aberrations such as RBBB + LAFB or RBBB + LPFB (see both sections 2.1 and 7.1 on idiopathic and fascicular VT).

iv. If the Q or QS pattern of MI in the previous ECG (without tachycardia or RBBB) does not or only minimally changes during the wide QRS tachycardia, showing an RBBB pattern, SVTab is very probable (although, statistically VT is much more probable in a patient with MI).

v. If the frontal QRS axis does not change between the *previous* ECG (*without* RBBB) and the first 60 msec of the QRS complex during wide QRS tachycardia with an RBBB pattern, SVTab is probable.

9.2 QRS Criteria

9.2.1 QRS Duration

A QRS duration ≥ 0.16 msec strongly favors the diagnosis of VT. In SVT with aberrations (SVTab), the QRS duration is generally below 0.15 sec.

Note: antiarrhythmic drugs (especially of class Ia), ventricular hypertrophy, and severe hyperkalemia may prolong QRS duration considerably, e.g. from 100 to 140 msec or more (Chapter 16 Electrolyte Imbalances and Disturbances).

9.2.2 Frontal QRS Axis

In RBBB-like patterns, the frontal QRS axis ($\mathring{A}QRS_F$) does not allow distinction between VT and SVTab. In LBBB-like patterns a frontal axis in the upper right quadrant (between – 90° and + 180°) favors the diagnosis of VT. Differential diagnosis:

i. SVT with RBBB + LAFB, SVT with LBBB
ii. SVT in the WPW syndrome (antidromic type or BBB).

9.2.3 Morphologic QRS Criteria

Morphologic criteria are used preferentially for differentiating between VT and SVTab, and they often represent the *climax* of teaching courses about arrhythmias. However, the patterns of MI and left and/or right ventricular hypertrophy are generally *not* integrated in these criteria. Used in isolation, these criteria lack sufficient accuracy. Also very experienced rhythmologists reach an accuracy of only about 80% if they do not consider other ECG features mentioned (e.g. AV dissociation, fusion beats, second degree VA block) and anamnestic and clinical findings.

The following rule is often proposed: a *typical* RBBB or LBBB pattern favors SVTab, whereas an *atypical* mono- or bifascicular bundle-branch block pattern favors VT. This rule is valid about 80% of the time.

The ECG signs, provided in Table 26.2, for differentiating between VT and SVTab are based on the literature and on our experience. Points 9.2.3a to 9.2.3g present typical features of VT and possible different diagnosis.

9.2.3a Negative QRS in All Precordial Leads

ECG 26.22a shows an example of negative QRS in all precordial leads. ECG 26.22b shows the QRS configuration of the same patient in sinus rhythm.

9.2.3b Positive QRS in All Precordial Leads

See ECG 26.23. Differential diagnosis: SVT in the WPW syndrome with antegrade activation of the ventricles, over the accessory pathway (rare).

9.2.3c High Voltage of QRS in Precordial Leads $V_2/V_3/V_4$

Besides giant QRS amplitude in V_1 to V_3 the ECG 26.24 provides other typical signs for VT. Differential diagnosis in other cases: WPW.

9.2.3d Pre-existing Bundle-Branch Block

Alteration of BBB indicates VT; unchanged configuration indicates SVT.

9.2.3e Cases with LBBB-like QRS Configuration

i.   r wave in $V_1/V_2 \geq$ 0.03 sec or/and
ii. duration of onset QRS to nadir of S wave $\geq$ 0.07 sec (Nadir sign)
iii. Q wave in V_6. Differential diagnosis: SVTab with extensive lateral MI.

9.2.3f Cases with RBBB-like Configuration

QS in V_6 and/or aVF. This sign is very reliable for the diagnosis of VT. However, no rule without exception (see Short Story/Case Report 2).

9.2.3g QRS configuration in RBBB, in lead V_1

The proposed different QRS morphologies that should allow differentiation between VT and SVTab are unreliable in many cases, because the QRS configuration is variable in the aberrations. The QRS morphologies are:

i.   A monophasic notched purely positive QRS does *not* exclude SVTab. About 30% of common RBBB aberrations show this pattern, that is also seen if lead V_1 is attached somewhat too high and too far to the right.
ii. A qR complex does *not* exclude SVTab and is encountered in anteroseptal MI, in RVH, and in acute pulmonary embolism.
iii. An Rs complex may be observed in VT *and* in SVTab.
iv. Only in the presence of an *rsR'* configuration (typical for an antegradely blocked right bundle) can VT be excluded reliably.

Table 26.2
ECG differentiation between ventricular tachycardia (VT) and supraventricular tachycardia with aberration (SVTab)

VT	SVTab
• AV dissociation	• No AV dissociation
• Fusion beats	• Rarely fusion beats in WPW tachycardia
• Retrograde AV block (VA block) 2° (2 : 1 block or Wenckebach)	• No VA block 2°
QRS	
• Purely negative QRS in V_1 to V_6	• Never seen in SVTab
• Purely positive QRS in V_1 to V_6	• Only in antidromic WPW tachycardia
• QRS amplitude strikingly high	• Very high QRS amplitude only in rare cases of WPW tachycardia
• QRS duration $\geq$ 160 msec	• QRS $\geq$ 160 msec only in severe LVH or RVH or hyperkalemia
• Superior QRS axis	• Other than superior QRS axis (exception: LBBB, RBBB+LAFB, antidromic WPW)
• In the presence of BBB pattern in sinus rhythm: different BBB pattern during tachycardia	• In the presence of BBB pattern in sinus rhythm: identical BBB pattern in tachycardia
• QRS in VT similar to VPB in sinus rhythm >>> unreliable (see 9.1.6.i)	
LBBB-like morphology	
• Nadir sign $\geq$ 70 msec (lead V_1/V_2)	• Nadir sign $\leq$ 60 msec
• Q wave in lead V_6	• No Q wave in lead V_6
RBBB-like morphology	
• QS configuration in leads V_6 and aVF	• No QS in V_6 and aVF
• Mono- or biphasic QRS in lead V_1 (R, QR, RS) >>> unreliable (see 9.2.3g)	• Any QRS configuration in V_1 (rsR' type strongly favors SVT!)
Note: The signs for VT are highly specific but show *low* sensitivity (see text)	Note: Many signs for SVT do *not* exclude VT (see text)

LAFB, left anterior fascicular block; LBBB, left bundle-branch block; LVH, left ventricular hypertrophy; RBBB, right bundle-branch block; RVH, right ventricular hypertrophy; SVT, supraventricular tachycardia; VPB, ventricular premature beat; VT, ventricular tachycardia; WPW, Wolff-Parkinson-White syndrome.

Short Story/Case Report 2

In December 2000 a 71-year-old man was admitted to hospital after several episodes of syncope. He had a regular pulse of 180/min and suffered from mild dyspnoea at rest, due to a lung disease. The ECG showed a regular wide QRS tachycardia with a rate of 180/min. The clinical diagnosis was pulmonary hypertension due to severe obstructive lung disease (due to heavy smoking). The patient had amiodarone for intermittent atrial fibrillation. There was no history for CAD; the coronary angiogram 4 years previously was normal. Based on the RBBB-like pattern with a purely positive deflection in V_1 and – especially – a QS complex in V_6 (and V_5) and aVF, the diagnosis of VT was made (ECG 26.25). Lidocaine was without effect, and carotid sinus massage did not influence the tachycardia. Electroconversion was successful after the third attempt, with 360 Joules. The echo showed severe hypertrophy and dilatation of the right ventricle, and LV function was normal. During electrophysiologic investigation, no VT could be induced. However rapid atrial stimulation provoked atrial flutter type II with 1:1 conduction and a rate of 180/min, but without aberration. During catheter manipulation at the right side of the interventricular septum, functional RBBB was induced. The ECG then showed exactly the same QRS configuration in leads V_1, V_6/V_5 and aVF as during spontaneous pseudo-VT, that was unmasked as atrial flutter with 1:1 AV conduction and RBBB aberration. The AV node was ablated and a pacemaker implanted.

Discussion: retrospectively, the QS complex in the lateral leads (and in aVF) was explained by the combination of severe RVH (and dilatation) and complete RBBB, both reducing the amplitude of the R wave in these leads – in this case up to zero.

Especially in very fast tachycardias, differential diagnosis may be very difficult or impossible, e.g. the differentiation between VT and SVT in the WPW syndrome. In some cases of VT at a high rate (≥ 220/min), depolarization and repolarization cannot be distinguished any more, the morphology is equal to ventricular flutter. Although this pattern is very suspicious for VT, it is also seen in SVT in association with the WPW syndrome, e.g. in 1:1 conducted atrial flutter over the accessory pathway.

The currently used flow diagram by Brugada et al [26] for differentiation between VT and SVTab is based on 384 patients with VT and 170 patients with SVTab, investigated with electrophysiology. Grimm et al [27] investigated 240 cases with wide QRS tachycardias, comparing those 'new' criteria with the 'old' ones published by Wellens et al in 1978 [28] and found identical results. The specificity in RBBB-like QRS was 72% with Brugada's criteria, and 70% with Wellens' criteria, and in LBBB-like QRS 87% with both methods.

A critical analysis was recently published by Alberca et al [29]. Based on the results of 232 patients with wide QRS tachycardias, they found a specificity of $\geq 90\%$ in only 5 of 12 criteria analysed:

i.   triphasic QRS in V_1 (rsR', also including Rr') in an RBBB-like pattern (for SVTab)
ii. QS, QR or R pattern in V_6 in an RBBB-like pattern (for VT)
iii. any Q wave in V_6 in an LBBB-like pattern (for VT)
iv. a concordant pattern in all precordial leads (for VT)
v. absence of RS complex in all precordial leads (for VT). The 'Nadir sign' had a specificity of only 66%, however, due to the low limit of 0.06 sec, instead of > 0.07 sec (in our opinion).

Griffith et al [30] have chosen another diagnostic approach in 102 patients with wide QRS tachycardias (QRS ≥ 0.11 sec). They classified a tachycardia as SVTab if a typical bundle-branch block was present. VT was diagnosed in the cases with different patterns. The criteria and results are not completely convincing however.

10   Misdiagnoses of Wide QRS Tachycardias

10.1 VT Misdiagnosed as SVTab

Several publications illustrate that drug therapy of a VT misdiagnosed as SVTab may be deleterious [31,32].

10.2 Differentiation Between Wide Complex Tachycardias (especially VT) and Artifacts

Misdiagnosis of artifacts mimicking VT has been known about since 1970 at least [33]. In a recent publication Knight et al [34] demonstrated the true size of this problem. The authors sampled 12 cases of artifacts that more or less simulated a VT, which had partially erroneous diagnostic and therapeutic consequences, culminating in the implantation of a cardioverter defibrillator (ICD) device in a 41-year-old woman with presyncope but no heart disease.

Table 26.3

Differentiation of VT (without artifacts) from pure artifacts (simulating VT)

Signs for VT

ECG:

- No interference with other rhythms (during tachycardia)
  >>> Absence of 'notches' (see Signs for Artifacts (below))
- Depolarization and repolarization distinguishable in most cases
- Beginning of the tachycardia with a VPB with:
  - configuration similar or equal to the following QRS
  - onset at a reasonable distance from the last SV beat (especially not falling into the absolute refractory period)
- Post-tachycardia pause

Clinical and general conditions:

- Often symptoms during tachycardia
- Often presence of heart disease
- No simultaneous mechanical maneuver
- Well-fixed electrodes

Signs for Artifacts (simulating VT)

ECG:

- Continuous basic rhythm during artifacts
  >>> Presence of 'notches' at identical intervals, corresponding to basic rhythm (detectable best with the help of dividers)
- Depolarization and repolarization not clearly detectable
- Beginning of the 'tachycardia' (unphysiologically) with:
  - a pseudo VPB (1) atypical morphology; (2) onset often too early, falling into the absolute refractory period
  - without VPB
- End of the 'tachycardia' (unphysiologically) with:
  - the first supraventricular beat after the 'VT' often falls into the 'absolute refractory period' of the last 'VT' beat. The post-tachycardia pause is often lacking
- Often excessive rate

Clinical and general conditions:

- No symptoms during 'tachycardia'
- Often absence of heart disease
- Often simultaneous mechanical maneuver
- Occasionally inconstant electrode-skin contact

SV; supraventricular; VPB, ventricular premature beat.

The reason for artifacts that consist in formally wide 'QRS' sequences often remains unclear. However in a substantial number of cases the artifacts are produced by teeth-brushing and physiotherapeutic manipulations or by inconstant skin–electrode contact. ECG 26.26 and ECG 26.27 show a pseudo-VT of two patients, while brushing their teeth, with an astonishingly high rate of about 300/min. Table 26.3 lists the ECG signs and general conditions that allow differentiation between VT and artifacts. The main characteristic is the presence of a basic rhythm during 'VT', recognizable by regular 'notches' (ECG 26.28). In particular, the beginning and end of the 'tachycardia' should be examined with caution. In doubtful cases, e.g. in the case of an irregular basic rhythm (as in atrial fibrillation) and in the absence of 'notches', a cautious evaluation is needed. It is bad enough to mistake an artifact for a VT – it may be deleterious to take a VT for an artifact.

11   Final General (and Therapeutic) Considerations

In spite of the considerable progresses during the last two decades, in the differentiation between VT and SVTab, on the bases of morphologic criteria in the 12 leads ECG, we would like to state:

i.   The accuracy of the 'morphologic' method hovers around 85%. Would the reader be happy to be treated for a potentially life-threatening arrhythmia based on a probability of 85%?

ii. It is mandatory to consider criteria other than morphologic ones, such as the history and clinical findings of each patient. Comparing the tachycardic ECG with a previous ECG without tachycardia is very helpful.

iii. Long rhythm strips sometimes allow detection of VA block 2°, fusion beats, or capture beats.

iv. The presence or absence of AV dissociation can easily be determined using an oesophageal or an intra-atrial electrode.

v.   In selected cases the correct diagnosis is made by electrophysiologic testing.

vi. If the diagnosis cannot be made with 100% reliability, DC conversion is preferred as a first therapeutic approach – no drug-cocktails, please.

vii. Let us enjoy future lectures by arrhythmia experts about morphologic criteria. *We* know that *they* know the true diagnosis already (based on previous electrophysiologic investigations). Anyway, we will continue to study these ECGs with passion and enjoyment. Dealing with complex arrhythmias is an *intellectual* challenge; cardiology images (coro, echo, CT, MRI) are useful and often important, but generally boring (intellectually).

References

1. Tchou P, Young P, Mahmud R, et al. Useful clinical criteria for the diagnosis of ventricular tachycardia. Am J Med 1988;84:53–6
2. Gettes L. ECG Tutor (CD ROM). Armonk NY: Futura Publishing Company 2000
3. Coumel P. Cardiac arrhythmias and the autonomic nervous system. J Cardiovasc Electrophysiol 1993;4:338–55
4. Fontaine G, Guiraudon, Frank R, et al. Stimulation studies and epicardial mapping in ventricular tachycardia: study of mechanism and selection for surgery. In: Kulbertus HE (ed). Re-Entrant Arrhythmias: Mechanisms and Treatment. Lancaster PA: MTP Publishers 1977, pp 334–50
5. Fontaine G, Fontaliran F, Hebert JL, et al. Arrhythmogenic right ventricular dysplasia. Annu Rev Med 1999;50:17–35
6. Fontaine G, Fontaliran F, Frank R. Arrhythmogenic right ventricular cardiomyopathies: clinical forms and main differential diagnoses (Editorial). Circulation 1998;97:1532–5
7. Altemose GT, Buxton AE. Idiopathic ventricular tachycardia. Annu Rev Med 1999;50:159–77
8. Lerman BB, Stein KM, Markowitz SM, et al. Ventricular arrhythmias in normal hearts. Cardiol Clin 2000;18:265–91
9. Belhassen B, Shapira I, Pelleg A, et al. Idiopathic recurrent sustained ventricular tachycardia responsive to verapamil: An ECG-electropysiologic entity. Am Heart J 1984;108:1034–7
10. Zipes DP, Foster PR, Troup PJ, Pedersen DH. Atrial induction of ventricular tachycardia: reentry versus triggered automaticity. Am J Cardiol 1979;44:1–8
11. Dessertenne F. Ventricular tachycardia with 2 variable opposing foci. Arch Mal Coeur Vaiss 1966;59:263–72
12. Romano C. Congenital cardiac arrhythmia. Lancet 1965;1:658
13. Ward OC. A new familial cardiac syndrome in children. J Ir Med Assoc 1964;54:103
14. Jervell A, Lange-Nielsen F. Congenital deaf-mutism, functional heart disease with prolongation of Q-T interval and sudden death. Am Heart J 1957;54:59–68
15. Viskin S. Long QT syndromes and torsade de pointes. Lancet 1999;354:1625–33
16. Kastor JA, Goldreyer BN. Ventricular origin of bidirectional tachycardia. Case report of a patient not toxic from digitalis. Circulation 1973;48:897–903
17. Castellanos A, Ferreiro J, Pefkaros K, et al. Effects of lidocaine on bidirectional tachycardia and on digitalis-induced atrial tachycardia with block. Br Heart J 1982;48:27–32
18. Eldar M, Belhassen B, Hod H, et al. Exercise-induced double (atrial and ventricular) tachycardia: a report of three cases. J Am Coll Cardiol 1989;14:1376–81
19. Gorgels AP, Vos MA, Letsch IS, et al. Usefulness of the accelerated idioventricular rhythm as a marker for myocardial necrosis and reperfusion during thrombolytic therapy in acute myocardial infarction. Am J Cardiol 1988;61:231–5
20. Gertsch M, Fuhrer J. Gefährliche Rhythmusstörungen. Schweiz Med Wochenschr 1993;123:833–43
21. Easly RM, Goldstein P. Differentiation of ventricular tachycardia from junctional tachycardia with aberrant conduction: The use of competitive atrial pacing. Circulation 1968; 37:1015
22. Swerdlow C, Winkle R, Mason J. Determinants of survival in patients with ventricular tachyarrhythmias. N Engl J Med 1983;308:1436–42
23. Graboys T, Lown B, Podrid P, DeSilva R. Long-term survival of patients with malignant ventricular arrhythmia treated with antiarrhythmic drugs. Am J Cardiol l982;50:437–43
24. Akhtar M, Shenasa M, Jazayeri M, et al. Wide QRS complex tachycardia. Reappraisal of a common clinical problem. Ann Intern Med 1988;109:905–12
25. Wellens HJJ, Lie KI. Ventricular tachycardia: The value of programmed electrical stimulation. In: Krikler DM, Goodwin JF (eds). Cardiac Arrhythmias: The Modern Electrophysiological Approach. Philadelphia: WB Saunders 1975, p 182
26. Brugada P, Brugada J, Mont L, et al. A new approach to the differential diagnosis of a regular tachycardia with a wide QRS complex. Circulation 1991;83:1649–59
27. Grimm W, Menz V, Hoffmann J, Maisch B. Value of old and new electrocardiography criteria for differential diagnosis between ventricular tachycardia and supraventricular tachycardia with bundle-branch block. Z Kardiol 1996;85:932–42
28. Wellens HJJ, Bar FW, Lie KI. The value of the electrocardiogram in the differential diagnosis of a tachycardia with a widened QRS complex. Am J Med 1978;64:27–33
29. Alberca T, Almendral J, Sanz P, et al. Evaluation of the specificity of morphological electrocardiographic criteria for the differential diagnosis of wide QRS complex tachycardia in patients with intraventricular conduction defects. Circulation 1997;96:3527–33
30. Griffith MJ, Garratt CJ, Mounsey P, Camm AJ. Ventricular tachycardia as default diagnosis in broad complex tachycardia. Lancet 1994;343:386–8
31. Stewart RB, Bardy GH, Greene HL. Wide complex tachycardia: misdiagnosis and outcome after emergent therapy. Ann Intern Med 1986;104:766–71
32. Dancy M, Camm AJ, Ward D. Misdiagnosis of chronic recurrent ventricular tachycardia. Lancet 1985;II:320–23
33. Arbeit SR, Rubin IL, Gross H. Dangers in interpreting the electrocardiogram from the oscilloscope monitor. J Amer Med Assoc 1970;211:453–6
34. Knight BP, Pelosi F, Michaud GF, et al. Clinical consequences of electrocardiographic artifact mimicking ventricular tachycardia. New Engl J Med 1999;341:1270–4

Further information see: Fromer M. Ventricular tachycardias (my hobby). Editor not yet determined. Publication: sometime this decade (when on earth will Doctor Fromer write this book?)

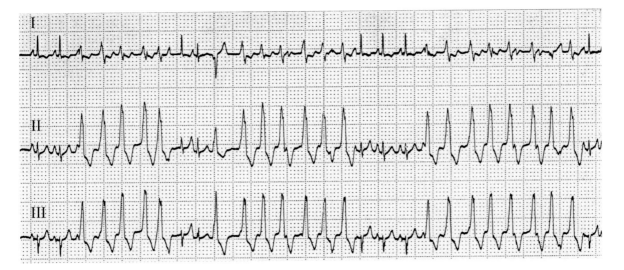

ECG 26.1
40 y/f. Palpitations. ECG (leads I, II, III; paper speed 10 mm/sec): *non*sustained (monomorphic) VTs.

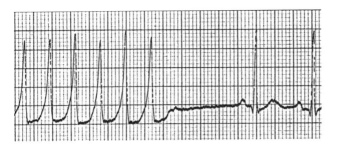

ECG 26.2a
72 y/m. Respiratory insufficiency. Monitor lead (lead II): VT, rate 220/min. Note the post-tachycardia pause.

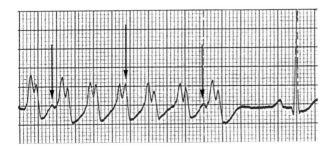

ECG 26.2b
Same patient. Monitor lead: VT, rate 182/min, with different QRS morphology and shorter post-tachycardia pause. AV dissociation: before the second and before the last VT QRS, a *p wave* is detectable; another is hidden within the second (higher) deflection of the forth QRS (arrows).

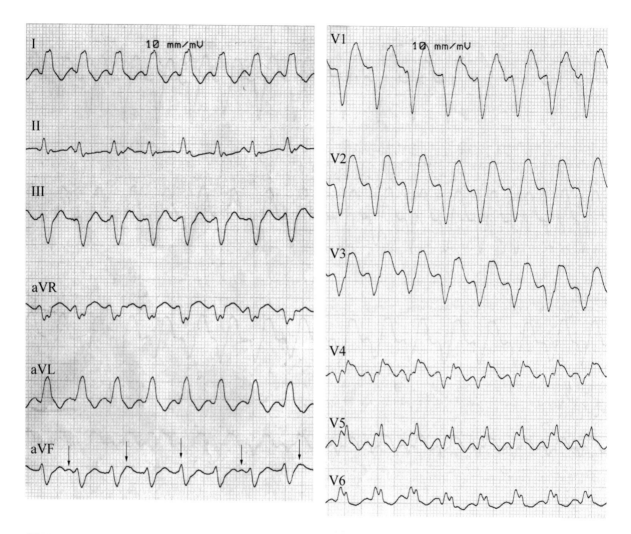

ECG 26.3a

70 y/m. Old anterior infarction with aneurysm. VT with LBBB-like QRS. QRS duration 160 msec. Ventricular rate 143/min. AV dissociation, best recognizable in lead aVF (arrow), atrial rate 85/min. 'Nadir' sign in lead V$_1$ is 90 msec. Note: the transition zone is similar to aberration, with quite abrupt change of negative to positive QRS in V$_4$/V$_5$, possibly due to old anterior infarct.

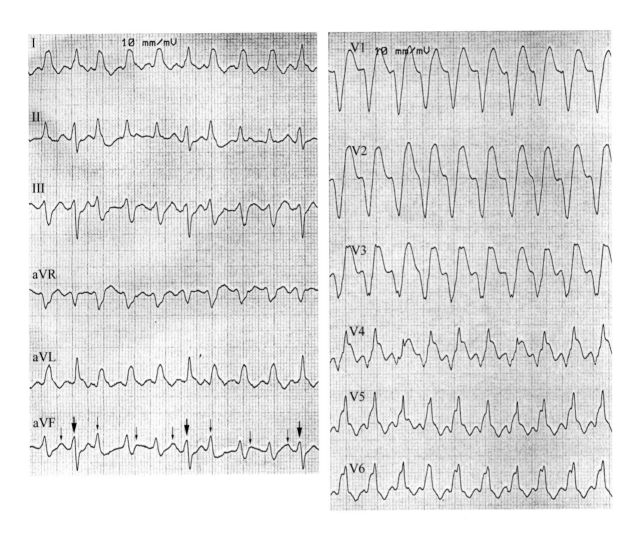

ECG 26.3b

Same patient, limb leads: VT with LBBB-like QRS. Ventricular rate 164/min. AV dissociation; atrial rate 123/min (small arrows). Fusion beats (big arrows), with shorter duration and different configuration, preceded by p waves (hidden within the T wave). Another proof for ventricular origin of the tachycardia is the LBBB-like pattern in this patient with RBBB+LAFB aberration in sinus rhythm (ECG 26.3c).

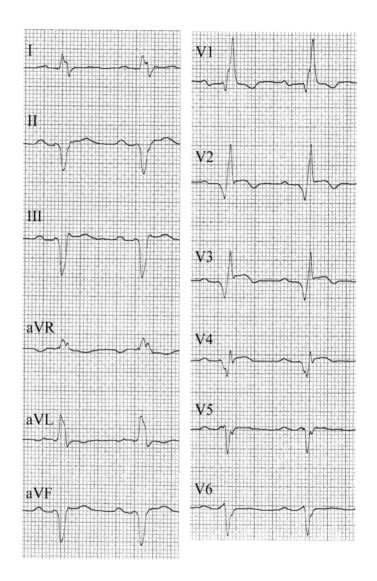

ECG 26.3c
**Same patient. Sinus rhythm (rate 69/min). LAFB +
RBBB. Extensive old anterior infarction, ST elevation
(V$_2$ to V$_4$) due to aneurysm.**

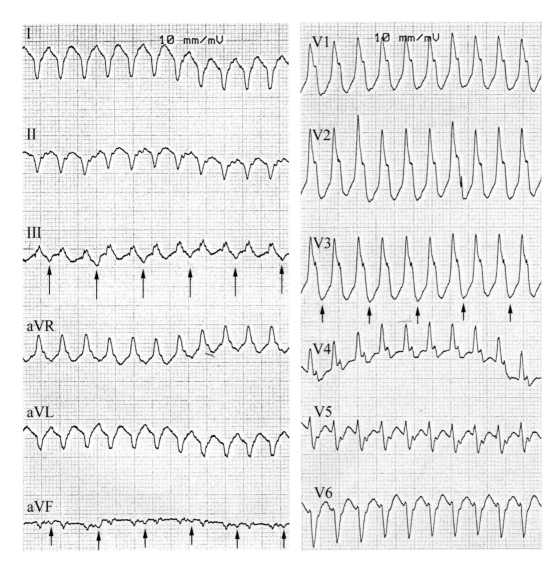

ECG 26.4a

76 y/m. CAD, history of two unlocalizable infarctions. VT with RBBB-like QRS. QRS duration 120 msec. Ventricular rate 236/min. Retrograde 2 : 1 AV block (2 : 1 VA block), best detectable in leads aVF and III (arrows). Atrial rate 118/min.

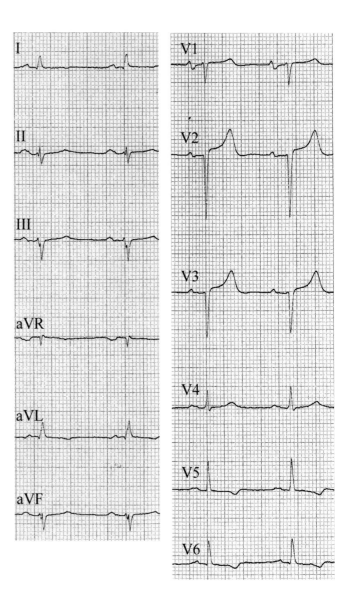

ECG 26.4b ▶
**Same patient. Sinus rhythm (rate 65/min). ÅQRS$_F$ - 30°.
Peripheral low voltage with slightly notched QRS. Absent
R progression V$_1$ to V$_3$. Negative symmetric T waves in
V$_5$/V$_6$. No distinct infarction pattern.**

ECG 26.5 ▼
**82 y/m. CHD. Monitor lead: VT, rate 172/min, with retro-
grade 2 : 1 AV block (2 : 1 VA block) (see arrows).**

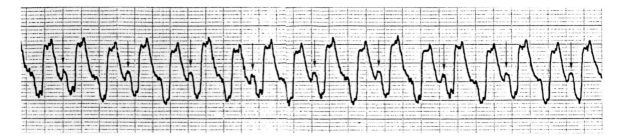

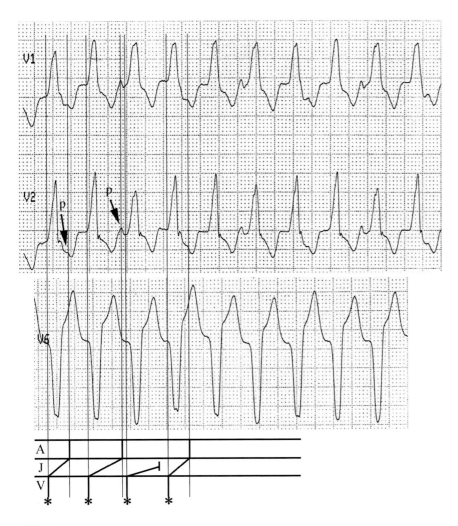

ECG 26.6
**92 y/f. CHD. Leads V₁, V₂, V₆. VT with RBBB-like pattern and QS complex in V₆. Retrograde AV block 2°
type Wenckebach.**

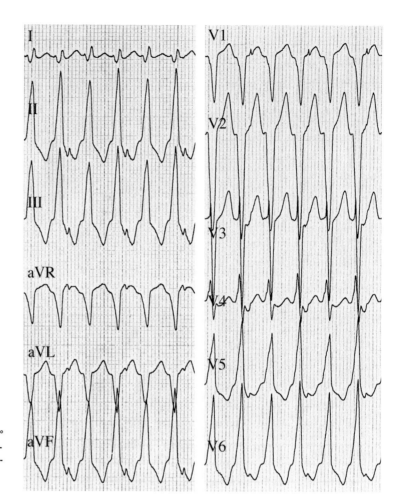

ECG 26.7

36 y/m. Presyncope episodes associated with palpitations. ECG: VT, rate 190/min. ÂQRS$_F$ + 100° and the LBBB-like QRS pattern suggest a VT arising in the *RV outflow tract* (confirmed by electrophysiologic testing). Note: retrograde AV block 2 : 1.

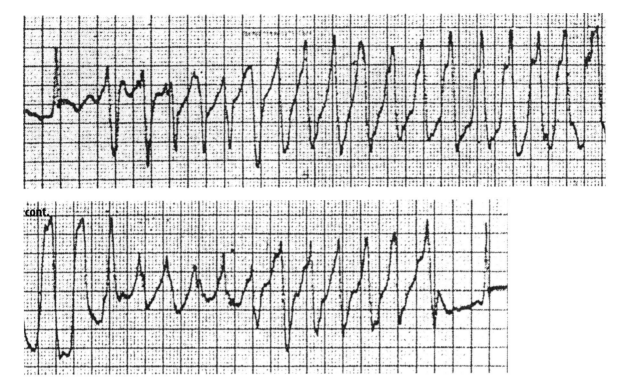

ECG 26.8
Self-limiting polymorphic VT of the type torsade de pointes, rate about 220/min (the first and last beat being normal).

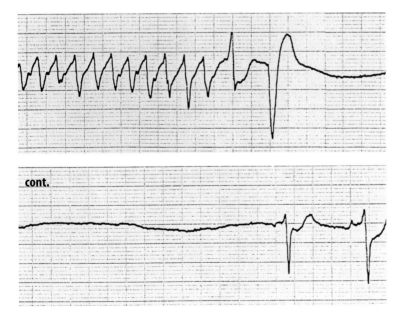

ECG 26.9
Rhythm strip: VT of type torsade de pointes (not clearly visible in this lead), rate > 300/min. Spontaneous conversion after two slower ventricular beats, followed by complete cardiac standstill of 4.16 sec, into a supraventricular rhythm.

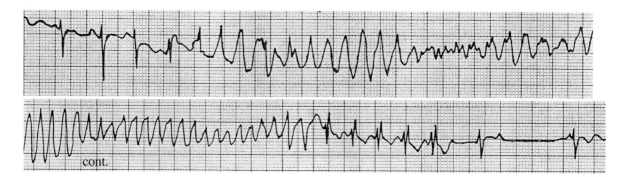

ECG 26.10

32 y/f. Anorexia nervosa. Potassium 2.2 mmol/l. ECG (continuous stripe): typical VT of the type torsade de pointes during 9.5 sec, with a maximal rate of 390/min(!), unusually changing into a supraventricular rhythm with RBBB (or to a regular VT?) at a rate of 176/min, before spontaneous conversion into a AV rhythm with AV dissociation, rate about 60/min.

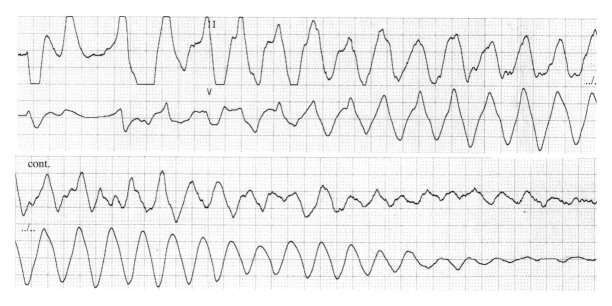

ECG 26.11

97 y/m. Terminal heart failure. ECG (continuous monitor stripes): after two slow beats, polymorphic VT without torsade de pointes. Rate about 130/min. Degeneration into ventricular fibrillation.

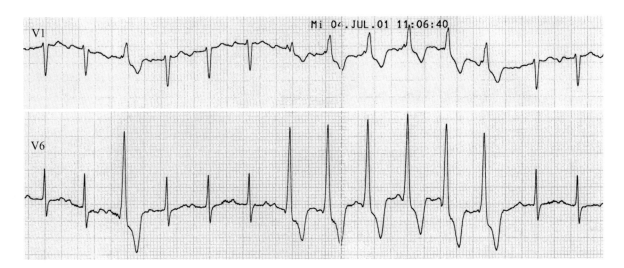

ECG 26.12

55 y/f. Aortic valve replacement 7 years previously. ECG (during exercise, 7 MET): sinus rhythm, rate 121/min. Third beat: late VPB. From beat 7 to beat 12: VT at a rate minimally superior to sinus rhythm, with purely positive QRS in all precordial leads. Beat 7 is a fusion beat, typical at the beginning (and/or end) of *accelerated* idioventricular rhythm. Differential diagnosis: parasystolic VT.

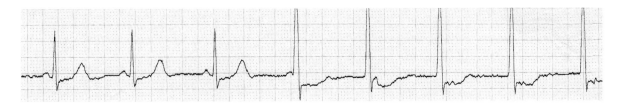

ECG 26.13

Accelerated idioventricular rhythm, beginning with the fourth beat. The p wave is visible either immediately before or after the QRS, or is hidden within QRS.

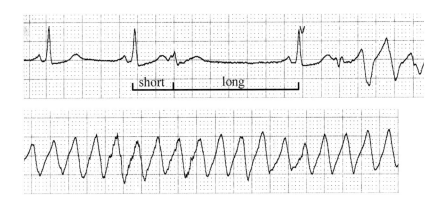

ECG 26.14
Monitor lead, coninuous stripe. VT preceded by *short–long* coupling intervals.

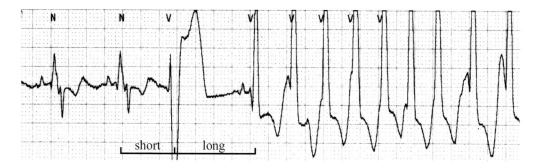

ECG 26.15
VT preceded by *short–long* coupling intervals.

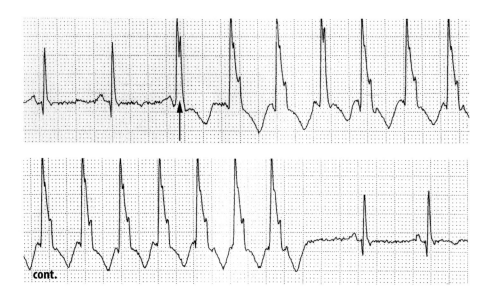

ECG 26.16
Nonsustained VT of 14 beats, beginning with a *fusion* beat (arrow) and ending after acceleration (R–R interval decreasing from 0.5 sec to about 0.4 sec).

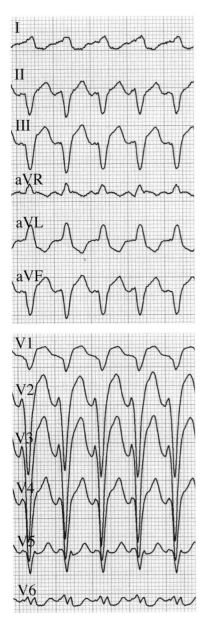

ECG 26.17
29 y/m. Arrhythmogenic right ventricular cardiomyopathy. ECG: VT, rate 150/min, LBBB-like QRS pattern.

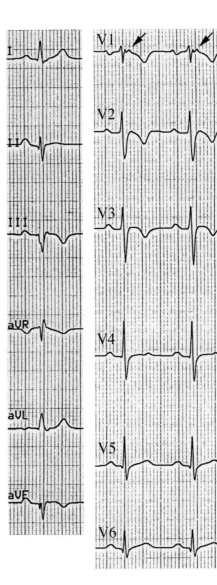

ECG 26.18
27 y/m. Sarcoidosis involving the right ventricle. ECG sinus rhythm: epsilon wave in lead V₁ (arrow).

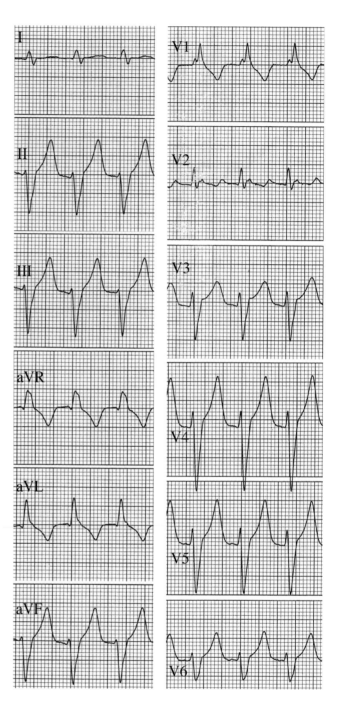

ECG 26.19

32 y/f. Palpitations. Normal echo/Doppler. ECG: left ventricular fascicular tachycardia, rate 116/min. Origin of VT in the left posterior fascicle (confirmed by electrophysiologic study). QRS left-axis deviation. Atypical RBBB pattern (courtesy of Reto Candinas MD).

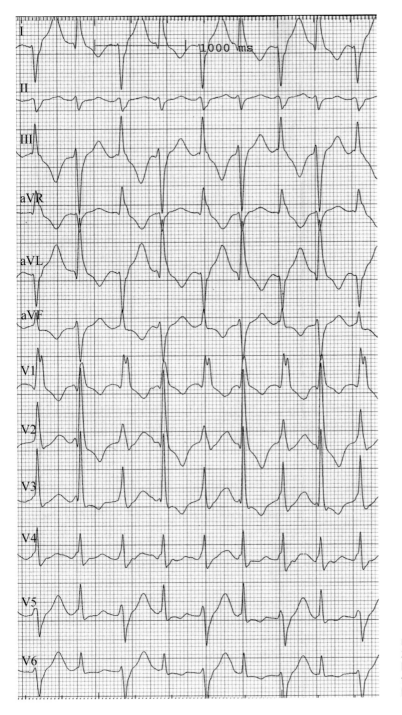

ECG 26.20

24 y/f. Palpitations. Normal echo/Doppler. ECG: bidirectional tachycardia (rate 137/min) with typical alternation of the QRS polarity, in most leads (courtesy of Thomas Cron MD).

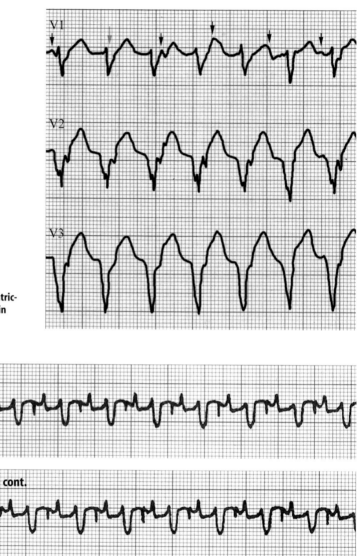

ECG 26.21a
Short Story/Case Report 1. 53 y/m. Accelerated idioventricular rhythm, rate 120/min. AV dissociation detectable in lead V$_1$ (arrow).

ECG 26.21b
Same patient. Atrial overpacing at a rate of 122/min (monitor lead).

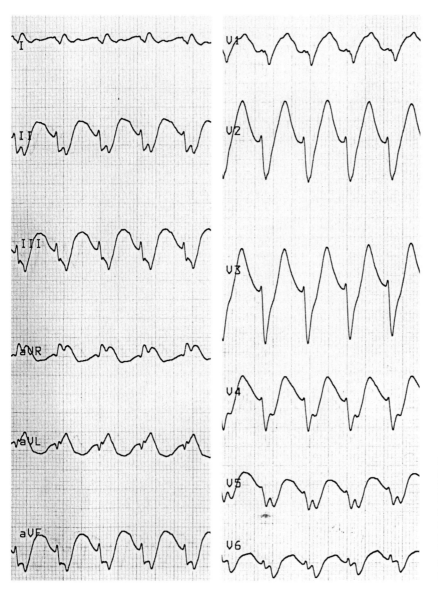

ECG 26.22a

55 y/f. CAD, CABG. High lateral and inferior akinesia. ECG: VT with LBBB-like QRS (see lead aVL/I) and additionally almost completely negative QRS in all precordial leads. QRS duration 200 msec. Ventricular rate 131/min. AV dissociation not detectable. Probable retrograde 1 : 1 conduction (peaked T waves in V_1).

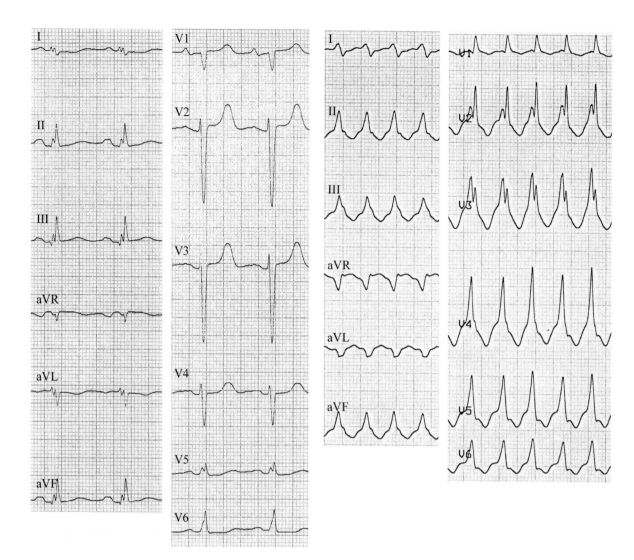

ECG 26.22b

Same patient. Sinus rhythm, rate 60/min. Notching of QRS in limb leads. Reduction of r wave from V_2 to V_4. Relatively small R waves with slurred R upstroke in V_5/V_6. No pathologic Q waves.

ECG 26.23

76 y/m. CAD, two-vessel disease with normal LV ejection fraction. Atrial fibrillation for years. ECG: VT, rate 180/min. Undefined BBB pattern with exclusively *positive QRS* deflections in the precordial leads. QRS duration 140 msec. Atrial fibrillation. Theoretic differential diagnosis: antidromic reentry tachycardia in WPW syndrome.

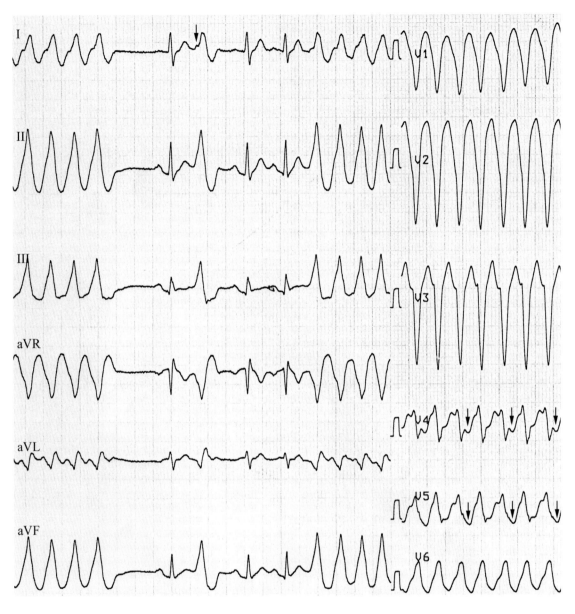

ECG 26.24

44 y/m. CAD without infarction. Presyncope during palpitations. ECG: VT, rate 210/min. Signs for VT: (1) broad QRS (VPB) without p wave before VT; (2) AV dissociation detectable during VPB (arrow); (3) retrograde AV block 2 : 1 (arrows); (4) giant QRS in V$_1$ to V$_3$ (half calibration!); (5) configuration of the first QRS in VT similar/equal to the VPB.

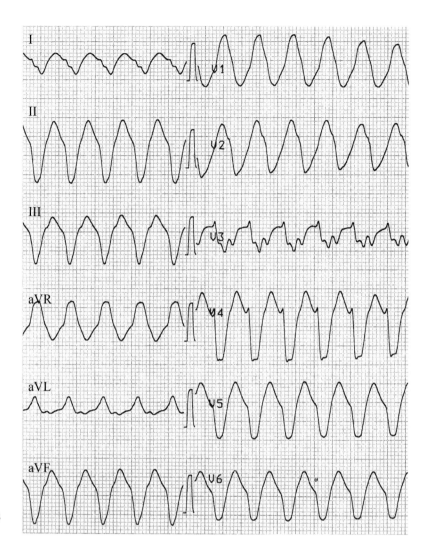

ECG 26.25
Short Story/Case Report 2. SVTab imitates VT.

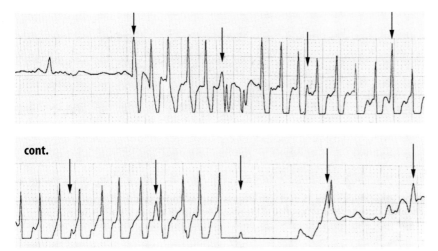

ECG 26.26
Continuous stripe. Pseudo-VT. Artifacts during teeth-brushing. Rate up to 300/min. The basic rhythm (sinus rhythm) is slightly irregular (arrow, indicating 'notches' that are scarcely visible). However, the *too* narrow 'R waves', the excessive rate and additional artifacts, for instance the shift of the curve off the paper, clearly indicate artifacts.

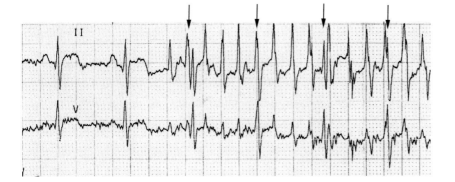

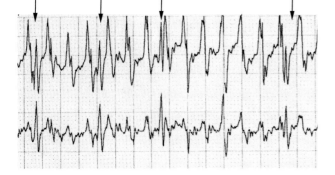

ECG 26.27
Continuous stripes. Pseudo-VT. Artifacts during teeth-brushing. Rate about 270/min. The real QRS are more distinctly detectable in the inferior stripe.

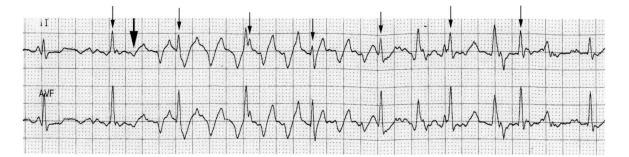

ECG 26.28

Pseudo-VT, due to artifacts. Signs for artifacts: (1) basic rhythm (rate 75/min) with obvious 'notches' during pseudo-VT (small arrows); (2) the first (abortive) 'beat' of pseudo-VT falls into the absolute refractory period of the sinusal beat (large arrow). (Details in Table 26.3.)

Chapter 27
Exercise ECG

At a Glance

In the exercise ECG ischemia is very easy detectable by significant ST depression in leads V_4 to V_6, with quite good reliability (in the condition of a normal ECG at rest). However, to conduct exercise testing professionally, the physician must be fully informed about the important basics – the instruments and equipment, indications and contraindications, possible limitations, about measurement of workload in watts or MET (metabolic equivalents), and about complications. Therefore, in this chapter the section At a Glance is larger than the section The Full Picture, and references to the literature are cited in both sections.

The exercise ECG is still the most widely used screening method for myocardial ischemia. A meta-analysis has revealed a specificity of 73% and a sensitivity of 68% [1].

Information from the Exercise Test

The exercise ECG represents the only single method that provides important results during physical *activity*. Besides ischemia, the exercise ECG can also be used to assess rhythm and conduction disturbances, the behavior of blood pressure, work capacity, and the state of body training. Moreover, the physician can directly recognize symptoms such as dyspnoea, paleness, cyanosis, sweating, and exhaustion. The patient is able to give a 'live' description of any sensations, such as chest pain, that may be typical or atypical for coronary heart disease (CHD), or cramps in the legs (Table 27.1).

1 Indications and Contraindications

1.1 Indications

According to the wide spectrum of results obtained by exercise testing, the indication for this procedure is not restricted to patients with present or suspected CHD (Table 27.2).

Table 27.1
Information gained from the ECG exercise test

1. General information
• Work capacity; state of body training
• Dynamic behavior of blood pressure and pulse
Symptoms
a. Objective
• Dyspnoea, paleness, cyanosis, sweating, exhaustion
b. Subjective (by 'live' description)
• Quality and intensity of chest pain and pain in the legs; dizziness and other symptoms
2. ECG
a. Direct signs of myocardial ischemia
• Depression of ST in leads V_4 to V_6
b. Possible signs of myocardial ischemia
• Arrhythmias
• Conduction disturbances

Table 27.2
Indications for exercise testing

1. Diagnostic (ischemia, arrhythmias)
• Differentiation of chest pains
• Validation of ischemia in patients with CHD
• Diagnosis of 'silent ischemia'
• Evaluation of ischemia after coronary revascularization
• Validation of arrhythmias
2. Prognostic; risk stratification; follow-up
• Evaluation of patients 5–10 days after uncomplicated MI: coronary revascularization necessary?
• Evaluation of work capacity in patients with CHD, valve disease, congenital heart disease, heart failure
• Preoperative risk stratification
• Evaluation of therapy in cardiac diseases
• Evaluation of patients with (rate responsive) pacemakers

Continued on next page

Table 27.2
(Cont.)

3. Noncardiac diseases

- Respiratory insufficiency
- Unexplained reduced work capacity

In these conditions the exercise test is combined with spirometry and blood gas analysis

CHD, coronary heart disease; MI, myocardial infarction.

1.2 Contraindications

All contraindications must be excluded *before* an exercise test is performed. The criteria for contraindications are quite well defined (Table 27.3). Nevertheless, the physician should never forget *common sense*.

Table 27.3
Criteria for contraindications for exercise testing

1. Absolute criteria

- AMI in the first 48 h (consider infarct size and cardiac state!)
- Unstable angina
- Arrhythmias with severe tachycardia or bradycardia (e.g. VT, SVT, AF with ventricular rate > 120/min, complete AV block with symptoms)
- Severe aortic valvular stenosis or HOCM
- Myocarditis, endocarditis (pericarditis)
- Severe heart failure (NYHA IV)
- Acute pulmonary embolism
- Chronic severe pulmonary arterial hypertension
- Severe arterial hypertension (systolic > 200, diastolic > 120 mmHg)
- Severely impaired general state of any origin

2. Relative criteria

- High arterial pressure (systolic > 180, diastolic > 110 mmHg)
- Arrhythmias (as salvos of VPBs)
- Medium degree valvular aortic stenosis and HOCM
- Left main coronary stenosis
- Medium degree chronic pulmonary artery hypertension
- Electrolyte imbalance

AF, atrial fibrillation; AMI, acute myocardial infarction; HOCM, hypertrophic obstructive cardiomyopathy; NYHA, classification of cardiac state/heart failure by the New York Heart Association, I being the slightest and IV being the most severe/worst; SVT, supraventricular tachycardia; VT, ventricular tachycardia.

2 Limitations

Other conditions that do not represent contraindications may limit considerably the validity of ischemic ECG response, such as pre-existing intraventricular conduction disturbances, or pre-existing ST/T alterations (Table 27.4).

Table 27.4
ECG conditions limiting validity of ischemic ECG response

1. Intraventricular conduction disturbances

- LBBB
- WPW pattern
- RBBB
- LAFB without or with additional RBBB

2. Pre-existing pathologic ST/T segment

- Systolic overload
- Ischemic
- Digitalis [2]
- Beta-blockers [3]
- Metabolic disorders
- Female gender?

3. Miscellaneous items

- Open heart surgery (during several months?)
- PTCA (first 48 hours)

LAFB, left anterior fascicular block; LBBB, left bundle-branch block; PTCA, percutaneous transluminal coronary angioplasty; RBBB, right bundle-branch block; WPW, Wolff-Parkinson-White syndrome.

3 Methods

There are two methods of exercise testing: bicycle exercise and treadmill exercise. In bicycle exercise, work is measured in watts. In treadmill exercise, it is measured in MET (metabolic equivalents). One MET corresponds to an oxygen uptake for a healthy individual at rest of 3.5 ml/kg bodyweight/min. Table 27.5 shows the relation between body activity and MET. Table 27.6 shows the corresponding values of MET and watts.

Table 27.5
Relation between activity and MET (metabolic equivalents)

1 MET	Rest
2 MET	Walking
4 MET	Fast walking
5 MET	Daily work at home
10 MET	Running
13 MET	Heavy working
18 MET	Athlete's activity
20 MET	World-class athlete's activity

Table 27.6
Corresponding values (approximate) of MET (metabolic equivalents) and watts

4 MET	50 watts
7 MET	100 watts
9 MET	150 watts
13 MET	200 watts
17 MET	250 watts

In treadmill exercise, the Bruce protocol [4] is used (Table 27.7): the workload is augmented by 2–3 MET every 3 min. With a reduction to 2 min or even 1 min, the steady state is not reached in every case.

Treadmill exercise is more physiologic than bicycle exercise and, due to a higher maximum volume of oxygen utilization, allows a higher workload [4,5] of 6%–25%. However, ECG artifacts are more frequent. To obtain a *valid* result, the conditions in Table 27.7 should be considered.

Table 27.7
Conditions for a valid exercise test

Exercise limited by symptoms/exhaustion
• High double product
• Duration of exercise at least 8 min
• Considering all exclusion criteria

3.1 Exercise Limited by Symptoms

In general the Borg scale [6] is used where the patient is workloaded up to *exhaustion*, but the patient is allowed to interrupt the exercise of *his own free will*. Table 27.8 shows a modified Borg scale, for a healthy 30-year-old man, and for a 70-year-old patient with CHD and a left ventricular ejection fraction of 50%.

With exercise limited by symptoms, most other important conditions assuring a valid exercise test are also fulfilled.

3.2 Heart Rate

The heart rate increases during exercise to the so-called *maximal heart rate* that depends on several factors (age, gender, stage of training, cardiovascular disease, other disease, drugs like beta-blockers).

As a general rule, maximal heart rate in healthy individuals is 220/min minus the age in years. However the maximal heart rate alone is no longer acknowledged as a valid criterion for the

Table 27.8
Subjective estimate of workload/symptoms in relation to 20 arbitrary steps of workload

Borg scale	Healthy 30-year-old man	70-year-old patient with coronary heart disease (ejection fraction 50%)
6		
7	very, very light	
8		very light
9	very light	
10		light to somewhat heavy
11	rather light	
12		
13	somewhat heavy	heavy
14		
15	heavy	very heavy
16		
17		
18	very heavy	
19		
20	extremely heavy	

exercise test. The submaximal heart rate is defined as 90% of the maximal rate.

3.3 Blood Pressure

Exercise leads to an increase in systolic blood pressure, but diastolic blood pressure remains more or less unchanged. A normal individual may reach a systolic pressure of up to 220 mmHg. An *insufficient* increase of systolic pressure is encountered in impaired LV ejection fraction, myocardial ischemia and obstructive LV cardiomyopathy. A *decrease* of systolic pressure during exercise is *dangerous* and suggests severely impaired LV ejection fraction or severe stenosis of the left main coronary artery.

3.4 Double Product

The double product is given by: heart rate × systolic blood pressure.

It is of outstanding importance in the exercise test. The higher the double product, the more valid the exercise test (Table 27.9). In the case of an insufficient double product without significant ST depression, the exercise test has to be interpreted as 'inconclusive' for ischemia, *not* as 'negative'.

At a Glance

Table 27.9
Quality of exercise in relation to the double product

Double product	Quality of exercise
< 20 000	Insufficient
20 000–25 000	Sufficient
25 000–30 000	Good
> 30 000	Very good

Another rule considers the individual double product at rest. A good double product at maximal workload is at least 2.5 times the double product at rest.

3.5 Workload and Exercise Capacity

The maximal workload is only reached in exercise limited by symptoms. The normal exercise capacity depends on age, gender, and stature (Figure 27.1). Its value is below that for maximal workload.

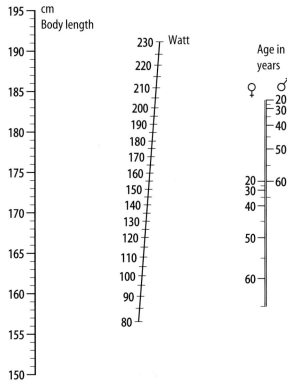

Figure 27.1
Nomogram of normal exercise capacity (Watt) based on age, gender and body length (derived from [7]). For nomogram based on metabolic equivalents (MET) and age in men see [8] and [9].

3.6 Duration of Exercise

To reach a 'steady state', exercise should last at least 8 min. In general an exercise test lasts 12–14 min.

3.7 Stepwise Exercise *versus* the Ramp Protocol

With the ramp protocol [4] the workload is increased *continuously*, thus allowing a higher oxygen uptake (and a higher workload). However, the difference from a stepwise exercise test is not decisively important.

3.8 Criteria for Interruption of the Test

Table 27.10 summarizes the absolute and relative criteria for interrupting the exercise test.

Table 27.10
Criteria for interrupting the exercise test

1. Absolute criteria
• Severe angina >>> possibly acute MI
• Systolic blood pressure below value at rest, or decreasing > 20 mmHg >>> suggesting left main coronary artery stenosis or severely impaired LV EF
• VT (≥ 6 beats and/or with symptoms)
• Has ventricular fibrillation to be mentioned?
• AV block 3°
• Ventricular asystole > 2 sec (extremely rare)
• Striking paleness or cyanosis
• Neurologic symptoms (dizziness, headache, and others)
• Technical problems (e.g. loss of ECG monitoring)
• Patient insists on interrupting

2. Relative criteria
• ST depression of 3 mm or more
• Increasing angina
• Rapid ventricular response in atrial flutter/fibrillation (> 180/min)
• VT < 6 beats
• Striking increase of VPBs

EF, ejection fraction; MI, myocardial infarction; VPBs, ventricular premature beats; VT, ventricular tachycardia.

4 Procedure

4.1 Exercise Preparation

Note: the exercise test begins *before* the exercise test! Before an exercise test is performed, some conditions related to technical material and to the patient must be fulfilled (Table 27.11). The patient's history, and especially the results of physical examination, allow estimation of the exercise capacity, or may indicate a contraindication.

Table 27.11
Preparation of the exercise test

1. Material
• Controlled *defibrillator*
• Drugs: adrenaline, lidocaine, atropine (infusion sodium chloride included)
• Oxygen mask; breathing bag; oxygen cylinder
2. Patient
• Estimation of general state
• Personal data; stature; weight
• Study of history: heart disease; other severe disease
• *Actual problem; indication for exercise test*
• Actual medication (digitalis, beta-blocker and other drugs)
• Auscultation of the heart and lungs
• ECG at rest
• Blood pressure at rest
3. Informing the patient of the procedure

4.2 Exercise Procedure

The procedure itself is performed in relation to the general state and cardiac condition of the patient (Table 27.12).

Table 27.12
Load in relation to individual state

Patient	Beginning load		Load increase/min	
NYHA III	10 watts	2 MET	10 watts	1 MET
NYHA I–II	20 watts	2 MET	20 watts	1–1.5 MET
Healthy; age < 60 years	25 watts	2 MET	25 watts	1.5–2 MET

NYHA, classification of the cardiac state by the New York Heart Association.

The patient undergoes the exercise up to the point of exhaustion or up to one of the criteria for interruption. For the practical procedure the physician's presence is mandatory (Table 27.13). By observing the patient and the ECG on the monitor, the presence of ischemia or arrhythmias can be detected instantly, and together with blood pressure measurements may give hints for interrupting the session and performing therapeutic intervention.

Table 27.13
Practical procedure of the exercise test

Patient's duty
• Doing the exercise following ramp protocol or stepwise, symptom-limited
Physician's duty
During exercise:
• Continuous observation of the patient
• Continuous observation of the monitored ECG
• Measurement of blood pressure at each load (every min)
• Registration and quick interpretation of the 12-lead ECG at each load (every min)
After exercise:
• Registration and quick interpretation of the ECG 2 min and 5 min later
• Measuring blood pressure 2 min and 5 min later

In patients who have had no physical training it is preferable to continue exercise at a minimal load for 1–2 min. A postexercise syncope (due to 'venous pooling' in the legs) can be avoided. The *postexercise* (recovery) ECG serves for the detection of ischemia occurring with latency (late ischemia) or, rarely, of late arrhythmias.

ECG

5 Validation

5.1 Ischemic Response

It should be remembered that the specificity and sensitivity of the exercise ECG for ischemia are about 73% and 68%, respectively. Consequently, there are false negative and false positive results in a substantial number of patients.

5.1.1 ST Segment

By far the most important marker of ischemia during exercise is significant ST depression in leads (V_4) V_5 and V_6, of which V_5 seems to be the most reliable lead. Isolated ST depressions in leads other than V_4 to V_6, especially in the inferior leads, do not indicate myocardial ischemia in most cases, and are often found in normal hearts.

The definition of *significant* ST depression (indicating ischemia) is given in Table 27.14 [7].

Table 27.14
Definition of significant ST depressions

- ST depression ≥ 1 mm (≥ 0.1 mV), if ST at rest is isoelectric
- *Additional* ST depression ≥ 1.5 mm (≥ 0.15 mV) if ST is *depressed* at rest
  ST depression is measured 0.08 sec after the J point (some authors prefer 0.07 sec at a rate between 120 and 160/min, and 0.06 sec at a rate > 160/min; so does also the author of this book)

A *false positive* result (significant ST depression that is *not* due to ischemia) is found in pre-existing ST/T alterations, occurring in patients with left ventricular hypertrophy (LVH), with digitalis treatment, or in intraventricular conduction disturbances such as the Wolff-Parkinson-White (WPW) pattern, and left bundle-branch block (LBBB). In these conditions, the pre-existing ST depression is generally accentuated during exercise (also *without* ischemia).

ECG 27.1 shows a normal finding at exercise. The ST segments in V_4 to V_6 remain isoelectric, and the exercise test is electrically *negative*.

ECG 27.2 shows that interpretation of the ST segment is sometimes quite difficult because of artifacts, more so with the treadmill test than the bicycle test.

In ECG 27.3 ST depression measures about 1 mm in V_5/V_6. This finding is called 'borderline'. What should be done in such a case?

i. Increase the workload, if possible
ii. In a person who is probably healthy (without risk factors), tested during a check-up, the test can be repeated after 6–12 months; in a patient with suspected CHD, stress echocardiography or stress scintigraphy should be performed.

ECGs 27.4, 27.5 and 27.6 show electrically *positive* exercise tests, all with signs of 'late ischemia'. Late ischemia is seen in about 30% of electrically positive exercise tests. ECG 27.6 represents a false positive result in a patient 1 day after successful two-vessel percutaneous transluminal coronary angioplasty (PTCA), controlled by repeated coronary angiography. (For exercise test after PTCA and coronary artery bypass grafting (CABG) see section The Full Picture.)

In *right bundle-branch block* (RBBB) pre-existing ST depression and T negativity in leads V_1 and V_2 mostly expand to V_3 and V_4 (rarely to V_5) during exercise, without ischemia. A significant ST depression in lead V_5 and V_6 in the presence of RBBB is specific in about 85%, whereas the sensitivity is poor (25%–35%). The same is true for RBBB associated with left ante-

rior fascicular block (LAFB) and for isolated LAFB. In the presence of *LBBB* it is impossible to confirm or to exclude ischemia.

Significant *ST elevation* of > 1.5 mm during exercise (not due to mirror image) is extremely rare in patients with a normal ECG at rest. The phenomenon has been observed in patients with exercise-induced coronary artery spasm (ECG 27.7).

ST elevation due to mirror image of ST depression in systolic overload or in LBBB may be accentuated in leads V_1 to V_3/V_4.

Significant ST elevation during exercise is commonly seen in patients with anterior Q wave infarction with aneurysm (ECG 27.8). This is *not* an ischemic response but represents an 'ECG bystander' of increased systolic expansion of the aneurysmic region during exercise.

In the case of persistent or new onset ST depression, and/or T negativity *after* exercise, late ischemia is suspected. It is therefore important to check the ECG for at least 6 min after exercise. Obvious alterations of repolarization during recovery generally confirm a positive test during exercise (ECGs 27.4, 27.5 and 27.6). In pre-existing abnormalities of repolarization (e.g. in LVH), similar ST/T alterations after exercise are difficult to interpret.

5.1.2 T Wave

Negative T waves at rest often become positive during exercise (ECG 27.9). This phenomenon is called 'pseudonormalization' of the T wave. Pseudonormalization may be an ischemic response, but in the majority of cases it is not. In patients with clinically suspected ischemia and pseudonormalization, a more specific test like scintigraphy or stress echocardiography should be performed.

The 'sign of Lepeschkin' (increase of T amplitude at exercise to ≥ three times T amplitude at rest) is very rare and is not reliable for ischemia detection.

5.1.3 Q Wave

Very rarely, in *normal* individuals, pre-existing Q waves may become deeper or new small Q waves may appear. In an rS complex with a very small r, the r wave may disappear, resulting in a QS complex (ECG 27.10). This can be explained by a shift of the QRS vector during exercise. Only in extremely rare cases does the exercise demasks the pattern of a Q wave infarction.

5.2 Arrhythmias and Conduction Disturbances

In general, arrhythmias and conduction defects during exercise may occur with or without ischemia. Ventricular tachycardia (and of course ventricular fibrillation) and *multiple,* especially *polymorphous,* ventricular premature beats (VPBs) are often of ischemic origin but may also be found in patients with other severe heart diseases. An increase of VPBs during exercise is generally associated with an impaired prognosis [10]. Supraventricular arrhythmias such as atrial flutter, atrial fibrillation, and supraventricular premature beats (SVPBs) may be combined with CHD. ECG 27.11 shows a ventricular tachycardia (VT) lasting for 12 sec in a young female patient without CAD. Conduction disturbances during exercise are rare but clinically important. Two cases of AV block 2° are demonstrated in ECGs 27.12 and 27.13. For LBBB, RBBB and fascicular blocks see section The Full Picture.

Short Story/Case Report 1

In 1993 a 42-year-old male technician told his family doctor about episodes of fatigue and dyspnoea during exercise. No explanation for these symptoms could be found. No exercise test was performed. During the next weeks the symptoms worsened and the patient was advised to visit a psychiatrist. After two sessions the psychiatrist (!) sent the patient to a cardiologist for an exercise test. The clinical findings at rest were normal, so was the echocardiogram. The ECG showed a complete RBBB. On bicycle exercise, at a load of 100 watts and a sinus rate of 146/min, the patient developed AV block 2 : 1 (drop of ventricular rate to 73/min), which progressed to 3 : 1 AV block at 150 watts and a sinus rate of 176/min, with a further slowing of ventricular rate to about 50/min (ECG 27.12). The patient complained about dyspnoea and weakness, the same symptoms usually experienced during exercise. Because there were no risk factors for CHD a coronary angiography was not performed. The etiology of the conduction disturbance was classified as 'unknown'. With a two-chamber (DDD) pacemaker the patient remained free of symptoms.

Another example of exercise-induced AV block 2° type high-degree is shown in ECG 27.13, in a patient who had received aortic valve replacement.

5.3 Pitfalls

Table 27.15 summarizes some of the pitfalls that may occur if the ECG is not cautiously observed and analysed before, during, and after exercise.

Table 27.15
Mistakes and misinterpretations caused by superficial analysis of the ECG

1. ECG at rest
• Acute myocardial infarction is overlooked! (This may happen)
• LVH is missed (due to half calibration?)
>>> false-positive result?

2. ECG during exercise
• Artifacts are misdiagnosed as arrhythmias
• Real heart rate is not recognized (because of false indication on the computer)
• SVT is overlooked (detectable by abrupt increase of the rate)
• VT is overlooked (detectable by abrupt increase of rate and QRS alteration)
• Intermittent RBBB or LBBB is overlooked
• Intermittent 2 : 1 AV block is overlooked

3. ECG during recovery
• Late ischemia is overlooked
• Intermittent 2 : 1 AV block is missed (rare)

AV, atrioventricular; LBBB, left bundle-branch block; LVH, left ventricular hypertrophy; RBBB, right bundle-branch block; SVT, supraventricular tachycardia; VT, ventricular tachycardia.

6 Complications

6.1 Severe Cardiac Complications

These are described in Table 27.16. The literature reports an incidence of 10 deaths or myocardial infarction in every 10 000 tests [11]. Stuart and Ellestad [12] calculated one myocardial infarction or sudden death per 2500 patients. During a period of 5 years in our clinic we observed over more than 7000 exercise tests; one patient had an acute anteroseptal infarction, and two had ventricular fibrillation (one after VT of the type torsade de pointes), with complete recovery of the VF patients. Two additional patients with acute inferior infarction and moderate chest pain were tested, because the ECG at rest was not analysed. Exercise was interrupted at 4 MET after severe chest pain and progression of ST elevation from 2–3 mm to 4 mm in the inferior leads.

Ventricular tachycardia is rare in its sustained form and rather common in its nonsustained form (salvos of VPBs). Sustained VT is *always* a reason (nonsustained VT is *often* a reason) for immediate interruption of the exercise, with close control of the patient.

Supraventricular tachycardias at excessively high rates (> 200/min) are encountered only exceptionally, e.g. in atrial flutter with 1 : 1 AV conduction, in atrial fibrillation, or in the WPW syndrome.

Decrease of arterial pressure (in some cases combined with bradycardia) is observed in patients with severely impaired LV function, significant left main coronary stenosis, or severe aortic stenosis, and may induce severe complications like syncope, cardiogenic shock, and ventricular fibrillation.

6.2 Severe Noncardiac Complications

These are listed in Table 27.16. Severe noncardiac complications are very rare and include cerebral insult and musculoskeletal trauma (the latter due to patients falling on the treadmill or off the bicycle). Such accidents can be avoided by giving good instructions and by closely observing the patient, and by conducting the exercise with common sense. A postexercise syncope must be prevented by a period of low-level exercise for the last few minutes.

Table 27.16
Severe complications

1. Cardiac
• Death due to acute infarction and/or lethal arrhythmia
• Acute infarction
• Cardiogenic shock
• High-rate ventricular tachycardia
• High-rate supraventricular tachycardia
2. Noncardiac
• Cerebral insult
• Musculoskeletal trauma

6.3 Common Nonsevere Complications

Multiple VPBs, isolated or in couplets are seen quite commonly. Polymorphous VPBs, associated with an impaired prognosis are also occasionally observed. The decision for continuing or interrupting exercise depends on the individual situation.

Elevation of systolic blood pressure to > 230 mmHg and/or diastolic > 120 mmHg is an indication for interrupting the exercise.

6.4 Rare Nonsevere Complications

Supraventricular arrhythmias with a relatively high rate (150–200/min) are occasionally seen in atrial fibrillation and in atrial flutter with 2 : 1 AV block. AV nodal reentry tachycardia is very rare.

AV block (in most cases 2 : 1) generally occurs in patients with pre-existing bundle-branch block.

A new bundle-branch block indicates CHD in about 50% of cases (see 'The Full Picture').

The Full Picture

7 Specificity and Sensitivity

Several meta-analyses reveal some differences in specificity and sensitivity, comparing the results of patients with or without LV hypertrophy, with or without ST depression at rest, and with or without digitalis. The highest specificity (84%) was found in patients without ST depression at rest, the lowest (69%) in patients with LV hypertrophy.

Patients without LV hypertrophy and without digoxin had a relative high sensitivity of 72%. Patients without myocardial infarction had the lowest sensitivity.

8 Exercise in Pre-existing Bundle-Branch Block and Left Anterior Fascicular Block

LBBB is generally acknowledged as exclusion criterion for the detection of ischemia in exercise. Recently Ibrahim et al [13] published a new index, based on 41 patients (34 with CHD): ST depression $\geq$ 0.5 mm (!) in II/aVF, measured at the J point, together with an increase of the R amplitude in lead II. In our opinion it would be surprising if a minimal ST alteration in lead II and/or aVF indicated ischemia, because of the variable frontal QRS axis ($\text{Å}QRS_F$) in LBBB and for other reasons.

In RBBB, all of the larger studies reveal good-to-excellent specificity and a sensitivity that is insufficient to very low. Yen et al [14] found a specificity of 87% and a sensitivity of 27% in 133 patients; Wangsnes and Gibbons [15] found values of 82% and 57%, respectively, in 82 patients. None of the 40 asymptomatic patients (all had coronary angiography; 12 had CHD) studied by Whinnery et al [16] showed a positive exercise test.

For the first time patients with pre-existing LAFB or LAFB + RBBB were recently studied by Rimoldi et al [17], with technetium-99m sestamibi as a 'gold standard'. In 41 cases with LAFB, specificity and sensitivity were 94.3% and 33.3% respectively, and in 28 cases with LAFB + RBBB they were 82.3% and 63.6% respectively. Similar to the condition of RBBB, the specificity was good and was associated with very low sensitivity in isolated LAFB. ECG 27.14 shows a *false negative* exercise test in the presence of LAFB (occurring *frequently*), ECG 27.15 a *true positive* exercise test (a *rare* result). False negative results were found in particular in cases with R ≤ S in V_5 and V_6 (a common finding in LAFB). A possible explanation for this is that the ischemic ST vector points in the opposite direction to the main QRS vector. At least partially, the same explanation could also apply for the false negative results seen in RBBB, with a small R wave in V_5/V_6. Indeed, we have seen cases with RBBB and/or LAFB and scintigraphically proven ischemia where the ST segment in V_5 and V_6 was slightly elevated during exercise.

9 New Bundle-Branch Block During Exercise

Opinions about the relation between exercise-induced bundle-branch block and coronary artery disease are contradictory. Williams et al [18] report a 70% incidence for LBBB and 100%

incidence for RBBB. Other authors found a significantly less strong relationship [19,20]. The prognosis of exercise-induced bundle-branch block depends, as in chronic bundle-branch block, on the underlying disease [21,22,23]. LBBB occurring during exercise may provoke chest pain [24]. Thallium-201 scintigraphy, technetium-99m sestamibi SPECT (single photon emission computed tomography), or N-ammonium positron emission tomography often show a perfusion defect, also in patients with normal coronary arteries. The defect is localized in the septum [25,26] or occasionally in the inferolateral wall [27].

10 Ventricular Premature Beats During Exercise

The incidence of VPBs increases with age [28]. It is probable – but not proven – that exercise-induced frequent VPBs are related to myocardial ischemia. Possibly they represent an independent predictor of future cardiovascular death. Jouven et al [10] recently found out in a cohort of 6101 men without known heart disease that the long-term risk of cardiovascular death in men with frequent VPBs during exercise is increased by a factor of 2.5 (frequent VPBs are defined as more than two VPBs in a row, or a proportion of VPBs that exceeds 10% of normal beats during a 30 sec period). But only 6% of these patients showed ischemic signs in the exercise test, while not more than 3% with a positive test showed frequent VPBs. However, other investigators have found a relation between exercise-induced VPBs and myocardial ischemia [29,30].

11 Alterations of QRS During Exercise, Without Intraventricular Conduction Disturbances

Bonoris et al [31] and others have found a good correlation between the increase in R wave amplitude in exercise, systolic LV dysfunction, and severity of coronary artery narrowing. With the so-called 'Athens QRS score' Michaelides et al [32] showed a significant correlation between QRS changes, the number of LV contraction abnormalities, and the number of diseased coronary vessels. Yet the method has not been accepted for practical use in general.

12 Right Precordial Leads in the Exercise Test

Michaelides et al [33] reported a significant increase of sensitivity and specificity in prediction of coronary artery disease using the right precordial leads V_3R, V_4R and V_5R. Their cohort included 85 patients with one-vessel disease, 84 with two-vessel disease, 42 with three-vessel disease, and 34 patients with normal coronary arteries. The new method was warmly appreciated in an editorial by Wellens [34], whereas Bokhari et al [35] could not confirm these favorable results. Further studies will reveal more definitive information on this interesting issue.

13 Exercise Test After Aortocoronary Revascularization

In patients after aortocoronary revascularization, exercise testing can be performed to evaluate the ultimate outcome of the operation. It may detect persisting ischemia due to incomplete revascularization, or new ischemia due to restenosis. However, abnormalities in the ECG at rest often limit the accuracy of the test. The prognostic value of performing the test after CABG is limited [36] (see section 17 below).

14 Exercise ECG After PTCA

The detection of ischemia shortly after successful PTCA (within about 2 weeks) in acute or chronic CAD may be misleading [37]. Occasionally, an obvious ST depression (with or without late ischemia) is seen, without remaining significant stenosis of the coronary arteries (ECG 27.6). Uren et al discuss a possible mechanism [38].

15 Exercise Training in Cardiac Rehabilitation After MI and Revascularization

An early meta-analysis of patients undergoing cardiac rehabilitation after myocardial infarction demonstrated a reduction in mortality [39]. Today this finding is doubted. In an extensive review article, Ades calculated that only 10%–20% of appropriate candidates in the USA currently benefit from a formal rehabilitation program. He emphasized supportive measures such as cessation of smoking, normalizing lipid levels, and weight loss (the latter improving lipid levels, insulin resistance, blood pressure and clotting abnormalities) [40].

16 Exercise Training in Heart Failure

In patients with heart failure, repetitive testing may be performed to check exercise capacity, to evaluating the effects of training and treatment. In this case, testing protocols have to

be modified [41]. For several years, exercise has been used as a therapeutic procedure in patients with and without CHD. Improved work capacity and positive effects on lifestyle and life quality have been reported. The responsible mechanisms are: increased peak oxygen consumption; improvement of the autonomic control of the circulation, including reduction in sympathetic activity and enhancement of vagal activity [42]; improvement in the process of LV remodeling after (even extensive) myocardial infarction [43,44]; enhancement of coronary collateralization [45]; improvement of endothelium-dependent vasodilatation in coronary vessels [46]. However, as pointed out in an editorial by Coats [42], until 1999 only about 600 patients with heart failure were enrolled in randomized trials of exercise training and the following issues are not (yet) definitively resolved:

i. Effects on mortality and morbidity?
ii. Can training effects be maintained over the long term?
iii. General practicability, outside of 'enthusiastic specialist clinics'?

Practical recommendations for exercise training in patients with chronic heart failure have recently been published [47].

17 Prognostic Impact of the Exercise Test

In an asymptomatic population an abnormal exercise test means a ninefold increase in the risk for future cardiac events such as angina, myocardial infarction, or death, in men. In women the prognostic value of an abnormal test lacks specificity [48]. In contrast, Younis and Chaitman [49] and Froelicher et al [50] have stated that silent ischemia induced by exercise testing in apparently healthy men is not as predictive as previously thought. They reviewed 24 studies of patients who had suffered myocardial infarction and concluded that ST segment shifts are not as predictive of high risk as abnormal systolic blood pressure response and a poor exercise capacity.

Studies in patients with stable CHD that consider angiographic findings, cardiac events, and the differential outcome of CABG, compared with medical therapy, have shown a prognostic power of exercise testing. In a study of 296 patients with exercise after CABG, Dubach et al [36] found the MET level and maximal heart rate to be significantly related to prognosis. No patient exceeding 8 METs died, compared to 15 patients with low MET levels who did die. Nevertheless, the authors estimate the predictive power of the exercise test to be low overall, and ST depression as not predictive at all. Studying 231 patients after CABG, Yli-Mayry et al [51] did not find any significant predictive value of exercise duration and workload, whereas a low postoperative ejection fraction and diuretic treatment were significant for predicting cardiac events.

In summary, in patients with CHD, ST segment changes during exercise have more diagnostic than prognostic value, while poor exercise capacity (< 75 watts) indicates a poor prognosis, and a good exercise capacity (> 200 watts) indicates a good prognosis [52].

As mentioned earlier, Jouven et al [10] reported that frequent VPBs and ST depression at exercise increase the risk for cardiovascular death by 2.5 times. More recently, Frolkis et al showed that frequent VPBs immediately after exercise are also a predictor of death [53].

References

1. Gianrossi R, Detrano R, Mulvihill D, et al. Exercise-induced ST depression in the diagnosis of coronary artery disease. A meta-analysis. Circulation 1989;80:87–98
2. Sketch MH, Mooss AN, Butler ML, et al. Digoxin-induced positive exercise tests: their clinical and prognostic significance. Am J Cardiol 1981;48:655–9
3. Herbert WG, Dubach P, Lehmann KG, Froelicher VF. Effect of beta-blockade on the interpretation of the exercise ECG: ST level versus delta ST/HR index. Am Heart J 1991;122:993–1000
4. Fletcher GF, Balady G, Froelicher VF, et al. Exercise standards. A statement for healthcare professionals from the American Heart Association Writing Group. Circulation 1995;91:580–615
5. Wicks JR, Sutton JR, Oldridge NB, Jones NL. Comparison of the electrocardiographic changes induced by maximal exercise testing with treadmill and cycle ergometer. Circulation 1978;57:1066–70
6. Borg GA. Psychophysical bases of perceived exertion. Med Sci Sports Exerc 1982;14:377–81
7. Bühlmann AA, Rossier PH. Klinische Pathophysiologie der Atmung. Berlin: Springer Verlag 1970
8. Gibbons RJ, Balady GJ, Beasley JW, et al. ACC/AHA guidelines for exercise testing. A report of the American College of Cardiology/American Heart Association Task Force on Practice Guidelines (Committee on Exercise Testing). J Am Coll Cardiol 1997;30:260–311
9. Morris CK, Myers J, Froelicher VF, et al. Nomogram based on metabolic equivalents and age for assessing aerobic exercise capacity in men. JACC 1993;22:175–82
10. Jouven X, Zureik M, Desnos M, et al. Long-term outcome in asymptomatic men with exercise-induced premature ventricular depolarizations. N Engl J Med 2000;343:826–33
11. Gordon NF, Kohl HW. Exercise testing and sudden cardiac death. J Cardiopulm Rehab 1993;13:381–6
12. Stuart RJ Jr, Ellestad MH. National survey of exercise stress testing facilities. Chest 1980;77:94–7
13. Ibrahim NS, Abboud G, Selvester RS, et al. Detecting exercise-induced ischemia in left bundle branch block using the electrocardiogram. Am J Cardiol 1998;82:832–5
14. Yen RS, Miranda C, Froelicher VF. Diagnostic and prognostic accuracy of the exercise electrocardiogram in patients with preexisting right bundle branch block. Am Heart J 1994;127:1521–5
15. Wangsnes KM, Gibbons RJ. Optimal interpretation of the supine exercise electrocardiogram in patients with right bundle branch block. Chest 1990;98:1379–82
16. Whinnery JE, Froelicher VF Jr, Longo MR Jr, Triebwasser JH. The electrocardiographic response to maximal treadmill exercise of asymptomatic men with right bundle branch block. Chest 1977;71:335–40
17. Rimoldi S, Fikrle A, DeMarchi S, et al. Electrocardiographic detection of ischemia in LAFB, isolated or in combination with RBBB, based on the results of bicycle exercise and scintigraphic findings. Kardiovask Med 2002;5:35 (abstract)
18. Williams MA, Esterbrooks DJ, Nair CK, et al. Clinical significance of exercise-induced bundle branch block. Am J Cardiol 1988;61:346–8
19. Wayne VS, Bishop RL, Cook L, Spodick DH. Exercise-induced bundle branch block. Am J Cardiol 1983;52:283–6
20. Vasey C, O'Donnell J, Morris S, McHenry P. Exercise-induced left bundle branch block and its relation to coronary artery disease. Am J Cardiol 1985;56:892–5
21. Grady TA, Chiu AC, Snader CE, et al. Prognostic significance of exercise-induced left bundle-branch block. J Amer Med Assoc 1998;279:153–6
22. Heinsimer JA, Irwin JM, Basnight LL. Influence of underlying coronary artery disease on the natural history and prognosis of exercise-induced left bundle branch block. Am J Cardiol 1987;60:1065–7
23. Hertzeanu H, Aron L, Shiner RJ, Kellermann J. Exercise dependent complete left bundle branch block. Eur Heart J 1992;13:1447–51
24. Virtanen KS, Heikkila J, Kala R, Siltanen P. Chest pain and rate-dependent left bundle branch block in patients with normal coronary arteriograms. Chest 1982;81:326–31
25. Munt B, Huckell VF, Boone J. Exercise-induced left-bundle branch block: a case report of false positive MIBI imaging and review of the literature. Can J Cardiol 1997;13:517–21
26. La Canna G, Giubbini R, Metra R, et al. Assessment of myocardial perfusion with thallium-201 scintigraphyon exercise-induced left-bundle branch block: diagnostic value and clinical significance. Europ Heart J 1992;13:942–6
27. Enseleit F, Kaufmann P, Ruschitzka F, et al. Retrosternale Schmerzen bei einer 55-jährigen Patientin. Kardiovask Med 2002;5:201–5
28. Busby MJ, Shefrin EA, Fleg JL. Prevalence and long-term significance of exercise-induced frequent or repetitive ventricular ectopic beats in apparently healthy volunteers. J Am Coll Cardiol 1989;14:1659–65
29. Drory Y, Pines A, Fisman EZ, Kellermann JJ. Persistence of arrhythmia exercise response in healthy young men. Am J Cardiol 1990;66:1092–4
30. Morrow K, Morris CK, Froelicher VF, et al. Prediction of cardiovascular death in men undergoing noninvasive evaluation in coronary artery disease. Ann Intern Med 1993;118:689–95

31. Bonoris PE, Greenberg PS, Castellanet MJ, Ellestad MH. Significance of changes in R wave amplitude during treadmill stress testing: Angiographic correlation. Am J Cardiol 1978;41:846–51

32. Michaelides AP, Triposkiadis FK, Boudoulas K, et al. New coronary artery index based on exercise-induced QRS changes. Am Heart J 1990;120:292–302

33. Michaelides AP, Psomadaki ZD, Dilaveris PE, et al. Improved detection of coronary artery disease by exercise electrocardiography with the use of right precordial leads. N Engl J Med 1999;340:340–5

34. Wellens HJ. The value of the right precordial leads of the electrocardiogram. N Engl J Med 1999;340:381–3

35. Bokhari S, Blood DK, Bergmann SR. Use of right precordial leads during exercise testing. N Engl J Med 2000;343:968–9 (letter)

36. Dubach P, Froelicher V, Klein J, Detrano R. Use of the exercise test to predict prognosis after coronary artery bypass grafting. Am J Cardiol 1989;63:530–3

37. Honan MB, Bengtson JR, Pryor DB, et al. Exercise testing is a poor predictor of anatomic re-stenosis after coronary angioplasty for acute myocardial infarction. Circulation 1989;80:1585–94

38. Uren NG, Crake T, Lefroy DC, et al. Delayed recovery of coronary resistive vessel function after coronary angioplasty. J Am Coll Cardiol 1993;21:612–21

39. Oldridge NB, Guyatt GH, Fischer Mary E, Rimm AA. Cardiac rehabilitation after myocardial infarction. Combined experience of randomized clinical trials. J Amer Med Assoc 1988;260:945–50

40. Ades PA. Cardiac rehabilitation and secondary prevention of coronary heart disease. New Engl J Med 2001;345:892–902

41. Larsen AI, Arsland T, Kristiansen M, et al. Assessing the effect of exercise training in men with heart failure. Comparison of maximal, submaximal and endurance exercise protocols. Europ Heart J 2001;22:684–92

42. Coats AJS. Exercise training for heart failure. Coming of age. Circulation 1999;99:1138–40

43. Giannuzzi P, Tavazzi L, Temporelli PL, et al. Long-term physical training and left ventricular remodeling after anterior myocardial infarction: Results of the exercise in anterior myocardial infarction (EAMI) study group. J Am Coll Cardiol 1993;22:1821–9

44. Giannuzzi P, Temporelli PL, Corrà U, et al. For the ELKVD Study Group. Attenuation of unfavorable remodeling by exercise training in postinfarction patients with left ventricular dysfunction. Results of the exercise in left ventricular dysfunction (ELVD) trial. Circulation 1997;96:1790–7

45. Zbinden S, Wustmann K, Zbinden R, et al. Increased coronary collateral flow after three month exercise in patients with stable angina. In preparation

46. Hambrecht R, Wolf A, Gielen S, et al. Effect of exercise on coronary endothelial function in patients with coronary artery disease. New Engl J Med 2000;324:454–60

47. Giannuzzi P, Tavazzi L, Meyer K, et al. Recommendations for exercise training in chronic heart failure patients. Working Group on Cardiac Rehabilitation and Exercise Physiology and Working Group on Heart Failure of the European Society of Cardiology. Europ Heart J 2000;22:125–35

48. Braunwald E (ed). Heart disease. A textbook of cardiovascular medicine, 5th edn. W.B. Saunders Company 1997, p 164

49. Younis LT, Chaitman BR. The prognostic value of exercise testing. Cardiol Clin 1993;11:229–40

50. Froelicher V, Duarte GM, Oakes DF, et al. The prognostic value of the exercise test. Dis Mon 1988;34:677–735

51. Yli-Mayry S, Huikuri HV, Airaksinen KE, et al. Usefulness of a postoperative exercise test for predicting cardiac events after coronary artery bypass grafting. Am J Cardiol 1992;70:56–9

52. Morris CK, Ueshima K, Kawaguchi T, et al. The prognostic value of exercise capacity. Am Heart J 1991;122:1423–31

53. Frolkis JP, Pothier CE, Blackstone EH, et al. Frequent ventricular ectopy after exercise as a predictor of death. N Engl J Med 2003;348:781–90

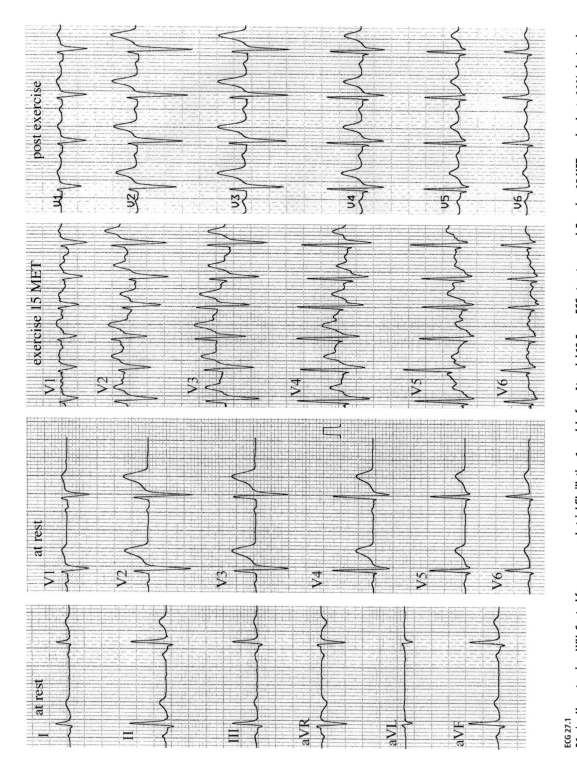

ECG 27.1

56 y/m. Hypertension. LVH. Control for paroxysmal atrial fibrillation 1 week before. Atenolol 12.5 mg. ECG at rest: normal. Exercise: 15 MET, maximal rate 166/min. Lead V_6: J point 0.5 mm below isoelectric line, ST isoelectric after 80 msec; V_4: ST normal; V_5: not conclusive. ECG postexercise: rate 115/min, normal. Normal exercise test. Echo/Doppler: LVH with mild diastolic dysfunction.

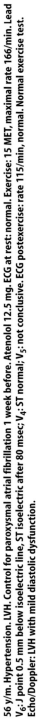

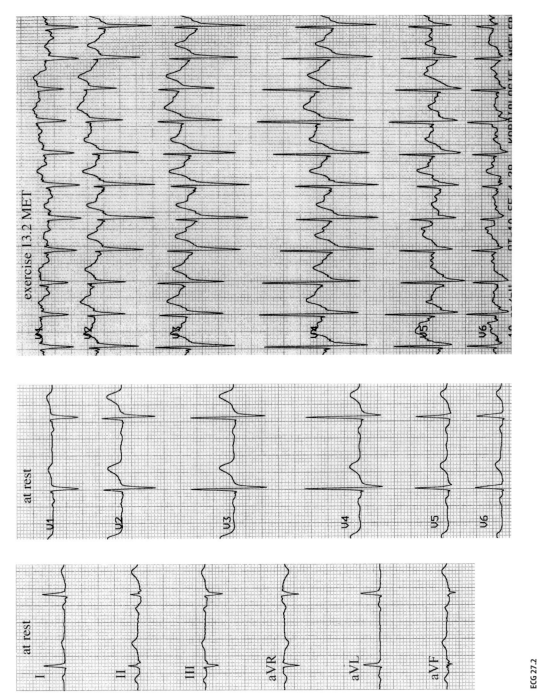
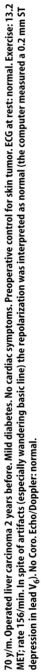

exercise 13.2 MET

at rest

at rest

ECG 27.2

70 y/m. Operated liver carcinoma 2 years before. Mild diabetes. No cardiac symptoms. Preoperative control for skin tumor. ECG at rest: normal. Exercise: 13.2 MET; rate 156/min. In spite of artifacts (especially wandering basic line) the repolarization was interpreted as normal (the computer measured a 0.2 mm ST depression in lead V_6). No Coro. Echo/Doppler: normal.

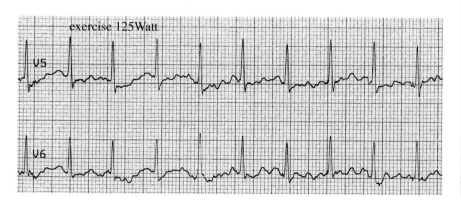

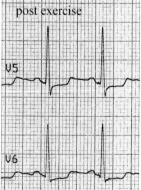

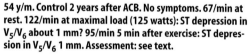

at rest

I

II

III

aVR

aVL

aVF

at rest

V1

V2

V3

V4

V5

V6

ECG 27.3

54 y/m. Control 2 years after ACB. No symptoms. 67/min at rest. 122/min at maximal load (125 watts): ST depression in V$_5$/V$_6$ about 1 mm? 95/min 5 min after exercise: ST depression in V$_5$/V$_6$ 1 mm. Assessment: see text.

exercise 125 Watt

V5

V6

post exercise

V5

V6

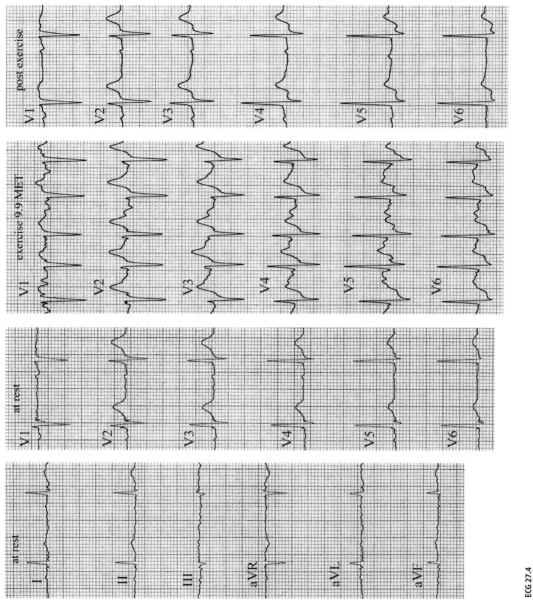

ECG 27.4

69 y/m. Mild angina at exercise. ECG at rest: normal (some artifacts). Exercise: 9.9 MET; rate 148/min, one atrial PB. ST depression 2 mm in V₆ (about 1 mm in V₅): ischemia. 6 min after exercise: rate 72/min: Descending/horizontal ST depression 1.5 mm in V₆/V₅(V₄), indicating 'late ischemia'. Coro: 80% stenosis of the great left anterior descending artery (LAD), 90% stenosis of small right coronary artery (RCA). Normal LV function.

494

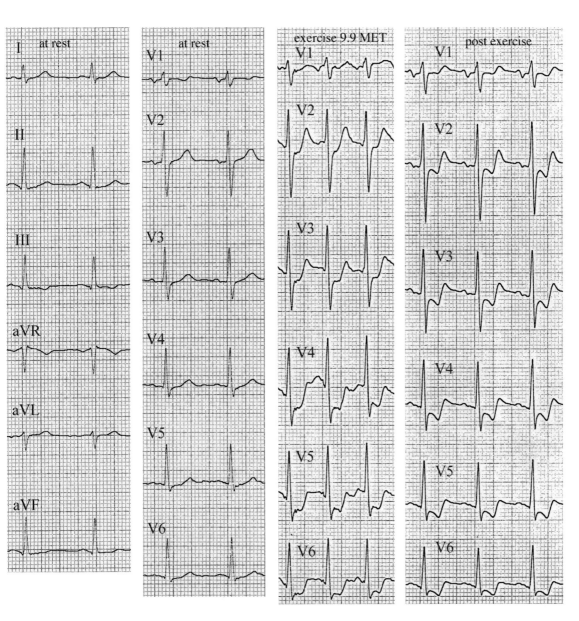

ECG 27.5

74 y/m. Preoperative risk stratification for operation of rectal carcinoma. No typical cardiac symptoms. Risk factor: smoking. ECG at rest: normal. Exercise: 9.9 MET; rate 142/min. Descending ST depression down to 3.5 mm in leads V_3 to V_6: ischemia. No symptoms! 6 min after exercise: descending ST depression in V_2 to V_6: 'late ischemia'. Coro: severe three-vessel disease, EF 67%, normal LV function. PTCA of LAD and RCA.

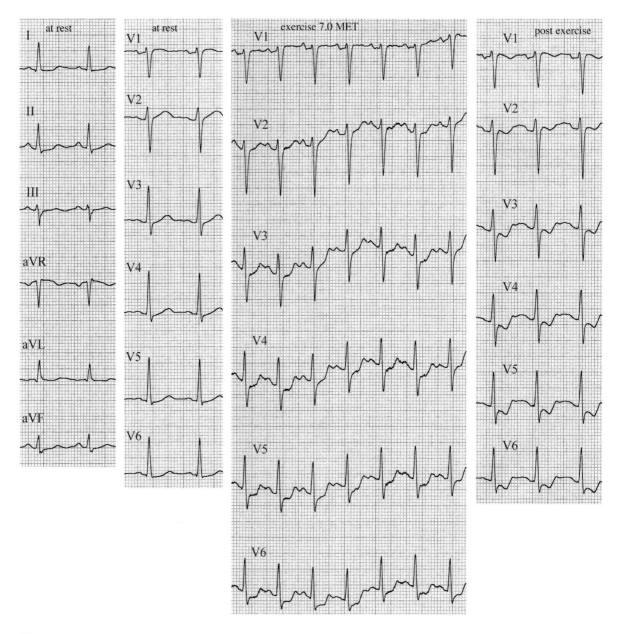

ECG 27.6

62 y/m. CHD. Coro: severe two-vessel disease. Normal LV function. PTCA of RCA and CX. ECGs 24 hours later. ECG at rest: Rate 91/min, ST depression 0.1 to 1 mm in V_5/V_6. Exercise: 7.0 MET; rate 136/min. Horizontal ST depression 1–2.5 mm in V_4 to V_6: ischemia. No symptoms. 4 min after exercise: Descending ST depression (up to 1.5 mm) and T negativity in V_2 to V_6: Late ischemia. Re-coro: no re-stenosis >>> false positive result, 24 hours after PTCA.

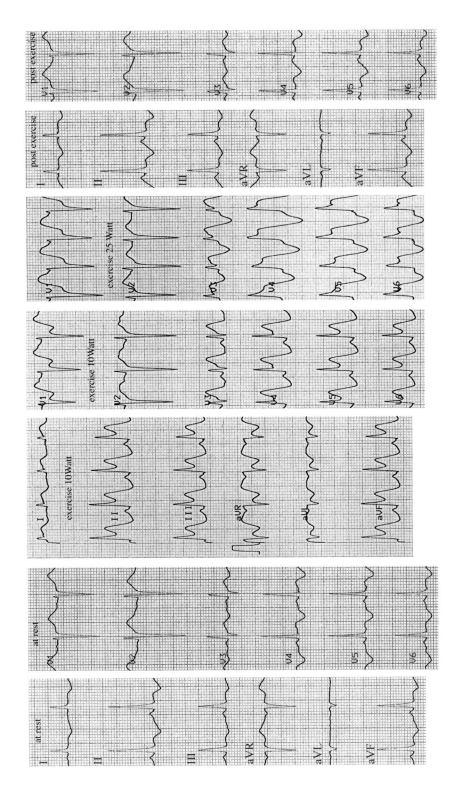

ECG 27.7

38 y/m. Typical attacks of angina at rest und during exercise. No Holter performed. Risk factors for CHD: smoking. ECG at rest: rate 99/min, negative symmetroid T waves in V$_3$ to V$_6$, I, II, aVF, III. Exercise: 10 watts; rate 128/min. No chest pain: ST elevation up to 5 mm in V$_1$ to V$_4$ and I, II, aVF, III. ST depression in V$_1$ (mirror image). Exercise: 25 watts, rate 147/min, mild typical pain. ST elevation up to 8 mm in the same leads: 'transmural lesion'. After exercise: rate 119/min, T negativity as before exercise. Coro: long 50% stenosis in the LAD (with ST elevation in III, aVF, II), reversible after nitroglycerine (spasm). Otherwise normal coronary arteries. Free of symptoms with nifedipine.

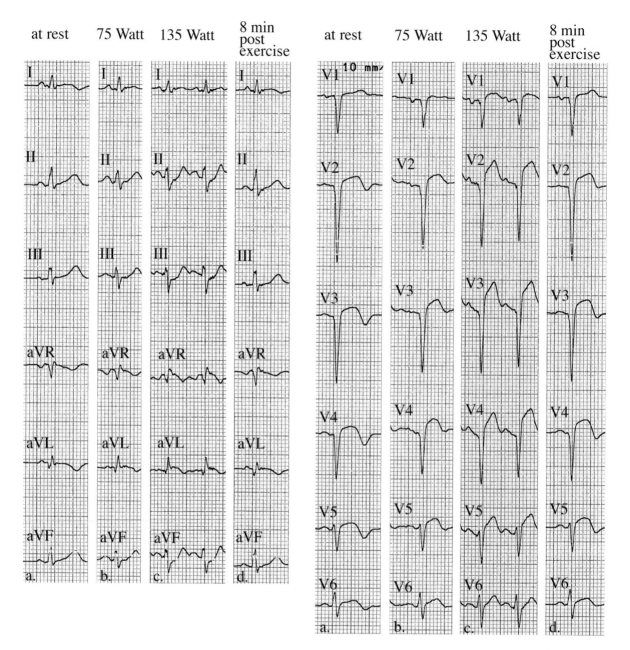

ECG 27.8

47 y/m. 6-month-old extensive anterior MI (ECG by courtesy of Paul Dubach, MD). a) ECG at rest: sinus rhythm, rate 63/min. ST elevation 1–1.5 mm in V$_1$ to V$_6$, terminal T negativity. b) Exercise: 75 watts, rate 107/min. Pronounced ST elevation (2–3 mm) in V$_1$ to V$_6$. c) Exercise: 135 watts, rate 148/min. Striking ST elevation (up to 5 mm) in V$_2$ to V$_5$ (also in aVL). T negativity disappeared. d) 8 min postexercise: rate 105/min. ST elevation regressed to 1 to 2 mm, reappearance of T negativity. The patient had no chest pain.

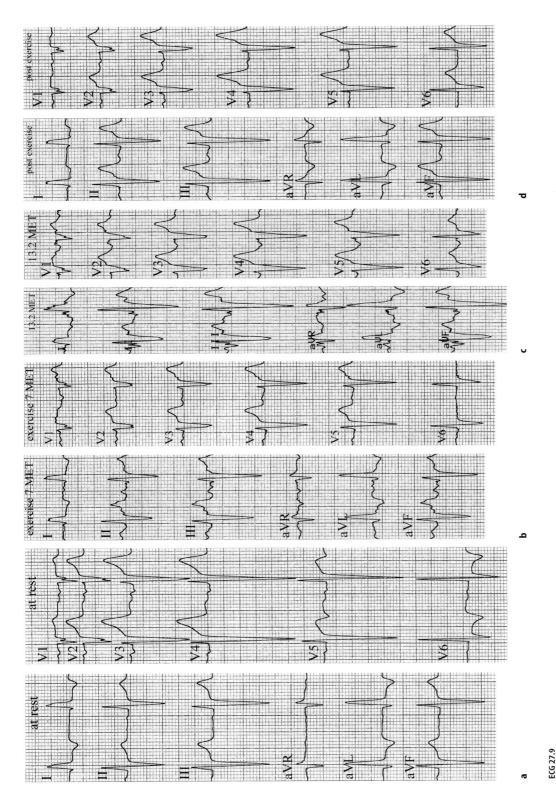

ECG 27.9

65 y/m. 5 years after heart transplant. Hypertension, LVH (LV mass 210 g/m²). a) ECG at rest: sinus rhythm, rate 82/min, LAFB, LVH. Negative T waves in I, aVL, V₆/V₅. b) Exercise 7 MET; rate 120/min, flat positive T in V₆/V₅. c) Exercise 13.2 MET; rate 156/min, positive T in V₅/V₆. d) Postexercise: rate 122/min, persistent positive T in V₆/V₅. Note: the negative T waves in leads I and aVL remain negative during and after exercise. Coro: no significant stenosis.

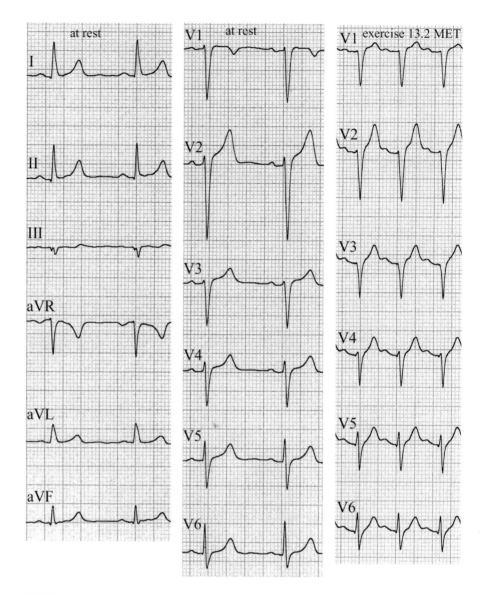

ECG 27.10

51 y/m. Preoperative risk stratification for cholecystectomy. Risk factors: positive family history, obesity, smoking. ECG at rest: QS in lead III, QRS clockwise rotation, mini q wave in V_6. Exercise: 13.2 MET; rate 132/min. QS in V_3, new small q waves in V_4 to V_6. Atypical chest pain. Coro: normal, normal LV function. The QRS alterations at rest (QS in III) and at exercise are classified as 'normal variants', retrospectively.

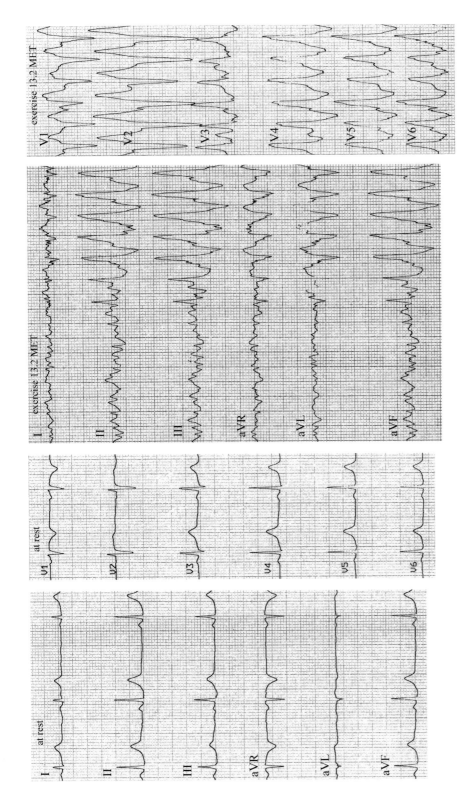

ECG 27.11

17 y/f. Palpitations at exercise. ECG at rest: sinus arrhythmia, rate about 54/min, normal ECG. Exercise: at the maximal workload (13.2 MET) with sinus rate 200/min ventricular tachycardia at a rate of 210/min develops, lasting 12 sec. Note: a) two or three fusion beats at the beginning of VT; b) the atypical LBBB pattern, with a change from a negative QRS to a positive one, already between V_2 and V_3. Electrophysiologic testing: 'focus' expected in the RV outflow tract but no VT inducible. Effective prophylaxis with atenolol.

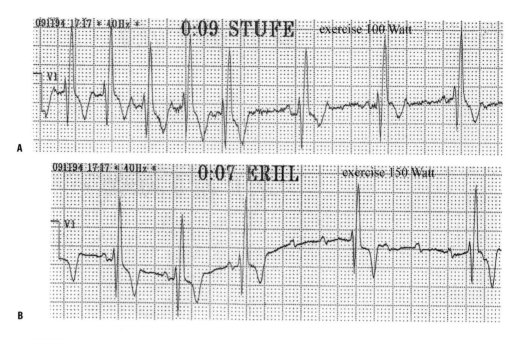

ECG 27.12

Short Story/Case Report 1. 42 y/m. Fatigue and dyspnoea during exercise. RBBB at rest. Exercise: stripe A: 100 watts, rate 146/min; AV block 2 : 1; fall of ventricular rate to 73/min. Stripe B: 150 watts, rate 176/min; progression from 2 : 1 to 3 : 1 and 4 : 1 AV block, with varying PQ interval (superimposed Wenckebach phenomenon); fall of ventricular rate to about 50/min.

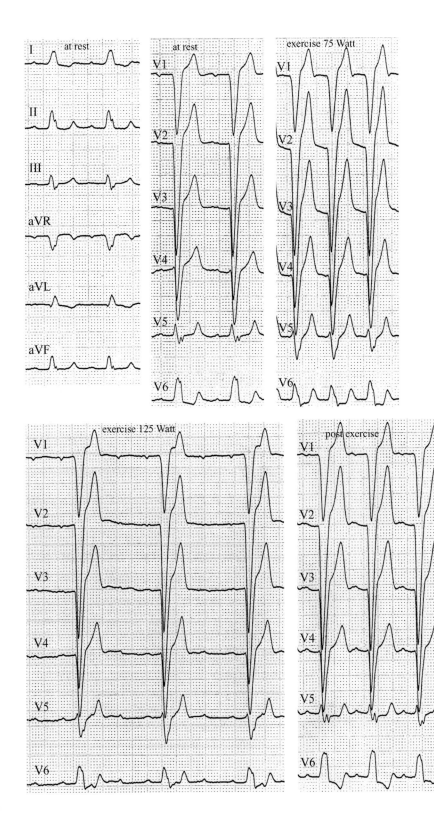

ECG 27.13
51 y/m. Dyspnea and fatigue during exercise, 2 months after aortic valve replacement. ECG at rest: sinus rate 78/min, AV block 1° (PQ 230 msec), LBBB. Exercise: 75 watts, rate 130/min (p partially hidden within the T wave, end of p only visible in V$_1$ as a negative wave). Exercise: 125 watts, sinus rate 156/min, AV block 3 : 1 (ventricular rate dropped to 52/min!). 3 min after exercise: sinus rhythm, rate 92/min, PQ 230 msec (1 : 1 AV conduction). Therapy with pacemaker.

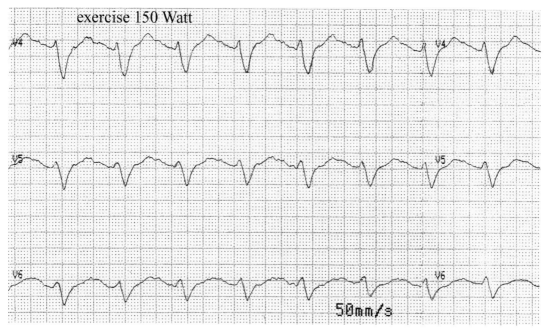

ECG 27.14

54 y/m. CAD with angina. LAFB with R < S in V_4/V_5/V_6. Exercise: 150 watts, rate 152/min, no ST depression in V_4 to V_6. False negative result. Coro: severe three-vessel disease, LV EF 60%. Technetium-MIBI: anterior ischemia (paper speed 50 mm/sec).

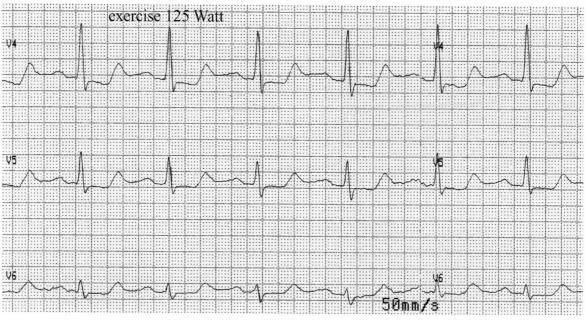

ECG 27.15

68 y/m. Hypertension, CAD. LAFB with R > S in V_4/V_5(V_6). Exercise: 125 watts, rate 103/min. ST depression 1.5 mm in V_4 to V_6. True positive result. Coro: 80% stenosis of LAD. Normal LV EF. Technetium-MIBI: anterior ischemia (paper speed 50 mm/sec).

Chapter 28
Pacemaker ECG

At a Glance

The first implantable cardiac stimulator device was used in humans in 1958. Since its introduction, this ingenious method for treating bradycardic arrhythmias has spread throughout the world; in 1998, 601 000 new pacemakers were implanted worldwide. The total number of people fitted with pacemakers is estimated at more than 4 million – and with a global population of some 8 billion this means approximately one person in every 2 million has a pacemaker. In some countries the ratio is about 1 : 600.

The first pacemaker (implanted by Senning in 1958) was a simple ventricular PM and had a fixed rate, with no sensing of spontaneous heart beats. The next stages in pacemaker evolution brought the 'on-demand' device that was able to sense spontaneous rhythm, the dual-chamber pacemaker that allowed atrioventricular sequential pacing, and the rate-responsive device that accelerated the pacing rate by analyzing body movement, respiration rate, and other parameters. In more recent years additional sophisticated functions have been integrated. These include mode switch (automatic change from two-chamber pacing to ventricular pacing after the onset of atrial fibrillation), sleep function, telemetry (including memory properties for counts of spontaneous and paced beats in detail), and programmed rapid atrial stimulation.

ECG

1 Single-chamber Pacemaker

The ECG pattern depends on the rate of the pacemaker on the one hand and on the spontaneous heart rate on the other. If the artificial pacing rate is greater than the spontaneous rate, every heart beat is paced.

The electric stimulus is mediated by an electrode localized in the right ventricle. The right ventricle is activated first, and the left ventricle over the septum, with latency. Consequently, we find a left bundle-branch block (LBBB) pattern in the ECG (ECG 28.1). In the rare cases of left ventricular pacing (through an electrode attached to the surface of the left ventricle) a right bundle-branch block (RBBB) pattern results. The electric stimulus itself manifests as a small and short spike immediately before the QRS complex. The stimulus is positive, negative, biphasic, or not visible – depending on its projection to the lead (ECG 28.1). Unipolar pacing results in markedly higher spikes than bipolar pacing.

The sensing mechanism of a pacemaker (on-demand function) inhibits pacing during and shortly after one or several premature beats (ECG 28.2).

Equally, the pacer function is inhibited if the pacing rate is lower than the spontaneous rhythm over a longer period. Thus there is no sign in the ECG that would identify the patient as having a pacemaker. It is possible in these cases to switch the on-demand mode to a fixed-rate mode with a magnet that is placed on the skin above the generator (ECG 28.3).

In cases with nearly the same rate of pacemaker and spontaneous rhythms, fusion beats or pseudofusion beats are detectable.

In a fusion beat the ventricles are activated in part by the pacer and in part spontaneously (ECG 28.4 and ECG 28.5). In a pseudofusion beat the stimulus occurs too late (during the absolute refractory ventricular period) and remains ineffective: the heart is exclusively activated by the pacemaker (ECGs 28.4 and 28.5).

Fusion beats and pseudofusion beats are normal features in a pacemaker ECG.

The pacing rate varies in all patients with a *rate-responsive* device, depending on the current activity. In general, the pacemaker rate is programmed to a maximum of 150/min and a minimum of 60/min. These pacing devices are called VVI(R) – only ventricular rate responsive pacing.

2 Dual-chamber Pacemaker

This device with double pacing and sensing properties has a ventricular electrode in the right ventricle and another electrode in the right atrium, allowing sequential atrioventricular pacing. The right atrium (and the left atrium shortly after) is only paced if the spontaneous atrial rate is lower than the pacing rate. As in ventricular pacing, in atrial pacing a pacemaker spike is visible – in this case at the beginning of the p wave. ECG 28.6 shows atrioventricular (AV) sequential dual-chamber pacing. In ECG 28.7 there is spontaneous activation of the atria by the sinus stimulus because the sinus rate is higher than the atrial rate of the pacemaker; therefore, the atrial spike is lacking. In both conditions (ECGs 28.6 and 28.7) the ventricles are activated by the pacemaker. This means that AV block is probably present – or at least that the spontaneous AV interval is longer than the programmed AV interval of the pacemaker.

3 Electric Complications and Failures

The complications are manifold and are due to generator or electrode problems. The majority of complications occur immediately after pacemaker implantation, or at 5–8 years later.

The *early* complications are mainly due to electrode displacement or incorrect connection of the electrode to the generator (this is not as rare as one would expect). These complications lead to loss of capture, and they are generally recognized during the postoperative period in the hospital, needing immediate revision. ECG 28.8 shows intermittent pacemaker failure during its implantation.

The *late* complications arise after several years. They are provoked either by depletion of the battery, or by critical rise of the stimulation threshold, or by both. Both conditions lead to loss of capture. The beginning of battery depletion is characterized by a decrease in the stimulation rate and/or a change to fixed-rate mode. In many cases of advanced depletion the pacemaker spike is still visible in the ECG, but without a consecutive QRS complex (ECG 28.9). In AV universal (DDD) pacemaker ECGs, battery depletion starts with a change of DDD-function to VVO-function, at a decreased pacing rate. ECG 28.10 shows intermittent nonfunction due to a manipulation during pacemaker control. In cases of battery depletion the generator must be replaced immediately. Fortunately, the best time for replacement of the generator can be estimated in advance with an accuracy of about 1 month. Most pacemaker control devices automatically indicate the life expectancy of a generator battery. At the same time the current pacing threshold is measured. A loss of capture may also occur during the measurement of the threshold, if the output of the pacemaker is decreased below the current threshold. However, in pacemaker-dependent patients a long ventricular pause (ECG 28.10) should be avoided.

Complications occuring between the early and late stages (*intermediate* complications) are relatively rare and generally involve other situations. Unexpected premature battery depletion or critical rises of the threshold have become rare.

The main intermediate complications are discussed in the following two paragraphs (3.1 and 3.2).

3.1 Undersensing and Oversensing

In *undersensing* the programmed sensing level of the generator (in mV) is too high – too 'insensitive' – for the normal sensing of the spontaneous QRS complex. Therefore, the pacer runs in a 'fixed-rate' mode. This may occur constantly or in isolated beats only. The ECG is characterized by spikes that fall into the spontaneous cardiac cycle at random (ECG 28.11). Of course, ventricular spikes falling into the refractory ventricular period of the spontaneous ventricular cycle do not result in stimulated beats, and may visually simulate a loss of capture. The same may occur with atrial spikes with respect to atrial cycles. Theoretically, undersensing can be a dangerous situation. A spike falling into the potentially vulnerable period of the ventricle ('spike on T' phenomenon) might induce ventricular fibrillation. However, this extremely rare complication will probably occur only in patients with severe ischemia. In practice, undersensing is harmless and does not induce symptoms.

Undersensing is eliminated by lowering the sensing threshold, perhaps from 2.5 mV to 1.5 mV. This represents a more or less cosmetic procedure, because complications are extremely rare. Moreover, lowering of the sensing level may induce oversensing, more often leading to dangerous situations.

In *oversensing* the programmed sensing level is too low – too 'sensitive'. Thus, small electric forces mainly arising in the upper thoracic skeleton muscles (pectoralis major, sternocleidomastoideus) are sensed, leading to inhibition of the pacemaker. In some cases, inhibition lasts for several heart cycles and may lead to syncope, in a currently pacemaker-dependent patient. The corresponding ECG may be detected in an ambulatory ECG and is characterized by multiple small spikes produced by skeletal muscles, absent pacemaker spikes, and ventricular asystole (ECG 28.12). Because oversensing occurs preferentially during extreme stress of these muscles in correlated activities (for instance chopping wood in younger patients or leaving the bathtub in older patients) a dangerous situation may arise, besides the loss of consciousness (see Short Story/Case Report 2).

Oversensing mainly occurs in patients with unipolar electrodes, where the sensed area is considerably greater than that with bipolar electrodes. Oversensing has become rare because of the better sensitivity of pacemakers, which can distinguish more precisely between heart potentials and skeletal muscle potentials. Oversensing is eliminated by increasing the sensing threshold (e.g. from 2 mV to 4 mV).

3.2 Lead Fracture and Lead Insulation Damage

Lead fracture and lead insulation damage may occur due to accidents, due to permanent wear and tear of the electrode, and due to the use of unsuitable insulation materials. The most current and dangerous result is a loss of capture. Electrode damage is often detectable in changes of lead parameters before a loss of capture arises.

The Full Picture

Out-of-hospital general practitioners, specialists in internal medicine, even those in cardiology, generally control only a few pacemaker patients. Pacemaker patients are regularly followed-up in the hospital by a specialized team. Due to the great variability of pacemaker generators, the complexity of control devices from different manufacturers, and the complexity of pacemaker arrhythmias, the members of this specialized team are obliged to undergo continuous education, regularly attending special courses organized by the National Associations of Cardiology and by the manufacturers. On top of this, it is essential for them regularly to consult the leading journals in this field such as *PACE* (published since 1978) and the *Journal of Cardiovascular Electrophysiology* (since 1989) which reflect the continuous progress in this field. A detailed presentation and discussion of the problems concerning pacemakers – com-

plex pacemaker arrhythmias included – is beyond the scope of this book.

4 Pacemaker Codes

Due to the development of simple single-chamber pacemakers into the complex devices seen nowadays, a pacemaker code was required for quick identification of the different functions. And as the devices became more sophisticated over the decades, the code underwent several modifications.

Every cardiologist concerned with the implanting and controlling of pacemakers is familiar with the current code, as shown in Table 28.1 [1].

The commonly implanted pacing devices nowadays are the DDD, DDD(R), VVI and VVI(R). Only dual-chamber pacemak-

Table 28.1
The revised NASPE/BPEG generic code for antibradycardic pacing

Position	I	II	III	IV	V
Category	Chamber(s) paced	Chamber(s) sensed	Response to sensing	Rate modulation	Multisite pacing
	O=none	O=none	O=none	O=none	O=none
	A=atrium	A=atrium	T=triggered	R=rate modulation	A=atrium
	V=ventricle	V=ventricle	I=inhibited		V=ventricle
	D=dual (A + V)	D=dual (A + V)	D=dual (T + I)		D=dual (A + V)
Manufacturers' designation only:	S=single (A or V)	S=single (A or V)			

ers guarantee AV sequential pacing – with one exception. In atrial inhibited (AAI) pacing the atrium is sensed and the ventricle is paced, also resulting in so-called physiologic pacing. Theoretically, VVI or VVI(R) devices should only be implanted in patients with atrial fibrillation, where atrial sensing or pacing is not possible. However, single-chamber ventricular pacing has not yet been abandoned worldwide, especially for economic reasons. The advantages of AV sequential pacing over single-chamber ventricular pacing are discussed below.

ECG Special _____

5　Morphologic Features

More than 98% of pacemakers are implanted transvenously, through the subclavian vein, with the electrode in the right ventricle. In about 30% of these cases an atrial electrode is also implanted in the right atrium. In common ventricular pacing the right ventricle is activated first and the left ventricle with latency over the septum, leading to an LBBB pattern. Depolarization and repolarization are uniform in the limb leads, with broad R waves in leads I and aVL, and wide QS complexes in leads II, aVF, and III. In the precordial leads we mostly miss a positive QRS deflection in leads V_5/V_6 as is commonly seen in LBBB aberration in a supraventricular rhythm. In most cases, after the stimulation spike we observe a QS complex in V_1 to V_5 and an rS complex in V_6. Due to a special position of the ventricular lead within the right ventricle, the rare pattern of Rs in lead V_1 may be detectable – a pattern never seen in LBBB aberration.

In the remaining 2% of patients with, for example, a single ventricle or severe tricuspid incompetence (in the latter case, if a screw-in electrode was not considered) the electrode is attached at the epicardium of the left ventricle by the surgeon. In this case the left ventricle is activated before the right ventricle, resulting in a more or less typical RBBB pattern.

Patterns of *old myocardial infarction* are easily detectable in rare conditions of epicardial left ventricular pacing with an RBBB pattern, but not in the vast majority of patients with endocardial right ventricular pacing and with an LBBB pattern.

ECGs 28.13 and ECG 28.14a (ECG 28.14b without pacing) illustrate that either inferior or anterior infarction are at least partially *masked* by the LBBB pattern, similar to LBBB aberration in patients without a pacemaker. A broad Q or QS wave in the inferior and anteroseptal leads, very common in right ventricular pacing with an LBBB pattern, may also imitate an infarction pattern. The QRS complex is wide, however.

Pacemaker spikes have greater amplitude in unipolar pacing compared to bipolar pacing. In bipolar pacing the spike may be so small that it is overlooked, especially in a generator output of 2.5 volts (ECG 28.13).

In 1969 Chatterjee et al described an interesting phenomenon [2,3] which is now unsurprisingly called the 'Chatterjee phenomenon'. If a spontaneous rhythm arises after right ventricular pacing (with a consecutive LBBB pattern) the T waves are negative in most cases in the precordial leads and eventually in the inferior limb leads. Ischemia may falsely be diagnosed (ECGs 31.10a–b in Chapter 31 Special ECG Waves, Signs, and Phenomena). The phenomenon has also been described after the disappearance of an LBBB (and to a minor degree of an RBBB) pattern without a pacemaker (ECG 31.11).

6　Pacemaker-Mediated Arrhythmia

Pacemaker-related arrhythmias include a vast number of arrhythmias that may be complex, especially in dual-chamber pacemakers. Analyzing those arrhythmias requires the knowledge of the technical properties of a generator and its programming.

The so-called 'pacemaker circus movement tachycardia' is based on the presence of retrograde atrial depolarization, detected by the atrial sensing component of a dual-chamber pacemaker. The following ventricular stimulus is delivered too early with the programmed AV interval. If this event repeats itself, a supraventricular reentry tachycardia results, also called 'endless loop' tachycardia, at a rate of about 130/min (ECG 28.15). Pacemaker circus movement tachycardia may be interrupted by increasing the atrial refractory period and/or by an increased AV interval. Nowadays, in all DDD devices a prolonged atrial refractory period after a sensed ventricular beat automatically inhibits the tachycardia.

In DDD(R) devices, pacing arrhythmias similar to AV block 2° (Wenckebach or 2 : 1 type) may arise, if the spontaneous sinus rate exceeds the programmed upper rate limit. The sensing of sinusal p waves inhibits atrial pacing, and ventricular pacing is delayed until the upper rate limit is reached. The degree of the AV interval is inversely proportional to the preceding AV interval. Consequently the prolongation of the PQ interval is progressive. A p wave falling into the postventricular atrial refractory period is not sensed and the ventricular impulse is not delivered. The next p wave is sensed again and with the correctly delivered ventricular impulse the AV block 2° episode may start again.

7 Pacemaker Malfunction

7.1 Battery Depletion

The first sign of 'normal' battery depletion is a fall in the stimulation rate. A decrease of more than three beats per minute in the automatic or magnet rate indicates the need for a battery exchange within 8 weeks, in most generators. If there is a switch from automatic to fixed-rate mode, and of course in incomplete and complete battery depletion (with ineffective or absent pacemaker stimuli), the replacement of the generator must be performed immediately. A progressive increase of the pacing rate (run-away) is very rare in the present pacemaker generation [4]. These have a programmer/interrogator device that determines the battery voltage by telemetry, so predicting future battery depletion accurately (in months) and allowing replacement in plenty of time.

Absent capture during implantation is due to electrode displacement, incomplete or inverse connection of the electrode(s) to the generator, and in rare cases to early and sudden battery depletion.

Short Story/Case Report 1

In 1988 the author implanted a VVI pacemaker in a 15-year-old girl for congenital complete AV block. The patient was anxious about the operation but proved to be very brave during the whole procedure. She and her mother, who was waiting outside the operating room, were warmly congratulated after the operation. Ten minutes later the nurse reported malfunction of the pacemaker. The ECG revealed complete AV block without any sign of pacemaker activity. X-ray examination showed an unchanged and good position of the electrode. However, the battery proved to be dead. The patient, the mother, and the cardiologist were terrified. The generator was immediately replaced. Some days later the patient and her mother were happy again. From the manufacturer of the pacemaker the girl received some CDs of her favorite artists and her mother received a huge bunch of flowers, the biggest she had ever received.

7.2 Electrode Problems

Persistent or intermittent failures of atrial or ventricular capture may also result from an increase of the stimulation threshold (mostly because of insulating fibrous tissue surrounding the tip of the electrode), very rarely due to drugs (e.g. flecainide [5]), wire fracture, or damaged electrode insulation. Again, analysis of malfunction is possible in most cases because of information about the battery and lead impedance through telemetry.

7.3 Oversensing and Undersensing

The signs of oversensing and undersensing are presented above in the first section of this chapter (ECGs 28.11–28.12). The following case report shows that oversensing may induce a life-threatening situation.

Short Story/Case Report 2

In 1978 a 79-year-old patient with a VVI pacemaker, implanted for complete AV block with syncopal attacks, wanted to leave his bathtub when it was still full of water. He heaved himself up by his arms but lost consciousness. He awoke to find himself lying in the bathtub with his head partially under water. He tried to get up two more times, with the same terrible result. Because he was panicking he did not think to let out the water. Through an extreme effort he catapulted himself out of the tub, and again lost consciousness. He then realized with great satisfaction that he was lying on the floor rather than the bathtub.

An inspection of the pacemaker revealed oversensing that was reproducible by strong straining of the muscles of the arm and thorax, with consecutive cardiac arrest lasting several seconds. The patient was enthusiastic about this test, asking for repetitions, up to short loss of consciousness. After changing the sensitivity of the pacemaker from 2.5 mV to 4 mV (the R wave reading was 7.4 mV) the patient remained free of symptoms.

8 Pacemaker Syndrome

8.1 Prevalence

The prevalence of the syndrome depends on its definition. The prevalence in patients with isolated ventricular pacing is about 2% if only serious symptoms are considered, and about 22% if all symptoms possibly related to the pacemaker syndrome are considered [6].

8.2 Condition

The pacemaker syndrome is not necessarily linked to VVI(R) pacing. It may also arise in patients with inappropriately programmed atrial pacing (AAI(R)) or dual-chamber pacing. In AAI(R) pacing, AV dysynchrony may result from a disproportionate increase of the atrial rate during exercise [7]. VDD(R) pacing may lead to the syndrome if the atrial rate falls below the lower programmed rate, resulting in VVI(R) pacing. In DDI(R) pacing the pacemaker syndrome arises if the spontaneous sinus rate exceeds the lower rate, or the sensor-indicated rate in patients with AV block because of continual AV dissociation [8]. Even in DDD pacing prolonged intra-atrial and/or interatrial conduction times, as well as pacemaker-mediated or endless-loop tachycardia, may induce AV dysynchrony or ventriculoatrial synchrony [9]. A pacemaker syndrome is easily overlooked in these conditions.

8.3 Pathophysiologic Mechanisms

The pathophysiologic mechanisms are more complex [7] than used to be assumed [10]. The absence of the atrial kick generally reduces arterial pressure to a modest degree. The atrial contraction against the closed atrioventricular valves may result in very high *venous a waves*, (atrial waves) up to 50 mmHg. These a waves may provoke an abnormal and exaggerated response of baroreceptors in the lung veins, resulting in a drastic fall of blood pressure, with syncope as a possible consequence. However, in recent times involvement of multiple reflex pathways has been postulated, including carotid and aortic baroreceptors, cardiopulmonary baroreflexes, and potentially inhibitory reflexes mediated by 'vagal afferents' present in the atria and the atrioventricular junctions [7]. Incidentally, Lüderitz described in an amusing article [11] a 'pacemaker syndrome' without a pacemaker that was observed by McWilliam as long ago as 1889 [12].

9 Indications for Pacing

The indications for implantation of cardiac pacemakers (and other antiarrhythmic devices) are presented in the ACC/AHA Guidelines of 1998 [13] with differentiation into three classes. A class I indication includes conditions for which there is evidence and/or general agreement that a given procedure or treatment is beneficial, useful, and effective. In Class II we find conditions with conflicting evidence and/or divergence of opinion about the usefulness/efficacy of treatment, subdivided into class IIa (weight of evidence/opinion in favor of usefulness/efficacy) and class IIb (usefulness/efficacy is less well established by evidence/opinion). Class III describes conditions with evidence/general opinion that a procedure/treatment is not use-

ful/effective and in some cases may be harmful [13]. The extensive review (333 references) provides detailed reasons for allocation of nearly all conditions to the three classes.

This book, therefore, presents only a short overview and two relatively new and interesting indications are discussed as follows.

Complete AV block and sinus node dysfunction (sick sinus syndrome) represent the most frequent reasons for chronic pacing, each condition responsible for about 40% of all pacemaker implantations. The remaining 20% are covered by bradycardic atrial fibrillation, so-called 'prophylactic' implantations in some forms of bifascicular and incomplete trifascicular blocks (Chapter 11 Bilateral Bifascicular Blocks), AV block 2° of high degree types or Mobitz type, and by rare conditions such as the carotid sinus syndrome, the long QT syndrome [14], sleep apnea [15], some cases of hypertrophic obstructive cardiomyopathy, and also heart failure in patients with wide QRS complexes. Also isolated AV block 1° may represent an indication for a pacemaker implantation in a few selected cases with heart failure and mitral incompetence. Shortening of the AV interval improves ventricular function [16].

9.1 Pacing in Hypertrophic Obstructive Cardiomyopathy

The first observations about the beneficial effect of pacing in patients with hypertrophic obstructive cardiomyopathy (HOCM) were reported from studies about acute pacing [17,18]. Thereafter, permanent dual-chamber pacing was applied in an attempt to avoid myectomy by open heart surgery. Shortening of the AV interval leads to a better left ventricular filling and consecutively to a significant reduction (at a mean of 50%) of the intraventricular systolic gradient and to significant improvement of symptoms [19–21]. So-called transcoronary alcohol septal ablation, introduced by Sigwart et al in 1995 [22], has proved to be as effective as a surgical septal resection [23,24]. Ethyl ablation, performed through a catheter introduced into the septal coronary artery branches, provokes necrosis of a portion of the hypertrophic interventricular septum with a dramatic reduction of the gradient, with a latency of several weeks. A recent study has shown minimal superiority of surgical myectomy over alcohol ablation [25].

Surgical resection results in an LBBB, whereas alcohol ablation provokes an RBBB in all cases, and complete AV block in more than 40% of cases. About 20% of patients need a dual-chamber pacemaker [24].

9.2   Pacing in Heart Failure

A prolonged QRS duration (> 0.12 sec) contributes to an additional impairment of ventricular function in patients with heart failure, by dysynchronous ventricular contraction. Moreover, it leads to inefficient use of energy in heart metabolism, called mechanoenergetic uncoupling [26]. It has been shown that synchronous pacing of the right ventricle (through a conventionally positioned electrode) and the left ventricle – through an electrode in the coronary sinus and in a coronary vein, thus stimulating the left ventricle from the epicardium – not only shortens the QRS duration but also improves ventricular function. The method is effective in patients with LBBB and, astonishingly, also in patients with RBBB. In the study by Abraham et al [26] with 228 patients randomly assigned to the resynchronization group, mortality was reduced by 40% compared with the control group (follow-up of 6 months). The NYHA functional class, the distance walked in 6 minutes, and the quality-of-life score were significantly improved. Large-scale controlled studies (the COMPANION trial and the CARE–HF study) are in progress. An overview of new pacemaker indications is presented in the article by Barold [27].

10   Prognosis of AV Sequential (Physiologic) Pacing *vs* Single-Chamber Ventricular Pacing

In physiologic pacing an AV sequential heart function is preserved. In patients with AV block the DDD(R) mode is used, whilst in sick sinus syndrome, with normal AV conduction, atrial pacing is sufficient. This statement is controversial and will be discussed later.

In single-chamber ventricular pacing, AV dissociation is present. The loss of the 'atrial kick' reduces cardiac output to a certain degree. More importantly, the additional synchronous atrial and ventricular contraction in many beats may provoke symptoms that are summarized in the term 'pacemaker syndrome'. Opinions about the significance of lacking AV sequential heart function for the most important endpoints such as mortality, thromboembolic events, and heart failure, have been controversial for many years.

The first larger studies involving limited cohorts of patients (168–215) [28–30] revealed clear superiority of physiologic pacing over single-chamber ventricular pacing with respect to mortality, prevalence of thromboembolic events, and heart failure. The risk for new AV block in patients with sick sinus syndrome was described as low (0.6% annual risk). These

results led to an increased enthusiasm in the 'western/developed' world for implanting AAI or DDD pacemakers for treating sick sinus syndrome and DDD devices in patients with complete AV block.

In recent multicenter studies with a considerably higher number of patients (407–2568) the (formerly postulated) clear superiority of physiologic pacing over single ventricular pacing has partially been revised.

In the 'Canadian' or CTOPP study (Canadian Trial of Physiologic Pacing [31]), 1474 patients were randomly assigned to receive a ventricular pacemaker and 1094 to receive a physiologic pacemaker. The annual rate of stroke or death due to cardiovascular causes was not significantly decreased in patients with physiologic pacing, with 5.5% *vs* 4.9% in patients with ventricular pacing after a follow-up of 3 years. Equally, the death from all causes, the incidence of new atrial fibrillation, and the number of hospitalizations showed small and statistically non-significant differences. Perioperative complications were more frequent in the group with physiologic pacemakers, in 9% *vs* 3.9% of cases in the group with ventricular pacemakers ($p < 0.001$). The authors concluded that the decision to use a physiologic or ventricular pacemaker should be based on the patient's individual needs.

The 'Elderly' or PASE study (Pacemaker Selection in the Elderly) included 407 patients at a mean age of 78 years (60% men), 204 patients with ventricular pacing, and 203 patients with dual-chamber pacing [32]. There were no differences between the two pacing modes in cardiovascular events or death. However, 26% of the patients assigned to ventricular pacing were crossed over to dual-chamber pacing because of symptoms related to the pacemaker syndrome. Patients with dual-chamber pacemakers had moderately better quality of life and cardiovascular functional status, but only in the presence of sick sinus syndrome and not in AV block. Strong trends of borderline statistical significance in clinical endpoints favoring dual-chamber pacing were only observed in patients with sick sinus syndrome. Regarding the relatively high number of patients with crossover from single- to dual-chamber pacing and a substantial improvement in quality of life by dual-chamber pacing, this pacing mode seems to be preferable, especially in the presence of sick sinus syndrome.

In the MOST study (Mode Selection Trial [33]), 2010 patients with sinus node dysfunction (sick sinus syndrome) were evaluated. The two groups with single-chamber (VVI(R), rate 60/min to $\geq$ 110/min) pacing (n=996) and dual-chamber (DDDR) pacing (n=1014) were followed for a median of 33.1 months and compared with respect to the following endpoints and parameters: death of any cause; cardiovascular death; non-fatal stroke; hospitalization for heart failure; heart failure score; atrial fibrillation; and health-related quality of life. Between the two groups no significant difference could be found for death of any cause, cardiovascular death, stroke, and hospitalization for heart failure. However, the patients with dual-chamber pacing accumulated fewer points on the heart failure score than patients with ventricular pacing. Patients receiving dual-chamber pacing and who had no history of atrial fibrillation had a lower incidence of atrial fibrillation after randomization than patients with ventricular pacing ($p < 0.001$), whereas patients with dual-chamber pacing and with a history of atrial fibrillation had a non-significant 14% reduction ($p=0.12$) of atrial fibrillation. Over a period of 4 years patients with dual-chamber pacing provided significant improvements in quality of life, compared with ventricular pacing, for six of eight SF-36 subclass in the carry-forward analysis. Summary scores for physical and mental components also improved significantly. If health status after crossover was included in the analysis, there were no significant differences between the two groups. The authors concluded that dual-chamber pacing in patients with sinus node dysfunction offers significant improvement over ventricular pacing, including a reduction of the risk of atrial fibrillation, a reduction of signs and symptoms of heart failure, and a slight improvement in the quality of life. Stroke-free survival was not improved by dual-chamber pacing compared to ventricular pacing.

The UKPACE (UK Pacing and Cardiovascular Events) trial [34] randomly allocated 2000 patients aged 70 years and over with high degree (second degree or complete) AV block undergoing first pacemaker implantation to receive a VVI (25%), VVI(R) (25%) or DDD (50%) pacemaker. The results are expected soon.

10.1 Conclusions

The later studies reveal no differences in all-causes or cardiovascular death or stroke between the two pacing modes. New onset atrial fibrillation is significantly reduced by dual-chamber pacing in patients with sinus node dysfunction. It is quite obvious that physiologic pacing reduces signs and symptoms of heart failure and improves quality of life in patients with sick sinus syndrome over ventricular pacing. It is also obvious that physiologic pacing has no disadvantage compared to single-chamber ventricular pacing, with the exception of increased perioperative complications and the increased costs of dual-chamber pacing. Because both disadvantages can be eliminated by atrial pacing in patients with sick sinus syndrome and normal AV conduction, this mode of pacing should also be considered in patients with this syndrome. Only a few patients need an upgrade to dual-chamber pacing because of new AV block. In 399 patients with sick sinus syndrome and atrial pacing the annual rate of new AV block requiring the implantation of a ventricular electrode was 1.7% [35]. However, a very cautious control is needed, because the lack of ventricular pacing may be deleterious in these cases. Moreover, single-chamber atrial pacing – in contrast to dual-chamber pacing – does not allow individual programming of the AV interval [36]. Overall the implantation of a single-chamber ventricular pacemaker in patients with AV block and also with sick sinus syndrome should not be regarded as an almost 'criminal procedure' – as it was some years ago. A better prognosis and a better quality of life is preferentially based on the pacemaker itself, independent of its mode [32]. However, physiologic pacing is preferable, especially in patients with sick sinus syndrome and in countries that are still able to pay the higher costs.

References

1. Bernstein AD, Daubert JC, Fletcher RD, et al. The revised NASPE/BPEG generic code for antibradycardia, adaptive-rate, and multisite pacing. PACE 2002;25:260–4
2. Chatterjee K, Harris AM, Davies JG, Leatham A. T-wave changes after artificial pacing. Lancet 1969;1(7598):759–60 (preliminary communication)
3. Chatterjee K, Harris A, Davies G, Leatham A. Electrocardiographic changes subsequent to artificial ventricular depolarization. Br Heart J 1969;31:770–9
4. Bohm A, Hajdu L, Pinter A, et al. Runaway pacemaker syndrome and intermittent nonoutput as manifestations of end of life of a VVI pacemaker. Pacing Clin Electrophysiol 2000;23:2143–4
5. Antonelli D, Freedberg NA, Rosenfeld T. Acute loss of capture due to flecainide acetate. Pacing Clin Electrophysiol 2001;24:1170
6. Ellenbogen KA, Stambler BS, Orav EJ, et al. Clinical characteristics of patients intolerant to VVI(R) pacing. Am J Cardiol 2000;86:59–63
7. Ellenbogen KA, Gilligan DM, Wood MA, et al. The pacemaker syndrome – A matter of definition. Am J Cardiol 1997;79:1226–9
8. Torresani J, Ebagosti A, Allard-Latour G. Pacemaker syndrome with DDD pacing. PACE 1984;7:1148–51
9. Barold SS. Repetitive reentrant and non-reentrant ventriculoatrial synchrony in dual-chamber pacing. Clin Cardiol 1991;14:754–63
10. Ausubel K, Furman S. The pacemaker syndrome. Ann Intern Med 1985;103:420–9
11. Lüderitz B. 'Pacemaker syndrome' 70 years before the first pacemaker was implanted. J Intervent Card Electrophysiol 2001;5:341

12. McWilliam JA. Electrical stimulation of the heart in man. Brit Med J 1889;1:348–50
13. Gregoratos G, Cheitlin MD, Epstein AE, et al. ACC/AHA Guidelines for Implantation of Cardiac Pacemakers and Antiarrhythmia Devices. J Am Coll Cardiol 1998;31:1175–209
14. Glikson M, Hayes DL, Nishimura RA. Newer clinical applications of pacing. J Cardiovasc Electrophysiol 1997;8:1190–203
15. Gottlieb DJ. Cardiac pacing – a novel therapy for sleep apnea? N Engl J Med 2002;346:444–5
16. Barold SS. Indications for permanent cardiac pacing in first-degree AV block: class I, II, or III? (Editorial). PACE 1996;29:747–51
17. Hassenstein P, Wolter HH. Therapeutische Beherrschung einer bedrohlichen Situation bei der idiopathischen hypertrophischen Subaortenstenose. Verh Dtsch Ges Kreisl 1967;33:342–6
18. Rothlin M, Moccetti T. Beeinflussung der muskulären Subaortenstenose durch intraventrikuläre Reizausbreitung. Verh Dtsch Ges Kreisl 1967;33:411–5
19. Jeanrenaud X, Goy JJ, Kappenberger L. Effects of dual-chamber pacing in hypertrophic obstructive cardiomyopathy. Lancet 1992;339(8805):1318–23
20. Kappenberger L, Linde C, Daubert C, et al. Pacing in hypertrophic obstructive cardiomyopathy. A randomized crossover study. PIC study group. Europ Heart J 1997;18:1249–56
21. Maron BJ, Nishimura RA, McKenna WJ, et al. Assessment of permanent dual-chamber pacing as a treatment for drug-refractory symptomatic patients with hypertrophic obstructive cardiomyopathy. A randomized, double-blind, crossover study (M-PATHY). Circulation 1999;99:2927–33
22. Sigwart U. Non-surgical myocardial reduction for hypertrophic obstructive cardiomyopathy. Lancet 1995;346(8969):211–4
23. Mazur W, Nagueh SF, Lakkis NM, et al. Regression of left ventricular hypertrophy after nonsurgical septal reduction therapy for hypertrophic obstructive cardiomyopathy. Circulation 2001;103:1492–6
24. Shamim W, Yousufuddin M, Wang D, et al. Nonsurgical reduction of the interventricular septum in patients with hypertrophic cardiomyopathy. New Engl J Med 2002;347:1326–33
25. Firoozi S, Elliott pacemaker, Sharma S, et al. Septal myotomy–myectomy and transcoronary septal alcohol ablation in hypertrophic obstructive cardiomyopathy. A comparison of clinical, hemodynamic and exercise outcomes. Europ Heart J 2002;23:1617–24
26. Abraham WT, Fisher WG, Smith AL, et al (for the MIRACLE study group). Cardiac resynchronization in chronic heart failure. New Engl J Med 2002;346:1845–53
27. Barold SS. New indications for cardiac pacing. In: Saksena S, Lüderitz B, eds. Interventional Electrophysiology – A Textbook. Mt Kisco, NY: Futura, 1996, pp 145–64
28. Rosenqvist M, Brandt J, Schüller H. Long-term pacing in sinus node disease: effects of stimulation mode on cardiovascular morbidity and mortality. Am Heart J 1988;116:16–22
29. Hesselson AB, Parsonnet V, Bernstein AD, Bonavita GJ. Deleterious effects of long-term single-chamber ventricular pacing in patients with sick sinus syndrome: the hidden benefits of dual-chamber pacing. J Am Coll Cardiol 1992;19:1542–9
30. Andersen HR, Thuesen L, Bagger JP, et al. Prospective randomized trial of atrial versus ventricular pacing in sick-sinus syndrome. Lancet 1994;344(8936):1523–8
31. Connolly SJ, Kerr CR, Gent M, et al. Effects of physiologic pacing versus ventricular pacing on the risk of stroke and death due to cardiovascular causes. Canadian Trial of Physiologic Pacing Investigators. N Engl J Med 2000;342:1385–91
32. Lamas GA, Orav EJ, Stambler BS, et al (for the Pacemaker Selection in the Elderly Investigators). Quality of life and clinical out-comes in elderly patients treated with ventricular pacing as compared with dual-chamber pacing. N Engl J Med 1998;338:1097–104
33. Lamas GA, Lee KL, Sweeney MO, et al (for the Mode Selection Trial in Sinus-Node Dysfunction). Ventricular pacing or dual-chamber pacing for sinus node dysfunction. N Engl J Med 2002;346:1854–62
34. Toff WD, Skehan JD, De Bono DP, Camm AJ. The United Kingdom pacing and cardiovascular events (UKPACE) trial. UK Pacing and Cardiovascular Events. Heart 1997;78:221–3
35. Kristensen L, Nielsen JC, Pedersen AK, et al. AV block and changes in pacing mode during long-term follow-up of 399 consecutive patients with sick sinus syndrome treated with an AAI/AAI(R) pacemaker. Pacing Clin Electrophysiol 2001;24:358–65
36. Barold SS. Permanent single-chamber atrial pacing is obsolete. Pacing Clin Electrophysiol 2001;24:271–5

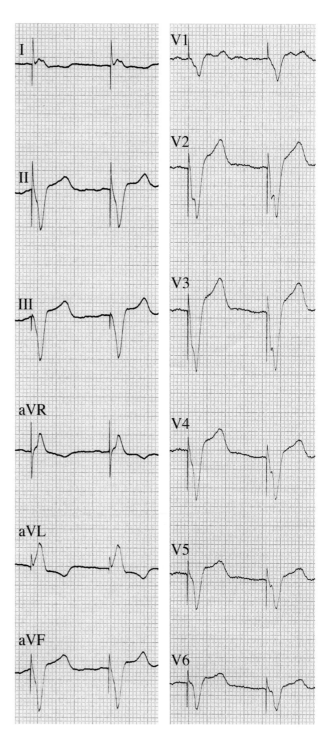

ECG 28.1

82 y/f. Bradycardic atrial fibrillation (mean rate 30/min), pre-syncope. ECG: VVI(R) pacemaker, rate 70/min (at rest). Every spike is followed by a wide QRS complex with LBBB pattern (endocardial right ventricular pacing). Atrial fibrillation. Note the different polarity of the pacemaker spikes (positive, negative, biphasic) in different leads.

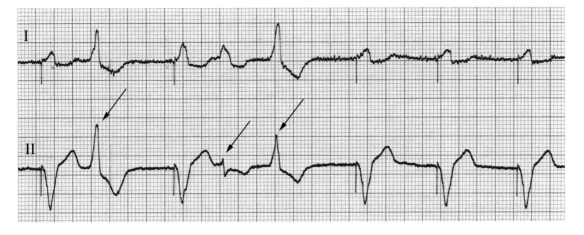

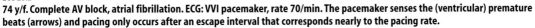

ECG 28.2

74 y/f. Complete AV block, atrial fibrillation. ECG: VVI pacemaker, rate 70/min. The pacemaker senses the (ventricular) premature beats (arrows) and pacing only occurs after an escape interval that corresponds nearly to the pacing rate.

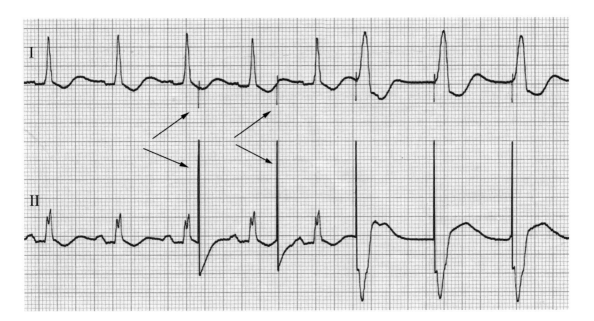

ECG 28.3

80 y/m. Sick sinus syndrome (with intermittent sinus arrest, not shown). VVI pacemaker (1974). ECG: sinus rhythm, rate 82/min. After positioning a magnet, the pacemaker delivers impulses at a rate of 71/min. The first two impulses are ineffective because they fall into the refractory period (arrows). After some beats the sinus node takes over the heart action again (not shown).

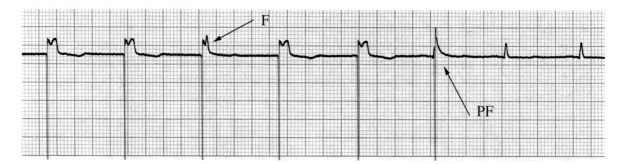

ECG 28.4

77 y/m. Sick sinus syndrome. VVI pacemaker (implanted in 1972). ECG: because of nearly the same rate of the pacemaker and the sinus node, the rhythms often change. The third beat is a fusion beat (↓), the sixth beat is a pseudofusion beat (↑).

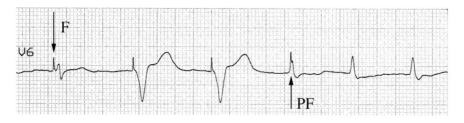

ECG 28.5

86/m. Bradycardic atrial fibrillation, presyncope. VVI(R) pacemaker. ECG: change between conducted and paced beats. One fusion beat (↓F) one pseudofusion beat (↑ PF).

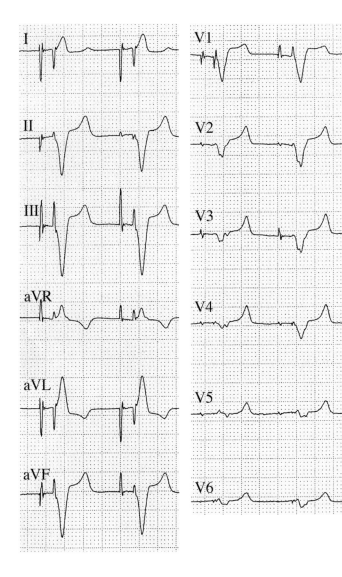

ECG 28.6

55 y/f. Complete AV block and sinus node dysfunction. DDDR pacemaker. ECG: AV sequential pacing of the atrium and the ventricle, at a rate of 70/min (note the pacemaker spikes before the (flat) p waves and QRS complexes).

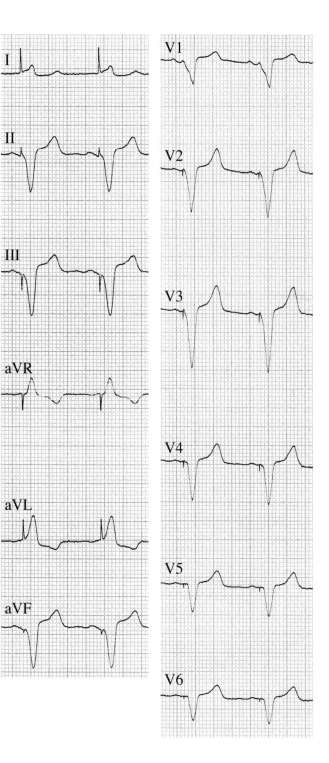

ECG 28.7

62 y/m. Sick sinus syndrome. DDDR pacemaker. ECG: the p waves are sensed and the ventricles stimulated AV sequentially, at the sinusal rate of 67/min in limb leads and 72/min in precordial leads.

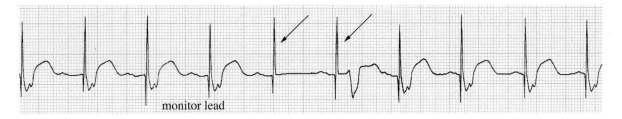

monitor lead

ECG 28.8
60 y/f. Sick sinus syndrome, AV block 1°. The ECG (monitor lead) during implantation of a DDD pacemaker shows intermittent pacemaker dysfunction, due to unstable position of the electrode tip. Two ventricular spikes are ineffective, the ventricular escape beat (↓) is not sensed.

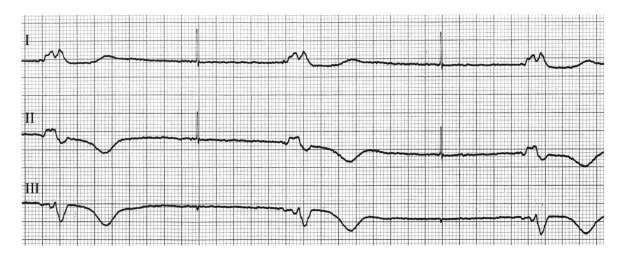

ECG 28.9
75 y/m. Complete AV block, atrial fibrillation. Generator depletion of a VVI pacemaker. ECG (50 mm/sec): ineffective pacemaker spikes (decreased rate of 44/min). Ventricular escape rhythm. Rate 44/min. The sensing function is still in action. The f waves are not visible in these leads.

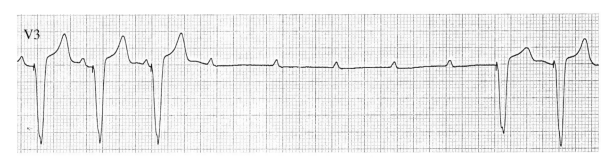

ECG 28.10
64 y/f. Complete AV block, Morgagni-Adams-Stokes attacks. VVI pacemaker. ECG: during pacemaker control the pacemaker was inadvertently inhibited for several seconds. A ventricular asystole of 4.2 sec occurred, without symptoms.

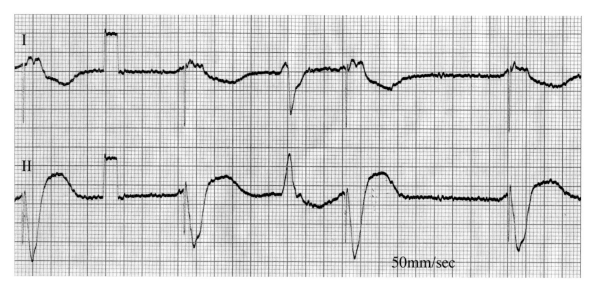

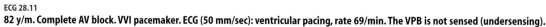

ECG 28.11

82 y/m. Complete AV block. VVI pacemaker. ECG (50 mm/sec): ventricular pacing, rate 69/min. The VPB is not sensed (undersensing).

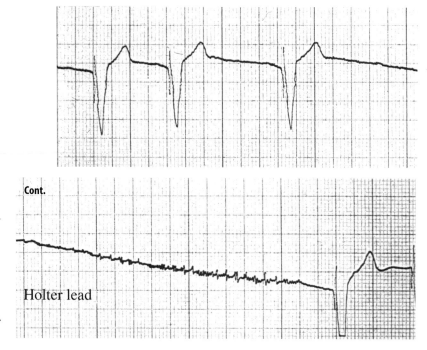

ECG 28.12

65 y/m. Complete AV block, syncope. Presyncope after VVI pacemaker implantation (1976), while chopping wood. ECG (Holter lead): the great pacemaker spikes suggest unipolar pacing. The third paced beat arises with small latency (inhibited for a very short period), then ventricular asystole occurs during 5 sec. The inhibiting muscle potentials are scarcely visible. Oversensing and the symptoms disappeared after programming the sensitivity from 2.5 mV to 5.0 mV.

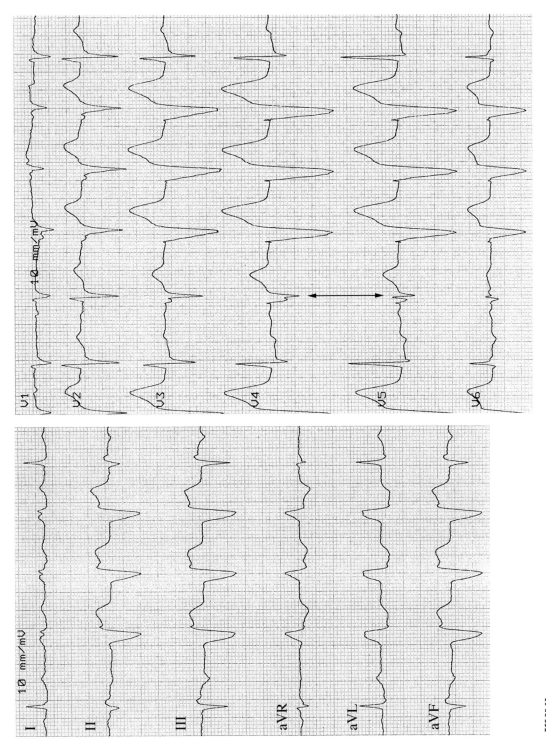

ECG 28.13

75 y/m. Old inferior MI with aneurysm. In SR leads II, aVF and III reveal old inferior MI, while during pacemaker rhythm there is the usual pattern of LBBB with QS complexes in these leads. The LBBB pattern in the precordial leads is common for paced beats, with a QS complex in all precordial leads (or a minimal R wave in lead V₆). The third QRS complex is a fusion beat (↓) and imitates a loss of anterior potentials. The second and the last (spontaneous) QRS complexes are normal.

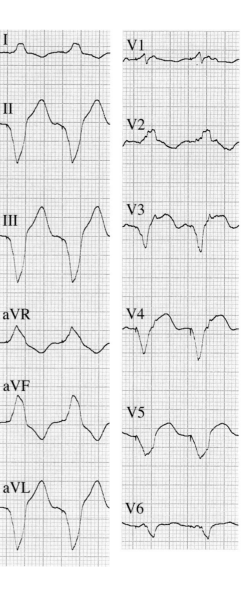

ECG 28.14a

69 y/m. Extensive anterior MI (left ventricular ejection fraction 30%) with intermittent complete AV block. ECG: DDD pacemaker. The anterior MI cannot be identified. However, this is a striking intraventricular conduction disturbance (additionally to the LBBB pattern) with a 'paradoxical' positive QRS complex in V$_2$ and a Qr complex in V$_3$. The sinusal p waves are very small.

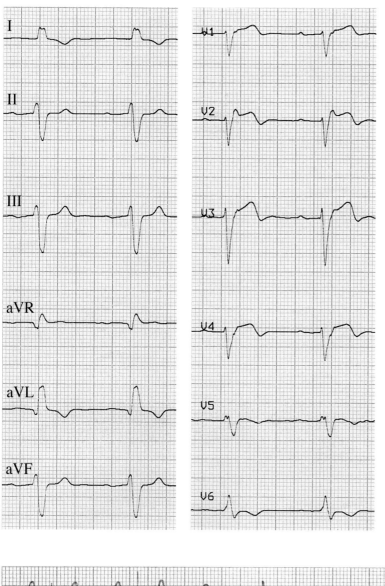

ECG 28.14b
Same patient. ECG (before pacemaker implantation): sinus rhythm, 57/min. AV block 1°, left anterior fascicular block. No pathologic Q waves, but unusual rSr' configuration in V$_2$ (and V$_3$) and reduction of the notched QRS complexes in V$_4$ to V$_6$ ('special infarction patterns' see Chapter 13 Myocardial Infarction).

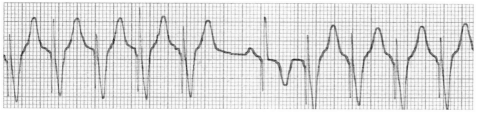

ECG 28.15
44 y/f. AV block 3° (congenital?), presyncope. DDD pacemaker (1972) at the age of 42 years. Palpitations during 1 week. ECG: 'endless loop' tachycardia at a rate of 125/min, interrupted by one sinus beat. The tachycardia could be abolished by increasing the atrial refractory period.

Chapter 29

Congenital and Acquired (Valvular) Heart Diseases

At a Glance

Until the introduction of heart catheterization in the 1950s, congenital heart disease was diagnosed by the interpretation of symptoms, heart auscultation, thoracic X-rays, and the ECG. In 1967 Burch and DePasquale [1] published a book of 773 pages entitled *Electrocardiography in the Diagnosis of Congenital Heart Diseases*; one detail of note in this book is that four forms of single ventricle were diagnosed (or suspected) on the basis of ECG features. However, modern diagnosis of congenital and acquired heart anomalies is made by heart catheterization and angiography, and even more often by echocardiogram and color Doppler.

Nevertheless, the first suspicion of a congenital heart anomaly is presently based on the patient's symptoms and on several clinical findings. Let us not forget heart auscultation. The ECG may be quite typical in some congenital heart diseases, perhaps allowing one to presume the disease, sometimes (in the case of Eisenmenger syndrome) allowing one to recognize important hemodynamic aspects.

ECG

1 Congenital Heart Diseases

Today we very occasionally meet *adult* patients who have had *no* surgical correction of their disease. The majority of *operated* patients reveal a pattern of complete right bundle-branch block (RBBB), due to incision of the right ventricle (that produces a similar pattern of RBBB to that due to proximal block of the right bundle branch).

1.1 Atrial Septal Defect of the Ostium Secundum Type

Atrial septal defect (ASD) of the ostium secundum type (II) is the most frequent congenital heart disease (14%–21%) of all

the significant ones. The ECG is quite uniform in about 90% of patients (ECG 29.1) with significant left-to-right shunt (> 50%), showing:

i.   frontal QRS axis ($\text{Å}QRS_F$) of about + 60°
ii. incomplete RBBB (iRBBB), generally with an r'>r
iii. slight clockwise rotation (especially in patients with a markedly dilated right ventricle)
iv. T wave negativity in V_2 (eventually up to V_3/V_4)
v.   in some cases there is a left axis of the frontal p wave, with a negative terminal part in III; generally the pulmonary artery pressure is normal.

The regression of ECG signs of right ventricular hypertrophy/dilatation after operation may last for years or may be incomplete. ASD II with small left-to-right shunt (and of course a patent foramen ovale) does not result in ECG abnormalities.

1.1.1 Differential Diagnosis

Abnormal drainage of the lung veins (into the right atrium or the cava veins) with a great left-to-right shunt shows a similar ECG pattern, more often without iRBBB.

Chronic pulmonary embolism or chronic cor pulmonale of the vascular type, due to intake of anorectic drugs (especially aminorex fumarate [2]) show an almost identical ECG pattern [3]. The diagnosis is made on the basis of anamnestic and other clinical findings.

In *acute* and *subacute* pulmonary embolism, the ECG may be similar to that of ASD II. The diagnosis is made on the basis of history, symptoms, clinical findings, echo, Doppler, and, if available, helical CT (Chapter 8 Pulmonary Embolism).

1.2 Atrial Septal Defect of the Ostium Primum Type

In atrial septal defect of the ostium primum type (ASD I) the ECG is characterized by left-axis deviation, due to absence or interruption of the left anterior fascicle (ECG 29.2). An iRBBB may or may not be present.

Major types of endocardial cushion defects (ASD I and ventricular septal defect (VSD) and complete atrioventricular (AV) channel) show similar ECGs, occasionally with RBBB, without operation.

1.3 Valvular Pulmonary Stenosis

In valvular pulmonary stenosis there is, in general, right-axis deviation. In about 60% of ECGs there is a tall R wave in V_1 (ECG 29.3); in about 40% rSr' configuration in V_1 (iRBBB), similar to ASD II. Signs of right atrial enlargement may be present.

1.4 Tetralogy of Fallot

Without surgical correction the ECG is similar to that of valvular pulmonary stenosis (ECG 29.4). *With* surgical correction the ECG has an RBBB pattern that is obligatory (ECG 29.5).

1.5 Ventricular Septal Defect

A small VSD generally does not alter the ECG. Left-axis deviation may be present. A great left-to-right shunt leads to biventricular overload and may show (in children) the 'Katz Wachtel sign' (Chapter 31 Special ECG Waves, Signs and Phenomena). Signs of left atrial enlargement may be present.

2 Acquired Valvular Diseases

There are no reliable ECG signs for differentiating between different acquired valvular diseases. However, a special constellation of p and QRS alterations may provide a hint for the diagnosis, e.g. atrial enlargement or atrial fibrillation combined with a vertical QRS axis suggests mitral stenosis. For more details see section 4.3 in ECG Special.

The Full Picture

ECG Special

This section briefly discusses some of the rarer congenital heart diseases, the Eisenmenger syndrome, and acquired valvular diseases.

3 Congenital Heart Diseases [1,4–6]

3.1 Ductus Arteriosus Botalli

In babies with great left-to-right shunt the rare pattern of left ventricular diastolic overload (Chapter 5 Left Ventricular Hypertrophy) may be observed.

3.2 Eisenmenger Syndrome

Eisenmenger syndrome may occur in patients with excessive left-to-right shunts that lead to alterations of the small pulmonary artery vessels with consecutive severe (fixed) pulmonary hypertension. The additional right-to-left shunt is a consequence of pulmonary hypertension. The ECG is characterized by (often extreme) right-axis deviation and a tall R wave in $V_1(V_2)$, with or without alterations of ST/T in the precordial leads (ECG 29.6).

3.3 Transposition of the Great Arteries

The frontal QRS axis depends on the mode of transposition. For all forms a huge R wave in lead V_1 is common (ECG 29.7). The ECG may be similar to that seen in Eisenmenger syndrome. For the ECG of congenitally corrected transposition of the great arteries, see ECG 14.17 in Chapter 14 Differential Diagnosis of Pathologic Q Waves.

3.4 Situs Inversus

Situs inversus without additional abnormalities leads to a very typical ECG. There is inversion of p and QRS in the limb leads and a decrease of the R voltage in V_4 to V_6 (ECG 29.8). See also Chapter 32 Rare ECGs.

3.5 Ebstein's Anomaly

The so-called typical Ebstein ECG consists of:

i.   extreme 'p pulmonale', with tall p waves in III and aVF and tall/peaky p waves in V_1/V_2
ii. right-axis deviation
iii. 'M' configuration of QRS in leads III and aVF. In 25 years we have seen this pattern only twice in about 30 cases of Ebstein's anomaly. The ECG alterations are often much more modest, or are absent or atypical (ECG 29.9). Even left-axis deviation may be present.

3.6 Complex Congenital Cardiac Diseases

ECG alterations in complex diseases often show QRS prolongation and signs of right ventricular hypertrophy. However, many other patterns occur, depending on the anomaly.

3.7 Mitral Valve Prolapse (Barlow's Disease)

Generally this disease is not connected with a typical ECG. In about 5%–10% negative asymmetric T waves in leads III/aVF and V_6 are present – a pattern rarely seen in other conditions. In inferolateral ischemia the T waves are mostly negative and symmetric.

3.8 Hypertrophic Obstructive Cardiomyopathy (HOCM)

Occasionally, the diagnosis is suspected by prominent Q waves in leads I, aVL, and V_4 to V_6 that may be combined with signs of left ventricular hypertrophy (LVH) (ECGs 5.11a–b, 5.12 and 5.13 in Chapter 5 Left Ventricular Hypertrophy). Other possible ECG patterns in hypertrophic obstructive cardiomyopathy are:

i.   signs of left ventricular hypertrophy without prominent Q waves
ii. LBBB pattern
iii. normal ECG (!)

4 Acquired Valvular Heart Diseases

On one hand, the ECG alterations generally depend on the severity of the anomaly. On the other hand, the ECG may completely fail to show typical alterations, as happens for instance in left ventricular hypertrophy.

4.1 Valvular Aortic Stenosis

About 60% of valvular aortic stenosis patients show classic signs of left ventricular hypertrophy, generally with a slightly prolonged QRS and discordant negative asymmetric T waves in leads I, aVL, and V_5/V_6 (systolic overload) (ECG 29.10). An $\mathring{A}QRS_F$ of between + 30° and + 60° is not uncommon (though not present in ECG 29.10), probably because of concentric left ventricular hypertrophy. Especially in young adults, the ECG can be normal – even in severe aortic stenosis.

4.2 Valvular Aortic Incompetence

The pattern of 'left ventricular diastolic overload' is seen very rarely:

1. tall R waves with deep Q waves in V_4 to V_6, without QRS prolongation
2. slight ST elevation and tall symmetric T waves in the same leads.

Generally the ECG pattern cannot be distinguished from that in valvular aortic stenosis: in advanced aortic incompetence we mostly find T inversion in the lateral leads (ECG 29.11). The $\mathring{A}QRS_F$ is generally more to the left than in valvular aortic stenosis, between + 30° and – 10°.

4.3 Mitral Stenosis

A pattern of extensive left atrial enlargement (p mitrale, with a peak-to-peak interval of > 40 msec) is found in > 60% of ECGs

(ECG 29.12). In advanced diseases atrial fibrillation is common. Right ventricular hypertrophy is often detectable by a vertical $\mathring{A}QRS_F$ and an incomplete RBBB (ECG 29.13) or a relatively high R wave in V_1.

4.4 Mitral Incompetence

There are no typical ECG signs of mitral incompetence. In longstanding mitral incompetence only, left atrial enlargement (of a lesser degree than that in mitral stenosis) and obvious left ventricular hypertrophy are found in only about 30% of cases. Surprisingly, we may find a QRS counter-clockwise rotation instead of an expected clockwise rotation in left ventricular dilatation.

For details about congenital heart disease see the book of Perlof (7).

References

1. Burch GE, DePasquale NP. Electrocardiography in the diagnosis of congenital heart disease. Philadelphia: Lea & Febiger, 1967
2. Gurtner HP, Gertsch M, Salzmann C, et al. Häufen sich die primär vaskulären Formen des chronischen Cor pulmonale? Schweiz med Wschr 1968;98:1579–94
3. Gertsch M, Kaufmann M, Althaus U. Zur Circumclusion des Ostium-secundum-Defektes. Schweiz med Wschr 1973;103:281
4. Gersony WM, Rosenbaum M. Congenital heart disease in the adult. New York: McGraw-Hill, 2002
5. Brickner ME, Hillis LD, Lange RA. Congenital heart disease in adults (first of two parts). N Engl J Med 2000;342:256–63
6. Brickner ME, Hillis LD, Lange RA. Congenital heart disease in adults (second of two parts). N Engl J Med 2000;342:334–42
7. Perlof JK. Clinical Recognition of Congenital Heart Disease. Philadelphia. Saunders, 5th edition 2003

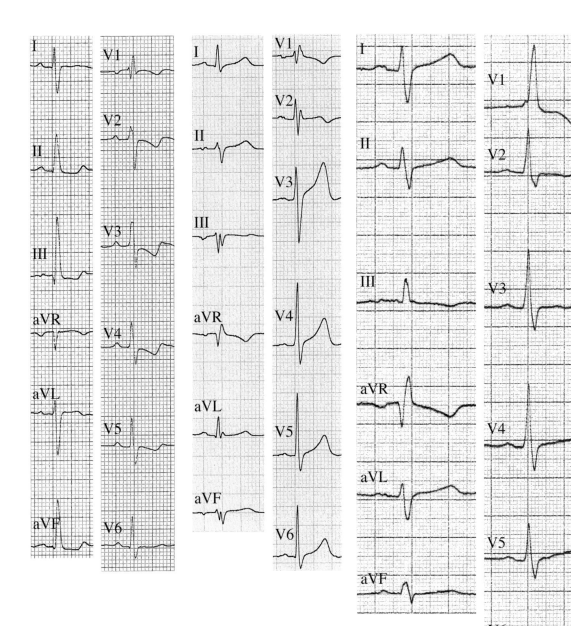

ECG 29.1

49 y/f. Atrial septal defect of the ostium secundum type (ASD II), left-to-right shunt > 60%. PA pressure normal. ECG: ÅQRS$_F$ + 105°. iRBBB with r' > r, T negative up to lead V$_5$.

ECG 29.2

25 y/m. Atrial septal defect of the ostium primum type (ASD I). Left to right shunt 60%. PA pressure minimally increased. ECG: sinus rhythm, left atrial overload (lead V$_1$: negative portion of the p wave greater than positive portion). ÅQRS$_F$ – 60°. iRBBB with r' > r (lead V$_1$). T negativity in V$_1$/V$_2$.

ECG 29.3

19 y/m. Severe pulmonary valve stenosis (gradient 90 mmHg). ECG (paper speed 50 mm/sec): ÅQRS$_F$ + 120°. Tall single R wave (15 mm), ST depression and negative T wave in V$_1$. R > S in V$_2$ to V$_4$. Note: about 40% of ECGs in pulmonary stenosis show the pattern of iRBBB and this is difficult to distinguish from that of ASD II. In ASD II a single R wave in V$_1$ is extremely rare.

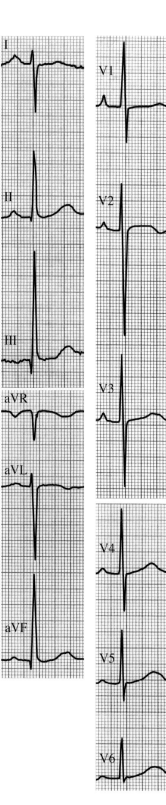

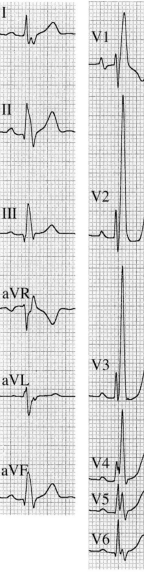

ECG 29.4
2 y/m. Fallot's tetralogy, not operated. ECG (50 mm/sec): QRS right-axis deviation. R > S in lead V$_1$, indicating RV hypertrophy.

ECG 29.5
26 y/m. Fallot's tetralogy operated 10 years previously. ECG: ÅQRS$_F$ (of the first 60 msec) + 75°. Direct pattern of RBBB in V$_1$ to V$_5$ (V$_6$), with giant amplitude of R' in V$_2$/V$_3$, corresponding to persisting severe RV hypertrophy, confirmed by echo.

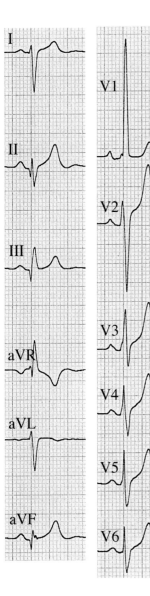

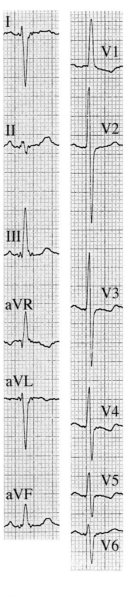

ECG 29.6
27 y/m. Huge ventricular septal defect
with early Eisenmenger reaction at the
age of 2 years. ECG: QRS right-axis deviation. Single R wave (30 mm) in V$_1$.
Positive T wave in all precordial leads.

ECG 29.7
14 y/f. d-transposition of the great arteries. Correction by Mustard operation
12 years previously. ECG: sinus rhythm.
ÅQRS$_F$ +160°. Huge R wave in lead V$_1$
(12 mm). High RS amplitude in V$_2$/V$_3$.
T negativity in V$_1$ to V$_5$.

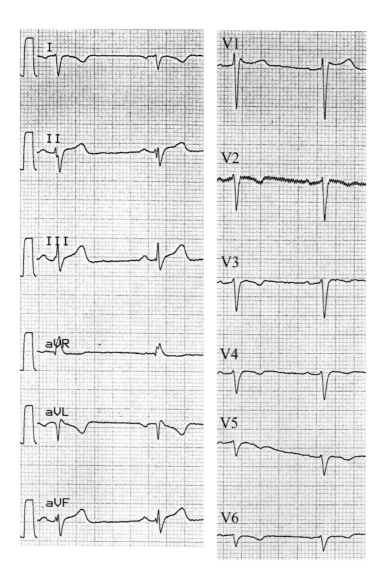

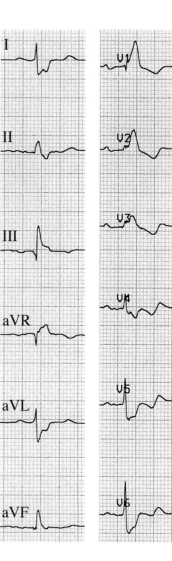

ECG 29.8

40 y/m. Situs inversus in an otherwise healthy man. ECG: typical inversion of p waves and QRS complexes (similar or identical to that in false poling of the upper limb leads). rS complex in all precordial leads, with decreasing r amplitude from V_1 to V_6. ST/T alterations.

ECG 29.9

60 y/m. Ebstein's anomaly of medium to a severe degree. Right ventricular failure. ECG: sinus rhythm. Left (!) atrial enlargement. AV block 1°. ÂQRS$_F$ (first 70 msec) + 70°. Complete RBBB. T negativity in V_1 to V_3 (to V_6). Note: the ECG does not suggest Ebstein's anomaly. Left atrial overload, rather than right, is unusual. Also the so-called typical M-configuration in lead III is missed. However, in our experience these ECG signs, that should be typical for the disease, are often missed.

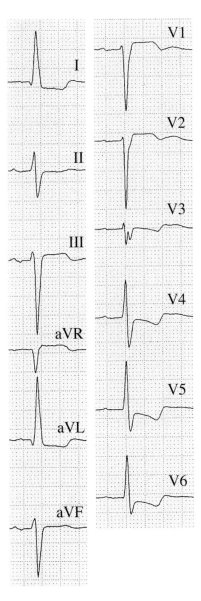

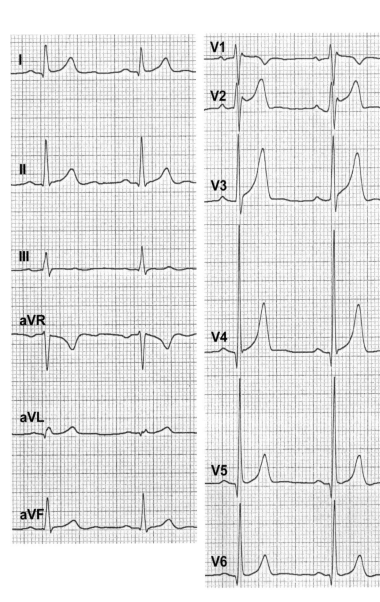

ECG 29.10

71 y/f. Severe valvular aortic stenosis, hypertension. ECG: $\text{ÅQRS}_F - 40°$ (due to LAFB or LV hypertrophy?). LV hypertrophy, Sokolow index negative, Lyon and Gertsch indices positive, R_{avL} 18 mm. Descending ST segment and preterminal asymmetric negative T waves in leads I, aVL, and (V_3) V_4 to V_6. Echo/Doppler: gradient 72 mmHg, LV mass 140 g/m².

ECG 29.11

64 y/m. Mild aortic valve incompetence. ECG: typical pattern of 'diastolic overload'. Relatively deep Q waves and tall, narrow R waves, slight ST elevation, and positive, high and peaked T waves in V_4 to V_6. The pattern is probably due to low rate sinus rhythm. In *severe* aortic incompetence the pattern of systolic overload is generally seen, like the pattern in valvular aortic *stenosis*. In valvular aortic stenosis a more 'rightward' ÅQRS_F is often observed.

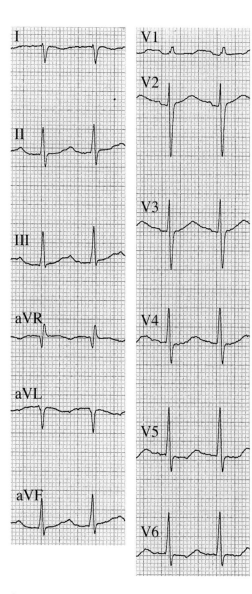

ECG 29.12

44 y/f. Severe mitral stenosis with pulmonary hypertension. ECG: probable p mitrale (T–P fusion). ÂQRS$_F$ about + 110°. Single R wave in V$_1$ (2 mm).

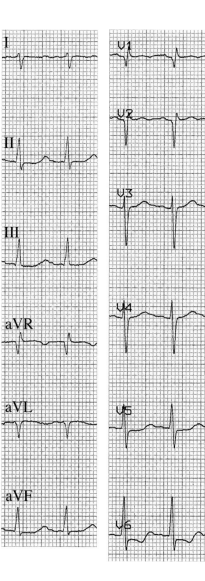

ECG 29.13

43 y/f. Severe mitral stenosis with tricuspid regurgitation. Mitral valve replacement and tricuspid de Vega plastic 2 years before. ECG: sinus rhythm 116/min. P duration > 200 msec. The first peak of the p wave is partially hidden within the T wave. AV block 1°. ÂQRS$_F$ + 115°. Qr in V$_1$ and V$_2$. Alteration of the repolarization. Coro: normal.

Chapter 30

Digitalis Intoxication

At a Glance

Digitalis intoxication in its chronic or subacute form occurs especially in old patients with reduced body weight and in patients with renal failure. Based on new data, intoxication is more frequent in women than in men, possibly due to relative overdose. Conditions that increase sensitivity to digoxin may also be important, such as hypothyroidism, hypokalemia, hypomagnesemia, and acute ischemia. Moreover, drugs such as quinidine, amiodarone and spironolactone increase the serum level of digoxin.

ECG

Digitalis intoxication leads to conduction disturbances and arrhythmias. It affects the sinoatrial (SA) conduction and the supra-His atrioventricular (AV) conduction system. AV block 1° often develops to AV block 2° of the Wenckebach type and may further progress to AV block 2 : 1, or in rare cases to complete AV block, always with a supra-His escape rhythm and small QRS complexes (Chapter 12 Atrioventricular Block and Dissociation). In patients with pre-existing atrial fibrillation, impaired AV conduction provokes bradycardia. Sinus bradycardia may also be present.

Many arrhythmias are due to increased automaticity in the atrium, the AV junction and the ventricles. The most common arrhythmias are frequent premature beats, especially ventricular premature beats (VPBs) in bigeminy. In severe life-threatening cases ventricular tachycardia (VT) is common. The VT is often irregular, monomorphic, or polymorphic without torsade de pointes (ECG 30.1) and rarely of the type 'torsade de pointes'. Ventricular fibrillation may occur, as well as cardiac standstill (ECG 30.2). A rare but quite typical arrhythmia – atrial tachycardia with AV block (generally 2 : 1) – is an example of enhanced automaticity and combined conduction impairment (ECG 30.3). It is worthwhile to note that digitalis intoxication may provoke nearly all cardiac arrhythmias, even tachycardic atrial fibrillation. ST depression is seen in patients with normal or pathologic digoxin levels, whereas a striking shortening of the QT interval is observed only in digitalis intoxication.

1   Extracardiac Symptoms

Most of the extracardiac symptoms are as common as they are unspecific, like fatigue, weakness, nausea, and vomiting. A combination of these symptoms with visual symptoms (such as enhanced perception of yellow and green and seeing haloes of light) may lead to the correct interpretation. In some cases, hallucinations and delirium have been described.

Severe, acute digitalis intoxication is an extremely dangerous condition and it needs complex emergency treatment (see 'The Full Picture').

The Full Picture

Chronic digitalis intoxication is not a rare situation, because the drug is still used frequently, and because the mainly unspe-cific symptoms may lead to misdiagnosis. The incidence of toxicity (of various degrees) in digitalized patients varies between

6% and 23% [1,2]. Most publications deal with digoxin. Results from a recent study suggest that digoxin increases mortality in women with heart failure and depressed left ventricular function, in contrast to men [3]. Eichhorn and Gheorghiade [4] believe this is due to a high digoxin serum level in women, and they propose giving a dose that will result in a serum concentration lower than 1.0 nmol/l – especially in women.

ECG Special

Besides common arrhythmias like VPBs (or supraventricular PBs) in bigeminy, VT and ventricular fibrillation, AV block of various degrees (especially of 2° Wenckebach type), and SA block, many other arrhythmias have been observed in digitalis toxicity. Atrial tachycardia with AV block is suspicious, in contrast to atrial flutter with AV block. However, this strict differentiation may be questioned in the light of recent progress regarding the electrophysiologic mechanisms and their capricious manifestations in the conventional ECG [5]. VT is generally more or less monomorphic. Polymorphic VT of the type torsade de pointes is seen preferentially in combination with a prolonged QT duration due to other drugs such as quinidine and sotalol, or due to hypokalemia (ECG 30.4).

Rare bradycardic arrhythmias include AV dissociation with and without interference and parasystole.

2   Electrophysiology and Pharmacokinetics

It is believed that digoxin increases myocardial contractility by inhibition of the sodium–potassium (Na^+–K^+) adenosine triphosphatase (ATPase) pump, and by increasing myocardial cellular calcium uptake. Digitalis glycosides increase SA and AV nodal refractory times and at the same time shorten the refractory periods of the atrial and ventricular muscle [6]. These changes are mediated by a reduction in duration of the action potential, by increased phase 4 depolarization and reduction in the resting membrane potential.

In the absence of severe malabsorption, digoxin is adequately absorbed from the intestinal tract even in the case of vascular congestion due to heart failure. Digoxin bioavailability is about 80% and protein-binding is about 25%. Digoxin has a half-life of 1.6 days. It is filtered in the glomeruli and excreted by the renal tubules, mostly in unchanged form. Renal excretion surpasses biliary excretion by a factor of 7 when there is normal renal function [7]. Consequently, significant reduction of the glomerular filtration rate reduces the elimination of digoxin, and may lead to toxic levels.

The development of a radioimmunoassay for digoxin in serum has considerably improved the management of therapy and has contributed to a declining incidence of toxicity [8]. However, there is no strong correlation between the serum level and the ECG changes or symptoms. Only very high levels of > 6.0 nmol/l correlate with an increased mortality rate of up to 50% [9].

3   Acute Digitalis Intoxication and its Therapy

Acute digitalis intoxication is much more often related to suicide than accidents. The lethal dose of digoxin is about 15 mg . Serum levels are only reliable after a lapse of 8 h from intake of the drug. In otherwise healthy individuals digitalis toxicity manifests as impaired AV conduction [10,11]. Conversely ventricular ectopic beats are frequent in a diseased heart [11]. In acute overdose the potassium serum level is at the upper limit of 'normal' or it is increased, whereas in chronic toxicity potassium is generally normal (in the absence of renal failure).

The emergency treatment consists of gastric decontamination with ipecacuanha, charcoal, and lavage (with atropine pretreatment). Digoxin-specific Fab antibodies should be administered as early as possible. The superb effectiveness of this treatment has been documented in multicenter studies and in many case reports [12]. Antman et al [13] have shown that 80% of 150 patients had complete remission within a short time and 54% of the 56 patients with cardiac arrest survived. Of 770 digitalis-intoxicated patients in the observational surveillance study of Smith [14] 74% had complete or partial responses to the antibodies. Side-effects of digoxin-specific Fab antibodies are rare and are generally harmless.

Severe hyperkalemia is treated with glucose, insulin and bicarbonate in order to shift potassium into the intracellular space. Lidocaine and phenytoin are used in the presence of ventricular arrhythmias due to enhanced automaticity, whereas pronestyl and quinidine should be avoided because of the depressant effect on SA and AV conduction.

A temporary pacemaker is mandatory for the treatment of bradycardic episodes that may arise inadvertently. Troester et al [15] describe the spectacular case of a 50-year-old woman with digitalis intoxication (1000 mg of oral digoxin) that was successfully treated.

References

1. Smith TW, Harker R. Digitalis. N Engl J Med 1973;289:1125–8
2. Sharff JA, Bayer MJ. Acute and chronic digitalis toxicity. Presentation and treatment. Ann Emerg Med 1982;11:327–31
3. Rathore MPH, Wang Y, Krumholz HM. Sex-based differences in the effect of digoxin for the treatment of heart failure. New Engl J Med 2002;347:1403–11
4. Eichhorn EJ, Gheorghiade M. Digoxin: New perspective on an old drug. New Engl J Med 2002;347:1394–5
5. Saoudi N, Cosio F, Waldo A, et al. A classification of atrial and regular atrial tachycardia according to electrophysiological mechanisms and anatomical bases. Eur Heart J 2001;22:1162–82
6. American Drug Association. American Drug Association Drug Evaluations, fifth edn. AMA 1985, p 602
7. Wilson JD, Braunwald E, Isselbacher KJ, et al (eds). Harrison's principles of internal medicine, twelfth edn. New York: McGraw Hill 1991, pp 98–9
8. Smith TW, Butler BP, Haber E. Determination of therapeutic and toxic serum digoxin concentrations by radioi mmunoassay. N Engl J Med 1969;181:1212–6
9. Ordog GJ, Benaron S, Bhasin V. Serum digoxin levels and mortality in 5100 patients. Ann Emerg Med 1987;16:32–9
10. Fowler RS, Rath L, Keith JD. Accidental digitalis intoxication in children. J Pediatr 1964;64:188–99
11. Smith TW, Willerson JT. Suicidal and accidental digoxin ingestion. Circulation 1971;44:29–36
12. Bayer MJ. Recognition and management of digitalis intoxication: implications for emergency medicine. Am J Emerg Med 1991;9(Suppl 1):29–32
13. Antman EM, Wenger TL, Butler VP Jr, et al. Treatment of 150 cases of life-threatening digitalis intoxication with digoxin-specific Fab antibody fragments: Final report of a multicenter study. Circulation 1990;81:1744–52
14. Smith TW. Review of clinical experience with digoxin immune Fab (ovine). Am J Emerg Med 1991;9(Suppl 1):1–6
15. Troester S, Bodmann KF, Schuster HP. Schwere Digitalis-Intoxikation nach Ingestion von 1g Digoxin. Deutsch Med Wschr 1992;117:1149–52

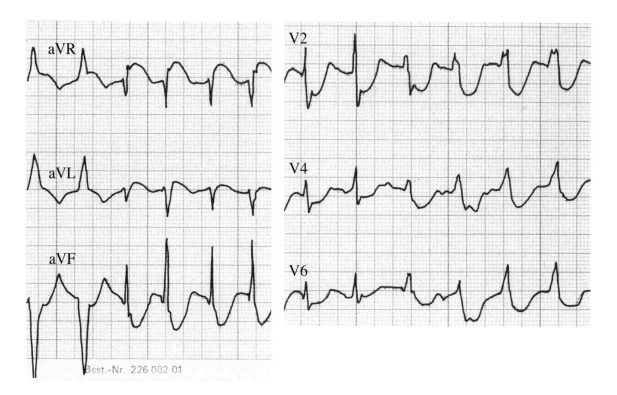

ECG 30.1
50y/f. Four hours after intake of 30 tablets digoxin 0.25 mg in a suicide attempt. Serum level 11 nmol/l. ECG (only Goldberger leads, V$_2$, V$_4$, V$_6$; other leads and rhythm strip lost): possible bidirectional ventricular tachycardia. Striking ST depression in some leads.

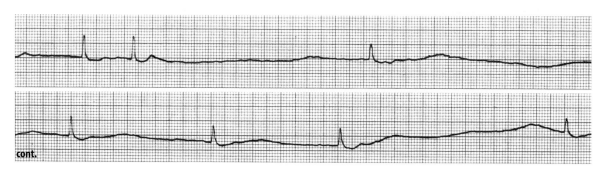

cont.

ECG 30.2
78y/f. Subacute overdose of digoxin. Serum level 9.4 nmol/l. ECG (continuous rhythm strip): no p waves detectable. Irregular AV junctional rhythm with several ventricular pauses up to 3.88 sec.

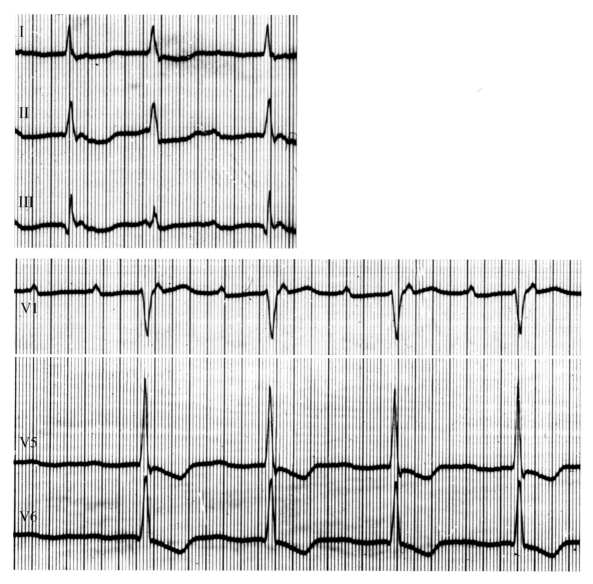

ECG 30.3

54y/m. Severe aortic and mitral valve disease. Subacute overdose of digoxin. Serum level 7.2nmol/l. ECG (paper speed 50 mm/sec): Atrial tachycardia (atrial rate 170/min) with high degree AV block 2°; ventricular rate about 85/min.

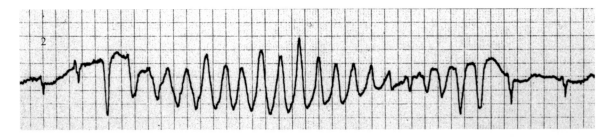

ECG 30.4

54y/f. 2 years after aortic and mitral valve replacement. Digoxin serum level 6.0 nmol/l. Potassium 2.0 mmol/l(!). VT of the type torsade de pointes, maximal instantaneous rate about 260/min. The VT is more likely due to hypokalemia than to digitalis intoxication.

At a Glance and The Full Picture

This chapter was designed to illustrate that there are still some *clinically relevant* ECG signs or phenomena that are often connected with the names of their 'inventors', while others are only of historical interest (or are ridiculous). It is likely that readers of both sections will be interested in this subject. The 'special waves' are listed in alphabetical order.

1   Ashman Phenomenon

The so-called *Ashman phenomenon* was first described by Lewis [1] in 1910 (!) and in 1943 by Gouaux and Ashman [2] and may occur intermittently in atrial fibrillation and other atrial supraventricular arrhythmias. After a relatively long R–R interval, the following beat (after a short interval) is conducted with *aberration*, more frequently with a right bundle-branch block (RBBB) pattern than with a left bundle-branch block (LBBB) pattern (ECG 31.1). If this constellation is observed several times and the BBB pattern shows the characteristics of aberration, ventricular premature beats can be excluded and this pseudoextrasystole should not be treated. But is this true? In a review by Chaudry et al [3] which relies on publications with His bundle derivations, the reliability of the Ashman phenomenon is more than doubted. The last sentence of the paper states 'The Ashman phenomenon should be taught as a reasonable historical attempt that ultimately failed'. Incidentally, Akiyama et al [4] described an isolated Ashman phenomenon of the T wave also.

2   Brugada Sign or Syndrome

An ECG pattern with ST elevations in the right precordial leads not related to myocardial ischemia was already described by Osher and Wolff [5] in 1953. In 1954 Edeiken qualified the pattern as 'probable normal variant' in the right precordial leads,

disappearing with leads attached 1 to 2 cm lower [6]. Only in 1992 was this ECG alteration identified as a distinct clinical entity associated with a high risk of sudden cardiac death by Brugada and Brugada [7]. Together with the congenital 'long QT syndrome' and the 'arrhythmogenic right ventricular cardiomyopathy', the Brugada syndrome represents the most important genetically determined arrhythmogenic substrate so far, and is linked to the SCN5A gene encoding the cardiac sodium channel. The ECG is characterized by *ST elevations* in leads V_1 to V_2 (V_3), also described as 'prominent J waves' (ECGs 31.2a–b, and 31.3a–b). An atypical pattern of incomplete RBBB (without right ventricular conduction delay) and AV block 1° with HV interval $\geq$ 55 msec are common. The QT interval may be prolonged.

Patients with the Brugada syndrome are at a high risk for ventricular arrhythmias, especially ventricular fibrillation. Generally no structural heart disease is detectable, but association with right ventricular myopathies has been described. Brugada et al published results from 334 members of 25 Flemish families with the syndrome; there were 42 sudden cardiac deaths, 24 of which were related to the syndrome, and all in symptomatic families [8]. The typical ECG may be unmasked by antiarrhythmic drugs (flecainide, ajmaline, procainamide, propafenone) and be masked by beta-blockers and other drugs. Patients with Brugada syndrome have been detected all over the world and it seems that this syndrome, together with the 'long QT syndrome', is one of the most frequent causes for sudden cardiac death in young otherwise healthy individuals. However, in a series of 39 consecutive patients (mean age 41 ± 15 years; 24 men) with idiopathic ventricular fibrillation, Viskin et al [9] found the Brugada sign in only eight patients (21%). Three patients had incomplete RBBB without ST elevation, and 28 had a normal ECG. In 592 healthy controls a 'definitive' Brugada sign was not seen in any case and a 'probable/questionable' sign in five individuals (1%). Unmasking of the Brugada sign was tried with class IA antiarrhythmic drugs (intravenously) in six patients and in 26 patients orally, but flecainide was not used and genetic determination was not performed.

Differentiation between 'definitive' Brugada sign and the 'questionable/borderline' Brugada sign is not always easy. ECGs 31.4, 31.5, 31.6 and 31.7 show examples of 'pseudo' Brugada signs. However, it is convenient to ask such patients about symptoms and about a family history of sudden death. Moreover, the typical ECG pattern may be mimicked by overdose of antidepressants such as clomipramine, and by poisoning with neuroleptic agents that block sodium channels [10–12].

It is also important to know that the Brugada sign may occur only intermittently (with a normal ECG in the intervals).

Sangwatanaroy et al [13] propose placing the leads V_1 to V_3 one and two intercostal spaces higher (the leads are then called $-V_1$ to $-V_3$, and $-2V_1$ to $-2V_3$, respectively) in order to unmask the syndrome in unclear cases. This new ECG method has been successful in several cases, and was warmly accepted by the 'Brugada family' [14].

Short Story/Case Report 1

In November 1999 a 62-year-old man with a history of diabetes and hypertension was admitted to hospital because of fever and short episodes of loss of consciousness. The ECG showed a typical Brugada pattern (ECG 31.3a) that was less typical 1 day later (ECG 31.3b). Creatine phosphokinase (CPK) and troponin were normal. Echo showed moderate left ventricular hypertrophy (LVH) and normal LV function. Holter ECG revealed some ventricular premature beats (VPBs), two episodes of supraventricular tachycardia (SVT) (up to 8 beats) with a maximal rate of 170/min. Electrophysiologic testing showed easy induction of ventricular fibrillation. There was an increase of ST elevation in V_2 from 2 mm to 5 mm after ajmaline. The fever was due to an urinary tract infection.

A diagnosis of Brugada syndrome was made. The short episodes of syncope were thought to be from VT or SVT (together with fever). Taking into account the age of this patient and the negative family history, implantation of an implantable cardioverter defibrillator (ICD) device was proposed, but not performed. Two years later the patient was well, without symptoms.

Diagnostic criteria for the Brugada syndrome were proposed in a 'Consensus Report' that presented three ECG patterns with different grades of junction-point elevation and ST segment elevation, as well as T wave morphology [15].

3   Cabrera Sign

In 1953 the Mexican cardiologist Cabrera [16] described a notch of the S upstroke in precordial leads (generally V_2 to V_4) that is quite specific (differential diagnosis: severe hypertrophic cardiomyopathy) but poorly sensitive for old (anterior) myocardial infarction, in the presence of LBBB (ECGs 31.8 and 31.9) [16].

4   Chatterjee Phenomenon

In 1979 Chatterjee et al [17,18] observed an interesting phenomenon. Thirty-one patients with a ventricular pacemaker showed striking inversion of the T wave in their ECGs after weaning from the pacemaker. The spontaneous rhythm was a ventricular or supraventricular escape rhythm. The T negativity was predominantly present in the chest wall leads but also in the inferior leads in some cases. The longer the time in which the patient had not been paced, the longer the T negativity persisted (up to years). The amplitude of the negative T wave was related to the voltage of the pacemaker. This type of 'electrical memory' is clinically important because these T alterations are much more frequently associated with post-pacing than with coronary ischemia (ECGs 31.10a–b). The phenomenon is also seen after reversion of spontaneous LBBB (ECG 31.11). Alessandrini et al [19] (and others) have shown that 'cardiac memory' is not only restricted to electric alterations, but also involves diastolic LV function for a certain time.

5   Delta Wave

Delta waves are the main signs for diagnosis of ventricular preexcitation in the Wolff-Parkinson-White syndrome and are combined with a shortened PQ interval (0.08–0.12 sec) in 99% of cases (ECG 31.12). The shortened PQ interval combined with a 'slurring' of the initial QRS was first described by Wilson in 1915 [20], the syndrome (in combination with tachycardias) was described by Wolff, Parkinson and White in 1930 [21], and the term 'delta wave' was introduced by Segers et al in 1944 [22], inspired by the Greek letter d (Δ), similar to the small initial deformation of the QRS complex (see Chapter 24 Wolff-Parkinson-White Syndrome).

6   Dressler Beat

In 1952 Dressler and Roesler published an observation of inter-mittent atrial captures during ventricular tachycardia present-ing as narrow QRS complexes [23]. Fusion beats are more often encountered than full capture with normal QRS configuration [24] (ECG 31.13).

7   Early Repolarization

This alteration of the repolarization is a rare normal variant (ECG 31.14). The mechanism is not clear. The ECG pattern may be misdiagnosed as acute MI (for details see chapter 3 The Normal ECG and its (Normal) Variants).

8   Epsilon Wave

The epsilon wave, a small delayed potential in lead V_1 in the region of the ST segment (ECGs 31.15a–b) was first described by Fontaine et al [25]. It represents delayed acti-vation of right ventricular portions by slow fractionated conduction in patients with right ventricular cardiomyopa-thy, often combined with ventricular arrhythmias. For this reason, the disease is also called 'arrhythmogenic RV dys-plasia' [26–29]. T negativity in V_2/V_3 is often observed and a QRS duration longer in V_1 than in V_6 may occasionally be seen [26].

9   McGee Index

The McGee index describes the duration of the p wave in rela-tion to the PQ interval (which must be normal). A p duration of > 60% of the PQ interval is an indicator for left atrial hyper-trophy. This index is no longer used. Today LA enlargement is diagnosed by p duration of ≥ 0.12 sec.

10   McGinn White Pattern (S$_I$/Q$_{III}$ Type)

A S_I/Q_{III} type (or a $S_I/Q_{III}/T_{III}$ type with a negative T wave in lead III), first described by McGinn and White [30], has dif-ferent levels of significance. In its acute form it is seen in many cases of major pulmonary embolism. In some cases, an S_I/rSr'_{III} type is observed. A slow evolution of the pattern may be a sign for right ventricular hypertrophy. Often a S_I/Q_{III} type is seen in normal hearts, especially in young peo-ple.

11   Katz-Wachtel Sign

In 1937 Katz and Wachtel [31] described in children with con-genital heart disease a diphasic QRS type, a huge RS complex in leads III and II or I, with the minor deflection ≥ 20% of the major one. Later, a 'Katz Wachtel variant index' (R + S > 40 mm in lead V_2 or V_3) was thought to be typical for biventricular hypertrophy, especially in children with ventricular septal defect. These rather vague signs are no more used.

12   Nadir Sign

In a premature beat or 'wide QRS complex' tachycardia with an LBBB-like pattern, a duration of ≥ 60 msec (or better ≥ 70 msec?) from QRS onset to the 'nadir' of the S wave in lead V_1 (ECG 31.16) strongly favors a ventricular origin of the arrhythmia (Chapter 26 Ventricular Tachycardia).

13   Osborn Wave

The Osborn wave (also called the 'J' wave, the 'J wave deflec-tion', 'the camel's hump' or the 'Dromedary wave'), is a positive short deflection in the region of the J point, with an amplitude of 0.5–2 mm, and is regularly seen in patients with hypother-mia [32] (ECG 31.17). The alteration is often present in most of the 12 standard leads but may also be restricted to the antero-lateral leads. In a prospective study, Vasallo et al [33] detected the Osborn wave in all 43 studied hypothermic patients. The amplitude of the wave was related to the grade of hypothermia. Occasionally an Osborn wave-like alteration was found in nor-mothermic patients also, e.g. in coronary heart disease (CHD) and pericarditis [34,35], after head injury [36] and after electric defibrillation. Kalla et al [37] described a 29-year-old man without structural heart disease, with recurrent ventricular fibrillation and 'J waves' in the inferior leads, combined with ST elevation. The authors presumed a possible variant of the Brugada syndrome.

In a more recent experimental study, a voltage gradient between the epicardial and endocardial action potential was detected as an explanation for the Osborn wave [38].

Minimal Osborn waves (< 1 mm) are occasionally seen as nor-mal variants, especially in leads V_5 to V_6 (ECGs 31.18 and 31.19).

14   Pardee Q Wave

In 1941 Pardee [39] described a Q wave with an amplitude 25% greater than the R wave in lead III as typical for old inferior MI.

Later a Q wave of > 0.04 sec duration in lead III was called 'Pardee Q'. Such a Q wave is found in many other conditions (e.g. in LV hypertrophy, pre-excitation or just as a normal variant), and inferior infarction often does not show a 'classical Q wave' (e.g. in combination with left posterior fascicular block or in 'unusual infarction patterns'; see The Full Picture in Chapter 13 Myocardial Infarction); thus the term 'Pardee Q' should no longer be used.

15   R-on-T Phenomenon

The R-on-T phenomenon is defined as a ventricular premature beat (VPB) following very early the preceding ventricular cycle. As the term indicates, the QRS ('R') falls into the preceding T wave, before 90% (or 85%?) of the preceding QT interval – into the so-called 'vulnerable period' of the repolarization. Forty years ago the R-on-T phenomenon was believed to be a dangerous and reliable precursor of ventricular fibrillation and took the highest ranking (class 5) in Lown's classification of VPBs [40]. In the late 1970s several authors could not find a correlation between the prematurity of VPBs and consecutive ventricular fibrillation in patients with and without acute MI [41–43]. This finding was confirmed more recently by Chiladakis et al [44]. The R-on-T phenomenon has apparently lost much of its previous importance and is not even mentioned in the 1997 edition of Braunwald's book *Heart Disease* [45].

On one hand, it is now generally accepted that the R-on-T phenomenon is not a reliable precursor of ventricular fibrillation, and is seen in many cardiac patients with VPBs and fast ventricular tachycardias, especially in polymorphous VT of the type 'torsade de pointes'. Rodstein et al [46] followed 59 individuals with 'R-on-T' VPBs; none of them died during a follow-up of 18 years. The grade of prematurity of VPBs was not clearly defined.

On the other hand, studies on patients with VF during ambulatory ECG have revealed an R-on-T phenomenon immediately inducing VF in a high percentage. Von Olshausen et al [47] combined the results of eight studies with 110 patients (CHD in 74%). In 43% an R-on-T phenomenon was found as a 'trigger' of VF. The authors pointed out that often the R-on-T phenomenon was *not* followed by VF. It is also known that *late* VPBs (falling in the late phase 4 of the cardiac cycle, e.g. in the region of the following p wave) may trigger ventricular tachycardia and fibrillation [41,47]. Tye et al [48] used the term 'R on P' for these late VPBs.

In our experience, a special form of VPB with the R-on-T phenomenon may be dangerous. If a single VPB occurs *extremely early* – that is, falling into the T wave at its apex or even slightly before – this represents a high-grade nonhomogeneity of repolarization. We have never observed this kind of VPB in healthy hearts, but have encountered it in several patients with acute or chronic CHD, and in isolated cases with hypertrophic left cardiomyopathy and arrhythmogenic right ventricular dysplasia. In these very rare patients, ventricular fibrillation occurred within minutes or days.

Short Story/Case Report 2

In April 2000 a 78-year-old patient had an acute anteroseptal infarction. Because of persisting angina despite adequate therapy he was transferred from a regional hospital to the university clinic 10 days later. Coronary angiography revealed severe three-vessel disease with proximal stenosis; the LV ejection fraction was moderately decreased (50%). Triple aortocoronary bypass operation was performed 1 day later. The postoperative course was uneventful, the monitored ECG showed only some banal VPBs. The patient was transferred to the general department. A 12-lead ECG on day 5 after the operation showed numerous monomorphic VPBs with an extremely short coupling interval, an excessive R-on-T phenomenon (ECG 31.20a). The patient was ECG monitored and oral amiodarone was given. During the following night, shortly after some fast ventricular runs (ECG 31.20b) he developed two episodes of ventricular fibrillation and had to be reanimated electromechanically. Amiodarone was given intravenously and orally. The re-coro revealed open bypasses but a new stenosis (plaque rupture?) of the CX artery, distally to the graft. Percutaneous transluminal coronary angioplasty (PTCA) was performed. Thereafter, relevant arrhythmias and R-on-T phenomena on the ECG monitor and in the Holter ECG disappeared. Five days later the patient was allowed home, with amiodarone 200 mg/day. Two years later he remained well (amiodarone 100 mg/day).

A 'visual' extreme R-on-T phenomenon is also seen in atrial fibrillation at a high instantaneous rate (more than 220/min). In these cases we have never observed ventricular fibrillation, except in the WPW syndrome.

If a VPB falls into the T wave later than 90% of the preceding QT interval, the term 'R-on-T' is fulfilled. However, in this case the VPB falls into the 'supernormal period' and *not* into the 'potential vulnerable period' of repolarization. Those 'R-on-T phenomena are always harmless and may also be seen in healthy individuals.

16 Shallow s Sign

This sign is better called 'shallow s in lead V_1/deep S in lead V_2'. It is occasionally seen in biventricular hypertrophy. The deep S wave in V_2 is a hint for left ventricular hypertrophy, whereas the s wave in V_1 is reduced by opposite vectors of the hypertrophied right ventricle. The sign is interesting for very enthusiastic ECG readers but is not reliable as also other criteria for biventricular hypertrophy are not convincing (Chapter 7 Biventricular Hypertrophy).

17 Stork Leg Sign

This sign is characterized by a small positive deflection at the J point and probably represents a variant of the Osborn wave, commonly seen in hypothermic patients (see section 13 above). In the context of acute pericarditis, it is called 'stork leg' sign in Europe; it is seen in about 25% of cases, together with other more reliable ECG findings (Chapter 15 Acute and Chronic Pericarditis).

Final Comment

Hurst produced an entertaining paper about the naming of normal ECG waves, which also covers some abnormal waves [49].

References

1. Lewis T. Paroxysmal tachycardia, the result of ectopic impulse formation, Heart 1910;1:262–82
2. Gouaux IL, Ashman R. Auricular fibrillation with aberration simulating paroxysmal tachycardia. Am Heart J 1947;34:366
3. Chaudry II, Ramsaran EK, Spodick DH. Observations on the reliability of the Ashman phenomenon. Review. Am Heart J 1994;128:205–9
4. Akiyama T, Richeson JF, Faillace RT, et al. Ashman phenomenon of the T wave. Am J Cardiol 1989;63:886–90
5. Osher HL, Wolff L. Electrocardiographic pattern simulating acute myocardial injury. Am J Med Sci 1953;226:541–5
6. Edeiken J. Elevation of the RS-T segment, apparent or real, in the right precordial leads as a probable normal variant. American Heart J 1954;38:331
7. Brugada P, Brugada J. Right bundle-branch block, persistent ST segment elevation and sudden cardiac death: a distinct clinical and electrocardiographic syndrome. A multicenter report. J Am Coll Cardiol 1992;20:1391–6
8. Brugada P, Brugada R, Brugada J. Sudden death in patients and relatives with the syndrome of right bundle-branch block, ST segment elevation in the precordial leads V(1) to V(3) and sudden death. Europ Heart J 2000;21:321–6
9. Viskin S, Fish R, Eldar M, et al. Prevalence of the Brugada sign in idiopathic ventricular fibrillation and healthy controls. Heart 2000;84:31–6
10. Bolognesi R, Tsialtas D, Vasini P, et al. Abnormal ventricular repolarization mimicking myocardial infarction after hererocyclic antidepressant overdose. Am J Cardiol 1997;79:242–5
11. Goldgrand-Toledano D, Sideris G, Kevorkian J-P. Overdose of cyclic antidepressants and the Brugada syndrome. N Engl J Med 2002;346:1591–2
12. Rouleau F, Asfar P, Boulet S, et al. Transient ST segment elevation in right precordial leads induced by psychotropic drugs: relationship to the Brugada syndrome. J Cardiovasc Electrophysiol 2001;12:61–5
13. Sangwatanaroy S, Prechawat S, Sunsaneewitayakul B, et al. New electrocardiographic leads and the procainamide test in the detection of the Brugada sign in sudden unexplained death syndrome survivors and their relatives. Europ Heart J 2001;22:2290–6
14. Brugada P, Brugada J, Brugada R. Dealing with biological variation in the Brugada syndrome (editorial). Europ Heart J 2001;22:2231–2
15. Wilde AAM, Antzelevitch C, Borggrefe M, et al. Proposed diagnostic criteria for the Brugada syndrome. Consensus report. Europ Heart J 2002;23:1648–54
16. Cabrera E, Friedland C. LA onda de activaciòn ventricular en el bloqueo de rama izquierda con infarto: un nuevo signo electrocardiografico. Arch Inst Cardiol Mex 1953;23:441–60
17. Chatterjee K, Harris AM, Davies JG, Leatham A. T-wave changes after artificial pacing (preliminary communication). Lancet 1979;1(7598):759–60
18. Chatterjee K, Harris AM, Davies JG, Leatham A. Electrocardiographic changes subsequent to artificial ventricular depolarization. Br Heart J 1979;31:770–9
19. Alessandrini RS, McPherson DD, Kadish AH, et al. Cardiac memory: a mechanical and electrical phenomenon. Am J Physiol 1997;272:1952–9
20. Wilson FN. A case in which the vagus influenced the form of the ventricular complex of the electrocardiogram. Arch Intern Med 1915;16:1008–27
21. Wolff L, Parkinson J, White PD. Bundle-branch block with the short P-R interval in healthy young people prone to paroxysmal tachycardia. Am Heart J 1930;5:685–704
22. Segers PM, Lequime J, Denolin H. L'activation ventriculaire précoce de certains coeurs hyperexitables: étude de l'onde δ de l'électrocardiogramme. Cardiologia 1944;8:113–67
23. Dressler W, Roesler H. The occurrence in paroxysmal ventricular tachycardia of ventricular complexes transitional in shape to sino-auricular beats. Am Heart J 1952;44:485–93
24. Young RL, Mower MM, Ramapuram GM, et al. Atrial fibrillation with ventricular tachycardia showing "Dressler" beats. Chest 1973;63:96–7
25. Fontaine G, Guiraudon G, Frank R, et al. Stimulation studies and epicardial mapping in ventricular tachycardia: study of mechanism and selection for surgery. In: Kulbertus HE (ed). Re-Entrant Arrhythmias: Mechanisms and Treatment. Lancaster PA: MTP Publishers 1977, pp 334–50
26. Jaoude SA, Leclercq JF, Coumel P. Progressive ECG changes in arrhythmogenic right ventricular diseases. Evidence for an evolving disease. Eur Heart J 1996;17:1717–21

27. Fontaine G, Gallais J, Fornesd P, et al. Arrhythmogenic right ventricular dysplasia/cardiomyopathy. Anaesthesiology 2001;95:250–4
28. Gemayel C, Pelliccia A, Thompson PD. Arrhythmogenic right ventricular cardiomyopathy. J Am Coll Cardiol 2001;38:1773–81
29. Marcus FI. Update of arrhythmogenic right ventricular dysplasia. Card Electrophysiol Rev 2002;6:54–6
30. McGinn S, White PD. Acute cor pulmonale resulting from pulmonary embolism. Its clinical recognition. J Amer Med Assoc 1935;104:1473–80
31. Katz LN, Wachtel H. The diphasic QRS type of electrocardiogram in congenital heart disease. Am Heart J 1937;13:202–6
32. Osborn JJ. Experimental hypothermia: Respiratory and blood Ph changes in relation to cardiac function. Am J Physiol 1953;175:389–98
33. Vassallo SU, Delaney KA, Hoffman RS, et al. A prospective evaluation of the electrocardiographic manifestations of hypothermia. Acad Emerg Med 1999;6:1121–6
34. Patel A, Getsos JP, Moussa G, Damato AN. The Osborn wave of hypothermia in normothermic patients. Clin Cardiol 1994;17:273–6
35. Martinez Martinez JA. Postoperative pericarditis and Osborn wave. Medicina (B Aires) 1998;58:428
36. Abbott JA. The nonspecific camel-hump sign. J Amer Med Assoc 1976;235:413–4
37. Kalla H, Yan GX, Marinchak R. Ventricular fibrillation in a patient with prominent J (Osborn) waves and ST segment elevation in the inferior electrocardiographic leads: a Brugada syndrome variant? J Cardiovasc Electrophysiol 2000;11:95–8
38. Yan GX, Antzelevitch C. Cellular basis for the electrocardiographic J wave. Circulation 1996;93:372–9
39. Pardee HEB. Clinical Aspects of the Electrocardiogram. London: Lewis 1941
40. Lown B, Wolf M. Approaches to sudden death by coronary heart disease. Circulation 1971;44:130–42
41. El-Sherif N, Myerburg RJ, Scherlag BJ, et al. Electrocardiographic antecedents of primary ventricular fibrillation. Value of the R-on-T phenomenon in myocardial infarction. Br Heart J 1976;38:415–22
42. Engel TR, Meister SG, Frankl WS. The 'R-on-T' phenomenon. An update and critical review. Ann Intern Med 1978;88:221–5
43. Chou TC, Wenzke F. The importance of R-on-T phenomenon. Am Heart J 1978;96:191–4
44. Chiladakis JA, Karapanos G, Davlouros P, et al. Significance of R-on-T phenomenon in early ventricular tachyarrhythmia susceptibility after acute myocardial infarction in the thrombolytic era. Am J Cardiol 2000;85:289–93
45. Braunwald E (ed). Heart Disease. A Textbook of Cardiovascular Medicine, 5th edn. Philadelphia: WB Saunders 1997
46. Rodstein M, Wolloch L, Gubner RS. Mortality study of the significance of extrasystoles in an insured population. Circulation 1971;44:617–25
47. Von Olshausen K, Treese N, Pop T, et al. Plötzlicher Herztod im Langzeit-EKG. Deutsch med Wochenschr 1985;110:1195–201
48. Tye KH, Samant A, Desser KB, Benchimol A. R-on-T or R on P phenomenon? Relation to the genesis of ventricular tachycardia. Am J Cardiol 1979;44:632–7
49. Hurst JW. Naming of the waves in the ECG, with a brief account of their genesis. Circulation 1998;98:1937–42

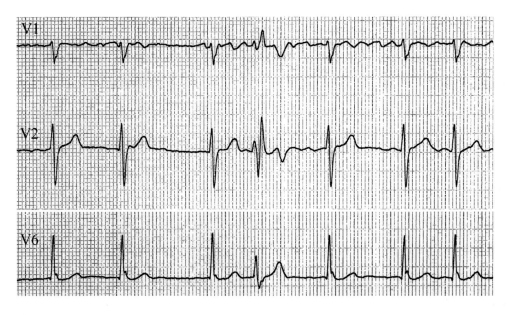

ECG 31.1

Ashman beat. 82 y/m. Chronic atrial fibrillation. ECG (V₁/V₂/V₆): after the longest R–R interval the next beat is conducted with RBBB aberration.

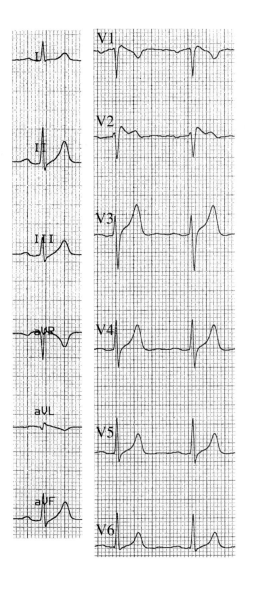

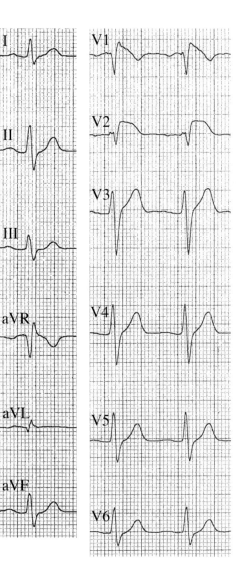

ECG 31.2a
Brugada syndrome. 53 y/m. No symptoms, ECG performed acciden-tally. ST elevation in leads V$_1$ and V$_2$ is compatible with the Brugada sign.

ECG 31.2b
Same patient. After intravenous flecainide the pattern in leads V$_1$ and V$_2$ is more typical for a Brugada sign. Considering the absence of symptoms, the absence of family history for premature sudden death (the patient had no children) and the normal ambulatory and exercise ECGs, no further investigations were performed.

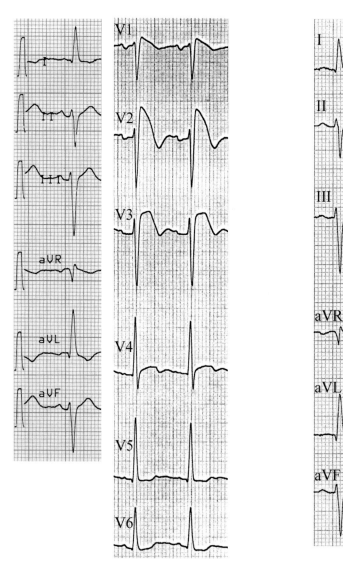

ECG 31.3a

Brugada syndrome. Short story/Case report 1. 62 y/m. QRS left-axis deviation (LAFB), LVH. Typical pattern of incomplete RBBB, ST elevation and negative T waves in leads V$_1$ to V$_3$ (V$_4$).

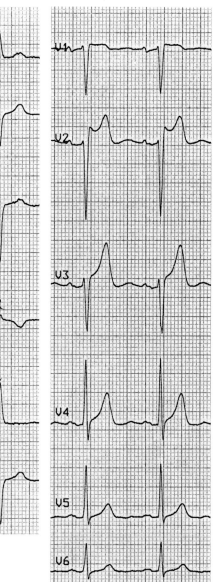

ECG 31.3b

Same patient, 1 day later. Less typical Brugada ECG pattern.

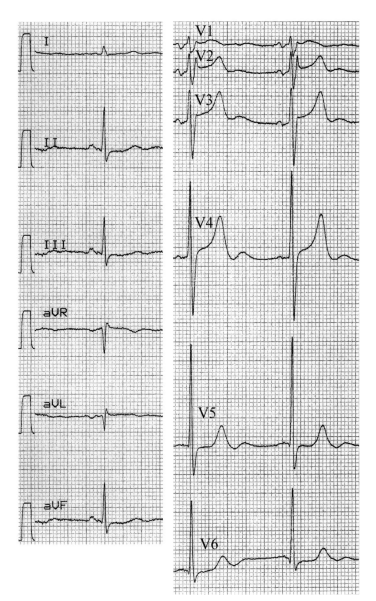

ECG 31.4
Pseudo Brugada ECG sign. 78 y/m. Hypertension, pulmonary emphysema. ECG: incomplete RBBB, ST elevation, and positive T waves in V_2/V_3. High amplitude of QRS in V_4 to V_6, suggestive for LVH. Echo: LV mass 152 g/m^2, normal systolic LV function.

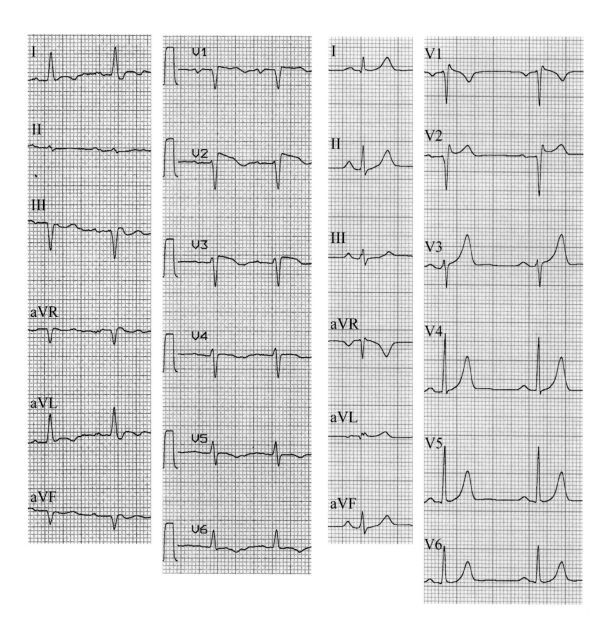

ECG 31.5

Pseudo Brugada ECG sign. 71 y/f. CHD with old inferior and anteroseptal MI and aortocoronary bypass operation. ECG: possibly incomplete RBBB (minimal r′ wave in V$_1$ to V$_3$, small r′ in aVR). ST elevation in V$_1$ to V$_4$, minimal T negativity in V$_2$.

ECG 31.6

Pseudo Brugada. 38 y/f. Normal heart, no family history. ECG: incomplete RBBB, ST elevation in V$_1$/V$_2$(V$_3$), negative T in V$_1$, positive T in V$_2$. The ECG was interpreted as normal variant.

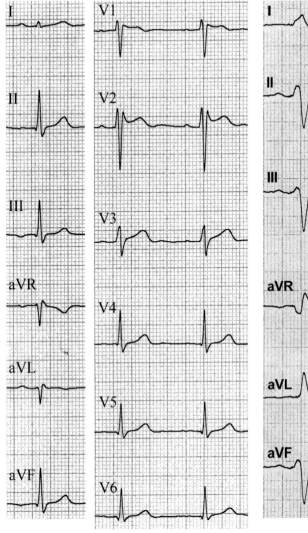

ECG 31.7
Pseudo Brugada ECG sign. 48 y/f. Lumbar disc prolapse. No cardiac symptoms, no family history. ECG: incomplete RBBB, ST elevation in $V_1/V_2(V_3)$, positive T waves.

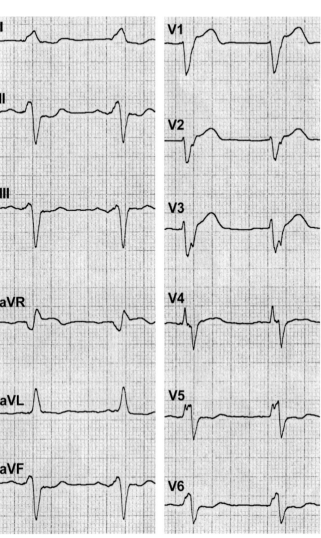

ECG 31.8
Cabrera sign. 75 y/m. 18-year-old extensive anterior MI. ECG: sinus rhythm, LBBB. Atypical increase of the R wave in V_1 to V_4. Pathologic notching in five precordial leads (V_2 to V_6), indicating anterior MI. Inferior MI not diagnosable. Echo: apical dyskinesia, lateral and inferior akinesia; ejection fraction 25%.

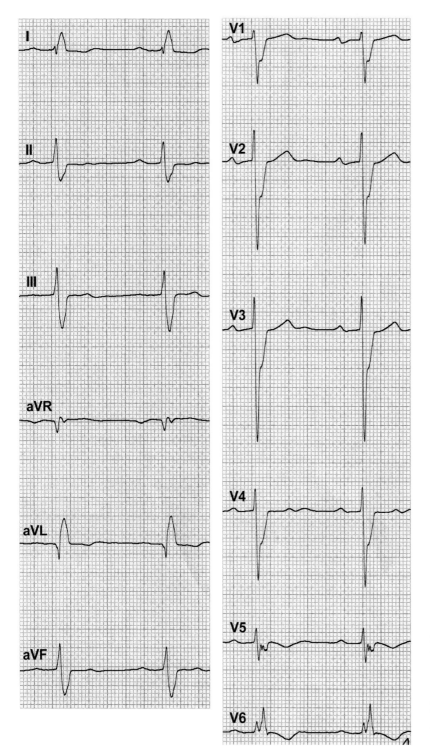

ECG 31.9
Cabrera sign. 67 y/m. Anterior, lateral, inferoposterior MI 20, 5 and 4 years ago. ECG: sinus rhythm, AV block 1°, LBBB. Q in aVL, rsR′ in I, notched QRS in V_5/V_6. Cabrera sign in V_1 to V_4. High R wave in V_2, decreasing in the leads up to V_5. Coro: severe three-vessel disease; LV ejection fraction 25%.

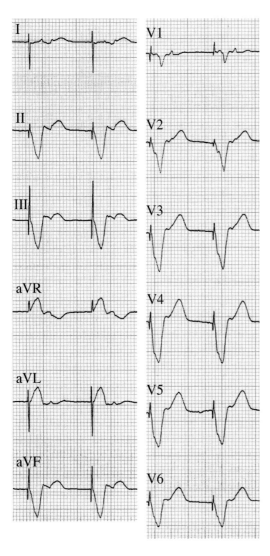

ECG 31.10a
Right ventricular pacing. 63 y/m. Sick sinus syndrome. ECG: LBBB pattern.

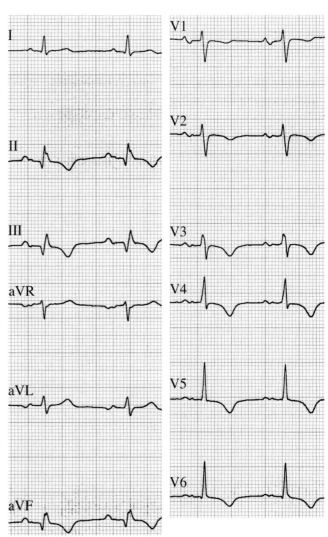

ECG 31.10b
Chatterjee phenomenon after *stopped pacing*. In sinus rhythm the T waves are inverted (negative) in the inferior and precordial leads.

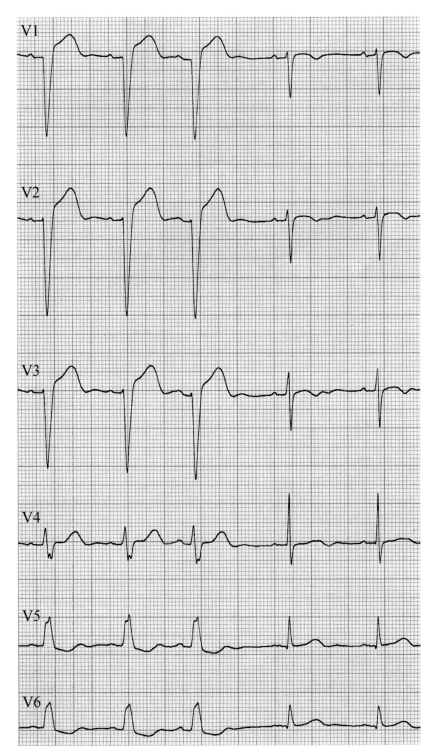

ECG 31.11

Chatterjee phenomenon after *sponta-neous LBBB pattern*. 82 y/f. Hyperten-sion. ECG: the last beat with LBBB aberration is an atrial PB. The follow-ing sinusal beats show slightly nega-tive T waves in V$_1$ to V$_4$.

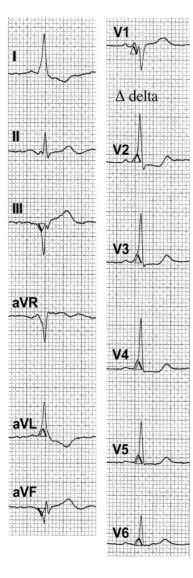

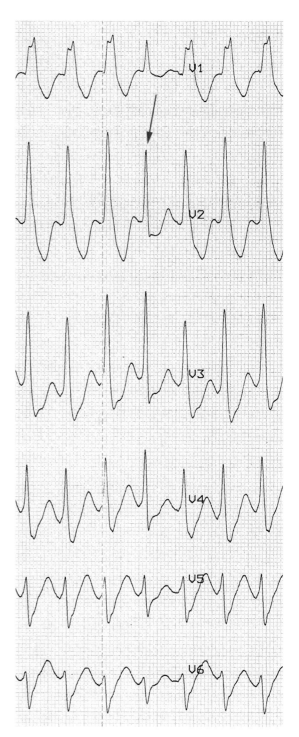

ECG 31.12 ▲
Delta wave. 60 y/f. Typical delta waves in several leads (see △). Note the negative delta waves in leads III and aVF.

ECG 31.13 ▶
Dressler beat. 44 y/m. Dilating cardiomyopathy. ECG (precordial leads): ventricular tachycardia, rate 140/min. RBBB pattern. The fourth QRS is smaller, corresponding to a fusion beat (arrow). Note: this QRS remains positive in leads V_1 and V_2 where it should normally be negative.

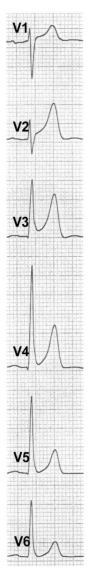

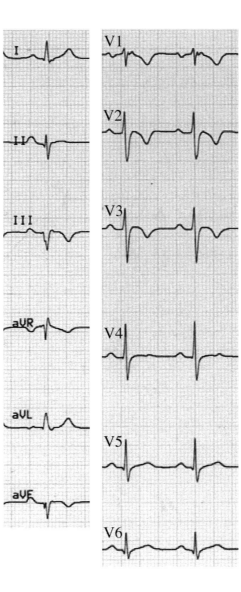

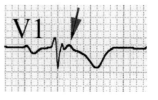

ECG 31.15b
**Same patient, ECG augmented.
Epsilon wave in lead V$_1$ (arrow).**

ECG 31.14
**Early repolarization. 31 y/m.
Normal heart. ECG (precordial
leads): ST elevation in leads V$_1$
to V$_4$ that is concordant with
the QRS in V$_3$ and V$_4$. See also
more spectacular cases in
Chapter 3 The Normal ECG and
its Normal Variants.**

ECG 31.15a
**Epsilon wave. 31 y/m. Histologically proved sarcoidosis
of several organs, also of the RV. Episodes of fast VT and
presyncope. ECG: sinus rhythm, ÅQRS$_F$ - 75°. Negative
(and symmetric) T waves in V$_1$ to V$_3$ and aVF/II. Epsilon
wave in lead V$_1$. The patient received an ICD device.**

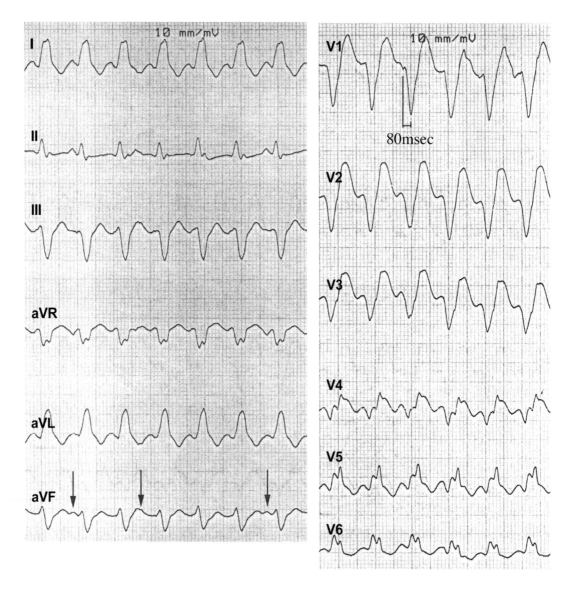

ECG 31.16

Nadir sign. 70 y/m. Old anterior infarction with aneurysm. VT with *LBBB-like QRS*. QRS duration 160 msec. Ventricular rate 143/min. AV dissociation, best recognizable in lead aVF (arrow), atrial rate 85/min. Nadir-sign (duration from beginning of QRS to the nadir of the S wave in lead V₁): 80 msec. Note: the transition zone is similar as in aberration, with quite abrupt change of negative to positive QRS in V₄/V₅, possibly due to old anterior infarction.

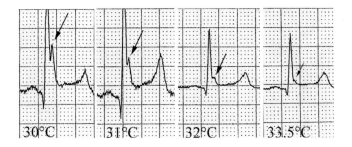

ECG 31.17
Osborn waves. 54 y/m. ECG stripe during open heart surgery: Osborn wave (arrow), decreasing during rising of body temperature.

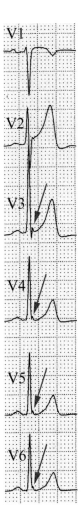

ECG 31.18
Osborn waves. 47 y/m. Erythrodermatitis, normal heart. ECG (precordial leads): Osborn waves in V_3–V_6 (arrows).

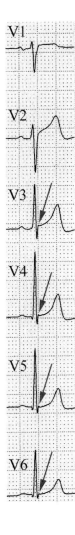

ECG 31.19
'Micro' Osborn wave. 32 y/f, normal heart. Very small Osborn wave in leads V_3–V_6 (arrows).

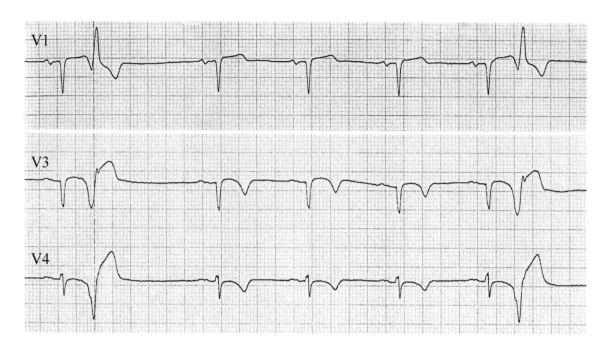

ECG 31.20a ▲
R-on-T phenomenon. 78 y/m. Short
Story/Case Report 2. ECG (leads V_1, V_3 and
V_4): sinus rhythm, 63/min. Single VPBs
falling into, or even slightly before, the apex
of the T wave.

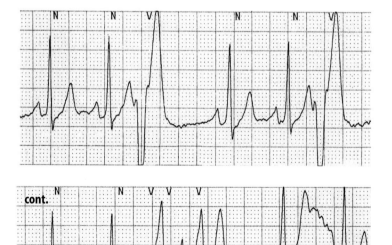

ECG 31.20b ▶
Same patient. Monitor stripe: sinus rhythm,
93/min. VPBs falling distinctly after the T
apex. The third VPB induces a short VT, with
'true R-on-T phenomena' at a maximal
instantaneous rate of about 280/min.
However, during fast VT, this phenomenon is
common, also without being a precursor of
ventricular fibrillation.

Chapter 32
Rare ECGs

At a Glance and The Full Picture

This chapter is not divided into two sections because everyone will be interested in this subject. Another purpose of this chapter is to entertain you – especially 'old ECG cracks' – and the author himself.

ECG and ECG Special

ECG 32.1
Multifocal or Chaotic Atrial Rhythm

Patient 60 y/m. Severe obstructive lung disease. Hypertension. Digoxin 0.125 mg/day, diuretics. ECG (V_1/V_2): instantaneous rate of 50–85/min. P wave morphology is always different, so are the PQ intervals. Consequently absolute irregularity of the ventricular action is present. Longer episodes of the arrhythmia persisted also after discontinuing with digoxin. The patient died 7 months later of pneumonia.

The arrhythmia is very rare if the strict definition is considered:

i. different morphology of p waves, *without* a regular basic rhythm. Generally there are innumerable different p configurations

ii. constantly different R–R intervals (completely irregular ventricular response='absolute ventricular arrhythmia' as in atrial fibrillation!)

iii. varying PQ intervals

iv. beats with AV block 1° may occur as well as AV escape beats and supraventricular premature beats

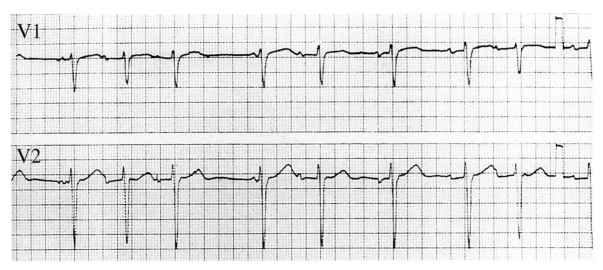

ECG 32.1

v. the rate is generally 80–100/min; tachycardia > 120/min is rare (in those cases the term 'multifocal' atrial tachycardia is used).

The arrhythmia lasts for minutes, hours, or days and has no hemodynamic consequences at a normal rate. However, due to frequent association (in about 50%) with severe chronic obstructive lung disease the prognosis is generally not good. About half of patients die within 6–12 months of the underlying disease. The association with digitalis intake has been described. In our experience degeneration into atrial fibrillation is rare but has occasionally been documented.

Differential diagnosis: sinus rhythm with multiple atrial premature beats (a generally harmless arrhythmia) [1,2].

ECG 32.2
Absent Pericardium

Patient 60 y/m. Severe two-vessel disease (left anterior descending coronary artery (LAD): 90% proximal stenosis; Circumflex (CX): 80% stenosis), normal LV function. ECG: sinus rhythm 58/min. Negative p in leads V_1/V_2, biphasic p in $V_3/V_4(V_5)$. Frontal QRS axis (ÅQRS_F) + 135°. Striking QRS clockwise rotation. Incomplete right bundle-branch block (iRBBB) with minimal first r wave in V_1. Negative T wave in V_2/V_3.

Short Story/Case Report 1

Although the cardiac surgeons were informed about the extensive anatomical clockwise rotation of the patient's heart (detected during coronary angiography), they performed a sternotomy. As only a part of the right atrium was visible, the patient was turned on his right side and two bypass grafts were attached to the LAD and CX through a left *posterior* thoracotomy. This operation lasted more than 5 hours instead of 2 hours. However, the patient was well 5 years later.

Congenital complete absence of pericardium is extremely rare and may be associated with diaphragmatic and other anomalies. Common ECG alterations are:

i. ÅQRS_F > + 60°
ii. QRS clockwise rotation
iii. incomplete RBBB
iv. peaked positive p waves in V_2/V_3 (in contrast to our case).

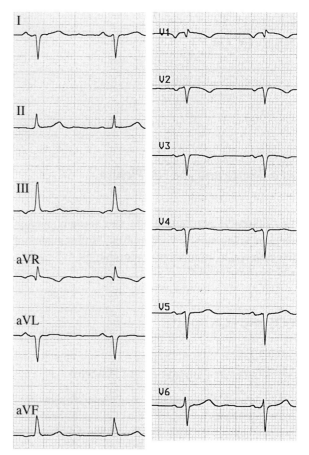

ECG 32.2

Thoracic X-rays show a blurred contour of the cardiac silhouette, and absence of a clear heart waist [3–5].

ECG 32.3
Right Ventricular Dysplasia (Arrhythmogenic Right Ventricular Cardiomyopathy)

Patient 40 y/m. Frequent ventricular premature beats (VPBs) with a left bundle-branch block (LBBB)-like pattern for 3 years. Intermittent therapy with amiodarone. After a short malaise the patient had severe syncope without a pulse. Fortunately, reanimation was begun after 2 minutes. The ECG showed ventricular fibrillation. After defibrillation the patient recovered. The echo revealed a severe dilatation and poor function of the

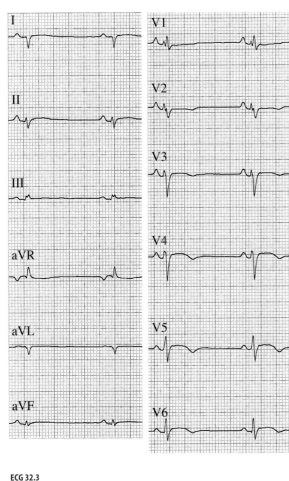

ECG 32.3

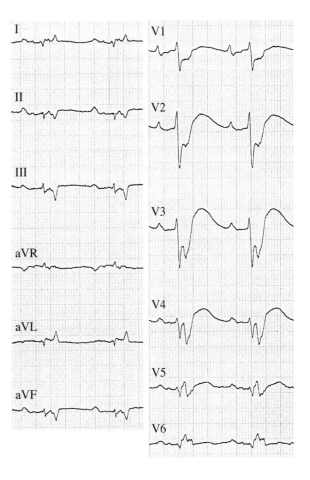

ECG 32.4

right ventricle. The coronary arteries were normal. An ICD device was implanted. Sinus rhythm 53/min. Tall and peaked p waves in V_1 to V_3. PQ 0.14 sec. ÅQRS$_F$ about + 180°. Peripheral low voltage. QRS clockwise rotation. Incomplete RBBB with rsR'S' type in V_1 (in this lead the QRS duration measures 20–40 msec more than in lead V_6! Slight ST depression in V_1/V_2, slight ST elevation in V_3 to V_6 (and I/II). Flat T waves in limb leads, negative T waves in V_2 up to V_6.

Right ventricular dysplasia (RVD) is a rare congenital disease. Together with the Brugada syndrome and the long QT syndrome, right ventricular dysplasia is responsible for *sudden death* in young people, due to ventricular fibrillation. In the ECG an incomplete RBBB and negative T waves in the right precordial leads (that may expand to the lateral wall) are common.

There is generally a frontal QRS right-axis deviation, but all other QRS axes may be seen. Incomplete RBBB may show three to five deflections (rsr's'r") and the QRS duration in V_1 may last 10–40 msec longer than in V_6 (as in our case). In rare cases an *Epsilon* wave is observed in lead V_1 (see Chapter 31 Special ECG Waves, Signs and Phenomena) [6–12].

ECG 32.4
Severe Hypertrophic Cardiomyopathy

Patient 34 y/m. Hereditary hypertrophic (non-obstructive) cardiomyopathy. Left ventricular wall thickness 3.8 mm. Severe diastolic dysfunction leading to disability and requiring heart transplantation. Sinus rhythm 62/min. Left atrial enlargement (p duration 0.18 sec). Peaked p waves in V_1/V_2 indicate also right atrial overload. AV block 1°. ÅQRS$_F$ about − 80°. Peripheral low voltage. Bizarre QRS complexes with multiple notches, duration 260 msec(!), with an abnormal LBBB-like pattern. No distinct ST segment. Deformation of T waves in V_2 to V_4. QT interval 630 msec(!). The rsR' complex in leads I, aVL and V_5/V_6 could reflect a special infarction pattern in the presence of LBBB. The enormous QRS duration is more consistent with a severe hypertrophic left ventricular cardiomyopathy, however.

ECG 32.5
Strange R Wave in Lead V₂ in a Patient with Severe Hypertrophic Cardiomyopathy

Patient 20 y/f. The patient was controlled for hereditary severe hypertrophic cardiomyopathy, surprisingly without obstruction. Septal diameter 40 mm(!), diameter of the free left ventricular wall 12 mm. ECG 32.5a shows a sinus rhythm of 58/min. Negative p wave in V_1, ÅQRS$_F$ − 60°. High QRS voltage. Minimal r wave in V_1/V_2. QRS clockwise rotation. Symmetric negative T waves in V_5/V_6. Striking *high positive* R wave in lead V_2.

The first interpretation was of an artifact. But what artifact? A control revealed that lead V_2 had been displaced erroneously at the fourth intercostal space 1.5 cm *to the left* and about 1 cm *too high*. On placing lead V_2 correctly, the ECG was nearly the same as one registered 1 year previously (ECG 32.5b). In conclusion and explanation: a modest displacement of lead V_2 provoked a bizarre alteration of the QRS vector. This is a beautiful example of the *magnifying glass* effect of a precordial lead. In a precordial surface area restricted to 2–3 cm² the QRS complex is completely dominated by the *vector* of the extremely thickened intraventricular septum, oriented *anteriorly*.

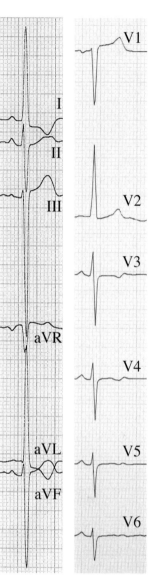

ECG 32.5a

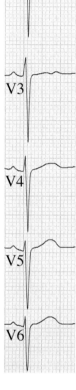

ECG 32.5b

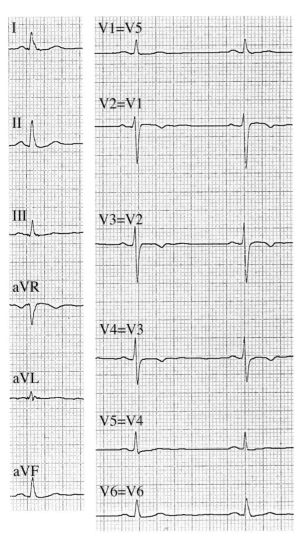

ECG 32.6

An analysis of the precordial leads revealed a misplacement of the leads. Lead V_5 was placed at V_1 and leads V_1 to V_4 were placed at V_2 to V_5. Only V_6 was placed correctly. An ECG control confirmed this opinion.

ECG 32.7
What is the Rhythm?

Short Story/Case Report 2

ECG courtesy of Armin Theler MD. One beautiful day a colleague and good friend of the author faxed an ECG with leads I, II, and III of a 72-year-old patient (ECG 32.7a). It was accompanied by a question: does this patient need a pacemaker?

At a first glance the ECG diagnosis is quite clear: sinus rhythm, rate about 63/min. AV block 2° with 4 : 1 block and aberrant ventricular conduction – probably RBBB + LAFB (left anterieor fascicular block). PQ interval of the conducted beats 560 msec. Ventricular rate only 16/min! However, some details are contradictory: the p waves are not of sinusal origin (negative in lead I). Conclusion: Ectopic atrial rhythm? False poling of limb leads? The p wave is missed at the end of the T wave and the p–p interval between the p wave before QRS, and the first p wave after QRS is less than twice the general p–p interval. Conclusion: premature p wave hidden within the T wave, due to atrial PB or to ventriculophasic 'sinus' arrhythmia? But does ventriculophasic arrhythmia exist in 'ectopic atrial rhythm'?

The author was quite troubled and phoned his friend to tell him the interpretation. The friend laughed and asked again 'Does this patient need a pacemaker?'

The reply was 'I think so – at a rate of 16/min!'

To which the friend responded: 'I have learned from you that one should never interpret an ECG without knowing the clinical situation! Why did you not ask "How is the patient?" To be honest, the patient has absolutely no limitations in his daily work!'

And he faxed the *precordial* leads (leads V_1 to V_3 are shown in ECG 32.7b) that resolved the enigma! The 'p waves' are unmasked as normally conducted beats, and the 'conducted beats with aberration' are unmasked as ventricular premature beats. The real p waves are scarcely visible (arrow); there is AV block 1°, with a shorter PQ interval after the VPB.

ECG 32.6
Strange R Wave in Lead V_1 in a Patient without Right Ventricular Hypertrophy or Posterior Infarction

Patient 72 y/f. A 1-week-old small non-Q wave infarction. Echo: left ventricular function slightly decreased. No right ventricular hypertrophy. Sinus rhythm 52/min. ÅQRS$_F$ + 50°. Strange positive QRS (pure R wave) in V_1. Negative T waves in V_2 to V_4.

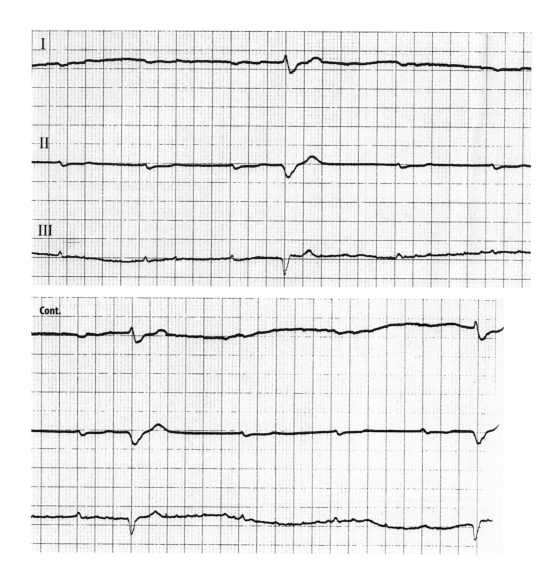

ECG 32.7a

In conclusion: misdiagnosis was due to a very rare projection on the limb leads resulting in *mini* QRS complexes (and due to a false conclusion by the temporarily absentminded author!).

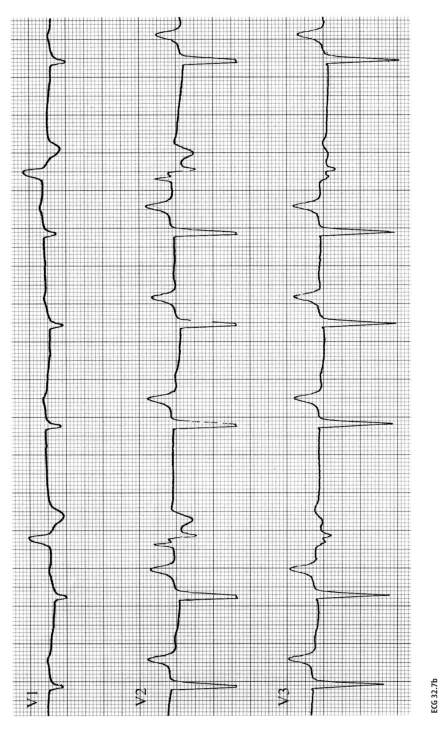

V1

V2

V3

ECG 32.7b

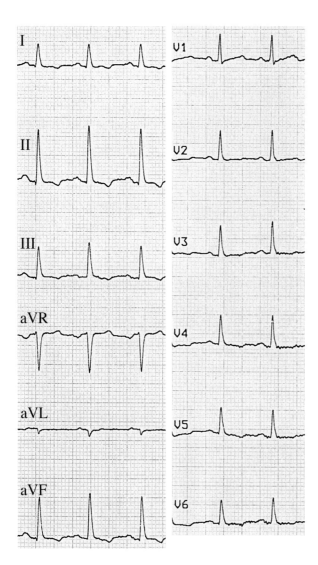

ECG 32.8

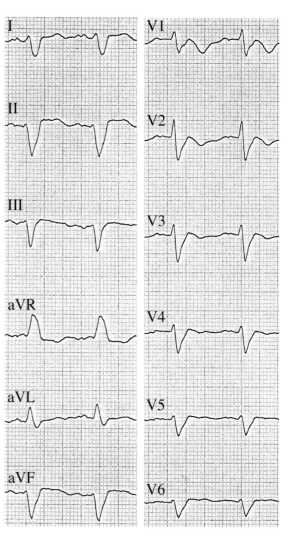

ECG 32.9

ECG 32.8
After Left Pneumectomy

Patient 77 y/m. Left pneumectomy 2 years previously because of lung carcinoma. Sinus rhythm 107/min. ÅQRS$_F$ about + 70°. Strikingly uniform positive QRS complexes in all precordial leads. Negative T waves in I, II, aVF, and III. Biphasic T waves in V$_3$ to V$_6$. Anatomically, the heart was displaced to the left.

ECG 32.9
After Right Pneumectomy

Patient 81 y/m. Right pneumectomy 6 years previously because of lung cancer. Sinus rhythm 82/min. Left atrial enlargement (p 160 msec). ÅQRS$_F$ – 130°. rS configuration in all precordial leads, with decreasing r waves from V$_1$ to V$_6$ (similar to situs inversus). ST/T alterations. Anatomically the heart was displaced to the right. As mentioned in Chapter 14 (Differential

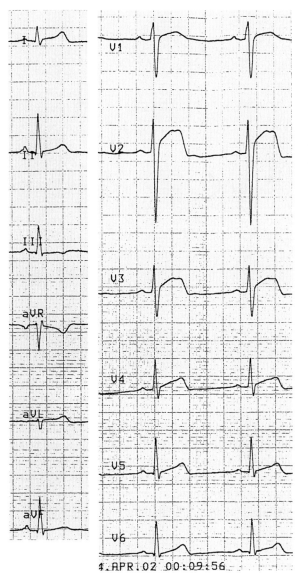

ECG 32.10

ECG 32.10
Pneumothorax

Patient 20 y/m. Admission to the emergency station because of dyspnoea and thoracic pain that varied during respiration. Striking ST elevations in leads V_2 and V_3 (V_1/V_4 to V_6) arising from the S wave. T wave with notches in V_2/V_3. Note also the minimal ST elevation in I and II *and* aVF combined with minimal PQ depression (frontal ST vector typical for pericarditis). Auscultation revealed a pericardial murmur. In the thoracic X-rays there was an extensive pneumothorax on the left side. Similar/identical ST alterations are described in pneumothorax without pericarditis.

Diagnosis of Pathologic Q Waves) the ECG after pneumectomy may reveal formally pathologic Q waves, thus suggesting myocardial infarction.

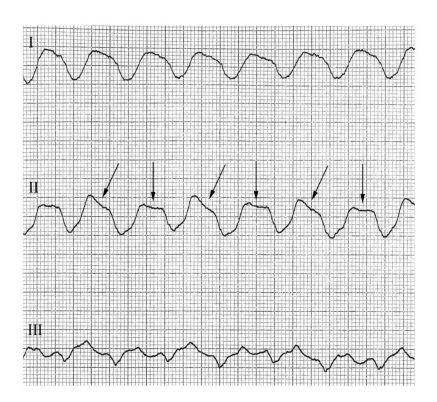

ECG 32.11

ECG 32.11
Electrical Alternans

ECG courtesy of Felix Frey MD. Patient 63 y/m. Terminal renal failure, patient under (insufficient) hemodialysis. Serum potassium 9.2 mmol/l. The ECG (leads I/II/III) shows sinus rhythm (without visible p waves) (see Chapter 16 Electrolyte Imbalances and Disturbances), rate 107/min. Bizarre prolongation of QRS duration (QRS about 230 msec) with LBBB pattern. Depolarization not clearly distinguishable from repolarization. *Alternation* of the repolarization wave, best seen in lead II (arrows).

After 10 mg calcium gluconate intravenously the ECG normalized within a few minutes and potassium reached normal levels after dialysis.

Electric alternans is occasionally observed in cardiac tamponade. In these cases the whole cardiac cycle is involved in general. However, the echocardiogram – instantaneously performed in this patient – revealed only a small pericardial effusion.

Overall, electrical alternans is not very rare [13] and is especially observed in AV and intraventricular conduction (for example alternating bundle-branch block). AV nodal alternans is due to dual pathway, concealed conduction, and other rare

reasons. Normal conduction alternating with bundle-branch block is based on conduction during the supernormal period of recovery. Alternation can also affect impulse formation or repolarization, inducing alternating ST segments [14], T waves (as shown in our example) [15], or even U waves. Alternating ST segments are seen in severe acute myocardial ischemia.

ECG 32.12
Common and Rare False Poling of the Limb Leads (Lead Displacement) in Frontal QRS Left Axis and in Frontal QRS Vertical Axis

False poling (lead displacement) of the limb leads occurs in about 1–2% of routine ECGs. Depending on the kind of displacement, the polarity of the whole electric cycle (p wave, QRS, and T wave) is influenced in a modest manner or a bizarre manner. If overlooked false poling may lead to false conclusions. In some false poling conditions a 'pathologic' Q wave may suggest an old myocardial infarction. The precordial leads do not confirm the diagnosis in these cases, however.

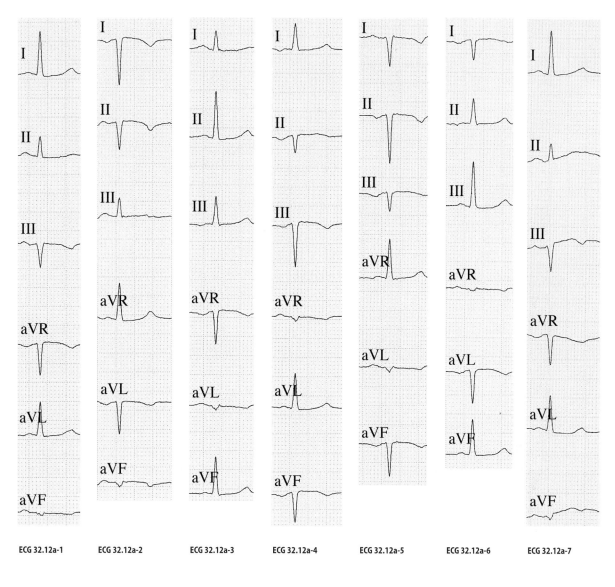

ECG 32.12a-1 ECG 32.12a-2 ECG 32.12a-3 ECG 32.12a-4 ECG 32.12a-5 ECG 32.12a-6 ECG 32.12a-7

ECG 32.12a
False Poling of Limb Leads in Frontal Left QRS Axis

Part 1 Correct poling

Part 2 Right arm → 'left arm', Left arm → 'right arm'
'I'=inversed I, 'II'=III, 'III'=II, 'aVR'=aVL, 'aVL'=aVR, 'aVF'=aVF

Part 3 Left arm →'left leg', Left leg → 'left arm'
'I'=II, 'II'=I, 'III'=inversed III, 'aVR'=aVR, 'aVL'=aVF, 'aVF'=aVL

Part 4 Right arm → 'left leg', Left leg → 'right arm'
'I'=inversed III, 'II'=inversed II, 'III'=inversed I, 'aVR'=aVF, 'aVL'=aVL, 'aVF'=aVR

Part 5 First clockwise rotation
Right arm → 'left arm', Left arm → 'left leg', Left leg → 'right arm'
'I'=III, 'II'=inversed I, 'III'=inversed II, 'aVR'=aVL, 'aVL'=aVF, 'aVF'=aVR

Part 6 Second clockwise rotation
Right arm → 'left leg', Left arm → 'right arm', Left leg → 'left arm'

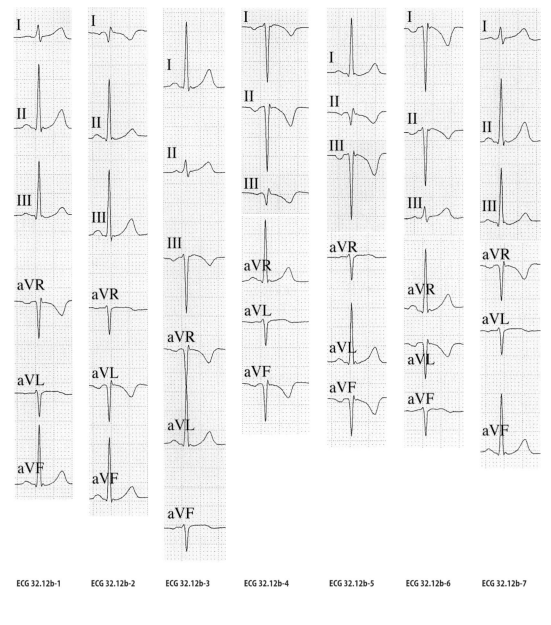

ECG 32.12b-1   ECG 32.12b-2   ECG 32.12b-3   ECG 32.12b-4   ECG 32.12b-5   ECG 32.12b-6   ECG 32.12b-7

'I'=inversed II, 'II'=inversed III, 'III'=I, 'aVR'=aVF, 'aVL'=aVR, 'aVF'=aVL

Part 7   Exchange of the leg leads
Left leg → 'right leg', Right leg → 'left leg'
'I'=I, 'II'=II, 'III'=III, 'aVR'=aVR, 'aVL'=aVL, 'aVF'=aVF

ECG 32.12b
False Poling of Limb Leads in Vertical QRS Axis

Part 1   Correct poling
Part 2   Right arm → 'left arm', Left arm → 'right arm'
'I'=inversed I, 'II'=III, 'III'=II, 'aVR'=aVL, 'aVL'=aVR, 'aVF'=aVF

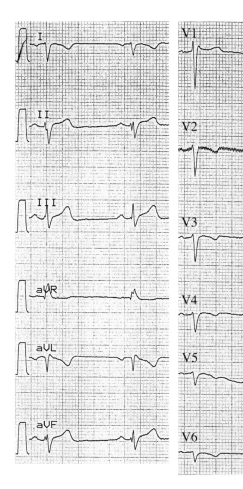

ECG 32.13

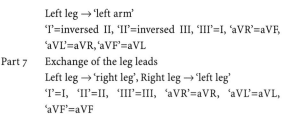

Left leg → 'left arm'

'I'=inversed II, 'II'=inversed III, 'III'=I, 'aVR'=aVF, 'aVL'=aVR, 'aVF'=aVL

Part 7   Exchange of the leg leads

Left leg → 'right leg', Right leg → 'left leg'

'I'=I, 'II'=II, 'III'=III, 'aVR'=aVR, 'aVL'=aVL, 'aVF'=aVF

The reader may note that the *most common* false poling, from exchange of the upper limb leads, results in a positive QRS deflection in lead 'aVR' ('aVR'=aVL) in the presence of a frontal *left* QRS axis. However, in the presence of a frontal *vertical* QRS axis, the QRS deflection remains negative. In both conditions lead 'I' leads to the detection of false poling, showing the mirror image of the original electric cycle.

ECG 32.13
Situs Inversus

Patient 40 y/m. The anomaly was detected at the age of 20, during a routine control. The patient never had cardiac symptoms. There is typical inversion of p waves and QRS complexes (similar or identical to false poling of the upper limb leads). rS complex in all precordial leads with decreasing r amplitude from V_1 to V_6 (a finding not seen in limb lead displacement). ST/T alterations. Exchange of the upper limb leads *and* placing of the precordial leads over the right hemithorax normalizes the ECG.

Part 3   Left arm →'left leg', Left leg → 'left arm'

'I'=II, 'II'=I, 'III'=inversed III, *'aVR'=aVR*, 'aVL'=aVF, 'aVF'=aVL

Part 4   Right arm → 'left leg', Left leg → 'right arm'

'I'=inversed III, 'II'=inversed II, 'III'=inversed I, 'aVR'=aVF, *'aVL'=aVL*, 'aVF'=aVR

Part 5   First clockwise rotation

Right arm → 'left arm', Left arm → 'left leg', Left leg → 'right arm'

'I'=III, 'II'=inversed I, 'III'=inversed II, 'aVR'=aVL, 'aVL'=aVF, 'aVF'=aVR

Part 6   Second clockwise rotation

Right arm → 'left leg', Left arm → right arm',

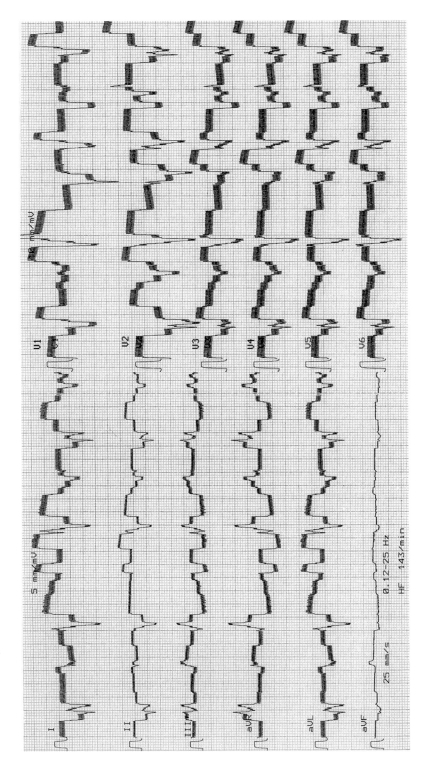

ECG 32.14

ECG 32.14
Epileptic Attack of the ECG Machine

The clinical status of the patient does not matter when the evidently sick ECG machine suffers from 'convulsions' of unclear origin, combined with artifacts caused by alternating current (AC).

ECG 32.15
Parasystole

Patient 66 y/m. Coronary heart disease, coronary artery bypass grafting 3 years previously. Left ventricular ejection fraction 40%, mild heart failure. A second (ventricular) rhythm at a rate of 45–47/min (arrows) interferes with sinus rhythm (rate 53–59/min). Ventricular impulses falling into the refractory period of the sinus beats are not conducted (arrows), and *vice versa* (not shown).

Parasystole occurs very rarely as tachycardia of a modest rate (up to 140/min), or more commonly at a rate of 50–90/min. Short episodes are often misinterpreted as VPBs with different coupling intervals. Parasystole is characterized by a regular interectopic interval, a variable interval of the parasystolic beats to the beats of basic rhythm, and fusion beats. Intermittent failure of parasystolic beats to manifest is due to exit block (type 1 or 2) and may make the diagnosis difficult.

Parasystole is generally associated with heart disease of any origin but is occasionally encountered also in healthy people [16]. For special practical diagnostic criteria see Ren et al [17], for irregular parasystole see Ren et al [17] and Kinoshita et al [18], for numerology see Castellanos et al [19], for association with VT see Singh [20], for a mathematical model see Itoh et al [21] and Castellanos et al [22], and for triple parasystole see Oreto et al [23].

Principally a parasystolic 'focus' may arise in any heart structure with electric properties, even in the sinus node. Supraventricular parasystole is only of theoretic interest, however [24,25].

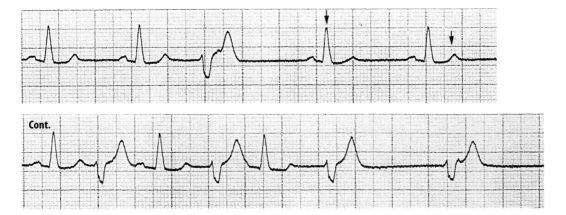

ECG 32.15

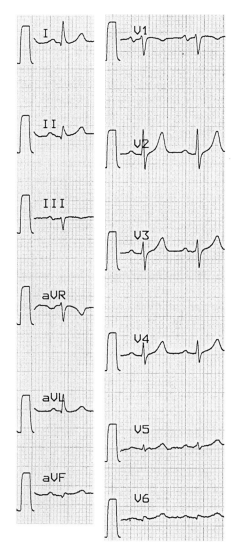

ECG 32.16

Of course the cardiologist did not tell his colleagues that he would never be able to diagnose a right-sided pleural effusion from the ECG!

ECG 32.17
So-Called Postsyncopal Bradycardia Syndrome

Patient 78 y/f. Hypertension with probable coronary heart disease. (Therapy with enalapril 5 mg, torasemide 5 mg, isosorbide dinitrate 80 mg, atenolol 25 mg, verapamil 80 mg, levothyroxin 0.05 mg (hypothyreosis)). The patient was admitted to the hospital because of the abnormal ECG, combined with mild vertigo.

Sinus rhythm? Ectopic atrial rhythm (p positive in aVR)? Rate 61/min. AV block 1°. ÅQRS$_F$ + 75°. Gigantically prolonged negative T waves in I, II, aVF, and V$_2$ to V$_6$. QT interval 0.76sec(!). Other findings: no recent syncope; blood pressure 95/70 mmHg; neurologic status normal. Laboratory findings were normal, including potassium.

By reduction of antihypertensive medication, blood pressure rose to 130/80 mmHg and the ECG normalized within 48 hours. A Holter ECG was normal. The further outcome was good.

The so-called *postsyncopal bradycardia syndrome* (an 'ECG syndrome') is a very rare ECG finding (the author has observed it about 30 times in 35 years). The bizarre ST/T alterations are generally associated with sinus bradycardia or with AV or ventricular escape rhythm in complete AV block. In about a third of the cases the ECG abnormality was preceded by a recent Morgagni-Adams-Stokes attack (see also Chapter 17 Alterations of Repolarization), in three cases after a cerebral insult. Potassium and other electrolyte levels were generally normal. The 'syndrome' is probably associated with cerebral alterations in most cases, but in some patients the etiology remains unclear. In any case, it is convenient to control the rhythm with repeated ambulatory ECGs to find out if asystole occurs during sleep. In our patient a bradycardiac arrhythmia or an excessive fall of blood pressure during sleep – caused by antihypertensive 'over-therapy' – could not be excluded (retrospectively).

ECG 32.16
Left Pleural Effusion

Patient 57 y/f. Pleuropneumonia. On the basis of the ECG alone, the cardiologist predicted a large left-sided pleural effusion – his colleagues in internal medicine were very impressed by this correct diagnosis. Sinus rhythm 105/min. The ECG is within normal limits, except leads V$_5$/V$_6$, where the amplitude of QRS and repolarization (damped by the left-sided pleural effusion) is very small.

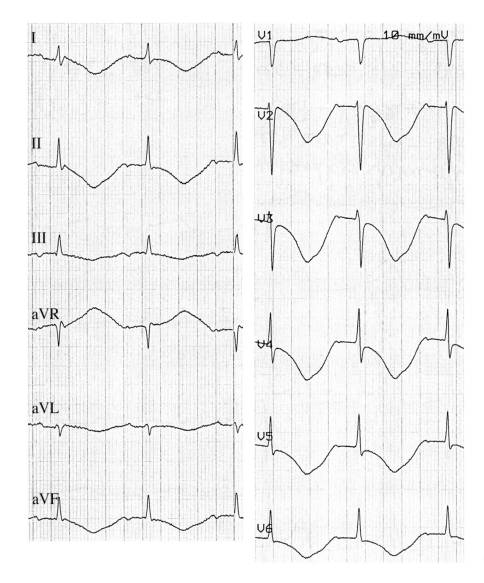

ECG 32.17

ECG 32.18
'Dying Heart'

Patient 50 y/m. Suicidal lethal intoxication with four different anti-depressant drugs.

ECG (paper speed 50 mm/sec): no distinct atrial activity. AV escape beats with polymorphous ventricular premature beats followed by ventricular standstill (not shown).

Several times we have seen dying patients (without drug intoxication) in whom, after episodes of similar arrhythmias and complete heart standstill, a normal sinus rhythm (with normal p waves, normal QRS, and near normal repolarization) suddenly arises for about 20 seconds, 5–10 minutes after the patient's last breath and an arrest of circulation.

The ECGs of dying patients are uncommon because they are rarely registered.

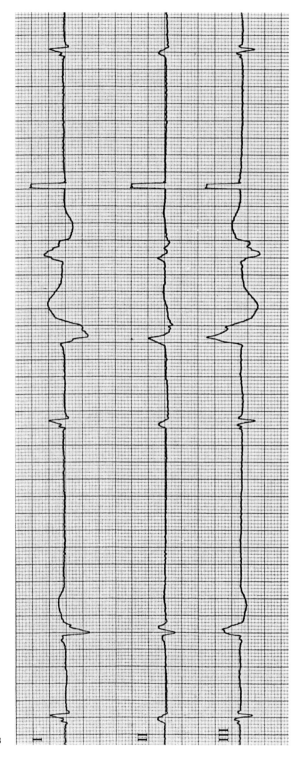

ECG 32.18

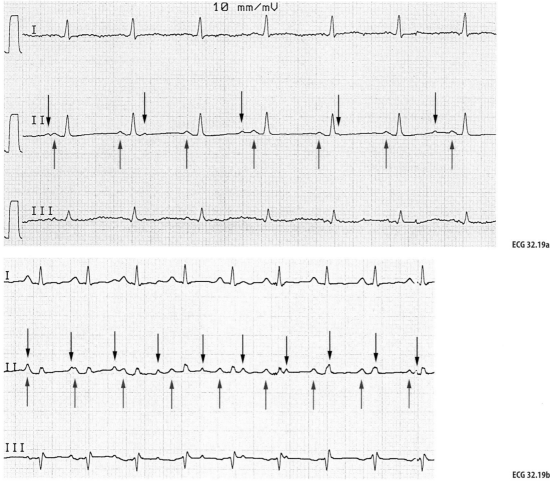

ECG 32.19a

ECG 32.19b

ECG 32.19
Two p Waves: Highly Specific for a Transplanted Heart

ECG 32.19a (patient 62 y/f) was registered 1 week after heart transplantation because of dilating cardiomyopathy. Besides flat T waves in some leads the ECG shows one abnormality: *two* p waves (best seen in lead II). The *normal* p wave (↑) corresponds to normal atrial activation by the *new* sinus node of the transplanted (new) heart and is responsible for ventricular activation: sinus rhythm, rate 83/min. The *other* p wave (↓) is due to activation of the remaining small portion of old right atrium by the *old* sinus node (rate about 55/min).

Of course this phenomenon is only seen in patients where a special surgical technique is used: a small portion of the old

right atrium, the old sinus node included, is left in place. The rhythm of the old sinus node is often irregular and often slower than the rhythm of the new sinus node (that activates the whole heart). This 'residual' p wave gets smaller from day to day and generally disappears after some weeks.

ECG 32.19b (patient 19 y/m) was registered 5 days after heart transplantation because of complex congenital heart disease associated with Ivemark syndrome (see also Short Story/Case Report 1 in Chapter 16 Electrolyte Imbalances and Disturbances). This ECG looks the same as ECG 32.19a because two p waves are visible. The p wave of the new sinus node activates the whole heart (rate 114/min (↑)), and the old p wave activates only a small right atrial portion of the old heart (rate 129/min (↓)).

ECG 32.20
Pseudo-p Waves in Precordial Leads V_3/V_4

Patient 78 y/f. Hypothyreosis treated with levothyroxin. At a first glance T alterations in leads V_3 and V_4 imitate p waves (↓) and the pattern of 2 : 1 AV block. However, p waves are missed in the other leads. The 'pseudo-p' waves are due to an alteration of the T wave. From our experience those T wave alterations have no special significance. However, similar patterns are occasionally seen in patients with hypothyreosis (as in our patient) and under medication with amiodarone.

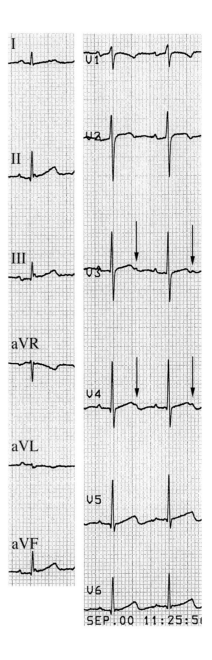

ECG 32.20

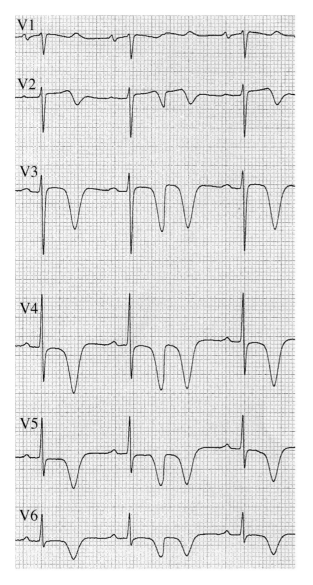

ECG 32.21

ECG 32.21
'Double Ventricular Repolarization'

ECG courtesy of Beat Meyer MD. Patient 72 y/f. Coronary heart disease without infarction. This phenomenon has been seen by the author only twice in 35 years. We hope that some clever electrophysiologist has a sophisticated explanation. For us it is a rare artifact that begins during the first T wave where the upstroke is unphysiologically steep. By some unclear mechanism the ECG machine fails to detect the next p and QRS (at the same time decreasing the registration speed).

ECG 32.22
T Wave without QRS Complex

The 'opposite' of double repolarization, namely a repolarization wave *without* a depolarization (T wave without QRS complex) is more often seen preferentially in Holter ECG stripes. The ECG machine fails to detect the QRS complex, but detects the following repolarization, without troubling the regular rhythm. This pattern always corresponds to an artifact that is generally confirmed by a preceding p wave.

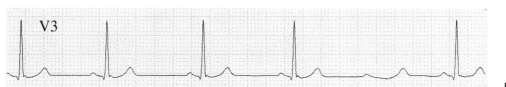

ECG 32.22

ECG 32.23
Double Ventricular Response to a Single Atrial Impulse. Another Artifact?

ECG courtesy of Marc Zimmermann MD. Patient 59 y/f. Supraventricular tachycardias (SVT) with palpitations. ECG 32.23a shows SVT, with a sinus rate of 63/min, and a ventricular rate of 126/min. This exciting ECG is *not* an artifact. On one hand, the sinus impulse travels along the fast AV nodal pathway and activates the ventricles. On the other, the sinus impulse is simultaneously conducted over a very slow AV nodal pathway and then depolarizes the ventricles for a second time. In Electrophysiology Studies (EPS) the phenomenon was proven (ECG 32.23b). Moreover, a complex supraventricular tachycardia was detected, probably based on *three* different nodal pathways [26].

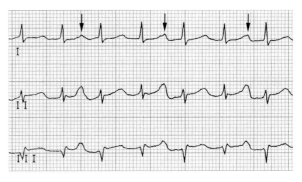

ECG 32.23a

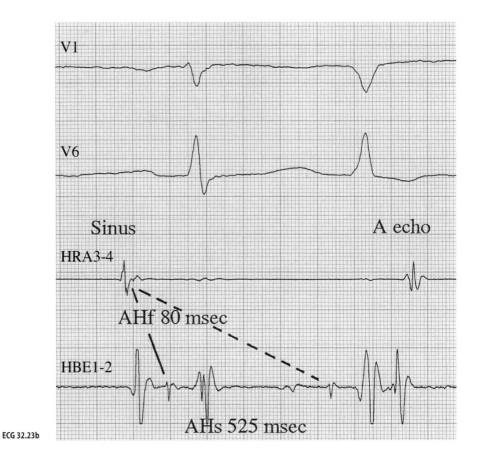

ECG 32.23b

ECG 32.24
Another Rare ECG

Short Story/Case Report 3

ECG courtesy of Andres Jaussi MD. In 1992 a dear friend sent this strange ECG with no details about the age and disease of the patient. The following assessment was made.

ECG: sinus bradycardia, rate 42/min. Left atrial enlargement. AV block 1°. ÅQRS$_F$ – 40°. QRS duration 120 msec.

Strange QRS configuration in precordial leads, with single R waves in V$_2$/V$_3$ and rS complexes in V$_3$ to V$_6$. Even stranger was repolarization with biphasic negative/positive T waves in leads II, aVF, III, and V$_3$ to V$_6$ (note the very unusual and *impossible* sharp T deflections).

The author gave the following interpretation 'A very strange ECG – never seen before. CHD with posterolateral infarction? Also – hypothyreosis or amiodarone?'

The friend laughed 'Your first impression is correct. It is a normal ECG – of my *horse*.'

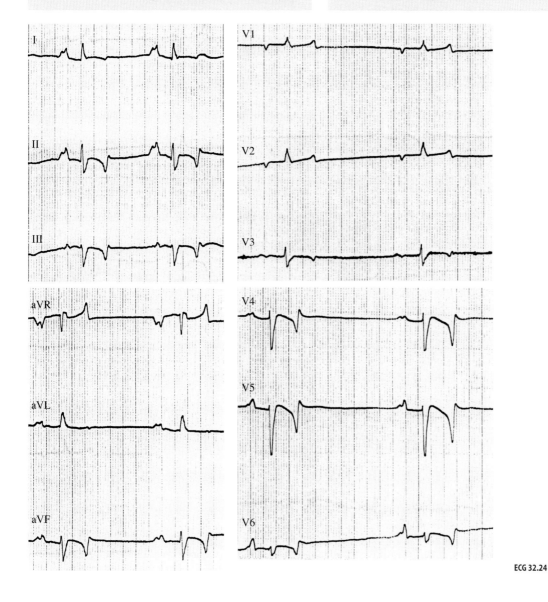

ECG 32.24

References

1. McCord J, Borzak S. Multifocal atrial tachycardia. Chest 1998; 113:203–9
2. Kastor JA. Multifocal atrial tachycardia. N Engl J Med 1990;322: 1713–7
3. Samuels LE, Sharma S, Kaufman MS, et al. Absent pericardium during coronary bypass. Arch Surg 1997;132:318–9
4. Deutsch AA, Brown KN, Freeman NV, Stanley DA. A case of diaphragmatic hernia, absent pericardium, and hamartoma of liver. Br J Surg 1972;59:156–8
5. Baim RS, MacDonald IL, Wise DJ, Lenkei SC. Computed tomography of absent left pericardium. Radiology 1980;135:127–8
6. Thiene G, Nava A, Corrado D, et al. Right ventricular cardiomyopathy and sudden death in young people. New Engl J Med 1988;318:129–33
7. Basso C, Thiene G, Nava A, Dalla Volta S. Arrhythmogenic right ventricular cardiomyopathy: a survey of the investigations at the university of Padua. Clin Cardiol 1997;20:333–6
8. Fontaine G, Guiraudon, Frank R, et al. Stimulation studies and epicardial mapping in ventricular tachycardia: study of mechanism and selection for surgery. In: Kulbertus HE, ed. Re-entrant Arrhythmias: Mechanisms and Treatment. Lancaster, PA: MTP Publishers 1977, pp 334–50
9. Fontaine G, Gallais Y, Fornes P, et al. Arrhythmogenic right ventricular dysplasia/cardiomyopathy. Anaesthesiology 2001; 95:250–4
10. Gemayel C, Pelliccia A, Thompson PD. Arrhythmogenic right ventricular cardiomyopathy. J Am Coll Cardiol 2001;38:1773–81
11. Marcus FI. Update of arrhythmogenic right ventricular dysplasia. Card Electrophysiol Rev 2002;6:54–6
12. Case Reports of the Massachusetts General Hospital: Case 20–2000. New Engl J Med 2000;342:1979–87
13. Fisch C, Knoebel SB. Electrocardiography of clinical arrhythmias. Armonk, NY: Futura Publishing Company 2000, pp 281–92
14. Kleinfeld MJ, Rozanski JJ. Alternans of the ST segment in Primzmetal's angina. Circulation 1977;55:574–7
15. Fisch C, Edmands RE, Greenspan K. T wave alternans: an association with abrupt rate change. Am Heart J 1971;81:817–21
16. Chung EK. Parasystole. Prog Cardiovasc Dis 1968;11:64–81
17. Ren Z, Zhou J, Xu G, et al. The diagnostic criteria for classic parasystole. Chin Med J 1999;112:992–4
18. Kinoshita S, Katoh T, Mitsuoka T, et al. Ventricular parasystolic couplets originating in the pathway between the ventricle and the parasystolic pacemaker: mechanism of 'irregular' parasystole. J Electrocardiol 2001;34:251–60
19. Castellanos A, Moleiro F, Guerrero J, et al. Intermittent parasystole with exit block. J Electrocardiol 1997;30:331–5
20. Singh VK. Numerology of ventricular parasytole. Chest 1996;109:1663
21. Itoh E, Aizawa Y, Washizuka T, et al. Two cases of ventricular parasystole associated with ventricular tachycardia. Pacing Clin Electrophysiol 1996;19:370–3
22. Castellanos A, Moleiro F, Interian A Jr, Myerburg RJ. A different approach to the analysis of ventricular parasystole. Chest 1995;107:1463–4
23. Oreto G, Satullo G, Luzza F, Saporito F. Triple ventricular parasystole. J Electrocardiol 1993;26:159–64
24. Manolas J, Rutishauser W, Holzmann M. Linksatriale Parasystolie. Z Kardiol 1975;64:919–25
25. Khan AH. Atrial dissociation. Brit Heart J 1972;34:1308–10
26. Maudry P, Zimmermann M, Metzger J, et al. Association between nonreentrant supraventricular and atrioventricular node reentrant tachycardia: a presentation of dual AV node physiology. PACE 1999;22:1410–5

Acknowledgment:
The idea for the figures 1.2, 1.3, 1.4, 1.5, 1.7, 1.8, 1.10, 1.11, 1.12, 1.13, and 1.14 is based on figures in the book Thomas Horacek, *Der EKG-Trainer. Ein didaktisch geführter Selbstlernkurs mit 200 Beispiel-EKGs.*

Subject Index

Purkinje fibers 3

ECG Index

N

ECG Index

ECG Index